Polyphenols-based Nanotherapeutics for Cancer Management

Shams Tabrez • Mohammad Imran Khan
Editors

Polyphenols-based Nanotherapeutics for Cancer Management

Springer

Editors
Shams Tabrez
King Fahd Medical Research Center
King Abdulaziz University
Jeddah, Saudi Arabia

Mohammad Imran Khan
Department of Biochemistry, Faculty of Science
King Abdulaziz University
Jeddah, Saudi Arabia

ISBN 978-981-16-4934-9 ISBN 978-981-16-4935-6 (eBook)
https://doi.org/10.1007/978-981-16-4935-6

This Springer imprint is published by the registered company Springer Nature Singapore Pte Ltd.
The registered company address is: 152 Beach Road, #21-01/04 Gateway East, Singapore 189721, Singapore

My beloved Mother
and
Sister
Whom we lost in the last one year

Preface

The contemporary medicines presently available to treat cancers are costly, toxic, and less potent. The increasing magnitude of the cancer problem and the failure of conventional chemotherapy to bring about significant reductions in the mortality rates demand the development of more effective novel therapeutics. Over the past few decades, polyphenols have risen as a standout amongst naturally occurring compounds with huge therapeutic perspectives. Despite giving positive results in pre-clinical studies, these polyphenols have met with limited success in clinics. Therefore, further research is required to improve their delivery to the specific sites of the body at particular times and an effective concentration.

Nanotechnology has evolved as an effective alternative approach for the delivery of chemotherapeutics and imaging. Over recent years, there have been several attempts to develop novel nanoparticle (NP)-based formulations on encapsulating different polyphenols as chemotherapeutic agents.

This book reviews various polyphenols for cancer management and evaluates current trends and challenges for developing polyphenols-based nano-chemotherapeutics in different cancer models. Different polyphenols, sources, and bio-physiological properties against multiple diseases, including cancer, have been discussed in the first chapter. The second chapter highlights the biomedical application of different polyphenols (flavonoids, non-flavonoids, and phenolic acids) through different intracellular/signaling pathways targeting specifically NF-κB, MAPKs, and PI3K/Akt. In the next chapter, the authors have covered well-known medicinal herbs and highlighted their antioxidant potential via the free-radical quenching mechanism. The beneficial role of long-term intake of these antioxidants on overall health and reduction in cancer risk has also been discussed.

The polyphenols have demonstrated the potential to modulate cancer-causing transcription factors and signaling molecules resulting in the regulation of cancer cell apoptosis, proliferation, invasion, and metastasis. In the next chapter, multiple cell signaling pathways for cancer treatment have been covered. The following chapter highlights the role of polyphenols as a modulator of oxidative stress. Several polyphenols have been suggested as a beneficial anti-cancer tool in combination therapy and standard chemotherapeutic agents leading to fewer side effects.

The next chapter is based on the epigenetic basis of different polyphenols in cancer treatment. The authors have listed the mechanism of polyphenols targeting various epigenetic landscape, their parameters, immunogenic responses, signaling pathways, and physiological barriers in cancerous cells.

Cancer stem cells (CSCs) are responsible for tumor growth, heterogeneity, relapse, and cancer progression. They play a role in developing chemotherapeutic resistance, promoting epithelial-mesenchymal transition (EMT), and metastasis in tumors. In this chapter, different flavonoids have been explored as potential candidates, targeting CSCs to treat various cancers. The following chapter highlights the possible usage of several non-flavonoids and their effect on the reduction/eradication of CSCs via attenuation of different signaling pathways. In the next chapter, the author explored polyphenol's role in nutrition, mainly focusing on fish and other seafood-based diets enhanced with polyphenols. The polyphenols as immune/chemotherapeutic agents have also been discussed in this chapter.

Polymeric and lipid nanoparticles are increasingly used for the encapsulation of different polyphenols for targeted delivery. This nanoformulation enhances the aqueous solubility, bioavailability, and protects polyphenols from degradation. In this chapter, the encapsulation potential of different nanoparticulate systems has been discussed. The next chapter highlights the recent advancement in polyphenols-based nanotechnology for pharmaceutical applications, mainly focusing on quercetin, resveratrol, epigallocatechin-3-gallate, and curcumin. The last chapter provides a comprehensive literature on the possible usage of green nanoparticles for the targeted delivery of natural therapeutics to manage glioblastoma multiforme (brain tumor). The latest knowledge and challenges for developing polyphenols-based nano-chemotherapeutics against different cancer are highlighted in these chapters. We hope that this book's will be a valuable source of information for students, academics, researchers, clinicians, and medical professionals working in the anti-cancer research field.

Jeddah, Saudi Arabia Shams Tabrez
Jeddah, Saudi Arabia Mohammad Imran Khan

Acknowledgments

The editors gratefully acknowledge the research facility provided by the King Fahd Medical Research Center (KFMRC) and Department of Biochemistry at King Abdulaziz University, Jeddah, Saudi Arabia.

Contents

About the Editors

Shams Tabrez is working as a Professor of Biochemistry at King Fahd Medical Research Center, King Abdulaziz University (KAU). Earlier, he has obtained Ph.D. in Biochemistry from Aligarh Muslim University (AMU), India. His research is focused on cancer chemoprevention using bioactive compounds and the improvement of their delivery by nanotechnology-based techniques. He also has a strong research interest in the field of metabolomics and enzymology. He has published more than 135 articles in journals of high repute. Prof. Tabrez is serving and/or served as an editorial board member of several journals, including Cells, Current Pharmaceutical Design, Current Clinical Pharmacology, Cells, Current Vascular Pharmacology, and Pharmacognosy Magazine.

Mohammad Imran Khan is an Associate Professor in the Department of Biochemistry at KAU, Saudi Arabia. He obtained his Ph.D. in Medical Biochemistry from CSIR-Indian Institute of Toxicology Research (CSIR-IITR) and Aligarh Muslim University (AMU), India, and did post-doctoral training from the University of Wisconsin, Madison. His research interest includes nano-chemoprevention, epigenetics, and metabolomics. He has published more than 70 research articles in the journals of international repute.

Introduction and Classification of Natural Polyphenols

1

Abrar Ahmad, Varish Ahmad, Mazin A. Zamzami, Hani Chaudhary, Othman A. Baothman, Salman Hosawi, Mohammad Kashif, Mohammad Salman Akhtar, and Mohd Jahir Khan

Abstract

Polyphenols are naturally found in plant-based meals, and these molecules come in a wide range of complex forms. The phenolic ring is the most basic monomer in polyphenols therefore phenolic alcohols are commonly classified as phenolic acids. Polyphenols are divided into numerous groups based on the strength of the phenolic ring, with phenolic acids, flavonoids, stiblins (a type of polyphenol), phenolic alcohols, and lignans being the most common. Bioactive substances are phytochemicals that protect human health from chronic degenerative disorders. Polyphenols are a class of biologically active chemicals found in plant-based diets. These chemicals are found in fruits, vegetables, grains, and coffee and are introduced into the human diet. Polyphenols are also thought to help inhibit the onset of degenerative illnesses. Polyphenol studies were postponed due to their unique structural complexity characteristics. Polyphenols are the most important

A. Ahmad (✉) · M. A. Zamzami · H. Chaudhary · O. A. Baothman · S. Hosawi
Department of Biochemistry, Faculty of Sciences, King Abdulaziz University, Jeddah, Saudi Arabia
e-mail: aaldin@kau.edu.sa; mzamzami@kau.edu.sa; hchaudhary@kau.edu.sa; oabaothman@kau.edu.sa; shosawi@kau.edu.sa

V. Ahmad
Department of Health Information Technology, Faculty of Applied Studies, King Abdulaziz University, Jeddah, Saudi Arabia

M. Kashif
CSIR-NBRI, Lucknow, India

M. S. Akhtar
Faculty of Medical Applied Studies, Al-Baha University, Al-Baha, Saudi Arabia

M. J. Khan
School of Biotechnology, Jawaharlal Nehru University, New Delhi, India

S. Tabrez, M. Imran Khan (eds.), *Polyphenols-based Nanotherapeutics for Cancer Management*, https://doi.org/10.1007/978-981-16-4935-6_1

antioxidants in our food. These obstruct the oxidative transition in the lipoprotein of low density, and this is the fundamental cause of atherosclerosis occurring in endothelial lesions. Polyphenols have been studied for their function in the treatment of cardiovascular disease, osteoporosis, neurodegenerative illness, cancer, and diabetes mellitus.

Keywords

Polyphenols · Structures · Classifications · Clinical uses · Food Sources · Bioavailability

1.1 Introduction

More than 2000 years ago, Hippocrates said, "Let your food be your medicines and your food be medicine," and the health advantages of natural foods have been studied since ancient times [1]. Plant food like fruits and vegetables provides the human body with calories and other critical nutrients and has a significant role in the health of people [2–5]. Over the last 16 years, secondary plant metabolites have been increasingly researched and their potential to promote human health has been substantiated [6]. It is recognized that these plant compounds play a crucial role in adapting to their environment [7], but they are also a source of active medicines [8]. The significance of primary metabolites in basic activities of life, such as growth and development, breathing, storage, and reproduction, has been clarified for almost 200 years in contemporary chemical and biology [9–11]. Kossel was the first scientist to find secondary metabolites compared with primary metabolites [12]. Czapek was the second person to identify novel actions for phytochemicals and coincide with the phrase "finished product" for these molecules because of the advancement in biochemical testing in the mid-twentieth century [13]. Polyphenols/ Phytochemicals (PCs) are a diverse, diverse, bioactive, and omnipresent group of secondary plant metabolites that form a major component of the human diet and are significantly important because of their biological characteristics [14–17]. Several studies have examined the health benefits of polyphenols during recent decades [18–20]. The risk of cardiovascular disease [21], colon cancer [22], liver disorders [23], diabetes [24], obesity [25, 26], and other diseases can be minimally reduced by the use of polyphenols-rich diet. In plants, these substances are usually produced as a protective agent for physiological and environmental stimuli [18, 27, 28]. Many features of the chemical and biological activity of these compounds were identified and analyzed in recent years with regard to the human health benefits of PCs [29] and many of their chemical and biological activity aspects were identified and evaluated [30, 31].

PCs have advantages such as their accessibility, reaction specificities, and low toxicity, whereas their rapid metabolism and their low bioavailability are the main disadvantages [28, 32]. Many factors, including environmental considerations (i.e., sunshine exposure, precipitation, diverse crop varieties, fruit yield from trees, etc.)

and biochemical considerations (e.g., degree of maturity, storage, and cooking) [33, 34] may have an impact on plant and food concentrations of PC [20].

PCs are the major secondary metabolites of plants in human diets, especially glycosides of these plants, which offer a wide variety of health benefits [35]. Natural source compounds appear in recent decades to have taken on a distinctive role in pharmacies and are now being used to create and produce new pharmaceutical medicines [36]. In addition, these compounds are often used to boost therapeutic effectiveness in pharmacological studies.

Polyphenols can boost the bio-efficacy and bioavailability of conventional drugs. More than half of these chemicals, according to a research of PC literature with over 20,000 published studies on the subject [37], show the broad benefit of PCs to human cultures [38] as antibacterial, antifungal, anti-inflammatory, and anticancer effects. There has been a great deal of study on computers around the world and several scientific publications have published and indexed them. What kinds of PCs are the most widely studied in the globe and which signaling pathways are being modified by PCs which offer health benefits to people? This analysis concentrates on the most researched PCs and nations with the highest interest in PC research, together with a complete overview of the biology and health benefits of the most sought-after Dietary PCs.

1.2 Polyphenols

Polyphenols are one of the most important, if not most, of the phytochemical groups found in plants. Polyphenols are thought to aid digestion, functioning of the brain, and to protect against cardiovascular disorders, type 2 diabetes, and various cancers when they are ingested daily. The most well-known sources are red wine, dark chocolate, tea, and berries. However, several additional meals contain significant levels of such chemicals [39]. More than 8000 phenolic structures, of which over 4000 are flavonoids and hundreds of which are found in food plants were identified. However, as many of the phenolic compounds contained in fruit, vegetable, and derivatives are unknown, the methods and analytical technologies utilized have been avoided, and in most fruits and certain cereal varying grades, their composition is still unknown in Fig. 1.1 [40].

1.2.1 Polyphenol's Chemical Structure

The term polyphenols refers to a vast collection of compounds that can, on the basis of their source, biological function, or chemical structure, be categorized into several subclasses or subdivisions. A range of organic acids and carbohydrates can chemically be combined with structural phenolic properties. The general structures of traditional flavonoids are illustrated in Fig. 1.2. As indicated in Fig. 1.3, many egg-like plants, fruits, and vegetables contain polyphenols and other chemicals, such as carotenoids, vitamin C, and vitamin E [24, 41]. These polyphenols are

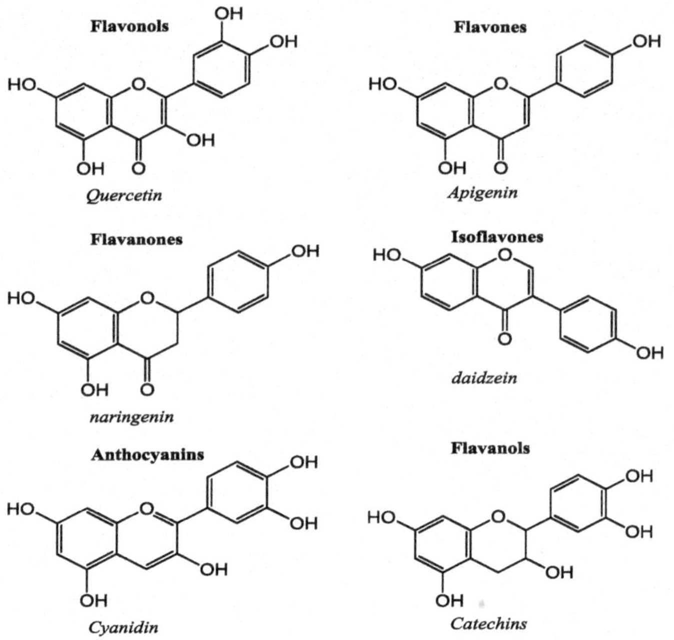

Fig. 1.1 Specific flavonoid structures [40]

Fig. 1.2 General Phenolic Acid Structural Formulae [40]

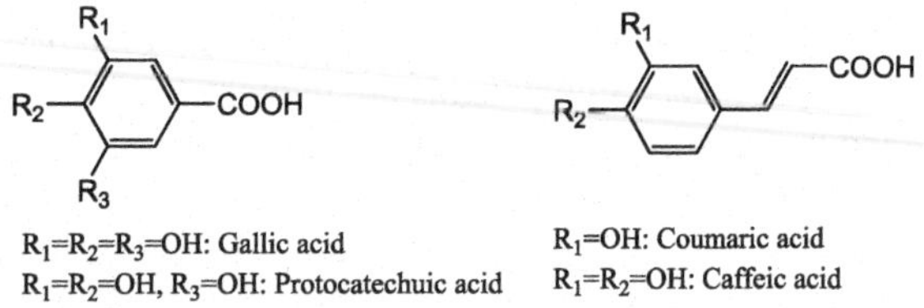

considered to have a health effect on both humans and animals. Other foods and drinks derived from these, such as red wine high in resveratrol, extra virgin olive oil high in hydroxytyrosol, chocolate, and tea, especially green tea high in epigallocatechin gallate (EGCG) [42] Fig. 1.4, are among the most abundant natural antioxidants to human diets but are also the most abundant natural antioxidants in human diets.

The term polyphenols refers to a large group of chemicals that can be classified into various subclasses, or subdivisions, based on their origin, biological function, or chemical structure. Compounds with structural phenolic characteristics can be coupled with a variety of organic acids and carbohydrates chemically. Figure 1.2 illustrates the general structures of typical flavonoids. Many edible plants, fruits, and vegetables contain polyphenols, as well as other compounds such as carotenoids, vitamin C, and vitamin E [24, 41], as illustrated in Fig. 1.3. These polyphenols are thought to be responsible for both human and animal health effects. Fruits, vegetables, and whole grains are the most abundant natural antioxidants in the

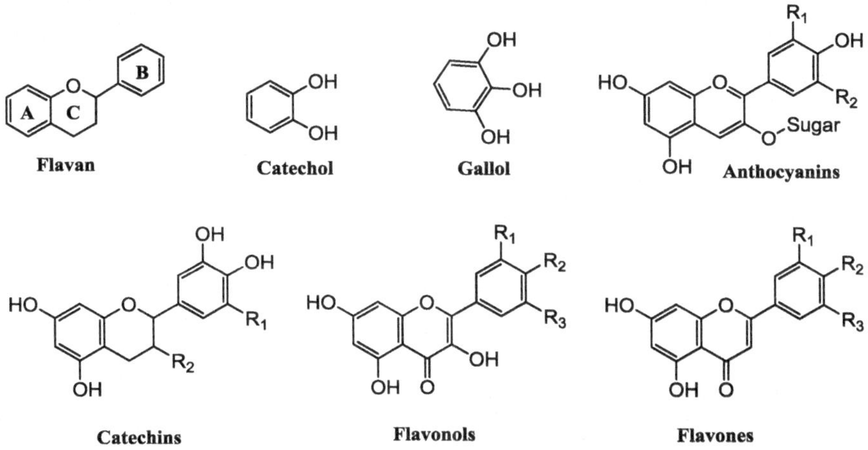

Fig. 1.3 Flavonoid derivatives with basic structures found most commonly [24]

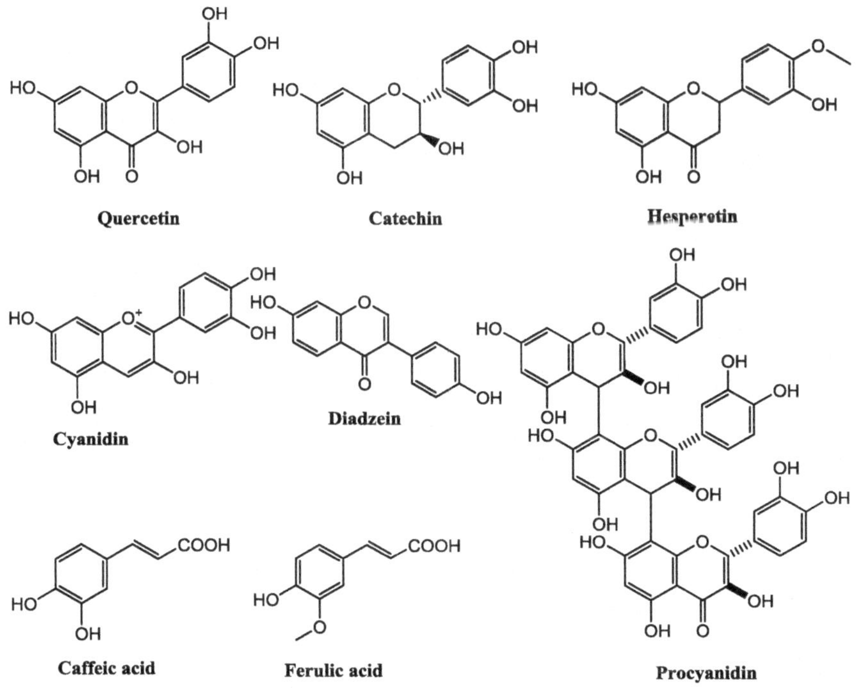

Fig. 1.4 Polyphenol commonly found in fruits and coffee with certain phenolic rings [41]

human diet, but so are other foods and beverages derived from them, such as red wine, which is high in resveratrol, extra virgin olive oil, which is high in hydroxytyrosol, chocolate, and tea, particularly green tea, which is high in epigallocatechin gallate (EGCG) [42] Fig. 1.4.

1.2.2 Ball-and-stick Model of Phenol

The majority of them are glycosides, which are related to sugars in plants. Carbohydrates and organic acids can be linked to the skeletons of polyphenols in a variety of ways. Polyphenols contain simple compounds like phenolic acids as well as complicated structures like proanthocyanins, which are highly polymerized molecules.

1.2.3 Classification

The structural components, which connect these rings to one other, and the corresponding substituents can therefore be separated into separate categories based on the number of phenolic rings in their arrangements. This can differentiate two primary groups: flavonoids and non-flavonoids. Flavonoids have a structure consisting of two aromatic rings, A and B, linked to the oxygenated C-ring, by three carbon atoms and subdivided into six subclasses according to the type of heterocycle involved (C-ring), which are: Non-flavonoids, Flavonols, flavonols, flavanols or flavanol-3-ols and/or flavan-3-ols, anthocyanins and isoflavones and flavanones, and flavanonolins, flavanonols, or catechins; Some of the easy phenols to be subdivided [24, 40–42] are benzoic aldehydes, phenolic acids, tannin hydrolyzable, acetophenones, and phenylacetic acids, coumarin, benzophenones, xanthones, stilbenes, lignans, and secoiridoids.

1.3 Variety of Plant, Plant Products, and Polyphenol Content

While several types of phenol, such as quercetin (flavonole, see figure), are found in the bulk of vegetable products (tea, wine, cereals, legumes, fruit, juices, etc.) (e.g., flavanones in citrus, isoflavones in soya, phloridzin in apples, etc.). Apples had among other polyphenols for instance flavanols, chlorogenic acid, hydroxycinnamic acid, phloretin glycosides, and anthocyanins. Other influencing elements include environmental and harvest maturity conditions, domestic or industrial processing, storage, and plant species. Factors that influence polyphenol concentration include Strawberries, lichi, and grapes have the highest concentration of Polyphenol among fruits, whereas artichokes, parsleys, and Brussels have the highest content of Polyphenol in fruits. Lowest concentration of polyphenol are found in melons and avocados [43].

1.4 Polyphenols' Various Health Benefits

1.4.1 It Can Decrease Blood Sugar Levels

Polyphenols can help to reduce blood sugar levels, lowering the risk of type 2 diabetes. This is largely due to polyphenols' ability to prevent starch from being broken down into simple sugars, lowering the risk of blood sugar increases after meals. These compounds can also help in stimulating the secretion of insulin, a hormone needed to transfer sugar into your cells from your bloodstream and maintain healthy blood sugar levels. Various studies further relate diets rich in polyphenol to lower levels of fasting blood sugar, higher glucose tolerance, and improved insulin sensitivity, all important factors that reduce the type 2 diabetes risk. In one study, persons who ate the most polyphenol-rich foods had a 57% lower risk of acquiring type 2 diabetes over the course of 2–4 years than those who ate the least. According to studies, anthocyanins have the most anti-diabetic effect of all polyphenols. They are commonly found in red, purple, and blue foods including berries, currants, and grapes [44–46].

1.4.2 Your Risk of Heart Disease Could Be Diminished

Adding polyphenols to your diet will increase the health of your heart. Experts agree that this is partially attributable to the antioxidant effects of polyphenols, a risk factor for cardiac disease that helps minimize chronic inflammation. Polyphenol supplements are related to lower blood pressure and LDL (bad) cholesterol levels, as well as greater HDL (good) cholesterol in two recent reviews. Another research showed that in those with higher levels of enterolactone, which is a measure of lignan intake, a 45% lower risk of death from heart disease was found. In flax seeds and whole grains, lignans are a type of polyphenol usually found [47].

1.4.3 Blood Clots Can Be Avoided

Polyphenols may reduce your chances of forming a blood clot. Blood clots occur when platelets circulating in your bloodstream start clumping together. Platelet aggregation is a technique for controlling excessive bleeding that works well. Excess platelet accumulation, on the other hand, can lead to blood clots, which can result in serious health problems such as deep vein thrombosis, stroke, and pulmonary embolism. According to test-tube and animal studies [48], polyphenols can help inhibit platelet aggregation, decreasing the formation of blood clots.

1.4.4 It Can Protect You from Cancer

Research consistently tries diets high in plant foods to a lower risk of cancer, and polyphenols are partly responsible for this, as assumed by many experts. Polyphenols, both of which can be helpful for cancer prevention, have significant antioxidant and anti-inflammatory impacts [49]. A recent analysis of test-tube studies indicates that polyphenols can block the development and growth of different cancer cells [50]. In humans, some studies have related high polyphenol intake blood markers to a lower risk of breast and prostate cancer, while others have no effects [51, 52]. Therefore, before firm conclusions can be made, further studies are needed.

1.4.5 It Can Encourage Good Digestion

Polyphenols can help digestion by stimulating the growth of healthy gut bacteria while fending off toxic ones [53]. For example, evidence indicates that extracts of polyphenol-rich tea can foster the growth of beneficial *bifidobacteria*. Similarly, polyphenols from green tea can help in combat against harmful bacteria, like *E. coli*, *Salmonella,* and *C. difficile*. As well as improving the symptoms of peptic ulcer disease (PUD) and inflammatory bowel disease (IBD) [54]. In addition, emerging research suggests that polyphenols can assist probiotics to flourish and survive. These are beneficial bacteria that exist and can be taken in supplement form in some fermented foods. More research however is required.

1.4.6 Brain Function Can Be Encouraged

Foods rich in polyphenols can improve your concentration and memory. One study showed that in older adults with moderate mental illness, drinking grape juice, which is naturally abundant in polyphenols, helped to dramatically improve memory in as little as 12 weeks [55]. Others believe that cocoa flavanols can increase blood flow to the brain and have related these polyphenols to enhanced memory and concentration at work [56]. Similarly, *Ginkgo biloba*, a polyphenol-rich plant extract, seems to improve memory, learning, and concentration. In those with dementia, it has also been related to improved brain function and short-term memory [57]. Polyphenols can prevent blood clots, lower the level of blood sugar, and lower the risk of heart disease. While more research is required, they can also promote brain activity, improve digestion, and give some protection against cancer.

1.5 Polyphenol-rich Foods

Although the best-known sources of polyphenols are currently tea, dark chocolate, red wine, and berries, many other foods also contain high concentrations of these beneficial compounds. Here are the 60 polyphenol-richest foods, classified by category [58].

S. no.	Name of fruit
1.	Apples
2.	The Apricots
3.	Chokeberries in black
4.	Red and black currants
5.	Elderberries in black
6.	Yellow grapes
7.	Bromberries
8.	Blueberry
9.	The Quarries
10.	Grapes
11.	Grapefruit
12.	Lemon
13.	Nectarines
14.	Peaches
15.	Pears
16.	Grenade
17.	Pens
18.	Framboises
19.	Strawberry
	Vegetables
20	Asparagus
21	Carrots
22	Endive
23	Potatoes
24.	Red Chicory
	Seeds and nuts
25.	Yogurt soy
27	White Beans
28	Milk soybeans
29	Meat from soy
30	Sprouts from soybeans
31	Tofu
32	Tempeh
33	Black beans
34	Lettuce in red
35	Yellow and red onions
36	Spinach

(continued)

S. no.	Name of fruit
37	Shallots
	Legumes
38	Almonds
39	Chestnuts
40	Rye
41	Oats
42	Hazelnuts
43	Seeds of flax
44	Pecans
45	Walnuts
46	Cereals
47	Capers
48	Vinegar
49	Red wine
50	Oil from rapeseed
51	Ginger
52	Tea
53	Olive oil
54	Dark Cake Chocolate
55	Powdered Cocoa
56	Dehydrated peppermint
57	Thyme
58	Rosemary Marriage
59	Oregano from Mexico
60	Cinnamon Dried Out

Having ingredients from each of these groups in your diet gives you a wide range of polyphenols. Many foods from plants are naturally rich in polyphenols. A smart way to improve your consumption of these beneficial nutrients is to include a number of these foods in your diet.

1.6 What Are Supplements of Polyphenols?

Supplements have the advantage of delivering polyphenols at a stable dosage. They still have some possible disadvantages, however. First, it has not been reliably shown that supplements provide the same benefits as foods rich in polyphenols and do not contain any of the additional beneficial plant compounds usually found in whole foods. In addition, when interacting with the many other nutrients naturally present in foods, polyphenols appear to function best. Whether isolated polyphenols, such as those in supplements, are as effective as those contained in foods is currently uncertain [59]. Lastly, polyphenol supplements are not regulated, and many contain doses that are more than 100 times greater than those in foods. In order to determine safe and efficient dosages, further study is needed, and it is uncertain if these large doses are beneficial. Polyphenol supplements do not offer the same health benefits as polyphenol-rich diets. There were no effective or safe doses found [60].

1.7 Potential Risks and Adverse Reactions

For most individuals, polyphenol-rich foods are healthy. Supplements that appear to have much higher levels of polyphenols than those usually found in a balanced diet cannot be said the same. Animal studies indicate that high-dose polyphenol supplements can trigger thyroid hormone levels to cause kidney damage, tumors, and imbalance. They can cause an increased risk of stroke and premature death in humans. Some supplements rich in polyphenols can interfere with the absorption of nutrients or interact with medication. They can decrease the capacity of your body to absorb iron, thiamine, or folate, for example. If you have a nutrient deficiency diagnosed or are taking medicine, it might be safer to talk about polyphenol supplements with your healthcare expert before taking them. In addition, certain foods high in polyphenols, such as beans and peas, can be lectin-rich. Lectins can cause unpleasant digestive symptoms, such as gas, bloating, and indigestion, when consumed in large amounts. If this is a problem for you, before eating your legumes, consider soaking or sprouting them, as this will help to reduce the content of lectin by up to 50%. Polyphenol-rich foods are considered safe for most people, while supplements may cause more harm than good. Try soaking or sprouting polyphenol-rich legumes prior to consuming them to minimize gas, bloating, and indigestion [61].

1.8 Bioavailability

Polyphenols rely mostly on their bioavailability to express their biological characteristics. Defined by its chemical composition are the limit and speed of absorption in the intestines. A large source of flavanone is Citrus fruit, while Green Tea supplies catechins that are widely accessible [62]. The plasma antioxidant activity after the intake of meals rich in polyphenol offers the necessary data for the evaluation for phenolic composite absorption in the intestines when phenolic concentrations in urine and plasma are assessed [63]. When a number of flavonoids are absorbed into the intestines, plasma content gradually falls. Because of the strong affinity of plasma albumin to quercetin, it has a prolonged half-life for removal. Normal glycosylation is used to treat flavones, isoflavones, flavonols, and anthocyanin [64]. Glucose and rhamnoses, which are chemical-bonded, are prevalent, such as xylose, glucuronic acid, and Galactose.

Polyphenols typically comprise one sugar but may contain two or three sugar replacements and wide diversity. The malonic acid group can also replace sugars. Glycosylation determines both the chemical, physical and biological properties of polyphenols that explains why quercetin and quercetin-3-O-rhamnoglucoside are different in their hydrophilic qualities. The mucosal and colon-microflora of gastro-intestinal are two sites in which glycosidase can develop, which is endogenous, so that glycosidase is present in food. Human cells often release—glucosidases, and during development a tissue-specific model of expression is generally controlled. The latent substrates of each cell are combined to xylose and glucose by polyphenols [65].

The only enzymes that can split polyphenols that are linked to rhamnose, microflora-rhamnosidases, are human glucosidases. Acids such as gallic acid are often used for epicatechin acylation. Galloyl substitution does not appreciably modify the partition coefficient of flavanols, and bioavailability is not influenced in the form of glycosylation. Flavanols are absorbed independently of hydrolysis while passing through a cellular membrane. Caffeine is often esterified with fats, lipids, and organic acids. Chlorogenic acid, which is found in coffee in significant quantities, is generated if quinic acid is esterified with caffeic acid. Chlorogenic acid and caffeic acid cannot be separated from human tissue by esterases, and no chlorogenic acid can release caffeic acid. Only in the colon microbiota can chlorogenic acid be treated [66].

Polyphenols also pass through the small intestine without being absorbed, influencing the intestinal bacteria that colonize it. Two-dimensional reactions occur as a result of these transiting polyphenols [67]. First and foremost, polyphenols are physiologically transformed into their more accessible metabolites. Second, polyphenols are most likely to change the microbial community of the gut by blocking harmful bacteria and increasing beneficial bacteria. These can boost beneficial microorganisms by acting as a prebiotic metabolite in the latter. As a result, interactions between dietary polyphenols and gut microbiota can affect the health of the human host [68].

1.9 Conclusion

Polyphenols, which are divided into flavonoids, phenolic acid, polyphenolic amides, and other polyphenols, are beneficial substances found in a variety of plant diets [69]. Besides protecting against blood clots, heart disease, and certain cancers, they can improve digestion, brain function, and blood sugar levels [70]. In order to establish appropriate and safe dosages of polyphenol supplements, further research is required. It is therefore best to focus on foods for the time being rather than supplements to improve your intake of these safe compounds [71, 72].

References

1. Wegener G. 'Let food be thy medicine, and medicine be thy food': hippocrates revisited. Acta Neuropsychiatr. 2014;26(01):1–3. https://doi.org/10.1017/neu.2014.3.
2. Clydesdale FM, Francis FJ. Food nutrition and health. Netherlands: Springer Science & Business Media; 1985.

3. Bohn SK, Croft KD, Burrows S, Puddey IB, Mulder TP, Fuchs D, Woodman RJ, Hodgson JM. Effects of black tea on body composition and metabolic outcomes related to cardiovascular disease risk: a randomized controlled trial. Food Funct. 2014;5(7):1613–20. https://doi.org/10.1039/C4FO00209A.
4. Rasouli H, Hosseini-Ghazvini SM-B, Adibi H. Differential A-Amylase/A-glucosidase inhibitory activities of plant-derived phenolic compounds: a virtual screening perspective for the treatment of obesity and diabetes. Food Funct. 2017;8:1942–54. https://doi.org/10.1039/C7FO00220C
5. Akbari M, Rasouli H, Bahdor T. Physiological and pharmaceutical effect of fenugreek: a review. IOSR J Pharm. 2012;2(4):49–53. https://doi.org/10.9790/3013-24204953.
6. Valdés L, Cuervo A, Salazar N, Ruas-Madiedo P, Gueimonde M, González S. The relationship between phenolic compounds from diet and microbiota: impact on human health. Food Funct. 2015;6(8):2424–39. https://doi.org/10.1039/C5FO00322A.
7. Oh M-M, Trick HN, Rajashekar C. Secondary metabolism and antioxidants are involved in environmental adaptation and stress tolerance in lettuce. J Plant Physiol. 2009;166(2):180–91. https://doi.org/10.1016/j.jplph.2008.04.015.
8. Yue W, Ming Q-L, Lin B, Rahman K, Zheng C-J, Han T, Qin L-P. Medicinal plant cell suspension cultures: pharmaceutical applications and high-yielding strategies for the desired secondary metabolites. Crit Rev Biotechnol. 2016;36(2):215–32. https://doi.org/10.3109/07388551.2014.923986.
9. Bourgaud F, Gravot A, Milesi S, Gontier E. Production of plant secondary metabolites: a historical perspective. Plant Sci. 2001;161(5):839–51. https://doi.org/10.1016/S0168-9452(01)00490-3.
10. Montero R, Pérez-Bueno ML, Barón M, Florez-Sarasa I, Tohge T, Fernie AR, Flexas J, Bota J. Alterations in primary and secondary metabolism in Vitis Vinifera 'Malvasía De Banyalbufar' upon Infection with Grapevine Leafroll-Associated Virus 3. Physiol Plant. 2016; https://doi.org/10.1111/ppl.12440.
11. Okumoto S, Funck D, Trovato M, Forlani G. Editorial: amino acids of the glutamate family: functions beyond primary metabolism. Front Plant Sci. 2016;7:1–3. https://doi.org/10.3389/fpls.2016.00318.
12. Kossel A. Ueber Die Chemische Zusammensetzung Der Zelle. Du Bois-Reymond's. Archiv Arch Anat Physiol Physiol Abt. 1891;278:181–6.
13. Czapek F. Biochemie Der Pflanzen, vol. 2. Germany: G. Fischer; 1925.
14. Rasouli H, Farzaei MH, Mansouri K, Mohammadzadeh S, Khodarahmi R. Plant cell cancer: may natural phenolic compounds prevent onset and development of plant cell malignancy? A literature review. Molecules. 2016;21(9):1104. https://doi.org/10.3390/molecules21091104.
15. Villaño D, Vilaplana C, Medina S, Algaba-Chueca F, Cejuela-Anta R, Martínez-Sanz J, Ferreres F, GilIzquierdo A. Relationship between the ingestion of a polyphenol-rich drink, hepcidin hormone, and longterm training. Molecules. 2016;21(10):1333. https://doi.org/10.3390/molecules21101333.
16. Zhou Z-Q, Xiao J, Fan H-X, Yu Y, He R-R, Feng X-L, Kurihara H, So K-F, Yao X-S, Gao H. Polyphenols from Wolfberry and their bioactivities. Food Chem. 2017;214:644–54. https://doi.org/10.1016/j.foodchem.2016.07.105.
17. Farzaei H, Rahimi MR, Abdollahi M. The role of dietary polyphenols in the management of inflammatory bowel disease. Curr Pharm Biotechnol. 2015;16(3):196–210.
18. Khurana S, Venkataraman K, Hollingsworth A, Piche M, Tai T. Polyphenols: benefits to the cardiovascular system in health and in aging. Nutrients. 2013;5(10):3779–827. https://doi.org/10.3390/nu5103779. 30 H. Rasouli et al. Downloaded by [Kermanshah Uni of Medical Sciences] at 04:47 22 December 2017
19. Pinent M, Blay M, Serrano J, Ardévol A. Effects of flavanols on the enteroendocrine system: repercussions on food intake. Crit Rev Food Sci Nutr. 2015; https://doi.org/10.1080/10408398.2013.871221. (just-accepted), 00–00

20. Visioli F, Lastra CADL, Andres-Lacueva C, Aviram M, Calhau C, Cassano A, D'Archivio M, Faria A, Favé G, Fogliano V. Polyphenols and human health: a prospectus. Crit Rev Food Sci Nutr. 2011;51(6):524–46. https://doi.org/10.1080/10408391003698677.
21. McSweeney M, Seetharaman K. State of polyphenols in the drying process of fruits and vegetables. Crit Rev Food Sci Nutr. 2015;55(5):660–9.
22. Yang CS, Chung JY, Yang G-Y, Chhabra SK, Lee M-J. Tea and tea polyphenols in cancer prevention. J Nutr. 2000;130(2):472S–8S.
23. Bose M, Lambert JD, Ju J, Reuhl KR, Shapses SA, Yang CS. The major green tea polyphenol, epigallocatechin-3-gallate, inhibits obesity, metabolic syndrome, and fatty liver disease in high-fat–fed mice. J Nutr. 2008;138(9):1677–83.
24. Scalbert A, Johnson IT, Saltmarsh M. Polyphenols: antioxidants and beyond. Am J Clin Nutr. 2005;81(1):215S–7S.
25. Lu C, Zhu W, Shen C-L, Gao W. Green tea polyphenols reduce body weight in rats by modulating obesity-related genes. PLoS One. 2012;7(6):e38332.
26. Aviram M, Dornfeld L, Rosenblat M, Volkova N, Kaplan M, Coleman R, Hayek T, Presser D, Fuhrman B. Pomegranate juice consumption reduces oxidative stress, atherogenic modifications to LDL, and platelet aggregation: studies in humans and in atherosclerotic apolipoprotein E–deficient mice. Am JClin Nutr. 2000;71(5):1062–76.
27. Bravo L. Polyphenols: chemistry, dietary sources, metabolism, and nutritional significance. Nutr Rev. 1998;56(11):317–33.
28. Brglez Mojzer E, Knez Hrnčič M, Škerget M, Knez Ž, Bren U. Polyphenols: extraction methods, antioxidative action, bioavailability and anticarcinogenic effects. Molecules. 2016;21(7):901–39. https://doi.org/10.3390/molecules21070901.
29. Shao Y, Bao J. Polyphenols in whole rice grain: genetic diversity and health benefits. Food Chem. 2015;180:86–97. https://doi.org/10.1016/j.foodchem.2015.02.027.
30. Pereira DM, Valentão P, Pereira JA, Andrade PB. Phenolics: from chemistry to biology. Molecules. 2009;14(6):2202–11.
31. Zhang H, Tsao R. Dietary polyphenols oxidative stress antioxidant anti-inflammatory effects. Curr Opin Food Sci. 2016;8:33–42.
32. Moga M, Dimienescu O, Arvatescu C, Mironescu A, Dracea L, Ples L. The role of natural polyphenols in the prevention and treatment of cervical cancer-an overview. Molecules. 2016;21(8):1055.
33. Miglio C, Chiavaro E, Visconti A, Fogliano V, Pellegrini N. Effects of different cooking methods on nutritional and physicochemical characteristics of selected vegetables. J Agric Food Chem. 2007;56(1):139–47.
34. Napolitano A, Cascone A, Graziani G, Ferracane R, Scalfi L, Di Vaio C, Ritieni A, Fogliano V. Influence of variety and storage on the polyphenol composition of apple flesh. J Agric Food Chem. 2004;52(21):6526–31.
35. Xiao J. Phytochemicals in food and nutrition. Crit Rev Food Sci Nutr. 2016;56(1):S1–3.
36. Pangeni R, Sahni JK, Ali J, Sharma S, Baboota S. Resveratrol: review on therapeutic potential and recent advances in drug delivery. Expert Opin Drug Deliv. 2014;11(8):1285–98.
37. Scopus. Scopus Database, USA (20.10.2016); 2016.
38. Rendeiro C, Vauzour D, Rattray M, Waffo-Téguo P, Mérillon JM, Butler LT, Williams CM, Spencer JP. Dietary levels of pure flavonoids improve spatial memory performance, and increase hippocampal brain derived neurotrophic factor. PLoS One. 2013;8(5):e63535.
39. Dragovicuzelac V, Levaj B, Mrkic V, Bursac D, Boras M. The content of polyphenols and carotenoids in three apricot cultivars depending on stage of maturity and geographical region. Food Chem. 2007;102:966–75.
40. Archivio D, Filesi M, Di Benedetto C, Gargiulo R, Giovannini R, Masella CR. Polyphenols, dietary sources and bioavailability. Annali-Istituto Superiore di Sanita. 2007;43:348.
41. Marrugat J, Covas M-I, Fitó M, Schröder H, Miró-Casas E, Gimeno E, López-Sabater MC, de la Torre R, Farré M. Effects of differing phenolic content in dietary olive oils on lipids and LDL oxidation. Eur J Nutr. 2004;43:140–7.

42. Tapiero H, Nguyen Ba G, Tew KD. Estrogens and environmental estrogens. Biomed Pharmacother. 2002;56:36–44.
43. Pandey KB, Rizvi SI. Plant polyphenols as dietary antioxidants in human health and disease. Oxidative Med Cell Longev. 2009;2(5):270–8.
44. Georgé S, Brat P, Alter P, Amiot MJ. Rapid determination of polyphenols and vitamin c in plant-derived products. J Agric Food Chem. 2005;53:1370–3.
45. Lambert JD, Hong J, Yang G-Y, Liao J, Yang CS. Inhibition of carcinogenesis by polyphenols: evidence from laboratory investigations. Am J Clin Nutr. 2005;81:284S–91S.
46. Hussain T, Gupta S, Adhami VM, Mukhtar H. Green tea constituent epigallocatechin-3-gallate selectively inhibits COX-2 without affecting COX-1 expression in human prostate carcinoma cells. Int J Cancer. 2004;113:660–9.
47. Khurana S, Venkataraman K, Hollingsworth A, Piche M, Tai TC. Polyphenols: benefits to the cardiovascular system in health and in aging. Nutrients. 2013;5(10):3779–827.
48. James AH, Konkle BA, Bauer KA. Prevention and treatment of venous thromboembolism in pregnancy and patients with hereditary antithrombin deficiency. Int J Women's Health. 2013;5:233–41.
49. Madigan M, Karhu E. The role of plant-based nutrition in cancer prevention. J Unexplored Med Data. 2018;3:9.
50. Dinu M, Abbate R, Gensini GF, Casini A, Sofi F. Vegetarian vegan diets, and multiple health outcomes: a systematic review with meta-analysis of observational studies. Crit Rev Food Sci Nutr. 2017;57(17):3640–9.
51. Niedzwiecki A, Roomi MW, Kalinovsky T, Rath M. Anticancer efficacy of polyphenols and their combinations. Nutrients. 2016;8(9):552.
52. Wang J, Tang L, Wang JS. Biomarkers of dietary polyphenols in cancer studies: current evidence and beyond. Oxid Med Cell Longev. 2015;2015:732302.
53. Marin L, Miguelez EM, Villar CJ, Lombo F. Bioavailability of dietary polyphenols and gut microbiota metabolism: antimicrobial properties. Biomed Res Int. 2015;2015:905215.
54. Dryden GW, Song M, McClain C. Polyphenols, and gastrointestinal diseases. Curr Opin Gastroenterol. 2006;22(2):165–70.
55. Krikorian R, Nash TA, Shidler MD, Shukitt-Hale B, Joseph JA. Concord grape juice supplementation improves memory function in older adults with mild cognitive impairment. Br J Nutr. 2010;103(5):730–4.
56. Field DT, Williams CM, Butler LT. Consumption of cocoa flavanols results in an acute improvement in visual and cognitive functions. Physiol Behav. 2011;103(3–4):255–60.
57. Vauzour D. Dietary polyphenols as modulators of brain functions: biological actions and molecular mechanisms underpinning their beneficial effects. Oxid Med Cell Longev. 2012;2012:914273.
58. Perez-Jimenez J, Neveu V, Vos F, Scalbert A. Identification of the 100 richest dietary sources of polyphenols: an application of the Phenol-Explorer database. Eur J Clin Nutr. 2010;64(Suppl 3):S112–20.
59. Cory H, Passarelli S, Szeto J, Tamez M, Mattei J. The role of polyphenols in human health and food systems: a mini-review. Front Nutr. 2018;5:87.
60. Mennen LI, Walker R, Bennetau-Pelissero C, Scalbert A. Risks and safety of polyphenol consumption. Am J Clin Nutr. 2005;81(1 Suppl):326S–9S.
61. Last Updated on December 20, 2019 by Michael Joseph. The Top 100 Foods High in Polyphenols. https://www.nutritionadvance.com/nutrition/top-foodsources-polyphenols.
62. Srini SV. Bioavailability of ingredients in dietary supplements. In: Pharmaceutical dissolution testing. Cambridge: Informa Healthcare; 2005. p. 407–19.
63. Natsume M, Osakabe N, Oyama M, Sasaki M, Baba S, Nakamura Y, Osawa T, Terao J. Structures of epicatechin glucuronide identified from plasma and urine after oral ingestion of epicatechin: differences between human and rat. Free Radic Biol Med. 2003;34:840–9.
64. Zhang H, Wang L, Deroles S, Bennett R, Davies K. New insight into the structures and formation of anthocyanic vacuolar inclusions in flower petals. BMC Plant Biol. 2006;6:29.

65. Purushotham A, Tian M, Belury MA. The citrus fruit flavonoid naringenin suppresses hepatic glucose production from FAO hepatoma cells. Mol Nutr Food Res. 2009;53:300–7.
66. World Health Organization. Global health risks: mortality and burden of disease attributable to selected major risks. Geneva: World Health Organization, WHO Press; 2009.
67. Kim K, Vance TM, Chun OK. Greater flavonoid intake is associated with improved CVD risk Factors in US adults. Br J Nutr. 2016;115(8):1481–8.
68. Klinder A, Shen Q, Heppel S, Lovegrove JA, Rowland I, Tuohy KM. Impact of increasing fruit and vegetables and flavonoid intake on the human gut microbiota. Food and Function. 2016;7 (4):1788–96.
69. de la Rosa LA, Alvarez-Parrilla E, Gonzàlez-Aguilar GA. Fruit, and vegetable phytochemicals: chemistry, nutritional value, and stability. 11th ed. Hoboken: Wiley J. & Sons, Inc., Publication; 2010.
70. Han X, Shen T, Lou H. Dietary polyphenols and their biological significance. Int J Mol Sci. 2007;9:950–88.
71. Manach C, Scalbert A, Morand C, Remesy C, Jimenez L. Polyphenols: food sources and bioavailability. Am J Clin Nutr. 2004;79(5):727–47.
72. Tsao R. Chemistry and biochemistry of dietary polyphenols. Nutrients. 2010;2:1231–46.

Natural Polyphenols a New Paradigm in Treatment of Various Diseases

2

Ali Raza Ishaq, Tahira Younis, Ayesha Noor, Faiza Jabeen, and Chen Shouwen

Abstract

Natural products are infinite resources of phytochemicals which continue to serve humans as natural drugs since ancient times. Polyphenols are natural plant-derived pharmacologically active compounds which have potential therapeutic properties including antioxidant, anti-inflammatory, and antitumor. Edible plants particularly phytochemicals and their biological activity in the human body is a trending subject of scientific investigations. Polyphenols are divided into three categories: flavonoids, non-flavonoids, and phenolic acids. Flavonoids have been further categorized as flavones, flavanones, flavonols, flavanols, and isoflavones, even as phenolic acids are classified into hydroxybenzoic and hydroxycinnamic acids. Polyphenols are bioactive compounds to manage the several autoimmune disorder such as vitiligo, ulcerative colitis, and multiple sclerosis through eliciting various intracellular pathways specifically (NF-κB), signaling pathway, mitogen-activated protein kinases (MAPKs) pathway, and phosphatidylinositol 3-kinase/protein kinase B (PI3K/Akt) signaling pathway. This chapter tends to provide a new insight into biomedical application of polyphenol for cancer, UTIs, diabetes, cardiovascular disorders, and neurodegenerative disorders.

All Authors contributed equally.

A. R. Ishaq · C. Shouwen
State Key Laboratory of Biocatalysis and Enzyme Engineering, Environmental Microbial Technology Center of Hubei Province, College of Life Science, Hubei University, Wuhan, China
e-mail: chenshouwen@hubu.edu.cn

T. Younis (✉) · A. Noor
Departments of Zoology, Government College University Faisalabad, Faisalabad, Pakistan

F. Jabeen
Department of Zoology, University of Education, Lahore, Pakistan

S. Tabrez, M. Imran Khan (eds.), *Polyphenols-based Nanotherapeutics for Cancer Management*, https://doi.org/10.1007/978-981-16-4935-6_2

Keywords

Polyphenols · Classification · Biological activity · Nano polyphenol · Source

2.1 Introduction

Nature, the master craftsman of molecules, created almost an inexhaustible array of molecular entities. Polyphenols are the exclusively plant-derived compounds that have unique chemical makeup like phenolic compounds with powerful antioxidant features [1, 2]. Fruits, herbs, green tea, grains, and secondary metabolites are great source of polyphenols [3]. More than 8000 polyphenols are produced by plants as a secondary metabolites [4–6].

Nowadays, researchers are focusing on the identification of natural antimicrobial chemicals in food and developing new compounds for healthy nourishment from alcoholic products [7]. Because many of these compounds [5] are particularly meaningful among the entire group of "natural" beneficial compounds [8], the present literature would provide a quick summary of their classification.

Polyphenols are the best group of phenolic system that have at least two phenyl rings and one or more hydroxyl moieties [9]. This concept encompasses a wide range of heterogeneous compounds in terms of their sophistication. There are two major groups of polyphenols such as flavonoids and non-flavonoids or subdivided [10]. The phenolic ring is the fundamental monomer in polyphenols that are categorized as phenolic acids and phenolic alcohols [11]. Polyphenols are divided into several categories depending on the size of the phenolic ring, but perhaps the most prominent are phenolic acids, flavonoids, stiblins, phenolic alcohols, and lignans [12].

Polyphenols are widely present in plant-based foods which are leading ingredients of a healthy human diet due to their versatile chemical structures [13]. Bioactive compounds are phytochemicals that shield human lives from chronic degenerative diseases [14]. That is why polyphenols are often used as a degenerative disease preventative [15]. Polyphenols are a family of pharmacologically important plant derivatives and most frequent antioxidants in our diet [16]. These suppress the oxidative modification in low-density lipoproteins, which is the underlying premise in atherosclerosis endothelial lesions [17]. A huge body of growing literature supports the application of polyphenols in the treatment of cardiovascular disorder, osteoporosis, neurodegenerative disease, cancer, and diabetes mellitus [18]. The biological activities of bioactive polyphenolic compounds are shown in Fig. 2.1.

This chapter will explore the knowledge about recent advancements in polyphenols application, classification, and their bioavailability.

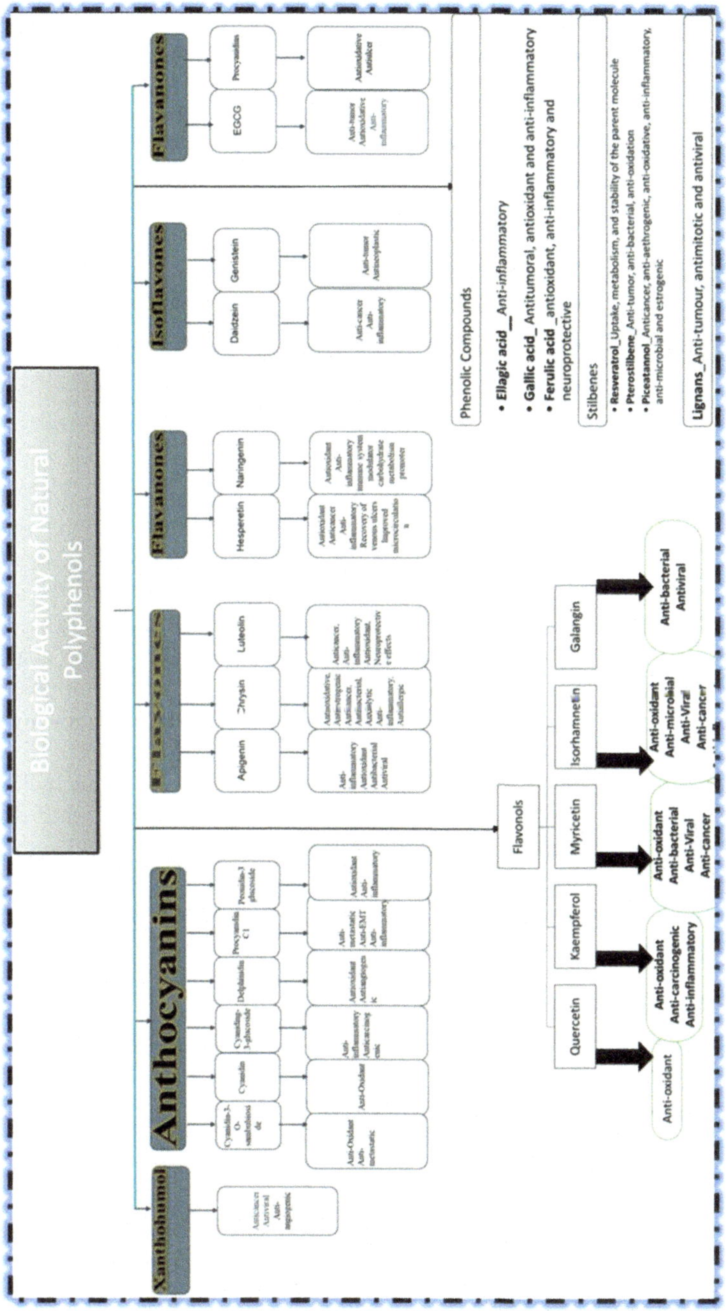

Fig. 2.1 Schematic representation of classification of polyphenol and their biological activity in the human body

2.2 Common Classification of Polyphenols

2.2.1 Non-flavonoids

The two major classes of polyphenolic compounds are hydroxycinnamic and hydroxybenzoic acids. Human diet has a very minute amount of hydroxybenzoic acids hence these are not really presumed to serve a key role in health [19]. The backbone of cinnamic acid and benzoic acid variants have C_1-C_6 and C_3-C_6, respectively [20]. Fruits and vegetables possess free-state phenolic compounds [21] while hull, bran, and seed have linked-form phenolic compounds [22]. Acid, alkali, and enzyme oxidation liberate linked phenolic acids from bran, hull, and seed [23]. These acids are rarely found in plant-based food despite blackberries and some red fruits that produce $<$270 mg/kg of fresh weight [24].

2.2.2 Flavonoids and Their Classification

Flavonoids comprise two benzene rings joined by three carbon chains from a near pyran ring which are widely disturbed in all vascular plants [25]. Over 4000 flavonoids have been discovered in plants which are divided into six classes based on the oxidation state of the central carbon [26]. These classes include flavanones, flavanols, flavonols, isofalvons, flavons, and anthocyanidins [27, 28]. The double bond can be seen among C_3 and C_2 in flavonols, and a hydroxyl group is connected at C_3 [29, 30]. Flavonols account for most flavonoids derived from various foods. Flavonols compounds are particularly abundant in onions [31], and they are often present in broccoli [32] and leeks [33].

Flavonoids have a specific backbone configuration of C_6-C_3-C_6, including two phenolic monomers (C_6). Flavonoids categorize into four subclasses based on their hydroxylation configuration: flavonols, flavones, flavanones, and anthocyanidins [34]. The C_2 of the third ring is linked with the second ring in several flavonoids, but C_3 and C_4 covalently bonded with each other. Although chalcones lack a third ring, they are as flavonoids and abundant in apples and hops [35]. Glycones (Sugar-moiety) form glycosidic linkage with non-sugar par (aglycone) to produce glycosides which have potential antidiabetic activity [36].

Isoflavones is a subclass of flavonoids that has a diphenyl-propane structure in which third ring (C-ring) is joined to second ring (B-ring) through its C_3 position [37]. Such compounds are ubiquitous in legumes, red clover, alfalfa, and kudzu [38]. Soybeans are the major source of isoflavones which have a stronger effect on the human body [38]. Daidzein and genistein, along with glycetein, are two main isoflavones, found in soy and red clovers which are potentially modulating the neutrophil recruitment to surgery site [39]. Most widespread isoflavone-aglycones are 7-O-glucosides and 6"-O-malonyl-7-O-glucosides in beans and soy plants which behave like anti-aging agent [40]. Mostly neo-flavonoids are not present in plants but dalbergin seems to be the most abundant neo-flavonoid occurring in plant-based foods [13].

Flavonols are present at fruit covering because their production is stimulated by light. As, the light to the various edges of the fruits on the same vine, and even on the same piece of fruit, is not equally falling that is why the flavonols content cannot be produced constantly [41]. Catechins and epicatechins have antioxidant properties which are chiefly present in wine and tea [42]. Flavones are far less abundant flavonoids with a double bond between the C3 and C2 carbon atoms [43]. Flavones (2-Phenyl-chromen-4-one) are widespread in the peel or skin of fruits such as berries, fruit peels, grape, parsley, olives, lettuce, and cranberries [44]. The flavone concentration of mandarin essential oil is 6.5 g/L. The classification and chemical structure of polyphenols and their types are shown in Table 2.1.

Flavonones have three saturated carbon rings and an oxygen molecule at C_4 [45]. Flavanones are quite typically present in citrus fruits as well as in aromatic plants [46]. Oranges, eriodictyol, and lemons produce a significant quantity of hesperidin approximately 470–761 mg/L [47]. Flavonones are abundant in hard parts of fruits and integument; entire foods have five times more amount of flavonones as compared to juices [48]. In isoflavones, the occurrence of –OH in between C4 and C7 just like in estradiol which is declared as the array of these compounds is associated with estrogens along with their ability to adhere to estrogen binding receptors. Due to their functional ability, these compounds are referred to as phytochemicals [49].

Soy and its ingredients, mainly glycitein and geinstein, are the major sources of isoflavones, that can be considered as aglycones or covalently linked with glucose monomer [50]. Soy milk has over 1530–130 mg/L of fresh soy which is sensitive to temperature and transforms to glycosides when heat is applied [51].

The existence of two double bonds in the heterocyclic rings of anthocyanidins and anthocyanins separates them from other flavonoids [52]. Glycosylated anthocyanins are water-soluble pigments that occur in vibrant color flowers and fruits; they are responsible for many of the colors which are used [53]. Fruit covering is the main source of anthocyanins, that are reported in the form of anthocyanidins and a moiety of sugar at C3 or at the 5, 7-position of the A-ring [54]. *Polyphenol Amides* Avenanthramides and capsaicinoids are reported to comprise significant features in terms of antioxidant and anti-inflammatory properties. Interestingly, these compounds are associated with peculiar foods: chili peppers when speaking of capsaicinoids and oat products with relation to avenanthramides [55].

2.3 Universe of Polyphenols and Their Bioavailability

Bioavailability of polyphenols is a measure of a significant amount of substance enter into circulation and get access to target organ to perform physiological function. Bioavailability mainly depends upon the two major factors; how much we get (absorption) and how much we exit out (Secretion). It seems to be important to know that polyphenols are most common in human diet but are not produced in human body. Their non-productivity confers due to narrow range of cellular activity,

Table 2.1 Polyphenols Classification, molecular Structure, and their source; Chemical Structure taken from Pubchem and ChemSpider

Polyphenols	Member	Chemical structure	Source
Anthocyanins	Peonidin-3 glucoside	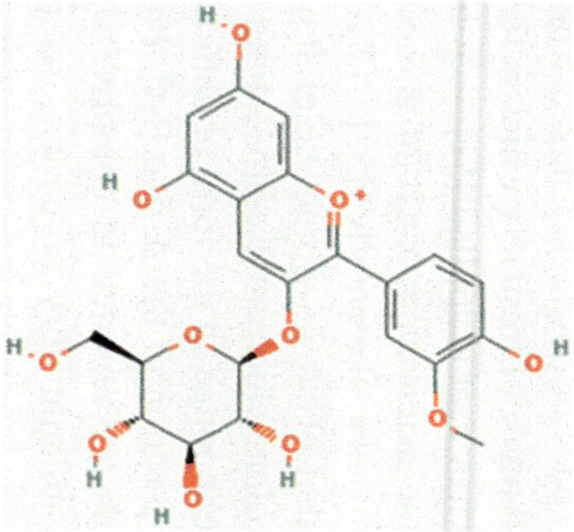	*Acanthopanax sessiliflorus*
	Procyanidin C1	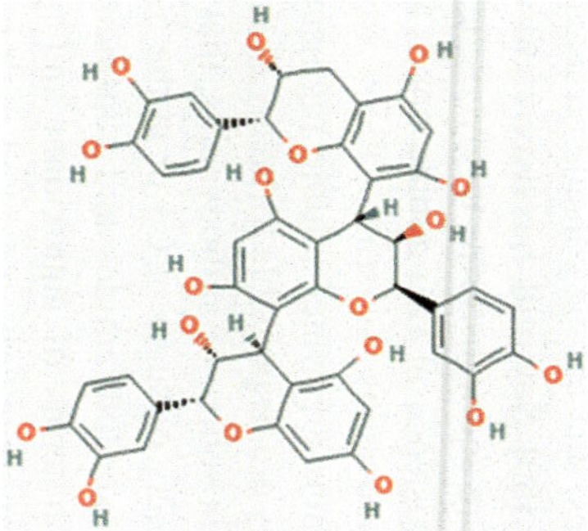	

	Delphinidin	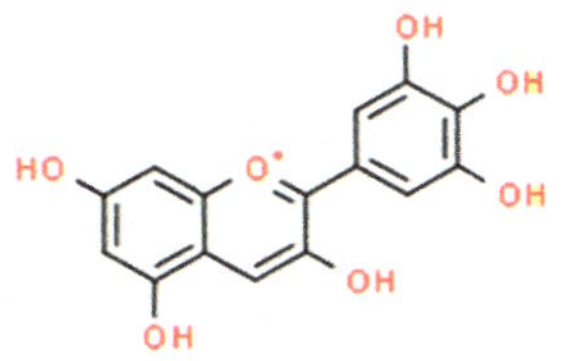	
	Cyanidin	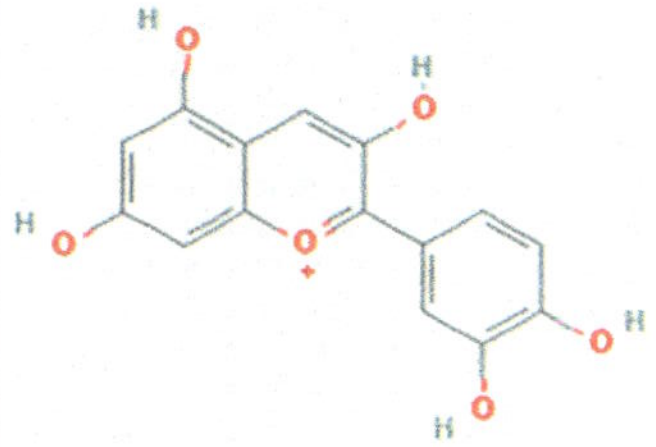	
	Cyanidin-3-O-sambubioside	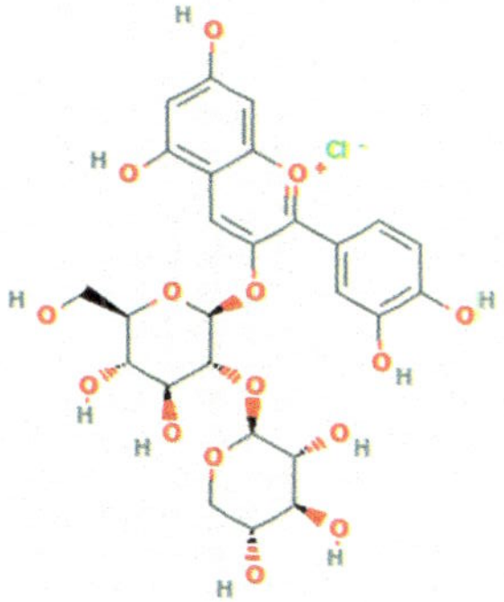	

(continued)

Table 2.1 (continued)

Polyphenols	Member	Chemical structure	Source
	Cyaniding-3-glucoside	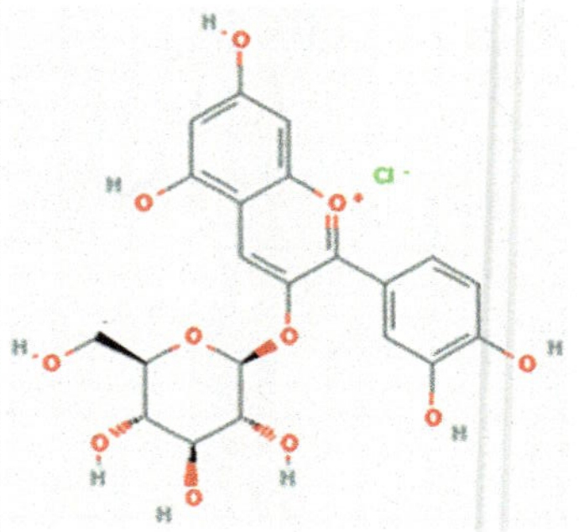	
Xanthohumol		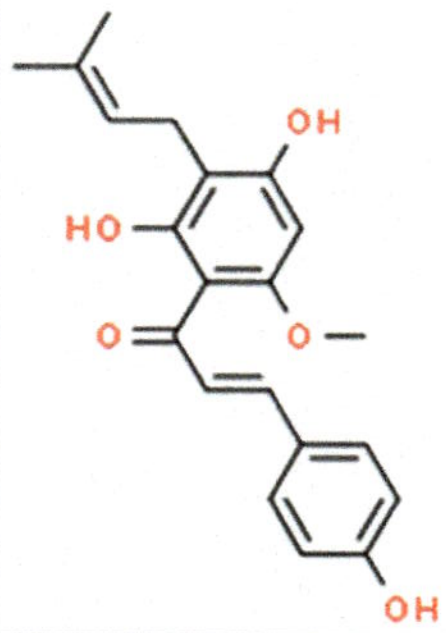	*Humulus lupulus* and beer

Flavanols	EGCG	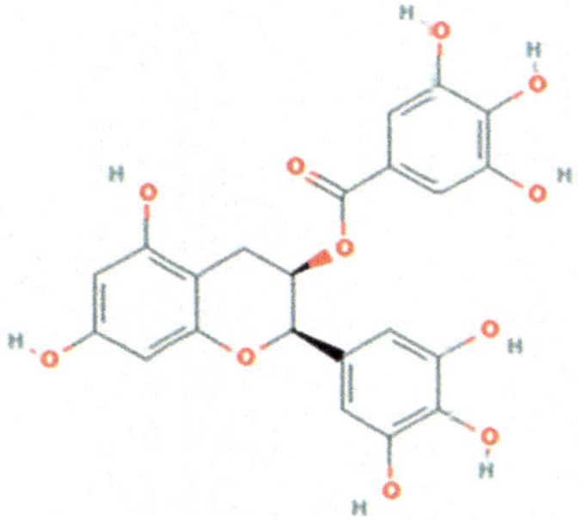	Green tea, apple skin, plums, onions, hazelnuts, pecans, and carob powder
	Procyanidins	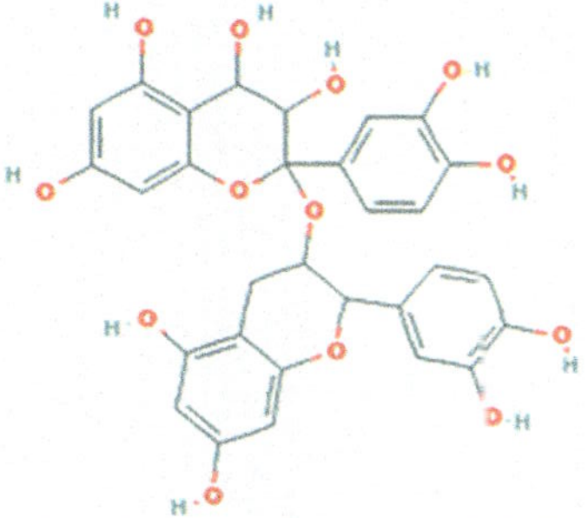	Blueberries, cranberries, black currant, and plums
Flavanones	Naringenin	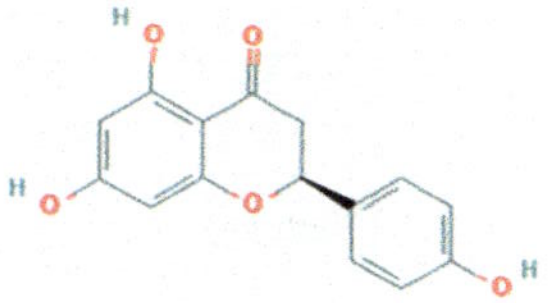	Citrus fruits, grapes, oranges

(continued)

Table 2.1 (continued)

Polyphenols	Member	Chemical structure	Source
	Hesperetin	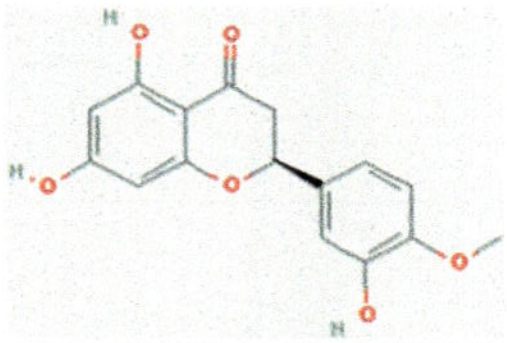	Citrus fruits
Flavones	Apigenin	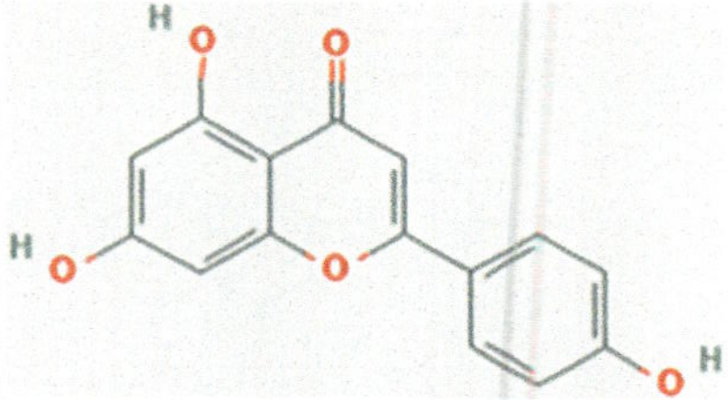	Orange, parsley, onion, tea, and wheat sprout
	Chrysin	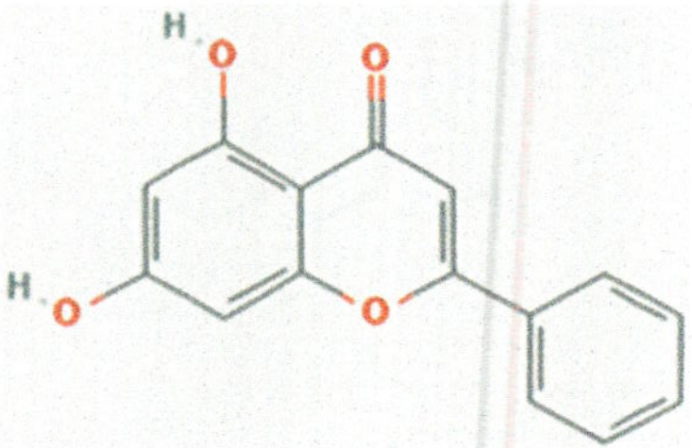	Honey, Propolis Passionflower (*Passiflora caerulea*)

	Luteolin	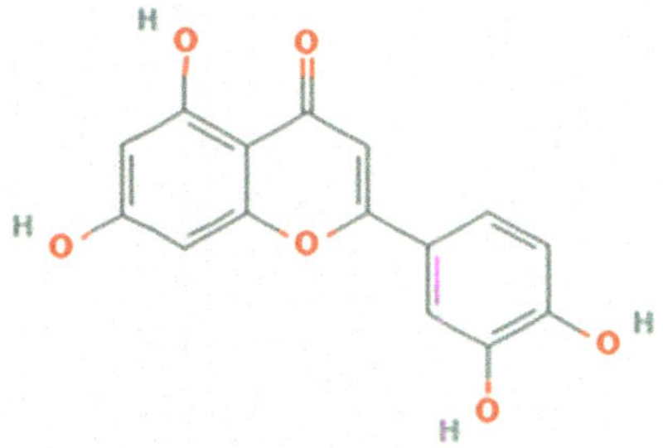	Artichoke, sage, thyme, oregano
Flavonols	Quercetin	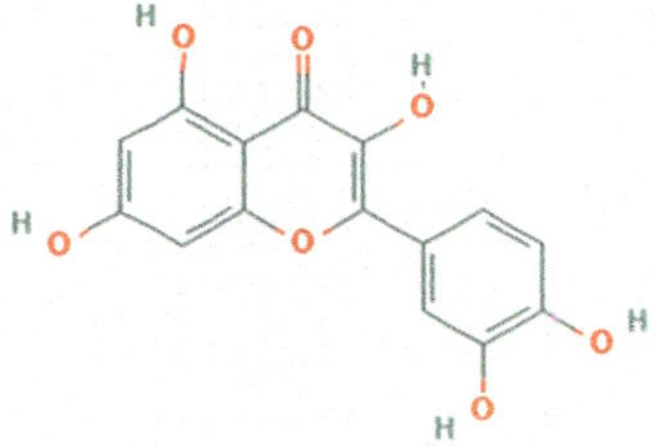	Fruits, vegetables, leaves, seeds, and grains; red onions and kale
	Kaempferol	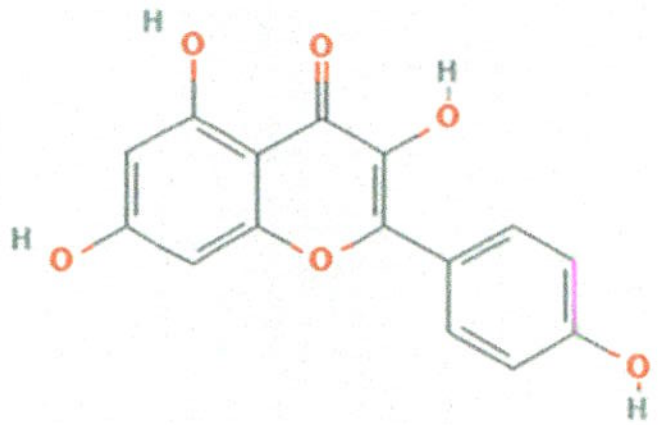	Kale, beans, tea, spinach, and broccoli

(continued)

Table 2.1 (continued)

Polyphenols	Member	Chemical structure	Source
	Myricetin	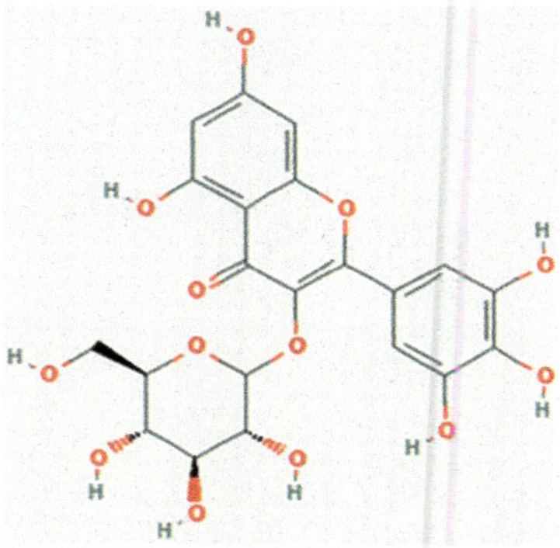	Tomatoes, oranges, nuts, berries, tea, and red wine
	Galangin	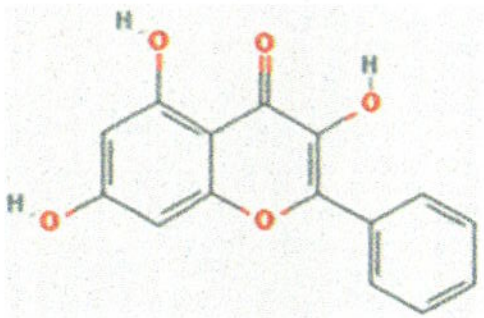	Lesser galangal *Helichrysum aureonitens* *Alpinia galanga* Propolis

	Isorhamnetin	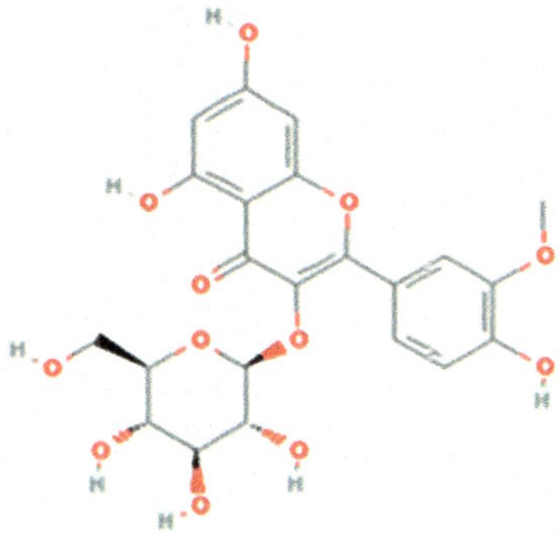	Pears, olive oil, wine, and tomato
Isoflavones	Daidzein	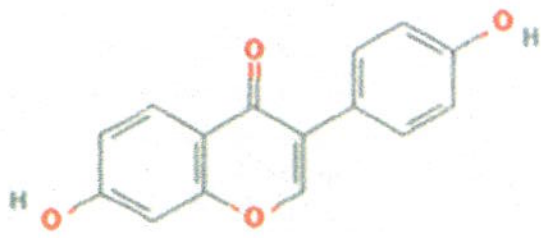	Kwao Krua *Pueraria lobata* *Maackia amurensis* Soybeans, soy products, tofu, textured vegetable protein.
	Genistein	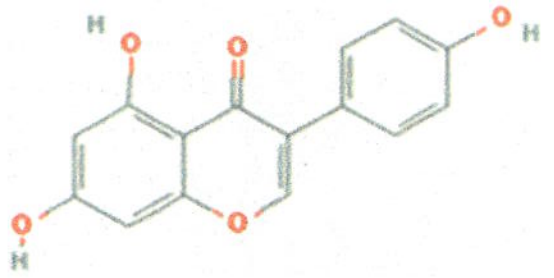	Lupin, fava beans, soybeans, kudzu, psoralea, medicinal plants, *Flemingia vestita*, F. *macrophylla*, coffee, and *Maackia amurensis*

(continued)

Table 2.1 (continued)

Polyphenols	Member	Chemical structure	Source
Phenolic acid	Ellagic acid	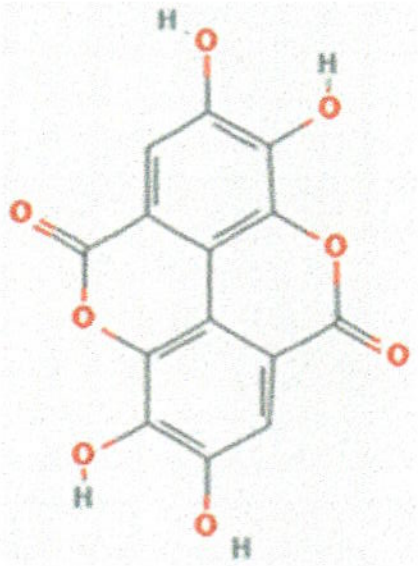	Chestnuts, walnuts, pecans, cranberries, raspberries, strawberries, grapes, distilled beverages, peaches, pomegranates, north American white oak European red oak *Myriophyllum spicatum* *Phellinus linteus*
	Gallic acid	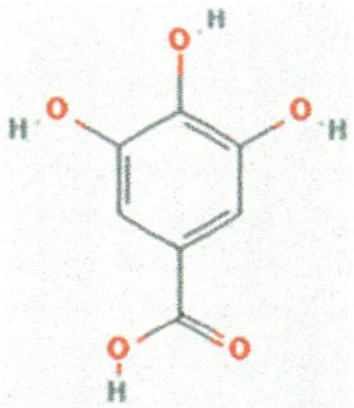	Gallnuts, sumac, witch hazel, tea leaves, oak bark,

	Ferulic acid	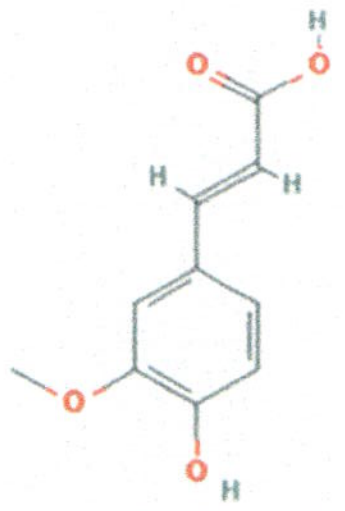	Popcorn and bamboo shoots, wheat, barley grains, legumes, navy bean, bread, Rye bread
Lignans		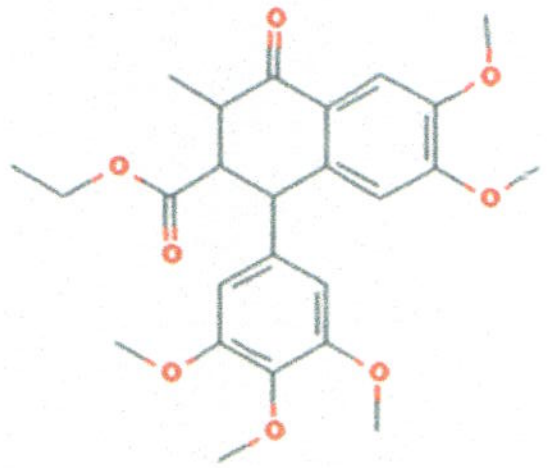	Flaxseed, sesame, and seeds of *Arctium lappa*

(continued)

Table 2.1 (continued)

Polyphenols	Member	Chemical structure	Source
Stilbenes	Resveratrol	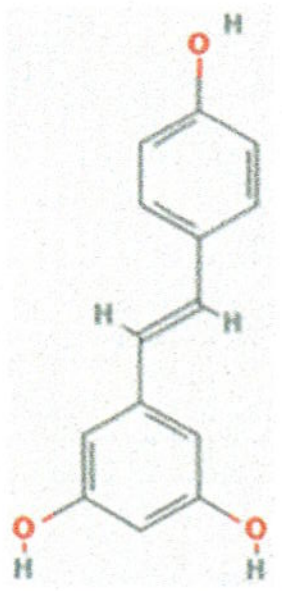	Grapes, blueberries, raspberries, mulberries, and peanuts
	Pterostilbene	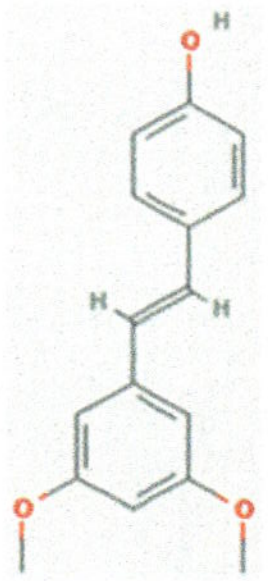	Almonds, Vaccinium berries, blueberries, grape leaves, vines, *Pterocarpus marsupium*

	Piceatannol	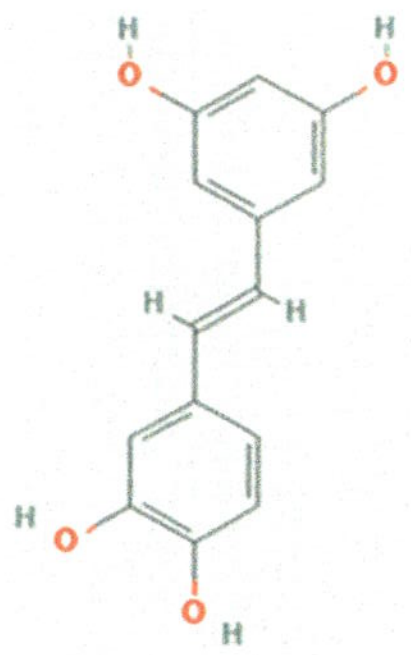	Red wine, grapes, passion fruit, white tea, Japanese knotweed, and Astringin

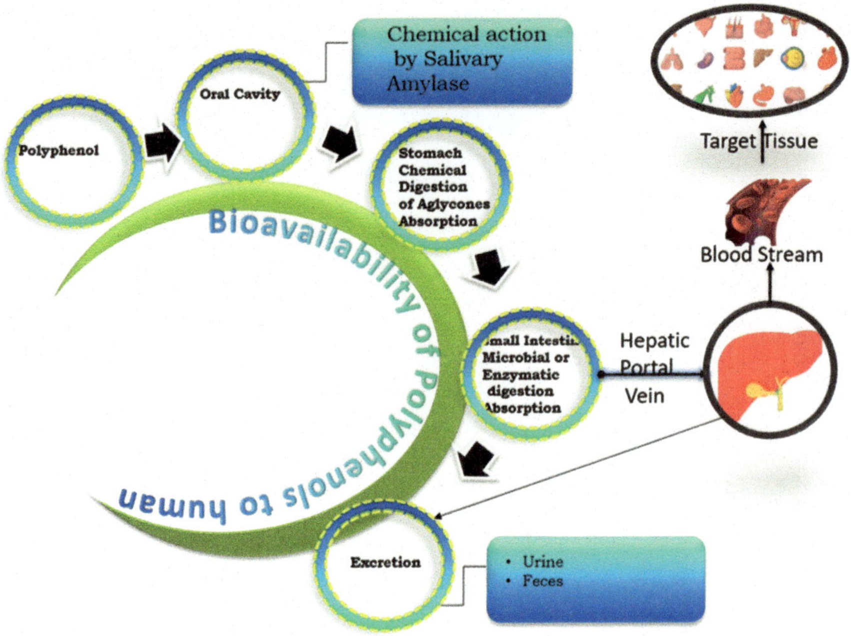

Fig. 2.2 Mechanism of polyphenol digestion in the human digestive system for the availability to target cells

poor absorption into small intestine, high metabolization, and quick excretion out of the body. Most common pathways of polyphenol metabolism are shown in Fig. 2.2.

Polyphenol's biological activities are strongly influenced by their bioavailability [56]. Their chemical makeup dictates their penetration capacity and frequency within the intestine [57]. Different food materials have different rate of bioavailability due to their unique molecular structure. Like green tea contains catechins with high bioavailability [58], while citrus fruits are rich in flavanones [59]. Although phenolic compound's concentration in plasma and urine can be examined during intake of a polyphenol-rich food. While the antioxidant potential of plasma supports clear evidence necessary to determine the absorption of such compounds in the intestine [60].

Flavonoids absorption into intestine gradually decreases the content of plasma into human body [61]. Because plasma albumin also has strong specificity for quercetin, which has a comparatively long dissolution half-life [62]. Glycosylation is typically the last phase in flavonoid biosynthesis, and it improves or facilitates flavonoid aglycone solubility, storage, and stabilization [63]. Glycosylation occurs in flavones, isoflavones, flavonols, and anthocyanins with the help of UDP-glucose glucosyltransferases (UGTs) [64]. Biologically, glucose and rhamnose, as well as xylose, glucronic acid, and galactose, are covalently linked to each other for the formation of complex bioactive compounds.

The variation in hydrophilicity of quercetin and quercetin-3-O-rhamnoglucoside is partly related to glycosylation, which further assesses the chemical, physical, and biological properties of polyphenols. Glycosidase action could be noticed within mucosa of the digestive tract and the microbiota of the large intestine and can also be observed in food [65].

Human cells naturally produce α-glucosidases on occasion, and the tissue-specific model of expression is usually controlled throughout development [66]. Individual cells have dormant substrates composed of xylose or glucose attached to polyphenols. Although human β-glucosidases can not break the polyphenol bound to rhamnose, microflora-rhamnosidase seem to be the only way to hydrolyze it. Epicatechins are acylated mainly with acids like gallic acid which promote the growth of muscle, brain, and heart. Galloyl replacement of flavanols seems to have no influence on glycosylation [67].

Caffeic acid is often used to esterify sugars, lipids, and organic acids. Once quinic acid and caffeic acid are esterified, chlorogenic acid is formed, which is found in significant amounts in coffee. Esterases present in human tissues never hydrolyze chlorogenic acid, and caffeic acid cannot be extracted from chlorogenic acid. The colon microbiota seems to be the only site where chlorogenic acid can be digested [68, 69].

Moreover, polyphenols migrate via the small intestine without even being consumed, which causes decolonization of gut microbiota. This action is achieved in two major steps; firstly, Polyphenols biologically transform into their more bioactive metabolites. Second, polyphenols switch the intestinal microbiota community's profile, quite probably via suppressing harmful bacteria whereas promoting healthy bacteria. These can serve only as prebiotic metabolites in the latter, enhancing the good bacteria. Consequently, dietary polyphenols and intestinal flora associations may have an impact on human host health [70].

2.4 Bioactivities of Polyphenols

Polyphenols are the most promising agents which have a wide range of biological activities including anti-inflammatory, antioxidant, anticancer, etc. They provide protection to the biological system from different diseases by boosting innate immunity. The role of polyphenol in different diseases is shown in Fig. 2.3.

2.4.1 Polyphenols and Cardiovascular Diseases

According to WHO, 17.5 million people died because of cardiovascular disease in 2005 and approximately 23.6 million people will die from CVDs, mainly from heart disease and stroke in 2030. Polyphenols are also known as cardioprotective which target different molecular pathways to lower the mortality rate.

Strokes and coronary heart disease are the key factors of death in advanced countries [71]. Exogenous and endogenous factors are also involved in the onset,

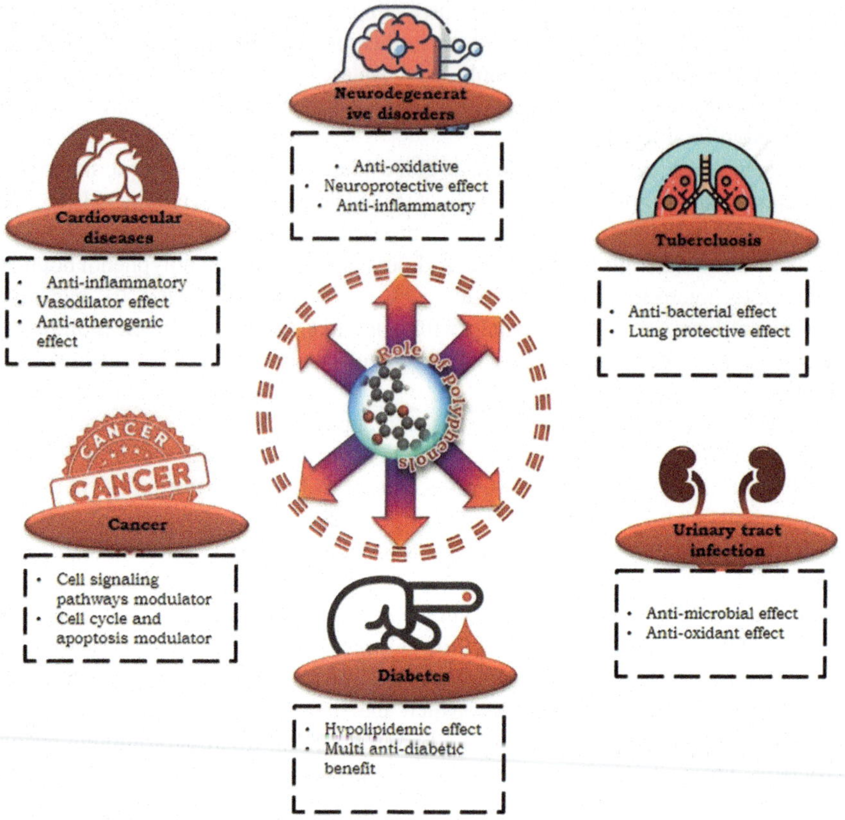

Fig. 2.3 Role of Polyphenols in different diseases

severity, and progression of cardiovascular disease [72]. Regular exercise, tobacco, dietary fat intake, and several other factors all play a significant role in the incidence of heart disease. It seems to be difficult to identify a single factor in this dynamic group that induces such disorders. Epidemiologists proved that a diet rich in polyphenols, including tea, vegetables, fruits, and cocoa, has been associated with a lower risk of cardiovascular disease. Polyphenols consumption is inversely proportional to the incidence of heart diseases [73].

The intake of flavanols, flavonols, and flavones was found to provide an opposite relation towards coronary disease. The ingestion of flavanones and anthocyanins minimize mortality because of cardiovascular disease. Drinking three cups of tea a day decreases the risk of heart disease by 11%. Despite cardiovascular disease, there seems to be some controversy about which polyphenols are more successful. Flavonoids present in cocoa and soy provide a detrimental effect on heart disease, but others are ineffective [74].

Flavonoids and flavonoid-rich ingredients ingestion can boost the recovery rate of endothelial function in humans as reported by a significant improvement in

NO-dependent flow-mediated dilation. Polyphenols are cardioprotective by performing following functions; Low blood pressure, enhanced endothelial function, and platelet aggregation (which are inhibited by the reduction in oxidation of low-density lipoprotein) [75] and minimal inflammatory response [76].

Cocoa, dark chocolate, and tea are the most promising agents to protect the human body from cardiac infections. Harvesting free radicals, chelating redox active transition metal ions, suppressing redox active transcription factors, retarding prooxidant enzymes, and triggering antioxidant enzymes are all methods of flavanols to show their magic antioxidant response [77]. High proportion of flavanol in diet lowers blood pressure, hypertension, and death rate of heart diseases. According to findings, an increase in the frequency of black tea intake decreases the risk of high blood pressure. Tea consumption for a brief period has no perceptible effect on blood pressure drop. Purple grapes, tea, and cocoa all have heart-healthy properties [78].

2.4.2 Polyphenol and Cancer

The mortality rate because of cancer is very high due to its contagious nature, approximately 18.1 million new cancer cases have been reported and 9.6 million cancer deaths. A case of breast cancer is diagnosed among women in every 19 s, and every 74 s a woman dies of breast cancer somewhere in the world [79, 80]. Cancer encompasses a range of diseases that are characterized by such a disruption in the regulation of cell growth and metabolism [81]. In addition, since the regulation of uncontrolled cell growth is just a main feature of cancerous cells, any agent which can prevent malignant cell growth can be used as a chemo-preventive agent. The anticancer activity of different polyphenols for different types of cancer is shown in Table 2.2.

There are also various types of cancer, such as breast cancer (which impacts mostly women), lung cancer, colorectal cancer, and prostate cancer, which further account for most of all newly diagnosed cases. A high dietary intake of fruits and vegetables is widely agreed to be beneficial in preventing the onset and development of cancer [82]. Studies conducted over the last 20 years have already shown that frequent intake of fruits and vegetables have a reciprocal association with the incidence of cancers, like prostate and colorectal cancer [83].

Polyphenols and bioactive compounds present in tea, red wine, chocolate, fruits, fruit juices, and olive oil are shown to manipulate cell proliferation and carcinogenesis at the cell level. Thus, bioactive compounds bind with nutrients, ROS metabolites, reactive carcinogens, and teratogens. These can also influence the sensitivity of many cancer-related genes through attenuating the activity of protein kinases associated with cell progression control. Green tea flavanols show anticancer potential in human cell lines as well as in human intervention trials. Green tea usage is also being associated with a lower risk of cancers of the bile duct, bladder, breast, and colon [84].

Many of the anticancer activities related to green tea are primarily mediated by the flavanol epigallocatechin gallate (EGCG), which is shown to trigger apoptosis

Table 2.2 Polyphenols and their anticancer activity

Polyphenols	Member	Cancer type	Action/effects on pathways	References
Anthocyanins	Peonidin-3 glucoside	Lung	⊥ Cancer cell invasion, motility, secretion of MMPs and u-PA	[14–18]
	Procyanidin C1	Lung	⊥ TGF-β-induced EMT	
		Colorectal	↥ Apoptosis and cell cycle arrest	
		Breast	↥ Apoptosis, ↓ Invasion and angiogenesis	
	Delphinidin	Colorectal	↥ Apoptosis, cell cycle arrest, oxidative stress	
		Prostate	↥ Apoptosis and cell cycle arrest	
	Cyanidin	Colorectal	↥ Oxidative stress	
	Cyanidin-3-O-sambubioside	Breast	⊥ Angiogenesis and invasion	
	Cyaniding-3-glucoside	Breast	⊥ Growth of HER2-positive tumor	
Xanthohumol		Lung	↑ Apoptosis and cell cycle arrest	[19–21]
		Liver	↥ Apoptosis ↑ NF-κB/p53 and Notch1 signaling pathways	
		Breast	↓ Expression of CXCR4 ⊥ Cell invasion, growth of ERα-positive breast cancer and estrogen singling pathway	
		Prostate	⊥ Tumor growth and progression	
Flavanols	EGCG	Lungs	⊥ Cancer cell invasion, migration, MMP-2, and nicotine-induced angiogenesis	[22–25]
		Gastric	↥ Apoptosis ↓ Surviving and β-catenin signaling pathway	
		Colorectal	↥ Epigenetic alteration, apoptosis, MAPK and Akt pathways activation	
		Breast	⊥ Estrogen-induced cancer cell proliferation and metastasis via MMP = TIMP ↓ERα	
		Prostate	Antagonizing androgen, ⊥ Tumor growth	
	Procyanidins	Breast	↓MMP, cell division, cell proliferation	[26, 27]
Flavanones	Naringenin	Lungs	↑ TRAIL-mediated apoptosis	[28–30]
		Gastric	↥ Apoptosis, ⊥ Cancer cell Proliferation, invasion, migration, and AKT pathway	

(continued)

Table 2.2 (continued)

Polyphenols	Member	Cancer type	Action/effects on pathways	References
		Colorectal	↕ Apoptosis	
		Liver	⊥ TPA-induced cancer cell invasion, ↕ Apoptosis and cell cycle arrest	
		Breast	⊥ Lung metastases by the host immunity	
	Hesperetin	Gastric	⊥ Tumor growth	[31, 32]
		Colorectal	⊥ Chemical-induced carcinogenesis	
		Breast	↕ Apoptosis, ROS production and activation of ASK1/JNK pathway ⊥ Glucose uptake	
		Prostate	↕ Apoptosis, ⊥ NF-κB pathway	
		Cervical	↕ Apoptosis	
Flavones	Apigenin	Lung	↕ Apoptosis and DNA damage	[33, 34]
		Gastric	↕ Apoptosis, preventing helicobacter pylori-induced atrophic gastritis and carcinogenesis	
		Colorectal	↕ Tumor growth and metastasis	
		Breast	⊥ Growth of cell ↕ Apoptosis possibly mediated by the STAT3 signaling pathway, cell cycle arrest through epigenetic change	
		Prostate	⊥ Tumor growth, angiogenesis, and metastasis	
	Chrysin	Lung	↕ Apoptosis, AMPK activation and ROS	[35, 36]
		Colorectal	↕ TNF-mediated apoptotic cell death	
		Breast	⊥ Cancer cell invasion and migration	
	Luteolin	Lung	↕ Apoptosis and cell cycle arrest ⊥ Monocyte recruitment, migration, EMT, and tumor growth	[33, 37, 38]
		Gastric	⊥ Tumor growth	
		Colorectal	↕ Apoptosis and cell cycle arrest	
		Breast	↓ ERα expression and tumor burden ↕ Apoptosis and cell cycle arrest	
		Prostate	↕ Apoptosis and cell cycle arrest ⊥ Cell invasion	
Flavonols	Quercetin	Lung	⊥ Tumor growth	[39–41]

(continued)

Table 2.2 (continued)

Polyphenols	Member	Cancer type	Action/effects on pathways	References
		Gastric	↨ Apoptosis and protective autophagy	
		Colorectal	⊥ Tumor growth by reducing AMPK activity ↑ Cachexia symptoms	
		Liver	⊥ Tumor growth	
		Breast	⊥ Tumor growth and angiogenesis	
		Prostate	⊥ Carcinogenesis induced by hormone and carcinogen	
		Cervical	↨ Apoptosis and cell cycle arrest	
	Kaempferol	Lung	⊥ TGF-β1-induced EMT and migration	[30, 42]
		Gastric	⊥ Tumor growth	
		Colorectal	↨ Apoptosis	
		Liver	↨ Cell cycle arrest and autophagy	
		Breast	↨ Apoptosis ⊥ Glucose uptake and preventing cancer development induced by estrogen	
	Myricetin	Gastric	↑ Apoptosis and cell cycle arrest	[43, 44]
		Colorectal	↨ Apoptosis	
		Liver	⊥ Chemical induced carcinogenesis	
	Galangin	Gastric	↨ Apoptosis	[45, 46]
		Liver	⊥ Chemical-induced cell invasion and metastasis ↨ ER stress	
	Isorhamnetin	Lung	⊥ Tumor growth	[47, 48]
		Gastric	↑ PPAR-γ ↓ Bcl-2 and CD31	
		Colorectal	⊥ Mortality, tumor number, tumor burden, and chemical-induced inflammatory responses	
		Breast	⊥ Cancer cell adhesion, migration, and invasion	
Isoflavones	Daidzein	Liver	↨ Apoptosis	
		Breast	↓ Invasion and MMP-2 expression ↑ Proto-oncogene BRF2 in ER-positive cancer cells	
	Genistein	Lung	⊥ Cancer cell proliferation and migration ↨ Apoptosis and cell cycle arrest	[49–52]
		Colorectal	↓ Weight and size of transplanted tumor ⊥ Angiogenesis and metastasis	

(continued)

Table 2.2 (continued)

Polyphenols	Member	Cancer type	Action/effects on pathways	References
		Liver	⊥ Intrahepatic metastasis	
		Breast	↨ Apoptosis, cell cycle arrest, drug resistance, tumor growth	
		Prostate	Different effects dependent on androgen receptor	
		Cervical	↨ Apoptosis, cell cycle arrest ⊥ Cell migration	
Phenolic acid	Ellagic acid	Colorectal	↨ Apoptosis	
		Liver	⊥ Chemical-induced carcinogenesis	
		Breast	↨ Cell cycle arrest ⊥ Tumor growth and angiogenesis	
		Prostate	↨ Apoptosis ⊥ Cell invasion and motility	
	Gallic acid	Gastric	↓ Tumor size and weight	[53–55]
		Colorectal	↑ Apoptosis	
		Liver	↑ Apoptosis	
		Breast	↑ Apoptosis	
		Prostate	⊥ DNA damage ↓DNA repair genes, invasion, and migration	
		Cervical	↓ Cell proliferation, invasion, and angiogenesis	
	Ferulic acid	Prostate	↑ Apoptosis and cell cycle arrest	[56]
		Cervical	↑ Efficacy of radiotherapy	
Lignans		Breast, Colon, prostate	↓ Cell division, cell proliferation	[57, 58]
Stilbenes	Resveratrol	Lung	↓ XRCC1 expression ↑ Chemosensitivity ⊥ Invasion and metastasis	[59, 60]
		Gastric	↑ Apoptosis, DNA damage, and ROS production ⊥ Tumor growth	
		Colorectal	↑ Apoptosis and DNA damage ⊥ Drug resistance and tumor development by modulation of Kras	
		Liver	⊥ Metastasis and chemical-induced carcinogenesis ↓ Expression of u-PA and SP-1 signaling pathway	

(continued)

Table 2.2 (continued)

Polyphenols	Member	Cancer type	Action/effects on pathways	References
		Prostate	↥ Autophagy-mediated cell death and apoptosis ⊥ Angiogenesis and metastasis	
		Cervical	↥ Apoptosis and cell cycle arrest	
	Pterostilbene	Breast	↥ Apoptosis ⊥ Tumor growth and metastasis	[61, 62]
		Prostate	↥ Apoptosis and cell cycle arrest ⊥ Tumor growth	
	Piceatannol	Colorectal	↥ Apoptosis mediated by miR-129	[7, 63]
		Prostate	↥ Apoptosis and cell cycle arrest ⊥ Lung metastasis	

"⊥" show Inhibit or suppress, "↓" Downregulation, "↑" Upregulation and modulating, "↥" Inducing, metalloproteinase (MMP), Cysteine X Cysteine chemokine receptor 4 (CXCR4), epithelial-mesenchymal transition (EMT), survivin, a potent anti-apoptotic protein, extracellular signal-related kinase (ERK) 1/2 and p38MAPK

and inhibit cancer cell growth via influencing the protein expression related to cell growth, transformation, and metastasis [85]. Olive oil contains a high number of flavonoids, phenolic alcohols, lignans, and secoiridoids. That is why olive oil have anticancer properties, which are used in animal and human models of large cell intestinal cancer. The behavior of phenolic compounds in olive oil is mainly suppression of the activation, progression, and metastasis in human colon adenocarcinoma cells, and decreased levels of expression of cyclooxygenase-2 (COX-2, an enzyme) protein, or Bcl-2 [86]. Such polyphenols do have the ability to impose antitumor activity via multiple mechanisms, along with the inhibition of cancer cell signaling, cell proliferation, apoptosis, and enzymatic activity manipulation.

Polyphenol can undo the damage of carcinogens by boosting the activity of glutathione peroxidase, catalase, nicotinamide adenine dinucleotide phosphate (NADPH), quinone oxidoreductase, glutathione-S-transferase, and/or activity of the P450 enzyme and also attenuate the action of signaling pathways associated with cancer cell proliferation [87]. With its central role in controlling cell survivability in a wide variety of human cancers, the mitogen-activated protein kinases (MAPK) signaling pathway is known as a promising target for anticancer therapies. Thus, it plays a crucial role mostly in transcriptional and posttranscriptional amplification of COX-2 [88].

2.4.3 Polyphenol and Diabetes

Type 2 diabetes is a rare disorder due to insulin resistance, cell dysfunction, lower insulin signaling, impaired fat and glucose metabolism, and increased oxidative stress. Almost all the preceding disorders result in infected cases containing neuropathy, nephropathy, macro and micro vascular obstacles, retinopathy, and a higher death risk and reduced quality of life. Nutrition is now the most important aspect which can be improved to minimize the incidence of degenerative diseases like diabetes.

Clinical studies showed that a diet high in total antioxidant potential, phytochemicals, and high phenolic content contributed to a reduced risk of diabetes as well as its incidence [89]. Numerous pharmacological therapies are employed in the treatment of diabetes and diet preventions to improve the glycemic index. Polyphenols can be used to treat diabetes due to various biological properties. Glycemic modulation can be optimized via four mechanisms; One of which is to shield pancreatic cells from glucose-induced toxicity and oxidative stress. Second, starch ingestion and oxidation is hindered; third, glucose secretion from the liver is restricted; so eventually, glucose endorsement in muscles and other adipose tissue is boosted [90]. Amplification in number and functional integrity of β-cells are the primary indications of diabetes [91]. In rats, a high phenolic content diet has been associated to protect from oxidative damage characterized by excessive glucose, and insulin secretion could also be monitored in humans. Many polyphenols with starch or sucrose are retained in the intestine and transferred to the colon without even being consumed.

Polyphenol-rich extracts reduce the function of enzymes involved in the release of glucose from starch in the gastrointestinal tract, such as α-amylase and glucosidase [92]. The communication between a sodium-dependent glucose transporter and a glucose transporter in the human digestive tract influenced the glucose uptake. Polyphenols boost insulin-stimulated glucose uptake as well as basal uptake. Phenolic compounds play a role in insulin sensing pathways, reducing glucose synthesis in the liver indirectly [93].

2.4.4 Polyphenol and UTI-Infections

The second most prevalent kind of infectious disease is urinary tract infection (UTI). Urinary tract infections affect about 150 million people worldwide per year [94]. Numerous categories of flavonoids, particularly pro-anthocyanidins, anthocyanidins, and flavonols, as well as phenolic acids and benzoates, are abundant in red cranberries [95]. Cranberry polyphenols to work as anti-adhesive agents in preventing/inhibiting pathogen adherence to uroepithelial cell receptors, which appears to be a major step in the pathogenesis of these infections, is one of the other possible mechanisms behind the protective effects of cranberries against UTIs [96]. Cranberry ingestion is shown to reduce the prevalence and intensity of UTIs in women and deter pathogenic bacteria from adhering to the urinary tract [97].

2.4.5 Polyphenols and Neurodegenerative Disorders

Neurodegenerative hallmarks are silent monsters resulting from imbalance in the nervous system. In the last few decades a growing interest is being paid to evaluate the potential benefits of polyphenols against neurodegenerative conditions [98, 99]. Alzheimer's disease, Parkinson's disease, stroke, Multiple sclerosis, and Huntington's disease are leading neurodegenerative disorders which all share a common mechanistic theme of genetics, mitochondrial dysfunction, cognitive impairment, and immune system deregulation, and oxidative stress [100]. Oxidative stress is a prime precursor of neurodegenerative disorders which cause damage to DNA and cause impaired function in the brain by affecting a broad range of brain activities [101].

It is well-established that polyphenols have a vital role in pathophysiology of neurodegenerative disorders due to their prominent antioxidant properties. Polyphenols modulate the activity of neuron cells by targeting antioxidant pathways, signaling pathways, and modulation of neuronal cell mediators, anti-amyloidogenic effects, and inhibition of NDMA neurotoxicity [102]. Epigallocatechin-3-gallate (EGCG), Berberine, Curcumin, Resveratrol, and Quercetin are major polyphenols which exert their neuroprotective effect mainly through inhibiting oxidative stress and effecting detoxifying enzymes to combat neurodegenerative disorders [103]. Among all polyphenols, EGCG has a prominent effect in oxidative stress by activation of SOD and catalase and metal ion chelation capacity [102].

2.4.6 Polyphenols and Tuberculosis

Tuberculosis is the deadliest, infectious pulmonary disease caused by *Mycobacterium tuberculosis* (MTB). Adverse side effects of anti-TB drugs have demanded the discovery of novel natural compounds [104]. Versatile photochemicals seem to be a good option due to their novel lead in disease management. Positive antimycobacterial activity of various phenolic compounds is supported by the number of publications. Pinocembrin, eupomatenoid-1, fargesin, (8R,8′R,9R)-cubebin, flavonoid 7-demethylartonol E, chromone artorigidusin, artonol B, artonin F, cycloartobiloxanthone, artoindonesianin C, (-)-butin, butein, butrin, cajanone, resveratrol, stipulin, afrormosin, apigenin, and monospermoside are some selected phenolic compounds which inhibit the growth of mycobacterium by targeting intrinsic and acquired resistance [104–107]. In intrinsic resistance, phenolic compounds cause Mycobacteria efflux system inhibition, Mycobacteria proteasome inhibition, mycolic acid biosynthesis inhibition, and nitric oxide inhibition to reduce the growth of mycobacterium [105, 108, 109].

Polyphenols possess a broad spectrum of pharmacological activities and therapeutic action, protect the human from autoimmune diseases as shown in Figure 2.4.

2.5 Nano Polyphenols

Nanoencapsulation is a process in which capsulation of active chemical material is done in the form of solid, liquid, and gas. This encapsulated material is called "core" which is covered by another secondary material called capsule or Nano capsule [110]. Nanotechnology represents a thrilling area of science which offers multiple

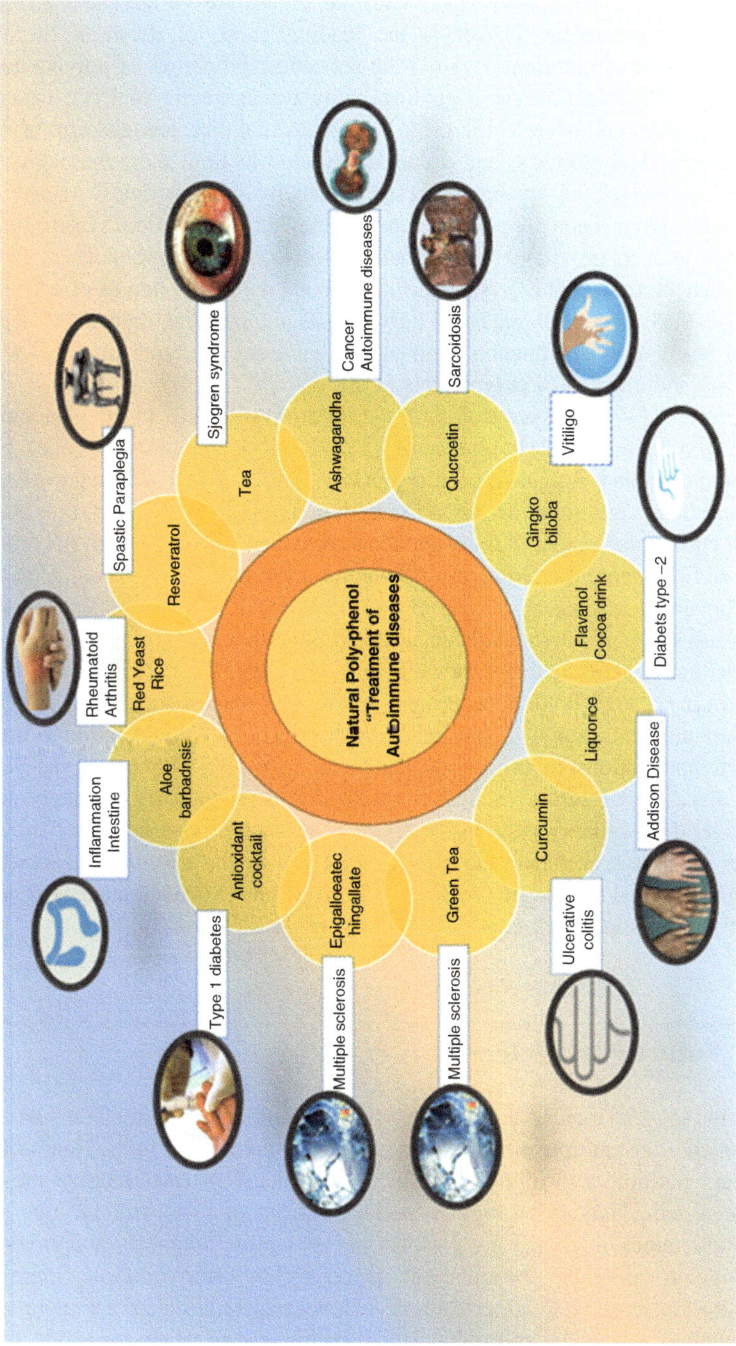

Fig. 2.4 Treatment options for autoimmune disease through magic bullet (Polyphenols)

valuable advantages such as nano polyphenols reducing the toxic side effects of drugs in cancer patients [111, 112]. Despite the extensive advances in cancer diagnostic and treatment, cancer is the leading cause of death in the world [113]. Rich body of literature suggests the anticancer properties of polyphenols by modulation of multiple cancer signaling pathways, targeting multiple cancerous agents, and arrest cell cycle [114, 115]. Poor bioavailability, low absorption, lower permeability, lower stability, and vulnerability tend to limit the administration of polyphenols in cancer treatment [116]. Recently nanoparticles loaded with polyphenols have been applied to overcome this restriction. Encapsulation techniques tend to provide a new paradigm for loading polyphenols to increase their anticancer activity [117]. Nanoparticles loaded with polyphenols offer multiple advantages such as control release of polyphenols at target site, reduce the degradation and reaction of polyphenols with outside environment, and improve the bioavailability and efficacy of polyphenols [118].

Curcumin [119], Resveratrol (3,5,4′-trihydroxystilbene) [120], Kaempferol (tetrahydroxyflavone) [121], Quercetin (3,3′,4′,5′-7-pentahydroxyflavone) [122], Apigenin [123] and Epigallocatechin gallate (EGCG) [124] are major phenolic compound with antitumor activity. Depending upon the nature of polyphenols different encapsulation methods are applied to provide a shield between polyphenols and the environment. The shift from convention methods (Spray drying, Coacervation, Emulsions, Microgels, Freeze drying, Co-crystallization, and Encapsulation within yeast cells) of polyphenols encapsulation to advanced nano delivery system represent more safe, active, and efficient targeting [125–127]. The fate of nanoliposomes, solid-lipid NPs, protein-based NPs, nanosuspensions, polymeric NPs, nanoemulsions, and cyclodextrins must be taken into consideration to investi gate their applications in the biomedical field [128–130]. Cancer is the second leading disease after cardiovascular diseases, so it is compulsory to deeply understand novel drug delivery systems for efficient loading of polyphenols as shown in Fig. 2.5. Multidrug resistance is a major problem in the treatment of cancer so randomized clinical studies are pressing the need of time to investigate the toxicity of nano polyphenols in novel natural drug discovery [127, 131, 132].

2.6 Future Prospective

Nanotechnology is rapidly developing science to produce materials at nanoscale range which offer multiple improved diagnostic and therapeutic tools. Nanotechnology offers multiple new dimensions in nanomedicine to revolutionize the drug delivery system. Nanotechnology is at the forefront of nanomedicine due to its novel applications in numerous prespectives of cancer diagnosis and treatment. Mind-boggling potential benefits of nanoparticles offer multiple innovative prespectives to improve treatment efficacy. Novel targeted drugs are a major scientific challenge especially as cancer is the leading cause of death in the world. Nanotechnology has facilitated the development of elegant diagnostic and treatment options which hold great potential to dramatically treat tumor cells.

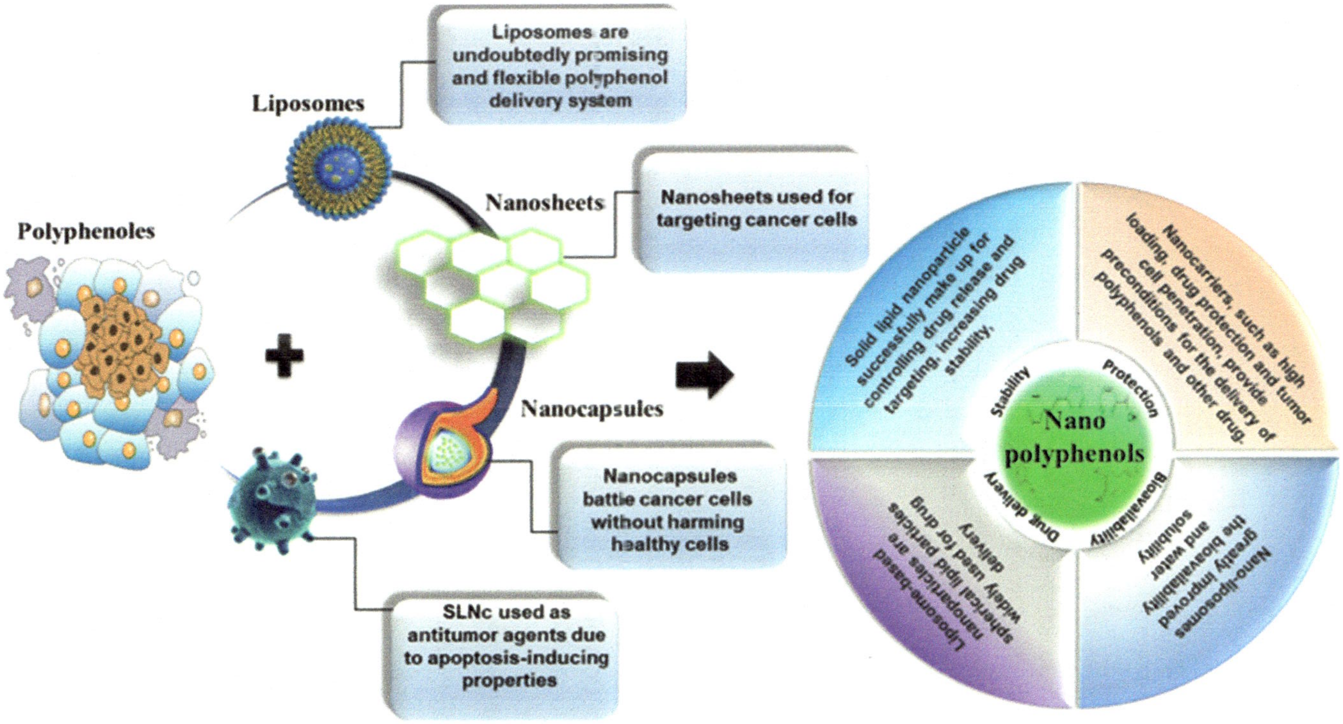

Fig. 2.5 Role of Nano polyphenol in different human diseases

Research involving the combination of nanoparticles and polyphenols for treating the cancer has attracted the interest of scientists due to their specificity, nontoxicity, and compatibility. A huge body of growing literature evidenced different types of polyphenols loaded with nanoparticles for efficient and targeted drug delivery to tumor cells. Thus, nano polyphenols have attracted a lot of interest for its promising future. Drug specificity is a major dilemma in cancer cell treatment as most anticancer agents also affect normal cells. Thus, as compared to conventional treatment methods nanoparticles allow more specific drug penetration and distribution to minimize the uptake of anticancer drugs by normal cells. So the combinational effect of nanoparticles and polyphenols are of great hope for cancer treatment due to reduced toxicity, control release, and improved activity. Thus, the nano polyphenols are appropriate candidates which offer a new spectrum of research in the field of oncology. Although there is extensively growing interest in the use of nano polyphenols for cancer treatment, however further clinical investigations are mandatory to validate their potential for pharmaceutical role.

2.7 Conclusion

Natural polyphenols are promising agents to treat various diseases. *G. biloba* and green tea show greater inhibitory response against the progression of vitiligo, ulcerative colitis, and multiple sclerosis. Cranberry polyphenols scavenge the microbial cloning in the urinary tract to stunt the development of microbes. Curcumin has shown strong antitumor activity in all types of cancer via regulating the cell signaling pathways. Consortia of nano polyphenol and polyphenols are the potential agents to stop the metastatic nature of cancer.

Ethics Approval and Consent to Participate Not applicable.

Consent for Publication Not applicable.

Availability of Data and Material Not applicable.

Competing Interests The authors declare that they have no competing interests.

Authors' Contributions All Authors contributed equally.

References

1. Satchanska G. Antimicrobial activity of natural polyphenols. Acta Microbiol Bulg. 2020;36 (4):132–8.
2. Dragovic-Uzelac V, Levaj B, Mrkic V, Bursac D, Boras M. The content of polyphenols and carotenoids in three apricot cultivars depending on stage of maturity and geographical region. Food Chem. 2007;102(3):966–75.
3. Long J, Guan P, Hu X, Yang L, He L, Lin Q, et al. Natural polyphenols as targeted modulators in colon cancer: molecular mechanisms and applications. Front Immunol. 2021;12 https://doi.org/10.3389/fimmu.2021.635484.

4. Jabir NR, Khan FR, Tabrez S. Cholinesterase targeting by polyphenols: a therapeutic approach for the treatment of Alzheimer's disease. CNS Neurosci Ther. 2018;24(9):753–62.
5. Ayissi VBO, Ebrahimi A, Schluesenner H. Epigenetic effects of natural polyphenols: a focus on SIRT1-mediated mechanisms. Mol Nutr Food Res. 2014;58(1):22–32.
6. Gormaz JG, Valls N, Sotomayor C, Turner T, Rodrigo R. Potential role of polyphenols in the prevention of cardiovascular diseases: molecular bases. Curr Med Chem. 2016;23(2):115–28.
7. Cao L, Park Y, Lee S, Kim D-O. Extraction, identification, and health benefits of anthocyanins in blackcurrants (*Ribes nigrum* L.). Appl Sci. 1863;11(4):2021.
8. Lopez-Velez M, Martinez-Martinez F, Valle-Ribes CD. The study of phenolic compounds as natural antioxidants in wine. Crit Rev Food Sci Nutr. 2003;43(3):233–44.
9. Baron G, Altomare A, Mol M, Garcia JL, Correa C, Raucci A, et al. Analytical profile and antioxidant and anti-inflammatory activities of the enriched polyphenol fractions isolated from bergamot fruit and leave. Antioxidants. 2021;10(2):141.
10. Mukherjee C, Chakraborty S. Study of dietary polyphenols from natural herbal sources for providing protection against human degenerative disorders. Biocatal Agric Biotechnol. 2021;33:101956.
11. Câmara JS, Albuquerque BR, Aguiar J, Corrêa RC, Gonçalves JL, Granato D, et al. Food bioactive compounds and emerging techniques for their extraction: polyphenols as a case study. Foods. 2021;10(1):37.
12. Gumul D, Berski W. The polyphenol profile and antioxidant potential of irradiated Rye grains. Int J Food Sci. 2021;2021:8870754.
13. Tsao R. Chemistry and biochemistry of dietary polyphenols. Nutrients. 2010;2(12):1231–46.
14. Ramirez DA, Altamirano JC, Camargo AB. Multi-phytochemical determination of polar and non-polar garlic bioactive compounds in different food and nutraceutical preparations. Food Chem. 2021;337:127648.
15. Giuliano C, Cerri S, Blandini F. Potential therapeutic effects of polyphenols in Parkinson's disease: in vivo and in vitro pre-clinical studies. Neural Regen Res. 2021;16(2):234.
16. Duthie GG, Gardner PT, Kyle JA. Plant polyphenols: are they the new magic bullet? Proc Nutr Soc. 2003;62(3):599–603.
17. El Gharras H. Polyphenols: food sources, properties and applications–a review. Int J Food Sci Tech. 2009;44(12):2512–8.
18. Murthy NTV, Agrahari V, Chauhan H. Polyphenols against infectious diseases: controlled release Nano-formulations. Eur J Pharm Biopharm. 2021;161:66–79.
19. Çelik EE, Rubio JMA, Andersen ML, Gökmen V. Interactions of dietary fiber bound antioxidants with hydroxycinnamic and hydroxybenzoic acids in aqueous and liposome media. Food Chem. 2019;278:294–304.
20. Balasundram N, Sundram K, Samman S. Phenolic compounds in plants and agri-industrial by-products: antioxidant activity, occurrence, and potential uses. Food Chem. 2006;99 (1):191–203.
21. Septembre-Malaterre A, Remize F, Poucheret P. Fruits and vegetables, as a source of nutritional compounds and phytochemicals: changes in bioactive compounds during lactic fermentation. Food Res Int. 2018;104:86–99.
22. Moreira AS, Nunes FM, Simões C, Maciel E, Domingues P, Domingues MRM, et al. Transglycosylation reactions, a main mechanism of phenolics incorporation in coffee melanoidins: inhibition by Maillard reaction. Food Chem. 2017;227:422–31.
23. Olech M, Pietrzak W, Nowak R. Characterization of free and bound phenolic acids and flavonoid aglycones in *Rosa rugosa* thunb. Leaves and achenes using LC–ESI–MS/MS–MRM methods. Molecules. 2020;25(8):1804.
24. Pedro AC, Maurer JBB, Zawadzki-Baggio SF, Ávila S, Maciel GM, Haminiuk CWI. Bioactive compounds of organic goji berry (*Lycium barbarum* L.) prevents oxidative deterioration of soybean oil. Ind Crop Prod. 2018;112:90–7.

25. Baranska M, Schulz H, Joubert E, Manley M. In situ flavonoid analysis by FT-Raman spectroscopy: identification, distribution, and quantification of aspalathin in green rooibos (*Aspalathus linearis*). Anal Chem. 2006;78(22):7716–21.
26. Kinoshita T, Lepp Z, Chuman H. Construction of a novel database for flavonoids. J Med Investig. 2005;52(Supplement):291–2.
27. Peterson J, Dwyer J. Flavonoids: dietary occurrence and biochemical activity. Nutr Res. 1998;18(12):1995–2018.
28. Khan AK, Kousar S, Tungmunnithum D, Hano C, Abbasi BH, Anjum S. Nano-elicitation as an effective and emerging strategy for in vitro production of industrially important flavonoids. Appl Sci. 2021;11(4):1694.
29. Krol W, Czuba Z, Scheller S, Paradowski Z, Shani J. Structure-activity relationship in the ability of flavonols to inhibit chemiluminescence. J Ethnopharmacol. 1994;41(1–2):121–6.
30. Kubina R, Iriti M, Kabała-Dzik A. Anticancer potential of selected flavonols: fisetin, kaempferol, and quercetin on head and neck cancers. Nutrients. 2021;13(3):845.
31. González-de-Peredo AV, Vázquez-Espinosa M, Espada-Bellido E, Carrera C, Ferreiro-González M, Barbero GF, et al. Flavonol composition and antioxidant activity of onions (*Allium cepa* L.) based on the development of new analytical ultrasound-assisted extraction methods. Antioxidants. 2021;10(2):273.
32. Paulsen E, Moreno DA, Periago PM, Lema P. Influence of microwave bag vs conventional microwave cooking on phytochemicals of industrially and domestically processed broccoli. Food Res Int. 2021;140:110077.
33. Shahrajabian MH, Sun W, Cheng Q. A Review of Leek (*A. ampeloprasum* L.), an important vegetable and food ingredient with remarkable pharmaceutical activities. Pharmacognosy Commun. 2021;11(1):9–12.
34. Tomas M, Zhang L, Zengin G, Rocchetti G, Capanoglu E, Lucini L. Metabolomic insight into the profile, in vitro bioaccessibility and bioactive properties of polyphenols and glucosinolates from four Brassicaceae microgreens. Food Res Int. 2021;140:110039.
35. Yu Z, Zhang P, Lin W, Zheng X, Cai M, Peng C. Sequencing of anthocyanin synthesis-related enzyme genes and screening of reference genes in leaves of four dominant subtropical forest tree species. Gene. 2019;716:144024.
36. Adki KM, Kulkarni YA. Glycosides from natural sources in the treatment of diabetes mellitus. structure and health effects of natural products on diabetes mellitus. New York, NY: Springer; 2021. p. 81–102.
37. Iannone M, Botrè F, Parenti S, Jardines D, de la Torre X. An investigation on the metabolic pathways of synthetic isoflavones by gas chromatography coupled to high accuracy mass spectrometry. Rapid Commun Mass Spectrom. 2019;33(19):1485–93.
38. Jung YS, Rha C-S, Baik M-Y, Baek N-I, Kim D-O. A brief history and spectroscopic analysis of soy isoflavones. Food Sci Biotechnol. 2020;29(12):1605–17.
39. Sarkar N, Bose S. Controlled release of soy isoflavones from multifunctional 3D printed bone tissue engineering scaffolds. Acta Biomater. 2020;114:407–20.
40. Sreenivasan L, Watson RR. Reduction is the new youth: the effect of polyphenols on brain aging and diseases. Bioactive Nutraceuticals and Dietary Supplements in Neurological and Brain Disease; 2015. pp. 137–140.
41. Tsanova-Savova S, Ribarova F, Petkov V. Quercetin content and ratios to total flavonols and total flavonoids in Bulgarian fruits and vegetables. Bulg Chem Commun. 2018;50:69–73.
42. Harada M, Kan Y, Naoki H, Fukui Y, Kageyama N, Nakai M, et al. Identification of the major antioxidative metabolites in biological fluids of the rat with ingested (+)-catechin and (−)-epicatechin. Biosci Biotechnol Biochem. 1999;63(6):973–7.
43. Tapas AR, Sakarkar D, Kakde R. Flavonoids as nutraceuticals: a review. Trop J Pharm Res. 2008;7(3):1089–99.
44. Kumar P, Kumar S, Tripathi M, Mehta N, Ranjan R, Bhat Z, et al. Flavonoids in the development of functional meat products: a review. Vet World. 2013;6(8):573.

45. Spiegel M, Andruniów T, Sroka Z. Flavones' and flavonols' antiradical structure–activity relationship—A quantum chemical study. Antioxidants. 2020;9(6):461.
46. LdLd O, Carvalho MV, Melo L. Health promoting and sensory properties of phenolic compounds in food. Revista Ceres. 2014;61:764–79.
47. Man M-Q, Yang B, Elias PM. Benefits of hesperidin for cutaneous functions. Evid Based Complement Alternat Med. 2019;2019:2676307.
48. Moldovan B, David L. Bioactive flavonoids from Cornus mas L. fruits. Mini-Rev Org Chem. 2017;14(6):489–95.
49. Domínguez-López I, Yago-Aragón M, Salas-Huetos A, Tresserra-Rimbau A, Hurtado-Barroso S. Effects of dietary phytoestrogens on hormones throughout a human lifespan: a review. Nutrients. 2020;12(8):2456.
50. Riswanto FDO, Desra A, Sari RM, Thomas V, Rohman A, Pramono S, et al. Employing an R software package rsm for optimizing of genistein, daidzein, and glycitein separation and its application for soy milk analysis by HPLC method. Indones J Chem. 2020; https://doi.org/10.22146/ijc.51669.
51. Ikya JK, Gernah I, Ojobo E, Oni K. Effect of cooking temperature on some quality characteristics of soy milk. Adv J Food Sci Technol. 2013;5(5):543–6.
52. Kasote DM, Duncan GJ, Neacsu M, Russell WR. Rapid method for quantification of anthocyanidins and anthocyanins in human biological samples. Food Chem. 2019;290:56–63.
53. Khoo HE, Azlan A, Tang ST, Lim SM. Anthocyanidins and anthocyanins: colored pigments as food, pharmaceutical ingredients, and the potential health benefits. Food Nutr Res. 2017;61(1):1361779.
54. Jiang W, Li N, Zhang D, Meinhardt L, Cao B, Li Y, et al. Elevated temperature and drought stress significantly affect fruit quality and activity of anthocyanin-related enzymes in jujube (*Ziziphus jujuba* Mill. cv.'Lingwuchangzao'). PLoS One. 2020;15(11):e0241491.
55. Kim B, Kang B, Vales TP, Yang SK, Lee J, Kim H-J. Polyphenol-functionalized hydrogels using an interpenetrating chitosan network and investigation of their antioxidant activity. Macromol Res. 2018;26(1):35–9.
56. Nagar EE, Okun Z, Shpigelman A. Digestive fate of polyphenols: updated view of the influence of chemical structure and the presence of cell wall material. Curr Opin Food Sci. 2020;31:38–46.
57. Hu X, Wang Y, Zhang L, Xu M. Construction of self-assembled polyelectrolyte complex hydrogel based on oppositely charged polysaccharides for sustained delivery of green tea polyphenols. Food Chem. 2020;306:125632.
58. Liu Z, Bruins ME, Ni L, Vincken J-P. Green and black tea phenolics: bioavailability, transformation by colonic microbiota, and modulation of colonic microbiota. J Agric Food Chem. 2018;66(32):8469–77.
59. Pereira-Caro G, Polyviou T, Ludwig IA, Nastase A-M, Moreno-Rojas JM, Garcia AL, et al. Bioavailability of orange juice (poly) phenols: the impact of short-term cessation of training by male endurance athletes. Am J Clin Nutr. 2017;106(3):791–800.
60. Henning SM, Wang P, Abgaryan N, Vicinanza R, de Oliveira DM, Zhang Y, et al. Phenolic acid concentrations in plasma and urine from men consuming green or black tea and potential chemopreventive properties for colon cancer. Mol Nutr Food Res. 2013;57(3):483–93.
61. Boyle S, Dobson V, Duthie SJ, Kyle J, Collins A. Absorption and DNA protective effects of flavonoid glycosides from an onion meal. Eur J Nutr. 2000;39(5):213–23.
62. Wang L, Morris ME. Liquid chromatography–tandem mass spectroscopy assay for quercetin and conjugated quercetin metabolites in human plasma and urine. J Chromatogr B. 2005;821(2):194–201.
63. J-r J, Yuan S, J-f D, Zhu S-c, Xu H-d, Chen T, et al. Conversion of puerarin into its 7-O-glycoside derivatives by microbacterium oxydans (CGMCC 1788) to improve its water solubility and pharmacokinetic properties. Appl Microbiol Biotechnol. 2008;81(4):647–57.
64. Xiao J, Muzashvili TS, Georgiev MI. Advances in the biotechnological glycosylation of valuable flavonoids. Biotechnol Adv. 2014;32(6):1145–56.

65. Ajmal G, Bonde GV, Mittal P, Khan G, Pandey VK, Bakade BV, et al. Biomimetic PCL-gelatin based nanofibers loaded with ciprofloxacin hydrochloride and quercetin: a potential antibacterial and anti-oxidant dressing material for accelerated healing of a full thickness wound. Int J Pharm. 2019;567:118480.
66. Lee B-H, Hamaker BR. Maltase has most versatile α-hydrolytic activity among the mucosal α-glucosidases of the small intestine. J Pediatr Gastroenterol Nutr. 2018;66:S7–S10.
67. Den Hartogh DJ, Tsiani E. Antidiabetic properties of naringenin: a citrus fruit polyphenol. Biomol Ther. 2019;9(3):99.
68. Kim K, Vance TM, Chun OK. Greater flavonoid intake is associated with improved CVD risk factors in US adults. Br J Nutr. 2016;115(8):1481–8.
69. Tapiero H, Tew K, Ba GN, Mathe G. Polyphenols: do they play a role in the prevention of human pathologies? Biomed Pharmacother. 2002;56(4):200–7.
70. Klinder A, Shen Q, Heppel S, Lovegrove JA, Rowland I, Tuohy KM. Impact of increasing fruit and vegetables and flavonoid intake on the human gut microbiota. Food Funct. 2016;7(4):1788–96.
71. Quiñones M, Miguel M, Aleixandre A. Beneficial effects of polyphenols on cardiovascular disease. Pharmacol Res. 2013;68(1):125–31.
72. Vita JA. Polyphenols and cardiovascular disease: effects on endothelial and platelet function. Am J Clin Nutr. 2005;81(1):292S–7S.
73. Visioli F, Davalos A. Polyphenols and cardiovascular disease: a critical summary of the evidence. Mini Rev Med Chem. 2011;11(14):1186–90.
74. Grassi D, Lippi C, Necozione S, Desideri G, Ferri C. Short-term administration of dark chocolate is followed by a significant increase in insulin sensitivity and a decrease in blood pressure in healthy persons. Am J Clin Nutr. 2005;81(3):611–4.
75. Mathur S, Devaraj S, Grundy SM, Jialal I. Cocoa products decrease low density lipoprotein oxidative susceptibility but do not affect biomarkers of inflammation in humans. J Nutr. 2002;132(12):3663–7.
76. Stocker R, O'Halloran RA. Dealcoholized red wine decreases atherosclerosis in apolipoprotein E gene–deficient mice independently of inhibition of lipid peroxidation in the artery wall. Am J Clin Nutr. 2004;79(1):123–30.
77. Ferri C, Grassi D, Grassi G. Cocoa beans, endothelial function and aging: an unexpected friendship? J Hypertens. 2006;24(8):1471–4.
78. Goldbohm RA, Hertog MG, Brants HA, van Poppel G, van den Brandt PA. Consumption of black tea and cancer risk: a prospective cohort study. J Natl Cancer Inst. 1996;88(2):93–100.
79. Bray F, Ferlay J, Soerjomataram I, Siegel RL, Torre LA, Jemal A. Global cancer statistics 2018: GLOBOCAN estimates of incidence and mortality worldwide for 36 cancers in 185 countries. CA Cancer J Clin. 2018;68(6):394–424.
80. Noor F, Noor A, Ishaq AR, Farzeen I, Saleem MH, Ghaffar K, et al. Recent advances in diagnostic and therapeutic approaches for breast cancer: a comprehensive review. Curr Pharm Des. 2021; https://doi.org/10.2174/1381612827666210303141416.
81. Estrela JM, Mena S, Obrador E, Benlloch M, Castellano G, Salvador R, et al. Polyphenolic phytochemicals in cancer prevention and therapy: bioavailability versus bioefficacy. J Med Chem. 2017;60(23):9413–36.
82. Mitsiogianni M, Koutsidis G, Mavroudis N, Trafalis DT, Botaitis S, Franco R, et al. The role of isothiocyanates as cancer chemo-preventive, chemo-therapeutic and anti-melanoma agents. Antioxidants. 2019;8(4):106.
83. Park Y, Subar AF, Hollenbeck A, Schatzkin A. Dietary fiber intake and mortality in the NIH-AARP diet and health study. Arch Intern Med. 2011;171(12):1061–8.
84. Cox S, Noronha L, Herald T, Bean S, Lee S-H, Perumal R, et al. Evaluation of ethanol-based extraction conditions of sorghum bran bioactive compounds with downstream anti-proliferative properties in human cancer cells. Heliyon. 2019;5(5):e01589.
85. Dobrzynska M, Napierala M, Florek E. Flavonoid nanoparticles: a promising approach for cancer therapy. Biomol Ther. 2020;10(9):1268.

86. Pelucchi C, Bosetti C, Negri E, Lipworth L, La Vecchia C. Olive oil and cancer risk: an update of epidemiological findings through 2010. Curr Pharm Des. 2011;17(8):805–12.
87. van Muiswinkel FL, Kuiperij HB. The Nrf2-ARE signalling pathway: promising drug target to combat oxidative stress in neurodegenerative disorders. Curr Drug Targets CNS Neurol Disord. 2005;4(3):267–81.
88. Achkar IW, Abdulrahman N, Al-Sulaiti H, Joseph JM, Uddin S, Mraiche F. Cisplatin based therapy: the role of the mitogen activated protein kinase signaling pathway. J Transl Med. 2018;16(1):96.
89. Gao Q, Zhong C, Zhou X, Chen R, Xiong T, Hong M, et al. Inverse association of total polyphenols and flavonoids intake and the intake from fruits with the risk of gestational diabetes mellitus: a prospective cohort study. Clin Nutr. 2021;40(2):550–9.
90. Dong Y, Yin J, Zhang Y, Chen JD. Electronic bypass for diabetes: optimization of stimulation parameters and mechanisms of glucagon-like peptide-1. Neuromodulation. 2021; https://doi.org/10.1111/ner.13367.
91. Jain C, Far FF, Homberg S, Wißmiller K, von Hahn FG, Raducanu A, et al. Inceptor counteracts insulin signalling in β-cells to control glycaemia. Nature. 2021;590(7845):326–31.
92. Ombra MN, d'Acierno A, Nazzaro F, Spigno P, Riccardi R, Zaccardelli M, et al. Alpha-amylase, α-glucosidase and lipase inhibiting activities of polyphenol-rich extracts from six common bean cultivars of southern Italy, before and after cooking. Int J Food Sci Nutr. 2018;69(7):824–34.
93. Forester SC, Gu Y, Lambert JD. Inhibition of starch digestion by the green tea polyphenol,(−)-epigallocatechin-3-gallate. Mol Nutr Food Res. 2012;56(11):1647–54.
94. Foxman B. Urinary tract infection syndromes: occurrence, recurrence, bacteriology, risk factors, and disease burden. Infect Dis Clin N Am. 2013;28(1):1–13.
95. Sánchez-Patán F, Bartolomé BA, Martín-Alvarez PJ, Anderson M, Howell A, Monagas M. Comprehensive assessment of the quality of commercial cranberry products. Phenolic characterization and in vitro bioactivity. J Agric Food Chem. 2012;60(13):3396–408.
96. Gonzalez de Llano D, Liu H, Khoo C, Moreno-Arribas MV, Ba B. Some new findings regarding the antiadhesive activity of cranberry phenolic compounds and their microbial-derived metabolites against uropathogenic bacteria. J Agric Food Chem. 2019;67(8):2166–74.
97. Kimble LL, Mathison BD, Kaspar KL, Khoo C, Chew BP. Development of a fluorometric microplate antiadhesion assay using uropathogenic Escherichia coli and human uroepithelial cells. J Nat Prod. 2014;77(5):1102–10.
98. Potì F, Santi D, Spaggiari G, Zimetti F, Zanotti I. Polyphenol health effects on cardiovascular and neurodegenerative disorders: a review and meta-analysis. Int J Mol Sci. 2019;20(2):351.
99. Scapagnini G, Caruso C, Calabrese V. Therapeutic potential of dietary polyphenols against brain ageing and neurodegenerative disorders. Bio-farms for nutraceuticals. New York, NY: Springer; 2010. p. 27–35.
100. Di Meo F, Valentino A, Petillo O, Peluso G, Filosa S, Crispi S. Bioactive polyphenols and neuromodulation: molecular mechanisms in neurodegeneration. Int J Mol Sci. 2020;21(7):2564.
101. Chandran R, Abrahamse H. Identifying plant-based natural medicine against oxidative stress and neurodegenerative disorders. Oxidative Med Cell Longev. 2020;2020:8648742.
102. Ebrahimi A, Schluesener H. Natural polyphenols against neurodegenerative disorders: potentials and pitfalls. Ageing Res Rev. 2012;11(2):329–45.
103. Uddin MS, Al Mamun A, Kabir MT, Ahmad J, Jeandet P, Sarwar MS, et al. Neuroprotective role of polyphenols against oxidative stress-mediated neurodegeneration. Eur J Pharmacol. 2020:173412. https://doi.org/10.1016/j.ejphar.2020.173412.
104. Mazlun MH, Sabran SF, Mohamed M, Abu Bakar MF, Abdullah Z. Phenolic compounds as promising drug candidates in tuberculosis therapy. Molecules. 2019;24(13):2449.
105. Gröblacher B, Kunert O, Bucar F. Compounds of Alpinia katsumadai as potential efflux inhibitors in Mycobacterium smegmatis. Biorg Med Chem. 2012;20(8):2701–6.

106. Jiménez-Arellanes A, León-Díaz R, Meckes M, Tapia A, Molina-Salinas GM, Luna-Herrera J, et al. Antiprotozoal and antimycobacterial activities of pure compounds from *Aristolochia elegans* rhizomes. Evid Based Complement Alternat Med. 2012;2012 https://doi.org/10.1155/2012/593403.
107. Namdaung U, Aroonrerk N, Suksamrarn S, Danwisetkanjana K, Saenboonrueng J, Arjchomphu W, et al. Bioactive constituents of the root bark of *Artocarpus rigidus* subsp. *rigidus*. Chem Pharm Bull. 2006;54(10):1433–6.
108. Chokchaisiri R, Suaisom C, Sriphota S, Chindaduang A, Chuprajob T, Suksamrarn A. Bioactive flavonoids of the flowers of *Butea monosperma*. Chem Pharm Bull. 2009;57(4):428–32.
109. Lechner D, Gibbons S, Bucar F. Plant phenolic compounds as ethidium bromide efflux inhibitors in *Mycobacterium smegmatis*. J Antimicrob Chemother. 2008;62(2):345–8.
110. Sharma A, Kaur M, Katnoria JK, Nagpal AK. Polyphenols in food: cancer prevention and apoptosis induction. Curr Med Chem. 2018;25(36):4740–57.
111. Blesso CN. Dietary anthocyanins and human health. Basel: Multidisciplinary Digital Publishing Institute; 2019.
112. Nasir A, Bullo MMH, Ahmed Z, Imtiaz A, Yaqoob E, Jadoon M, et al. Nutrigenomics: epigenetics and cancer prevention: A comprehensive review. Crit Rev Food Sci Nutr. 2020;60(8):1375–87.
113. Davatgaran-Taghipour Y, Masoomzadeh S, Farzaei MH, Bahramsoltani R, Karimi-Soureh Z, Rahimi R, et al. Polyphenol nanoformulations for cancer therapy: experimental evidence and clinical perspective. Int J Nanomedicine. 2017;12:2689.
114. Zhou Y, Zheng J, Li Y, Xu D, Li S, Chen Y, et al. Natural polyphenols for prevention and treatment of cancer. Nutrients. 2016;8(8):515.
115. Khan N, Mukhtar H. Tea polyphenols in promotion of human health. Nutrients. 2019;11(1):39.
116. Silva C, Correia-Branco A, Andrade N, Ferreira AC, Soares ML, Sonveaux P, et al. Selective pro-apoptotic and antimigratory effects of polyphenol complex catechin:lysine 1:2 in breast, pancreatic and colorectal cancer cell lines. Eur J Pharmacol. 2019;859:172533.
117. Lagoa R, Silva J, Rodrigues JR, Bishayee A. Advances in phytochemical delivery systems for improved anticancer activity. Biotechnol Adv. 2020;38:107382.
118. Esfanjani AF, Jafari SM. Biopolymer nano-particles and natural nano-carriers for nano-encapsulation of phenolic compounds. Colloids Surf B Biointerfaces. 2016;146:532–43.
119. Ghaffari S-B, Sarrafzadeh M-H, Fakhroueian Z, Khorramizadeh MR. Flower-like curcumin-loaded folic acid-conjugated ZnO-MPA-βcyclodextrin nanostructures enhanced anticancer activity and cellular uptake of curcumin in breast cancer cells. Mater Sci Eng C. 2019;103:109827.
120. Sznarkowska A, Kostecka A, Meller K, Bielawski KP. Inhibition of cancer antioxidant defense by natural compounds. Oncotarget. 2017;8(9):15996.
121. Imran M, Salehi B, Sharifi-Rad J, Aslam Gondal T, Saeed F, Imran A, et al. Kaempferol: a key emphasis to its anticancer potential. Molecules. 2019;24(12):2277.
122. Tang S-M, Deng X-T, Zhou J, Li Q-P, Ge X-X, Miao L. Pharmacological basis and new insights of quercetin action in respect to its anti-cancer effects. Biomed Pharmacother. 2020;121:109604.
123. Yan X, Qi M, Li P, Zhan Y, Shao H. Apigenin in cancer therapy: anti-cancer effects and mechanisms of action. Cell Biosci. 2017;7(1):1–16.
124. Kaur V, Kumar M, Kumar A, Kaur K, Dhillon VS, Kaur S. Pharmacotherapeutic potential of phytochemicals: implications in cancer chemoprevention and future perspectives. Biomed Pharmacother. 2018;97:564–86.
125. Jia Z, Dumont M-J, Orsat V. Encapsulation of phenolic compounds present in plants using protein matrices. Food Biosci. 2016;15:87–104.
126. Nedovic V, Kalusevic A, Manojlovic V, Levic S, Bugarski B. An overview of encapsulation technologies for food applications. Procedia Food Sci. 2011;1:1806–15.

127. Rahaiee S, Assadpour E, Esfanjani AF, Silva AS, Jafari SM. Application of nano/microencapsulated phenolic compounds against cancer. Adv Colloid Interf Sci. 2020;279:102153.
128. Liu C, Ge S, Yang J, Xu Y, Zhao M, Xiong L, et al. Adsorption mechanism of polyphenols onto starch nanoparticles and enhanced antioxidant activity under adverse conditions. J Funct Foods. 2016;26:632–44.
129. Albanese A, Tang PS, Chan WC. The effect of nanoparticle size, shape, and surface chemistry on biological systems. Annu Rev Biomed Eng. 2012;14:1–16.
130. Joye IJ, McClements DJ. Biopolymer-based nanoparticles and microparticles: fabrication, characterization, and application. Curr Opin Colloid Interface Sci. 2014;19(5):417–27.
131. Ramasamy T, Kim JH, Choi JY, Tran TH, Choi H-G, Yong CS, et al. pH sensitive polyelectrolyte complex micelles for highly effective combination chemotherapy. J Mater Chem B. 2014;2(37):6324–33.
132. Qiu L, Qiao M, Chen Q, Tian C, Long M, Wang M, et al. Enhanced effect of pH-sensitive mixed copolymer micelles for overcoming multidrug resistance of doxorubicin. Biomaterials. 2014;35(37):9877–87.

Role of Antioxidants Derived from Herbal Medicines: Potential Anticancerous Agents

3

Qazi Zaid Ahmad, Aziz Ur Rahman, Huda Nafees, and Zainab Zaki

Abstract

Phytochemicals as bioactive components of plants shows promising results in curing many diseases. Therefore, the demand for these natural medicines increases day by day. Phytochemicals such as phenols and flavonoids seem to act in various ways to protect health. Protection of cells can be done through different types of means such as change of reactive oxygen species to non-radicle type by breaking sequencing of auto oxidative reactions commenced by reactive oxygen species and by lowering the oxygen saturation of diseased area. Many phytochemicals balance antioxidants and free radicals in our bodies. Some recent studies have shown that intake of synthetic antioxidants for a long duration may cause many health problems, like allergies, digestive problems, and according to few studies may also increase the chances of cancer.

Therefore, as a result, there has been a substantial shift in recent years toward the usage of natural antioxidants. Many medicinal plants are good sources of antioxidants, which are divided into three categories: (1) phenolic compounds, (2) vitamins, and (3) carotenoids. Some researches show that the use of plant originated antioxidants reduces the risk of diseases linked with oxidative stress, such as cancer. Therefore, and especially due to its effectiveness against cancer, in the past few years, the popularity of herbal phenolic compounds along with their antioxidant properties rises among scientists and consumers. According to the recent studies many natural polyphenolic constituents or compounds depicted more efficacy than Vit. E and/or C as antioxidants.

Q. Z. Ahmad · A. Ur Rahman (✉) · H. Nafees · Z. Zaki
Department of Saidla (Pharmacy), Faculty of Unani Medicine, Aligarh Muslim University, Aligarh, India

S. Tabrez, M. Imran Khan (eds.), *Polyphenols-based Nanotherapeutics for Cancer Management*, https://doi.org/10.1007/978-981-16-4935-6_3

This chapter will present some well-known green medicines, i.e., medicinal plants that may add to the optimization of antioxidants status and therefore offer safe, effective, and significant preventive and curative values for overall health.

Keywords

Antioxidant · Anticancer · Phytochemicals · Phenols · Bioavailability

3.1 Introduction

There are many reasons for different human ailments but Oxidation of cells is one of the main causes of carcinoma. *"Reactive oxygen species" (ROS)* of different types caused oxidative stress thereby detrimental of *DNA* and many biological molecules. Excessive ROS generation is not only a major cause for the progression of malignancy, but may be the basis for the higher risk of it [1]. Oxidizing agents along with free radicals are unescapably end product of the many physiological and metabolic processes. Humans have a different antioxidant system for defense; in accordance with the type of the cell and tissue and may react adversely or in collaboration. Such types of antioxidants are enzyme generated and non-enzyme origin. The examples of enzyme generated antioxidants are *Catalase (CAT), Superoxide dismutase (SOD), and Glutathione peroxidase (GPx).* While the non-enzyme origin includes minerals, vitamins, polyphenols and many more, which have engrossed great interest in recent years. Antioxidants may protect damaging of cell *by the* conversion of *reactive oxygen species (ROS)* to non-radical *species* depending on the kind of associated antioxidant, or via limiting or inhibiting the auto-oxidative chain reactions started by ROS and by lessening O_2 concentration locally. Generally, antioxidants are found mainly in two major forms either synthetic or natural origin [2, 3]. Recently some published studies demonstrated the adverse effect caused by the synthetic origin antioxidants. Therefore, these findings have drawn the attention of the scientists to venture the natural sources to find out its antioxidant potential [4]. Besides, toxic effect of synthetic antioxidants the other reason for focussing on natural antioxidants is its economic importance and availability [5]. Moreover, researches on medicinal plants have drawn global attention; evidences have been gathered to establish the efficacy of plants having medicinal properties used in different indigenous systems of medicines such as Unani and Ayurveda. The herbs have abundant variety of secondary metabolites, such as alkaloids, glycosides, tannins, flavonoids, terpenoids and many more. These metabolites are tested for their efficacy as antioxidant and anticarcinogen and showed positive responses. Natural antioxidants have been divided into many subtypes. Although, the two main sources of antioxidants are from day-to-day diets (e.g., fruits, vegetables, cereals, etc.) and from plants, those have good antioxidant potential and they are not the part of routine diet. Many studies revealed that the herbs are one of the major source for the drugs developed for prevention of side effects of chemotherapy and can be used to treat different type of cancers because of their phytoconstituents which are present in high concentrations and have antioxidant properties.

Such phytoconstituents are polyphenols, carotenoids, catechin, epicatechin, resveratrol, flavonoids, glycosides, genistein, beicalein, cyanidin 3-glucoside, Vit. A and C, kaempferol, gallic acid, quercetin, curcumin, etc. Many studies depicted that these antioxidant phytochemicals are capable to prevent the cell propagation, viz., cancer of colon. Breast, cervix, skin, and hepatic cancers, etc., according to many researches the plant derived antioxidants may performed effectively as chemopreventives and can be used as significant inhibitors of cell propagation, helping caspase-mediated cell death, enhance enzymatic detoxification, and constraining gene expression along with ROS scavengers. There are several researches on herbal antioxidants specially for determining those antioxidants which could have significant efficacy against the cancer cells. Studies also depicted that these phytochemicals also have effective chemoprotective properties. This chapter dealt with the antioxidants derived from some well-known medicinal plants and herbs.

3.2 Cancer and Antioxidants

Cancer is an abnormal proliferation of the cell, and it can outspread through the blood in the body [6]. Among cancer, breast cancer has the highest death rate and can be easily diagnosed. Cancer is one of the major cause of death globally. As per WHO, nearly 1 crore deaths occurred in 2020 worldwide. They estimated the incidence of new cancer cases and found that, in 2020, lung cancer was the major cause of death and accounts 1.80 million deaths worldwide then colon and rectum accounts for 935,000 deaths then liver 830,000 deaths, respectively [7]. Oxidative Stress has a major role to develop cancer. Reactive oxygen species on reaction with metals such as with free Iron and Copper damages biomolecule like lipids and synthesize aldehydes and malondialdehyde which breaks double bond or induce mutation. It causes changes in guanine and thymine bases, as well as sister chromatid interactions. In result disruption occurs in signal transduction functions, transcription factors, and tumor suppressor genes like p53 that plays a key role in apoptosis and cell cycle control [8]. So, the inactivity may rise the expression of proto-oncogenes, that might cause significant harm. Some enzymes become dysfunctional due to Oxidative damages or genetic flaws and are unable to repair the degenerative changes which enhance the chances of senile malignancies [9, 10].

Further, use of anticancer medicines and radiations may increase reactive oxygen species along with reduction in antioxidant agents, causes rise in oxidative stress in result apoptosis occurs, which produces many unwanted effects [10]. The continuous oxidative stress at low levels can lead to apoptosis resistance. Some pathogens, such as bacteria and viruses, are also affecting through oxidative stress to develop certain cancers such as H. Pylori which may cause peptic and colon cancer. The studies revealed that low antioxidant levels may be the basis of cancer. Hence, the use of antioxidants can inhibit cancer or may cause damage to malignancy developing cells [8, 10].

Halliwell and others described antioxidants as "any substance that, when found in relatively small concentrations to oxidizable substrates (carbohydrates, lipids, proteins, and nucleic acids), remarkably retards/inhibits the oxidation of the given substances" [11]. There were some other definitions of antioxidants given, as "any substrate that avoids, postpones, or eradicates oxidative damage to a target molecule" [12] or any substrate capable of directly or indirectly eliminating reactive oxygen species, functioning as a regulator of antioxidant defense, or preventing the synthesis of those species." To maintain healthy cellular microenvironment, stability between oxidative agents and antioxidants (redox balance) is required [9, 13–17].

Antioxidants can protect damages due to free radicals. Free radicals are the type of molecules having incomplete electron shells due to this factor they are capable of being more reactive in comparison to those having complete electron shells. Free radicals can also be formed by exposure to many ecological factors such as smoking, tobacco chewing, and radiations. In living beings, the most prevalent kind of free radical is Oxygen, a charged or radicalized oxygen molecule that takes electrons from other molecules, resulting in damage to DNA and other substances which is often irreversible if persist and after prolong duration it may be the reason for the development of many chronic ailments and cancer. Antioxidants neutralize the free radicals that are generated through normal cell processes. Antioxidants can be characterized as "mopping up" free radicals, which means they balance the electrical charges and inhibit the free radicals from stealing electrons of other molecules.

In the 1920s, the first scientist who associated oxygen with cancer was Otto Warburg [18]. Though, the role of oxygen in carcinogenic process was unexplored for several decades. In 1968, the discovery of superoxide dismutase gives the idea about the relation of reactive oxygen species (ROS) to the pathogenesis of cancer in the living system. ROS is not precisely confined to cancer, but it can also connect with many other human diseases. Considerable laboratory evidence from a number of studies suggests that the antioxidants agents may reduce or perhaps prevent the occurrence of cancer. Several researches are ongoing to evaluate the possible role of antioxidants as anticancer agents for reducing the risk of development of cancer [19].

3.3 The Antioxidant Defense

Naturally, antioxidants are composed of endogenic and exogenic biomolecules. Endogenic antioxidants are synthesized by our body which are enzymatic and nonenzymatic in nature while the exogenic antioxidants can be obtained from herbs in the form of medicines, diet, and nutritional supplements.

As per the mechanism of action, antioxidants can be classified into three groups. First, those antioxidants which inhibit the development of new free radicals. It is a fairly varied category that consists of enzymes, proteins, and minerals, the examples of enzyme are superoxide dismutase (SOD), catalase (CAT), and glutathione peroxidase (GPX). Protein Antioxidants are those proteins which bind to the metals like ferritin and ceruloplasmin. Selenium, Copper, Zinc are minerals having antioxidant properties. Second, includes those antioxidants which prevent oxidative chain reaction by capturing free radicals, e.g., glutathione enzyme, albumin, vitamins C and E, carotenoids, and flavonoids. Third type of antioxidants includes those enzymes which manage harm done by free radicals to cells for instance lipases, proteases, DNA repair enzymes, transferases, and methionine-sulfoxide reductases [20–23].

3.4 Antioxidants in Unani System of Medicine

In Unani Medicine, the human system has been gifted with four natural faculties or powers which work in synchronization to maintain the functions of the organs at equilibrium. These faculties are Quwwat Hazima (Digestive Faculty), Quwwat Jāziba (Absorptive Faculty), Quwwat Māsika (Retentive Faculty), and Quwwat Dāfi'a (Excretory Faculty). The entire principle of treatment of the Unani medicine revolves around the concept of protection of the organ and the maintenance of its associated faculties (Quwā) at equilibrium. The balanced faculties are the assurance of normal functioning of related organ/system and make it immune to resist against unwanted or diseased elements. That is why for making faculties stable and at equilibrium and hence to assure the well-being of every organ/system many drugs have been proposed which are mainly antioxidants, stimulant, or tonic in nature. The sources of these drugs are purely natural. If due to any disease some derangement in the equilibrium or function of faculties or in organ/ system has occurred then these antioxidants or tonic drugs safeguards and bring it to its equilibrium, i.e., at healthy condition. Thus, It may be stated that the preservation of organs and systems in order to do prevention, treatment, or halt the progression of ailment is the characteristic feature of the Unani System of Medicine [23].

Muqawwīyat are medicines that restore an organ's normal function and temperament to the point where it can withstand diseased materials and toxins flowing toward it. This activity is carried out by either its attribute or temperament that neutralize the causative morbid material in terms of excessive bile, phlegm, black bile, etc., to produce the equilibrium or maintain the milieu interieur which is essential for the restoration of health. Quwwat Jāziba was created to attract what is beneficial matter and this is done by means of the absorptive power of the organs. If Quwwat Jāziba becomes weak, then all other three Quwā will also become effected, as metabolism is initiated by Quwwat Jāziba. Quwwat māsika retains the beneficial matters. If Quwwat māsika becomes weak then food will not retain in the organ and the desire nourishment of the body will be affected. Quwwat Hazima absorbs the material drawn by the Quwwat Jāziba and retains and transforms it into a consistency ready for the action of the other Quwwat Mughayyira (metabolism) and also modifies it according to the requirement of other associated Quwwah. If Quwwat Hazima becomes weak then nutrient may turn toxic and signs of indigestion will appear. Quwwat Dāfi'a expels the superfluous matter through the natural passages and orifices, which is the remnant of the nutriment, or excess quantity of the nutrition or is no more required by the organ or body. Some times Quwwat Dāfi'a diverts the superfluous matter from the superior organ to the inferior organ or from hard organ to a soft organ in result of some pathological conditions or due to effect of some medicines. If Quwwat Dāfi'a becomes weak then toxic substances will get accumulated and stored in the organ [24, 25]. Therefore, to maintain all Quwwah at equilibrium and improve the functioning of system or organs antioxidants have vital role.

3.5 Need of Natural Antioxidants

Natural antioxidants are the need of the hour because they are safe, effective, and abundantly available. There are many studies going on regarding natural antioxidants either obtained from plant or animal sources. Global acceptance of natural antioxidants increases day by day because of its higher safety index and natural occurrence. But due to higher stability, easy availability, cost-effectiveness antioxidants from synthetic origin have been used very much in place of plant origin antioxidants. There are many researches that show issues related to the safety of synthetic antioxidants in long-term use. Therefore, the paradigm is shifted toward the use of natural or naturally derived antioxidants. It is todays need to replace synthetic antioxidants with natural one (Fig. 3.1).

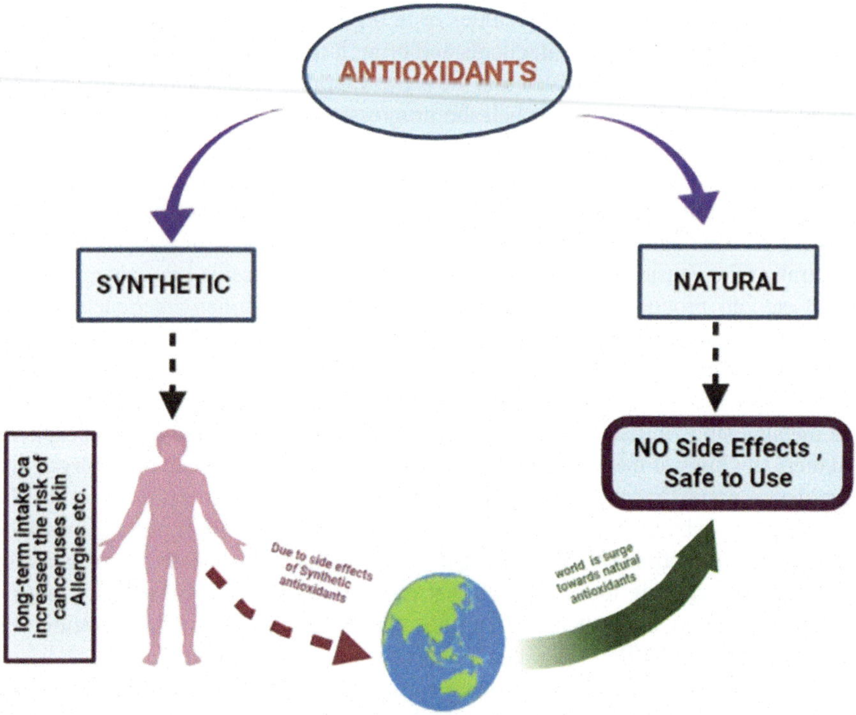

Fig. 3.1 Need of natural antioxidants

3.6 Phytochemicals as Antioxidants

Phytochemicals are the compound of plant origin with no nutritional value. Phytochemicals are classified into various categories and they are responsible for the major function of human biological system [26]. Medicinal herbs, cereals, fruits, and other food items are shown to have protection against various disorders, along with malignancy. This protective effect is mainly credited to phytochemicals present in them [27–30]. Approximately 10,000 phytochemicals have been discovered to date, with a major fraction of them remaining unknown. Alkaloids, Tannins, triterpenoids, steroids, flavones and saponins are among the phytochemicals discovered [31]. Excessive generation of oxidants (reactive oxygen and nitrogen species) is involved in the etiology of various ailments; therefore, phytochemicals' defensive role might be linked to their antioxidant activity [32].

Antioxidants found in plants are more than just backup in the fight against cellular damage and illness [33]. Cell proliferation is prevented by plant origin antioxidants thereby resulting in cancer cell death. Antioxidant phytochemicals including cyanidin, genistein, and keampferol may reduce the expression of gene causing cancer to inhibit cancer. Keampferol and cyanidin have the capacity to suppress the COX-2 gene expression, and therefore cancer-related genetic products. COX-2 activity increases in many malignancies, like lung, breast, and prostate cancers. The anticancer effect of a phytochemical namely "Genistein" on breast cancer is due to the reactivating and demethylating tumor suppressor genes which are through the direct interaction with the catalytic domain of DNA methyltransferase and also by inhibition of the DNA methyltransferase expression [34, 35]. The cancer-protective efficacy of phytochemicals found among plants has been proven in recent scientific studies. The antioxidant properties of many plant chemicals including ascorbic acid and polyphenols, the quenching of singlet oxygen and radicals by carotenoids, the suppression of activated enzymes by certain flavanols and tannins, and the stimulation of oxidation and conjugation (protective) enzymes by indoles, dithiothiones, and isothiocyanates, the protection of vulnerable structures by some polyphenols and the activation of DNA-repair caused by sulfur-containing compounds are among the mechanisms involved in preventing initiation. The antioxidant role of carotenoids and membrane stabilizing action described with polyphenols, the suppression of proteases induced by specific chemicals of soybeans, the activation of immunological responses shown with ascorbic acid and carotenoids, and the suppression of ornithine decarboxylase by carotenoids and polyphenols are all examples of biochemical mechanisms in antipromotion [36].

3.7 Classification of Antioxidants

The Antioxidants can be classified as shown in Fig. 3.2.

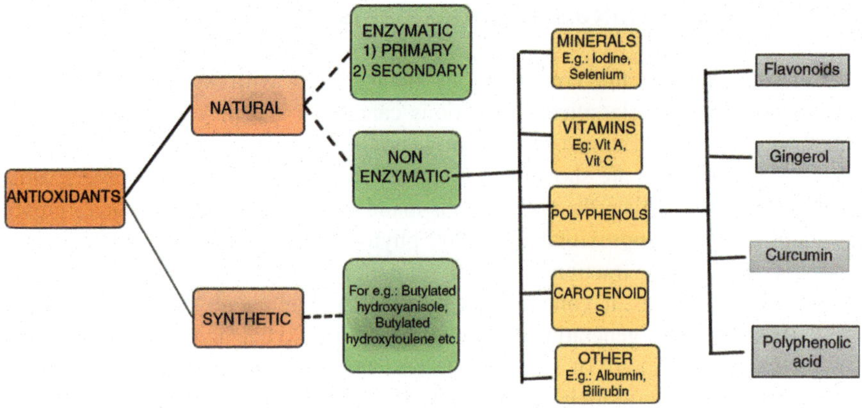

Fig. 3.2 Classification of antioxidants

3.8 Minerals as Antioxidants

3.8.1 Selenium

Selenium is one of the most important mineral elements responsible for the physiology of both plants and animals [37–39]. It is found in the atmosphere, lithosphere, hydrosphere, and biosphere, and among other places on the planet [40]. The areas which are having Se in abundant amount are known as seleniferous areas [41]. Usually, Se is taken into the body by consuming the animal products and also from the plants which are rich in Se. Se is taken by plants from the soil in the form of selenates [42], which are further transformed into the Se-Cys and Se-Met which are the organic forms [43]. Foods which are having abundant amount of Se are seafoods, eggs, mushrooms, chicken, nuts, and in green vegetables like cabbage, spinach, cauliflower, and the concentration of Se varies in humans according to their diet, and also with agro climatic conditions or regions. In water the amount of Se is minute and in the form of Selenites or Selenates.

The Prolonged deficiency of Selenium can lead to adverse effects on immunity and on cardiovascular system. It can also cause congenital hypothyroidism in fetuses and impair the nervous system [44]. Additionally, its deficiency has been associated with Alzheimer's disease, depression and anxiety [45]. Se low levels also increase the risk of some cancers [46] whereas, its over-sufficiency may result in anemia, bone stiffness, hair loss, or blindness [47].

Se. has numerous health benefits such as Se is a potent antioxidant that may contribute in fighting cancers, viral infections, and aging process. Se increases the quality of life for chemotherapy patients [48]. Chemotherapy side effects can be reduced by intake of Se [48–50]. Combs and Lu [51] have studied the effect of Se in preventing certain cancers. It is also important for the thyroid, brain, heart, and reproductive systems to function properly. It is the only micronutrient mentioned in the human genome (as the Se-Cys protein) [52].

The antioxidant mechanism of inorganic and organo-selenium in protection iron- and copper-induced oxidative DNA damage is because of the coordination of metal ions of selenium compounds [53–55]. Since fully coordinated $[Fe(EDTA)]^{2-}$ (400 μM) or $[Cu(bipy)_2]^+$ (500 μM) had no impact on DNA damage, fine tuning of Fe^{2+} or Cu^{2+} into an inorganic selenium compound is the primary mechanism for their activities as antioxidant as well as pro-oxidant [53, 56]. Similarly, organo-selenium compounds yielded similar findings. Though the exact mechanism for prevention of cancer through selenium compounds have not been found yet, the pro-oxidant seleno metabolites have direct action on the reactive oxygen species, resulting in cellular toxicity.

3.8.2 Zinc

It is considered as an important metal other than selenium and it is involved in a minimum of 200 enzyme antioxidant activities which are involved in several functions whether these functions are physiological and/or biochemical such as reproductive, cardiovascular, and nervous system [57]. It plays an important role in the regulation of carbohydrate and lipid metabolism [58]. Simultaneously its role is established for the immune system. Zinc also plays a role in managing the inflammatory responses. It also boosts up nutritional immunity and acts as an antioxidant [58]. Zinc is also useful to treat diarrhea in children and also in infants. Therefore, it is used to save millions of lives worldwide [59]. Approximately 2 billion people are having deficiency of zinc in developing countries; thisestimate is by WHO. The deficiency of Zinc shows several symptoms like its deficiency increase in the production of inflammatory cytokines, dysfunctions in the immune, hypo-fuctioning of testicular hormone, retardation in the development, and also its deficiency increases the oxidative stress [60].

Zinc exhibits antioxidant properties in a number of ways. The first and foremost activity is that zinc competes with the ions of Cu and Fe for binding to the proteins and cell membranes resulting in the displacement of the redox active metals which are responsible for the catalysis of the formation of ^{-}OH from H_2O_2. Secondly, Zinc also shows its antioxidant activity by the protection of biomolecules from oxidation by binding to their (SH) sulfhydryl group. Zinc also showed its antioxidant activity by enhancing the production of several enzymes, proteins, and molecules such as catalase enzyme and Glutathione and it also causes the reduction of the oxidant-promoting enzymes like NADPH oxidase, iNOS and inhibits the lipid peroxidation formation. The other mechanism behind the antioxidant activity is because it promotes the expression of metal-binding protein namely "Metallothionein" which is high in cysteine and it is a good excavator of ^{-}OH ions.

3.8.3 Iodine

Iodine is a micronutrient in chordates and is utilized by all living beings. In all vertebrates, it is a structural component of thyroid hormones and it is required for the proper functioning and development of many organs, mainly the Nervous System [61]. Although, a large portion of iodine in the body is not hormonal and contained in tissues also other than the thyroid, where its biological purpose is uncertain [62, 63]. According to various studies, from ancient algae to modern vertebrates, Iodine showed its antioxidant activity in all cells which concentrate it [64, 65]. Oxidized iodine can be utilized as an electron donor in these cells to neutralize reactive oxygen species (ROS) or to bind certain polyunsaturated fatty acids in cell membranes to double bonds, lowering ROS reactivity. [62, 66]. Iodine has also demonstrated a binding action with lipids like arachidonic acid (AA), apoptosis, and distinguishing properties on distinct epithelial cells [67–69]. Furthermore, immune cells absorb and metabolize iodine, depends on physiological functioning, and can play a role as a pro-inflammatory or anti-inflammatory agent [70, 71].

Iodine can cause scavenging activity for reactive oxygen species, such as superoxide anions (O_2) and hydroxyl radicals (OH), creating hypoiodous acid (HIO) and hydroiodic acid as neutral components (HI). Iodine reduces the activity of pro-inflammatory enzymes including cyclooxygenase type 2 (COX2) and nitric oxide synthase (NOS) when it is combined by "Arachidonic acid" to form the "iodolipid 6-iodolactone" (6-IL). Furthermore, iodination of the cysteine-rich protein Keap1 stimulates nuclear translocation of nuclear factor erythroid2-related factor-2 (Nrf2), which in turn result in the activation of antioxidant response element with Maf, resulting in the overexpression of antioxidant enzymes type II for instance catalase (Cat) and superoxide dismutase (SOD).

3.9 Carotenoids

Carotenoids (Crts) comes under the category of polyene-type natural pigments that are both structurally and functionally complex [72, 73]. Carotenoids are found within cell membranes because they are extremely lipophilic molecules. Carotenoids are abundant in fruits and vegetables, yellow-orange-red vegetables and fruits, and also in vegetables which are green in color. More than 700 Crts have been identified till date [73], with about 50 being part of the human food and barely 20 being included in the tissues and blood of humans [74]. Important are lycopene, α-carotene, β-carotene, lutein, β-cryptoxanthin, phytofluene, zeaxanthin, γ-carotene, α-cryptoxanthin, neurosporene, phytoene, and ζ-carotene and each are found in plasma of human [75, 76]. Their primary role appears to be protection from light in all non-photosynthetic species. They are considered as effective quenchers both physical and chemical of single oxygen ($^1O_2$), and reactive oxygen species scavengers (ROS) [77–79]. Carotenoids are effective at preventing although treating cancer, and their anticarcinogenic mechanisms vary. Carotenoids can induce their anticancer properties through a number of mechanisms, includes anti-inflammation, pro-oxidant and antioxidant, anti-proliferation, immunomodulation, anti-angiogenesis, and cell differentiation [80, 81].

Carotenoids are thought to be beneficial to one's well-being due to its antioxidant effect. The major carotenoids such as β-cryptoxanthin, lycopene, and β-carotene were widely investigated for their chemo-preventive capability to avert cancer as a result of antioxidant characteristics through peroxyl radicals, ROS quenchers and inducing phase II enzymes for instance NADPH, glutathione S-transferases, heme oxygenase-1, and quinone oxidoreductase [82]. Additionally, carotenoids can act as pro-oxidants and exert the processes for inducing the free radicals [83]. These compounds can produce oxidative stress depending on their concentration, composition, oxygen tension, arrangement in interactions in redox agents, cell redox state, and cell membranes. According to certain research, large dosages of crocetin and β-carotene can effectively raise intracellular oxidative stressors by increasing the rate of ROS formation in tumor cells; as a result, carotenoids can cause apoptosis and arresting cell cycle, resulting in the death of tumor cells [72, 83]. The immune system is important in the prevention of cancer cell growth. Carotenoids have no doubt influenced the role of our body's immune cells. As an immunomodulatory factor, β-carotene reduces the incidence of several malignancies by improving immune cell functioning [83]. Chronic inflammation is associated with the development of cancer cells, implying that it is the main risk factor for the growth of thecancer cells. As a result, reducing inflammation is an effective way to prevent and treat cancer. Inflammatory cytokine production is reduced as a result, and the carcinogenesis process is stopped. Astaxanthin, lycopene, and lutein have been shown in studies to have important anticancer effects, likely due to their anti-inflammatory properties [82, 84]. Angiogenesis characterized as the development of new vessels in previously avascular tissue as a result of endothelial cell proliferation and plays a major role in the progression of tumor and metastasis. As a result, in cancer diseases, avoiding the formation of feeding blood vessels is an effective way to monitor and/or eradicate them. In male C57BL/6 mice and B16F-10 cells, β-carotene has been found to have anti-angiogenic effects, which is advantageous for cancer prevention. Furthermore, because cancer cells comprise a low differentiation rate, encouraging them to develop into mature cells with a range of capabilities comparable to normal cells can help with chemoprevention. As a result, different mechanisms, such as cell growth regulation, are used to demonstrate carotenoids' anticancer capabilities. Growth factor, cell cycle development, and Gap junctional intercellular communication (GJIC) signaling could all be involved in this process. "Gap junctions," which are passageways between cells, carrying molecules having a low molecular weight (such as nutrition or signaling molecules). GJIC deficiency may be linked to malignant transformation. Lycopene, a carotenoid that is not a provitamin A, has been shown to raise GJIC and to be an anticarcinogenic agent in oral carcinogenesis [83]. Development factors are essential for tumor growth and have been related to a number of cancer risk factors. For instance, increased levels of (IGF)1 in blood, which may occur before many years of the diagnosis of cancer like

Table 3.1 List of some medicinal plants containing minerals with their pharmacological activities [85–128]

S. no	Mineral	Plant	Pharmacological effects
1.	Selenium (Se)	Quinoa *(Chenopodium quinoa) f-Chenopodiaceae*	Antioxidant activity, allergic effects, anti-obesity, and blood-fat reducing effects
		Mustard *(Brassica Juncea)* *f*-Brassicaceae	Anticancer, Antioxidant, Antitumor activity
		Radish *(Raphanus sativus)* *f*-Brassicaceae	Anti-inflammatory, Anticancerous activity, antioxidant
		Onion *(Allium cepa)* *f*-Amaryllidaceae	Antioxidant activity, anticancer activity, anti-inflammatory activity,
		Garlic *(Allium sativum)* *f*-Lillaceae	Antitumor, antioxidant
		Mint *(Mentha spicata)* *f*-Lamiaceae	Antioxidant activity, antimicrobial activity
2.	Zinc (Zn)	Stinging nettle *(Urtica dioica)* *f*-Urticaceae	Antioxidant, immunomodulatory, anti-inflammatory
		Cumin *(Nigella sativa)* *f*-Apiaceae	Antioxidant activity, Anticancer activity, analgesic effect, antimicrobial properties
		Mint *(Mentha piperita)* *f-Lamiaceae*	Antioxidant activity, antimicrobial activity, cytotoxic
		Basil *(Ocimum basilicum)* *f*-Lamiaceae	Antioxidant activity, anti-bacterial, anti-fungal, anti-inflammatory, antitumor
		Saffron *(Crocus sativus)* *f-Iridaceae*	Antioxidant, Anticarcinogenic
3.	Iodine (I)	Barbary *Berberis vulgaris* *f-Berberidaceae*	Anticancer, anti-inflammatory, antioxidant
		Bitter-apple *(Citrullus colocynthis)* *f*-Cucurbitaceae	Antioxidant, Anticancer, Anti-inflamatory
		Cocklebur *(Xanthum strumarium)* *f*-Asteraceae	Anticancer, anti-inflammatory
		Ajowain *(Carum copticum)* *f*-Umbelliferae	Antioxidant properties, Anti-inflammatory

breast, lung, prostate cancers have been related to it [82]. Some medicinal plants containing minerals with their pharmacological activities are given in Table 3.1.

3.10 Vitamins

3.10.1 Vitamin C

One of the most commonly supplemented Vitamin is Ascorbic acid. The preservative and antioxidative properties of this compound are used in the food industry [129]. Mangoes, oranges, brussels sprouts, kiwi, cantaloupe, strawberries, cranberries, papayas, melons, spinach, asparagus, and tomatoes are all high in vitamin C [130]. On an average, a daily recommendation of Vitamin C intake for women is 90 mg and for men 75 mg approximately [131]. The deficiency of Vitamin C is rare these days owing to appropriate nutrition, and only happens in rare circumstances such as malabsorption, malnutrition, renal illness, and smokers. Vitamin C needs to increase during breastfeeding, during severe physical activity, in smokers, drinkers, the elderly, and people who are hypertensive and diabetic and these individuals can cosume the Vitamin C in high quantity and can take more than 120 mg per day. Although the amount of vitamin C upto 3 g is recommended and the excessive intake of Vitamin C causes adverse effects such as nausea, vomiting, and diarrhea. Vitamin C is absorbed as ascorbate and dehydroascorbate in the entire length of the human intestine (DHA). Vitamin C overload can lead to increased iron absorption as well as vitamin B12 and copper absorption impairment [132].

As a water-soluble antioxidant, ascorbate is important in cellular oxidative metabolism, as it effectively scavenges "ROS" and "RNS" formed under a variety of stress conditions [133, 134]. Since ascorbate (and glutathione) are involved in the reduction in the radical tocopheroxyl into tocopherol, tocopherol-mediated defense against lipid peroxidation may be significantly enhanced [133, 135]. In addition, ascorbate is an important cofactor intended for multiple enzymes involved in the biosynthesis of carnitine and catecholamines (0). Ascorbate also maintains the catalytic activity of diverse Fe(II)-2-oxoglutarate-dependent dioxygenases throughout the posttranslational modification and folding of extracellular matrix proteins like collagen [136].

3.10.2 Vitamin E

"Vitamin E" is an important micronutrient which is made up of eight different compounds, i.e., 4 compounds of Tocopherols and 4 compounds of Tocotrienols. Tocopherol is the most important active component of vitamin E. Vitamin E is mostly obtained from fat-rich foods, particularly edible oils and nuts [137]. This Vitamin is a fat-soluble antioxidant which preserves the oxidizable lipids present in foods, cosmetics, and medications (Fats and oils are kept from going rancid). The lipids present in the body fluids and cells are also protected by the same antioxidant process, making it a natural anti-aging component of tissues of humans [138]. It also affects the gene expressions in the liver, blood, immune system, and central nervous system that are important in physiological processes. Humans require vitamin E as a free radical-scavenging antioxidant [139]. Cancer survivors frequently use them as well.

Due to the presence of a phenol group, the chromanol head group of vitamin E avoids damaging peroxidation [140] and it is the initial line of resistance against fatty acids peroxidation which are not saturated. When the acidic H from vitamin E's OH is converted to peroxy radicals (ROO), the radical chain is prevented from spreading inside the lipid domains [141]. Other oxidizing reagents that TP can trap include singlet oxygen, superoxide anion, ozone, peroxynitrite, and nitrogen dioxide radicals [137]. In an in vivo study, the deficiency of Vitamin E inhibited lipoperoxidation,

Table 3.2 Some medicinal plants containing vitamins [143–169]

S. no	Vitamin	Plants	Pharmacological study
1.	Vit C	Arabi *(Colocasia esculanta)* *f*-Araceae	Anticancer, Antioxidant, anti-inflammatory, probiotic
		Indian licorice *(Abrus precatorius)* *f*-Fabaceae	Antioxidant activity, Anti-inflammatory
		Roselle *(Hibiscus sabdariffa)* *f*-Malvaceae	Anti-inflammatory, Antioxidant activity
		Hogweed *(Boerhavia diffusa)* *f*-Nyctaginaceae	Antioxidant, Anti-inflammatory activity
		Turmeric *(Curcuma longa)* *f*-Zingiberaceae	Antioxidant, Anticancer, Anti-inflammatory agent
2.	Vit E	Silk cotton seed *(Gossypium herbaceum) f-Malvaceae*	Anticancerous, Dietetic, Antioxidant
		Fenugreek *(Trigonilla foenum-graecum)* *f*-Fabaceae	Anticancer, anti-inflammatory
		Lettuce *(Lactuca sativa)* *f*-Asteraceae	Antioxidant effects, Anticancer activity, analgesic
		Aloe vera *(Alove barbedensis)* *f*-Liliaceae	Antioxidant, Anticancer
		Amla *(Phyllanthus emblica)* *f*-Euphorbiaceae	Antioxidant effect, anti-inflammatory Anticancer effect, immunomodulatory effect

which is associated with the increase in lipoperoxides which are circulating [137]. Vitamin E inhibits lipoperoxidation, which affects the oxidation of cholesterol because of the blocking of sterol5,6-epoxidation [142]. Some Medicinal Plants containing Vitamins with their pharmacological actions are given in Table 3.2.

3.11 Polyphenols

Among all phytochemicals, phenolic compounds (PCs) play a very significant role in health benefits. The category of "organic compounds" known as Phenolic compounds are at number second as the most plentiful and after cellulose in the plant kingdom. Besides health benefits, they perform various activities in plants like protect them against ultraviolet (UV) solar radiation and provide structural support, biotic or abiotic stress, and many more. Phenolic compounds directly act as antioxidants because they have a significant role in neutralizing and adsorbing free radicals and they also reduces the decomposing of peroxides or triplet or singlet oxygen. As Phenolic compounds have hydroxyl group which is responsible for exerting powerful scavenging activity, due to this activity phenolic compounds are considered as important plant constituents and are also known as "potent chain breaking antioxidants." As anticancerous action, Polyphenols plays a significant role in all phytochemicals. The Polyphenols, such as ellagitannins and epicatechin gallate, exhibited anticarcinogenic properties [170, 171]. The existence of polyphenols in food gives significant organoleptic features in color, flavor, acrimony, etc. Polyphenols play a significant impact on health and have been utilized as a therapeutic agent for centuries.

In past decades, great interest has been developed between the users and researchers for the use of phenolic compounds because of their antioxidant activity as many epidemiological studies have been done which shows the linking between the use of natural antioxidants in diet having abundant quantity of these natural antioxidants, which in turn decreases the risk of those diseases which mainly occur and associated with the oxidative stress like "cancer."

It is expected that the global phenolic antioxidant market may reach up to 1.83 billion USD by 2023 due to wide applications of phenolic antioxidants other than therapeutic applications including cosmetics, plastic, rubber, fuel, lubricant, etc. [172]. In plants, these substances are obtained from different pathways like, "pentose phosphate-pathway," "shikimate-pathway," and "phenylpropanoid-pathway." The chemical structure of polyphenols contains an "aromatic compound," comprising at least one or more than one "hydroxyl" compound. There is an extensive diversity of "phenolic compounds" (PCs), which are present naturally, due to their structural diversity. As part of the phenylpropanoid pathway, cinnamic acid is formed due to the deaminization of Tyrosine and Phenylalanine. Though these organic constituents having a mutual carbon (C6-C3) phenylpropanoid element however an indispensable phase in their biosynthesis reaction is the addon of one or more than one –OH groups to the phenyl ring, increase to the variability of molecules, such as stilbenes, proanthocyanidins, cinnamic acids, lignans, flavonoids, lignins, coumarins, and benzoic acids.

At Present, minimum "8000" structures of "Phenolic compounds"(PCs) have been recognized, which further characterized into several classes [173]. Studies have exposed that polyphenols can reduce the amount of O^{-}_2 in vascular endothelial cells by inhibiting the production of NADPH (Nicotinamide adenine dinucleotide phosphate hydrogen) and also NOX (oxidase). They can also reduce the ATP synthesis in mitochondria by hindering the ATPase and mitochondrial respiratory chain. The polyphenols exert these effects because of the acceptance of electron by phenolic hydroxyl to have a more stable "phenoxy radical", which prevent "Cellular Components" from OS (Oxidative stress), further they decrease the risk of several ailments.

The classification of polyphenols has been given in Fig. 3.1, and among them the most significant PCs (Phenolic Compounds) are found in the human food and they are "Flavonoids," "Phenolic Acids" (PA), and "Tannins".

3.11.1 Phenolic Acids

The Chemical structure of "Phenolic Acids" contains at the minimum of "one" aromatic ring where a minimum of one Hydrogen atom is relieved by hydroxyl groups [174]. They comprise of two groups: the one is the "Hydroxybenzoic Acids"

(HBAs) and the other group is the "Hydroxycinnamic Acids" or HCAs, these are formed from "non-phenolic" molecules of "cinnamic" and "benzoic" acids and are produced by the pathway namely "Shikimate pathway," where"l-tyrosine" also known as "l-phenylalanine" is the premonitory constituent [175].

The responses involved in the synthesis of phenolic acids are "Methylation," "Hydroxylation," and "Deamination." Initially, Tyrosine or Phenylalanine undergo Deamination reaction, resulting in the formation of "p-coumaric acids" and/or "Cinnamic acid," respectively. Then Hydroxylation and methylation of "Aromatic rings" of "p-coumaric"or/and "Cinnamic acid" takes place and the resultant outcome is the formation of "Ferulic" and "Caffeic acid." Then degradation of the "Cinnamic acid" side chain occurs ensuing in formation of benzoic acid. Further, the processes "Hydroxylation" and "Methylation" of benzoic acid give rise to protocatechuic and p-hydroxybenzoic acids [176].

3.11.1.1 Hydroxybenzoic Acids (Hbas)

The Basic structure of hydroxybenzoic acids is C6–C1. Variation in their aromatic rings which is a basic structure leads to the formation of number of compounds. HBAs are "Gentisic Acid," "Vanillic Acid," "Protocatechuic," "Ellagic," "Syringic," "Gallic," "Salicylic," and 4-hydroxy Benzoic acids. These compounds are found in both the forms in plants in conjugated form and in free form and some compounds formed while processing [177].

3.11.1.2 Hydroxycinnamic Acids (Hcas)

The Basic structure of hydroxycinnamic acids is "C6–C3" where side chain having a double bond might be having "cis or a trans configuration" and occurs in the form of "Polymers," "Dimers," or "Monomers" can occur in precipitate form with acids of hydroxyl group, alcohols, and also monosaccharides or disaccharides forming "Esters," or they can be amino after precipitation with amines. While in the free form they are rarely found but as processed food they can be found in free form by freezing, or fermentation and sterilization processes [177].

3.11.2 Flavonoids

"Flavonoids" is the another most significant antioxidant compound. It is a subdivision of polyphenols present in abundant quantity in most of the herbal medicines. They contain nearly two-thirds of dietary "Phenolic Compounds" (PCs) or out of 8000 polyphenolic compounds 6000 are flavonoids. Their molecular weight is low, categorized by a 15-carbon structure, organized as "C6–C3–C6," with diverse characteristics like arrangement of the basic structure and unsaturation degree, subsequent in diverse subdivisions. Basically, the structures of Flavonoid are made up of two aromatic rings, i.e., ring A and ring B, amalgamated by a three carbon link, regularly in the form of a Heterocyclic ring, i.e., ring C. The formation of a molecule of flavonoid is from a pathway known as "Acetate/Malonate pathway" where A ring is formed and in the "Shikimate pathway" the "B Ring" is formed from "phenylalanine" [178]. Variation in the pattern of C rings produces a variety of sections like "Flavonols," "Flavanonols," "Flavanones," "Isoflavones," "Flavones," and "Anthocyanidins." These differences occur due to a number of reactions like "Oxygenation," "Glycosylation," "Sulfation," "Alkylation," and "Acylation" [178].

3.11.2.1 Flavones

They are categorized as the primary form of "Flavonoids." They comprise of a "Keto Group" in C4, and a covalent bond in between the ring C2 and C3 and "Ring B" is connected with C2. The utmost plentiful Flavones in vegetables and fruits contain "Luteolin," "Apigenin," and their Glycosides. The "Polymethoxylated Flavones" (like tangeretin and nobiletin) present in abundant amount in citrus peel have powerful bioactivities. They possess antioxidant benefits and also playing a role in delaying the metabolizing of drugs [177].

3.11.2.2 Isoflavones

Isoflavones are the kinds of flavones where ring "B" is adhered to "C3" at the place of "C2" because of the specific structural feature the isoflavones having resemblance to estrogens which is a female sex hormone having mild estrogenic activity due to which Isoflavones are also called as Phytoestrogens. The main Isoflavones are daidzein, glycitein, and genistein.

Researchers suspect that isoflavone may have a valuable role in decreasing the risk of cancers related to hormones, like Breast Cancer, Endometrial Cancer, and Prostate cancer. However, the mechanisms and outcomes of the studies are not clear until now. Though, The effect of Isoflavones on cancer is not clear yet because in some studies it is found that Isoflavones act as antioxidants while in some studies it is found that it acts as oxidant.

3.11.2.3 Flavonols

It is the extensively distributed subclass of flavonoids which includes "Quercetin" and "Kaempferol." Flavonols are flavones hydroxylated in C3. They are found in many foods and ensue in many medicinal herbs having anticancer potential. Such as, *"Alpinia officinarum" rhizomes* and flowers of "*Rosa chinensis*." [179].

Quercetin mainly exhibits its antioxidant activity due to several mechanisms like the effects of quercetin on activity of glutathione enzyme, reactive oxygen species, and the pathways of signal caused by several factors including toxicological and environmental. Its potent antioxidant activity is found because it maintains oxidative balance [180].

To slow down the purification in a system of "Human Neutrophil Myeloperoxidase" Quercetin plays its role by using undamaged "Human Neutrophils"; at this stage, it is found more powerful than "methimazole," which is definite "Myeloperoxidase-inhibitor." This kind of Flavonol was invented to be an influential constraint of "human neutrophil degranulation" and O_2 creation tempted by diverse secretagogues. The processes of "Phosphorylation of neutrophil proteins inhibition" and activation of neutrophil by "phorbol 12-myristate 13-acetate" occurs due to quercetin. Phosphorylation as a significant intracellular occurrence correlated with activation of Neutrophils because of Phosphorylation of a definite "Neutrophil protein" with some concentration of quercetin, in addition to abridged neutrophil degranulation and O2 production [181]. The result of some researches have found that quercetin provides prevention against various diseases, like osteoporosis, and also it helps in prevention of some forms of cancers and tumors. The preventive effect of quercetin for such diseases is due to its antioxidant activity [182].

3.11.2.4 Flavanones

The flavanones and dihydroflavonols (or flavanonols) are the compounds of flavonoids where C ring grants a saturated "Pyrane group" having no covalent bond in between the "C2" and "C3," and also holds "keto group" in "C4" and "Dihydroflavonols" contains OH in "C3." The important flavanones present are namely "Eriodictyol," "Naringenin," and "Hesperetin." They possess antioxidant, anti-inflammatory like pharmacological activities and are also helpful in maintaining the health of CVS (Cardiovascular System) [177].

3.11.2.5 Flavan-3-ols

The covalent bond between the rings of "C2" and "C3," and also the "Oxo group" in "C4" is absent in Flavan-3-ols, and keep OH in C3. These structural features develop in "C2" and "C3" at ring "C" in "chiral centers," meanwhile 4 diverse divisions are involved in every carbon atom, due to this Flavan-3-ols exhibits numerous diverse conformations [177].

The foremost types of Flavan-3-ols are "Catechin," "Gallocatechin," "Epicatechin," "Epigallocatechin," their "3-O-gallates," oligomers, polymers. They are considered as good antioxidants, specifically those containing "galloyl moieties." While "Oligomeric flavan-3-ols" also known as "Proanthocyanidins" is among the most copious component found in food which are occupied regularly. The capability to prevent the dermis from the several side effects or adverse effects which are caused due to ultraviolet radiation (UV radiation) present in them, decreases the chances of skin cancers. This property of protectiveness is primarily through 4 mechanisms, which are, protection against inflammation caused by UV radiations, secondly prevents oxidative stress, thirdly prevent the damage of DNA, and then the inhibition of immune responses [183].

3.11.2.6 Anthocyanidins

They do not have "Keto Group" in 'C4," but having an OH group in "C3," and two covalent bonds in ring "C"; owed to these specific characteristic features, they are the only "Ionic Flavonoids." Nearly all "anthocyanins" are "glycosylated" byproducts of "anthocyanidins" like, "Peonidin," "Petunidin," "Cyanidin," "Delphinidin," "Pelargonidin," and "Malvidin."

3.11.3 Curcumin

It is a phytochemical (dietary phenols) mainly present in *Curcuma longa* rhizome, commonly known as Turmeric or *Haldi*. The earliest research studies have shown that curcumin has preventive and curative effects against several diseases like carcinoma, neurological, autoimmune, cardiovascular diseases, etc. According to some anticancerous studies it was found that the antioxidant phytochemicals prevented cell proliferation thereby caused cancer cell death. Curcumin directly induces its effect on "Targeted Cancer Stem Cells" to produce anticancerous activity [184] and if combines with catechin then it exhibits "Synergistic" Anticanceorous activity in different cell lines for Cancer of Larynx and Colon Adenocarcinoma [185].

3.11.4 Tannins

They are commonly referred to as tannic acid. They are the plant phenolics having relatively high molecular weights (>1000) and precipitate protein from solution. As a large number of hydroxyl groups and other functional groups are present, these compounds are present as esters or "heterosis." Therefore, they are able to condense proteins and salivary glycoproteins which may lead to the loss or decrease in lubrication action which in turn is responsible for the astringency action of many plants [186]. The Hydrogen link in between the "Phenolic groups" and the "Site-Specific protein" of tannins play a role in binding between proteins and Tannins and the stability of this binding depends on the molecular weight of tannins. They have been chemically categorized into two classes: One is Hydrolyzable Tannins and the other is Nonhydrolyzable Tannins or also called Condensed tannins. The "Tannins" which are hydrolyzable composed from the shikimate pathway lead to the formation of "Gallic acid esters" or Gallotannins, esterified by glycosylated ellagic acid (ellagitannins) and gallic acid partially or completely. Glucose and gallic acids are yielded after the hydrolyzation by some specific enzymes, Bases, Acids, and also Gallic Acid Esters. However, Condensed tannins have more complex structure and uniform hydrolyzable tannins [177, 187]. List of some Tannin containing plants and their pharmacological activities are given in Table 3.3.

3.11.5 Stilbenes

Stilbenes have shown a promising effect to combat challenging diseases like cancer, because of its anti-inflammatory action, cell death activation, and antioxidant activity, which is coupled with reduced toxicity under in vivo conditions. Now the concept of chemoprevention is popular globally which promotes the administration of agents which have potent to protect or prevent, inhibit, or delay the progression process of carcinogenesis [200, 201]. Stilbenes have the potential to trim down the tumorigenesis by interacting with all stages of carcinogenesis at molecular level.

Table 3.3 List of some tannin containing plants and their pharmacological activities [188–199]

S. no	Plants	Pharmacological activity
1.	Black plum *(Eugenia jambolana) f*-Myrtaceae	Anti-inflammatory effects, Antioxidant, Antineoplastic effect, Chemopreventive effect, Radioprotective effects
2.	Arjun *(Terminalia arjuna) f*-Combretaceae	Anticancer activity, Antioxidant Anti-inflammatory, immunomodulatory
3.	Pomegranate *(Punica granatum) f*-Lythraceae	Antioxidant, Anticancer, Anti-inflammatory
4.	Sebastan *(Cordia latifolia) f*-Boraginaceae	Anticancer, Anti-inflammatory, Antioxidant
5.	Acacia *(Acacia Arabica) f*-Leguminosae	Antioxidant, Antimutagenic

Moreover, the limited concentration in the plant and low bioavailability limited its benefits [202]. The bioavailability of many phenolic compounds greatly depends upon their morphology, molecular size, administration site, metabolism, and absorption processes. These factors are also associated with the basic structure of the compound including Glycosylation or Acylation degree and conjugation with other phenolics, polymerization, solubilty, etc. [203, 204]. This is the major cause due to which the bioavailability of many phenolic compounds greatly differs [204].

3.11.6 Curcuminoids

Curcuminoids are defined as the derivatives of ferulic acid, contain two molecules of ferulic acid attached with a "β-diketone" in a highly conjugated form by methylene. They have been used since antiquity for different cultural, culinary, cosmetics, and medicinal purposes. Earlier its therapeutic potential was revealed through many researches. This phytochemical comes under the group of Phenolic compounds known as "Diarylheptanoids." The main chemical compounds of curcuminoids include curcumin, demethoxycurcumin, and bisdemethoxycurcumin [205]. All three chemical compounds of curcuminoids possess significant yellow color to turmeric, particularly to its rhizome. Furthermore, the antioxidant property is also found in curcuminoids which are isolated from species of Zingiber or Curcuma, such as *Curcuma domestica, Curcuma xanthorrhiza, Curcuma zedoaria, and Zingiber cassumunar* [206–208]. Curcuminoids have been reported for its antioxidant, anticancer [209], and antimicrobial activities. [210]. Curcumins have shown their antioxidant potential by transferring hydrogen atoms to make it larger than that of "α–tocopherol" and which is considered as more powerful natural antioxidant [211] which is related to the ability for inhibition of carcinogenic reactive oxygen species like "Nitrite Radicals", "Peroxides," "Superoxide Anions,"and "Hydroxyl radicals" [212]. The pathophysiology of Inflammatory disorders and also certain types of cancer have been associated with the improper upregulation of cyclooxygenase-2 or COX-2 and also iNOS enzymes. Curcumin exhibits its anti-inflammatory action most likely by inhibiting enzymes like "Lipooxygenase," "COX-2," and also "iNOS" as these are the enzymes which have a significant role in mediating inflammatory processes. Hence, Curcumin exhibits preventive effects on cancer because tumor progression is more likely to be closed with inflammation [213].

3.11.7 Coumarins

Plants contain coumarins in free form as well as in the form of glycosides. They are categorized on the basis of their oxygenation degree of their benzopyrane moiety and also on their large chemical diversity [179]. Up till now, using natural sources specifically from green plants more than 300 coumarins have been isolated and identified. A maximum number of compounds are having coumarins. These compounds include anticoagulant agents like Dicoumarol [214], Photosensitizing agents like psoralens, etc. The coumarins which are having pyrone rings and benzene rings in fused form comes under the group of phenolics having low molecular weight and these coumarins are extensively used for preventing and treating several diseases. On the basis of substitution pattern coumarins exhibits their pharmacological actions, therapeutic uses, and biochemical properties. Coumarins possess a number of important pharmacological actions like antioxidant action, anticancer, anti-inflammatory, antiviral, etc. [215–218]. They also possess its effect on "Central Nervous System" (CNS). In many researches, the effect of 7-hydroxycoumarin has been determined as antioxidant. In a study, the effects of 6–7 hydroxycoumarin also known as esculetin and 7-hydroxycoumarin on cellular metabolism of A431 cells for a time period of 24 h were investigated. Results showed that the 7-hydroxycoumarin exhibits the inhibition on the activity of "Succinate Dehydrogenase" at a concentration of more than 10μg/ml [219]. In another study the antioxidant namely "Auraptene" or 7-geranyloxycoumarin [220], which have been isolated from citrus fruits peel "*Citrus natsudaidai Hayata*" was determined for its effect as chemoprotective agent against chemically induced carcinogenesis [221]. The results of the study revealed that this antioxidant, i.e., auraptene having preventive effect through enrichment of immunity. Moreover, auraptene also possess antitumor effect in skin of mouse and in the rat tongue, colon, and esophagus it possess anticancerous activity [222]. The coumarins which are present naturally exhibit their anticancerous activity by inducing several enzymes which are responsible for detoxifying carcinogens like S-Transferase, Glutathione, etc. [223].

3.11.8 Lignans

Lignans are phytoestrogens, and their metabolites are worked as antioxidants and free radical scavengers, decreases the chances of cancer development [224]. These are polyphenols obtained as secondary metabolite of phenylanaline. Bacteria present in the intestine can metabolize Polyphenols or plant lignans and form "Mammalian lignans" namely enterolactone and enterodiol. Lignans bind with oestrogen receptors in the breast cells. Mammalian lignans, i.e., enterolactone and Entroldiol are having involvement in the cystostatic activity against cancer cell line of colon [225].

3.11.9 Quinones

The structure of quinones comprising of benzene ring where 2 carbonyl bonds are formed by substituting of 2 hydrogen atoms by 2 oxygen atoms. Among all quinones, the most important is the benzoquinone ($C_6H_4O_2$) and it is further categorized into other types like 1,2-benzoquinone, 1,4-benzoquinone, parabenzoquinone, and orthobenzoquinon. Herbal anthraquinones produce antitumor effects and also inhibiting carcinogenesis. In a study it was found that these "anthraquinones" eradicate cancer cells in the lungs of human and colon by blocking the benzo[a]pyrene mediated DNA damage in the cell line of human hematoma and showed high suppressing activity on proliferation of mesangial cells of humans, In addition, also have a specific antitumor activity of neuroectodermal tumor, this activity is due to the immune cytochemical response of this phytochemical to neutralizing the specific antigen of neuroendocrine and epithelial [226, 227].

Quinones also act effectively in colon cancer chemotherapy by inducing toxicity to the cancer cell line namely "MCF-7" which is involved in cancer of breast and also to the T-Lymphocytic Leukemia cell line which is CEM-SS to restrain telomerase and to possess powerful activity as antineoplastic. Furthermore, some of the furano naphtha quinones showed effects on toxic cells in mammalian species and also on the factors which damage DNA. The antitumor activity of quinones is mainly attributed on the nucleus of hydroxy bonds which are associated with inhibition of cell growth [226, 227].

3.11.10 Bioavailability of Phenolic Compounds (PCs)

The rate of absorption of Phenolic Compounds (PCs) across the intestine affects its bioavailability. Taguchi et al. have been reported the bioavailability of many polyphenols ingested in pure form or in foods, when reaching plasma varies from 0.072 to 5 μM [228]. Figure 3.3 demonstrates the bioavailability of phenolic compounds.

3.12 Conclusion and Future Perspective

The major causes of mortality and mental and physical disability are many chronic diseases including cancers, diabetes, and other related problems. The oxidative damage of biomolecules like protein, lipid, and DNA is caused by oxidative stress which occurs due to the reactive oxygen or nitrogen species in some conditions. Chronic inflammation and excessive production of oxidants are responsible for the

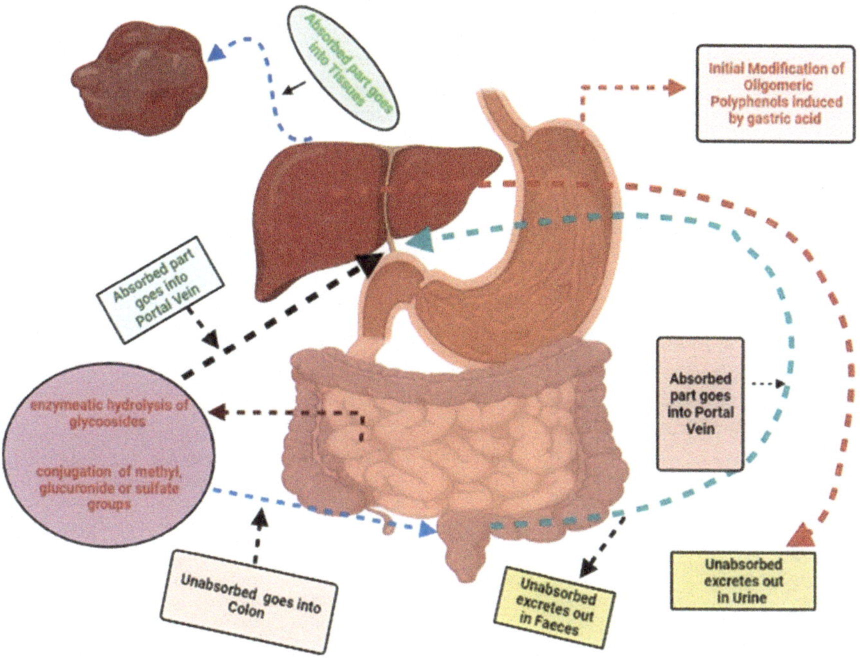

Fig. 3.3 Schematic representation for the bioavailability of phenolic compounds

derangement of normal physiological function resulting in pathogenesis of many diseases. Antioxidants have the potential to prevent cells from damage due to free radicals. Natural antioxidants have advantages over synthetic one as it has been mentioned in several studies that the continuing use of synthetic antioxidants can cause many side effects. Therefore, nowadays the world is venturing toward natural antioxidants due to their safe and effective status. The natural antioxidants can be derived from fruits, vegetables, medicinal plants, and other natural sources. The plant-derived antioxidants are among the most promising agents to combat chronic disorders. Many antioxidant phytochemicals consist of multifaceted effect, such as a phytochemical resveratrol, which is having preventing role in several diseases like Obesity, Diabetes, Cancers, Cardiovascular diseases, and also in Alzheimer disease.

Several experimental studies have been depicted that the antioxidants exhibit anticancerous activities and these antioxidants can be present in functional foods as well as nutritional supplements.

Therefore, it is advised to take in our daily routine a balanced diet which consists of fruits, vegetables, grains, and medicinal plants recommended by the experts because they contain many phytochemicals having antioxidant property, which helps to combat various chronic disorders. The traditional system of medicine, viz., Ayurveda and Unani has a vast treatise of natural products which have antioxidant property and a number of chronic disorders are successfully prevented/cured by them. There is a sire need to identify the leads from this rich heritage and develop

Table 3.4 A brief description of common antioxidant plants [229–251]

S. no	Medicinal plant	Part used	Chemical constituent responsible for antioxidant activity
1.	Turmeric *(Curcuma longa) f*-Zingiberaceae	Rhizome	Curcumin, 4-hydroxycinnamoylmethane
2.	Nutmeg *(Myristica fragrans) f*-Myristicaceae	Fruit	Myristphenone, phenolic volatile oils, phenolic acid (caffeic acid), flavanols (catechin)
3.	Acacia *(Acacia Arabica) f*-Fabaceae	Gum	Flavonoid, phenols
4.	Cobra saffron *(Mesua ferra) f*-Calophyllaceae		Phenols, flavonoid
5.	Ginger (Zingiber Officinale) *f*-Zingiberaceae	Rhizome	Gingerol
6.	Clove *(Eugenia Caryophyllata) f*-Myrtaceae	Bud	Phenolic acids (gallic acid), flavonol glucosides, phenolic volatile oils (eugenol, acetyl eugenol), Tannins
7.	Dodder *(Cuscuta reflexa) f*-Convolvulaceae	Seeds	Flavonoids, dulcitol, bergenin, coumarins, glycosides, lactone
8.	Carrot *(Daucus carota) f*-Apiaceae	Root	Carotenes, carotenoids, glycosides, flavonoids, sugars, quaternary bases
9.	Gooseberry *(Emblica officinalis) f*-Phyllanthaceae	Fruit	Polyphenols (ellagic acid, gallic acid,), tannins
10.	Fennel *(Foeniculum vulgare) f*-Umbelliferae	Fruit	Volatile oil, fenchone, anethole, limonene, anisaldehyde, estragole
11.	Licorice (*Glycyrrhiza glabra) f*-Fabaceae	Root	Glycyrrhizin, flavonoids
12.	Mango *(Mangifera indica) f-Anacardiaceae*	Fruit	polyphenols, vitamin A and C, quercetin, ellagic acid, gallic acid
13.	Nightshade *(Solanum nigrum) f*-Solanaceae	Fruit	Polyphenolic compounds, flavonoids
14.	Male fern *(Dryopteris. filix-mas) f*-Dryopteridaceae	Root/ Rhizome	Phenolic acids, Aspidinol, Filicinic acid
15.	Bayberry *(Myrica nagi thumb) f*-Myricaceae	Bark	Flavonoid, phenolic
16.	Arjun *(Terminalia arjuna) f*-Combretaceae	Bark	Phenols, flavonoids
17.	Monkhood *(Aconitum heterophyllum) f*-Ranunculaceae	Root	Phenolic, saponins
18.	Belleric myrobalan *(Terminalia bellirica) f*-Combretaceae	Fruit	Phenolics, tannin
19.	Rose *(Rosa damascene) f*-Rosaceae	Flower	Flavonoid, phenols

(continued)

Table 3.4 (continued)

S. no	Medicinal plant	Part used	Chemical constituent responsible for antioxidant activity
20.	Black myrobalan *(Terminalia chebula) f*-Combretaceae	Fruit	Flavonoid, phenols
21.	Black plum *(Eugenia jambolana) f*-Myrtaceae	Fruit	Phenolics, flavonoids, saponins
22.	Oak *(Quercus infectoria) f*-Fagaceae	Fruit	Flavonoids, phenols
23.	Pomegranate *(Punica granatum) f*-Lythraceae	Peel	Flavonoid, phenol
24.	White Rhapontic *(Centaurea behen) f*-Compositae	Root	Phenols, flavonoid

formulation with the help of reverse pharmacology to combat the challenging disorders which may not only be promising against various noncommunicable disorders (NCD) but ultimately it will escape the huge amount, very prolonged duration, and tedious process of drug discovery and development. Nowadays, the Antioxidants synthesized from natural sources like from food and medicated herbs have been investigated for their benefits in health and nutritional values in reference to medicinal uses mentioned in Unani and other classical literature, e.g., Al Hawi by Zakariya Razi (Rhazes), Ilaj al Amraz by Hakeem Shareef Khan and many more. The plant-derived medicines are a good source of phytoconstituents to combat cancer, but only limited aspects have been investigated so far. Hence, the screening and isolation of active constituents having no or less side effects should be a major task to combat cancer.

There is a need for identification and extraction of more phytochemicals having antioxidant properties from medicinal plants. Further to investigate their pharmacological functions with the mechanism of actions of these phytochemicals must be investigated for their safety studies, adverse or side effects to make safe and effective use of them (Table 3.4).

References

1. Valadez-Vega C, Delgado-Olivares L, González JA, García EA, Ibarra JR, Moreno ER, Gutiérrez MS, Martínez MT, Clara ZP, Ramos ZC. The role of natural antioxidants in cancer disease. In: Oxidative stress and chronic degenerative diseases-a role for antioxidants. IntechOpen: London; 2013.
2. Shahidi F, Zhong Y. Novel antioxidants in food quality preservation and health promotion. Eur J Lipid Sci Technol. 2010;112(9):930–40.
3. Embuscado ME. Spices and herbs: natural sources of antioxidants–a mini review. J Funct Foods. 2015;1(18):811–9.

4. Ramalakshmi K, Kubra IR, Rao LJ. Antioxidant potential of low-grade coffee beans. Food Res Int. 2008;141(1):96–103.
5. Asif M. Chemistry and antioxidant activity of plants containing some phenolic compounds. Chem Int. 2015;1(1):35–52.
6. Maxmen A. The hard facts: breast cancer. Nature (London). 2012;485(7400).
7. Ferlay J, Ervik M, Lam F, Colombet M, Mery L, Piñeros M, et al. Global cancer observatory: cancer today. International Agency for Research on Cancer: Lyon; 2020. https://gco.iarc.fr/today, accessed February 2021
8. Brown NS, Bicknell R. Hypoxia and oxidative stress in breast cancer Oxidative stress-its effects on the growth, metastatic potential and response to therapy of breast cancer. Breast Cancer Res. 2001;3(5):1–5.
9. Halliwell B. Oxidative stress and cancer: have we moved forward? Biochem J. 2007;401 (1):1–1.
10. Noda N, Wakasugi H. Cancer and oxidative stress. J Jpn Med Assoc. 2000;124(11):1571–4. 1356-8650
11. Halliwell BA, Gutteridge JM, Cross CE. Free radicals, antioxidants, and human disease: where are we now? J Lab Clin Med. 1992;119(6):598–620.
12. Halliwell B, Gutteridge JM. The antioxidants of human extracellular fluids. Arch Biochem Biophys. 1990;280(1):1–8.
13. Hekimi S, Lapointe J, Wen Y. Taking a "good" look at free radicals in the aging process. Trends Cell Biol. 2011;21(10):569–76.
14. Khlebnikov AI, Schepetkin IA, Domina NG, Kirpotina LN, Quinn MT. Improved quantitative structure–activity relationship models to predict antioxidant activity of flavonoids in chemical, enzymatic, and cellular systems. Bioorg Med Chem. 2007;15(4):1749–70.
15. Halliwell B. Antioxidants in Human Health and Disease. Annu Rev. 1996;16:1550–8382. 33-50
16. Halliwell B. The antioxidant paradox. Lancet. 2000;1:1179–80.
17. Halliwell B. Free radicals in biochemistry and medicine. Rev Cell Biol Mol Med. 2006;
18. Warburg O. On the origin of cancer cells. Science. 1956;123(3191):309–14.
19. Valadez-Vega C, Delgado-Olivares L, González JA, García EA, Ibarra JR, Moreno ER, Gutiérrez MS, Martínez MT, Clara ZP, Ramos ZC. The role of natural antioxidants in cancer disease. In: Oxidative stress and chronic degenerative diseases-a role for antioxidants. London: IntechOpen. p. 2013.
20. Mut-Salud N, Álvarez PJ, Garrido JM, Carrasco E, Aránega A, Rodríguez-Serrano F. Antioxidant intake and antitumor therapy: toward nutritional recommendations for optimal results. Oxid Med Cell Longev. 2016;1:2016.
21. Shetti A, Keluskar V, Aggarwal A. Antioxidants: Enhancing oral and general health. J Indian Acad Oral Med Radiol. 2009;21(1):1.
22. Irshad M, Chaudhuri PS. Oxidant-antioxidant system: role and significance in human body
23. Sindhi V, Gupta V, Sharma K, Bhatnagar S, Kumari R, Dhaka N. Potential applications of antioxidants–A review. J Pharm Res. 2013;7(9):828–35.
24. Ibn Rushd. Kitabul Kulliyat (Urdu translation). New Delhi: CCRUM; 1987.
25. Ibrahim AS. Kitab al-Fath fi al-Tadawi (Urdu Translation by Hakeem Abdul Bari). New Delhi: CCRUM; 2007.
26. Abbas ZK, Saggu S, Sakeran MI, Zidan N, Rehman H, Ansari AA. Phytochemical, antioxidant and mineral composition of hydroalcoholic extract of chicory (Cichorium intybus L.) leaves. Saudi J Biol Sci. 2015;22(3):322–6.
27. Yamada T, Hayasaka S, Shibata Y, Ojima T, Saegusa T, Gotoh T, Ishikawa S, Nakamura Y, Kayaba K. Jichi Medical School cohort study group. Frequency of citrus fruit intake is associated with the incidence of cardiovascular disease: the Jichi Medical School cohort study. J Epidemiol. 2011;21(3):169–75. https://doi.org/10.2188/jea.je20100084.

28. Mursu J, Virtanen JK, Tuomainen TP, Nurmi T, Voutilainen S. Intake of fruit, berries, and vegetables and risk of type 2 diabetes in Finnish men: the Kuopio Ischaemic Heart Disease Risk Factor Study. Am J Clin Nutr. 2014;99(2):328–33.
29. Kruk J. Association between vegetable, fruit and carbohydrate intake and breast cancer risk in relation to physical activity. Asian Pac J Cancer Prev. 2014;15(11):4429–36.
30. Kyrø C, Skeie G, Loft S, Landberg R, Christensen J, Lund E, Nilsson LM, Palmqvist R, Tjønneland A, Olsen A. Intake of whole grains from different cereal and food sources and incidence of colorectal cancer in the Scandinavian HELGA cohort. Cancer Causes Control. 2013;24(7):1363–74.
31. Barbosa AP, Silveira GD, de Menezes IA, Rezende Neto JM, Bitencurt JL, Estavam CD, de Lima AD, Thomazzi SM, Guimaraes AG, Quintans-Junior LJ, dos Santos MR. Antidiabetic effect of the Chrysobalanus icaco L. aqueous extract in rats. J Med Food. 2013;16(6):538–43.
32. Zhang YJ, Gan RY, Li S, Zhou Y, Li AN, Xu DP, Li HB. Review antioxidant phytochemical for the prevention and treatment of chronic disease. MDPI. 2015;20:21138–56.
33. Alok S, Jain SK, Verma A, Kumar M, Mahor A, Sabharwal M. Herbal antioxidant in clinical practice: a review. Asian Pac J Trop Biomed. 2014;4(1):78–84.
34. Kumar M, Kumar S, Kaur S. Role of ROS and COX-2/iNOS inhibition in cancer chemoprevention: a review. Phytochem Rev. 2012;11(2-3):309–37.
35. Xie Q, Bai Q, Zou LY, Zhang QY, Zhou Y, Chang H, Yi L, Zhu JD, Mi MT. Genistein inhibits DNA methylation and increases expression of tumor suppressor genes in human breast cancer cells. Genes Chromosomes Cancer. 2014;53(5):422–31.
36. Lee MT, Lin WC, Yu B, Lee TT. Antioxidant capacity of phytochemicals and their potential effects on oxidative status in animals—A review. Asian Australas J Anim Sci. 2017;30(3):299.
37. Kieliszek M. Selenium–fascinating microelement, properties and sources in food. Molecules. 2019;24(7):1298.
38. Hossain A, Skalicky M, Brestic M, Maitra S, Sarkar S, Ahmad Z, Vemuri H, Garai S, Mondal M, Bhatt R, Kumar P. Selenium biofortification: roles, mechanisms, responses and prospects. Molecules. 2021;26(4):881.
39. Galan-Chilet I, Tellez-Plaza M, Guallar E, De Marco G, Lopez-Izquierdo R, Gonzalez-Manzano I, Tormos MC, Martin-Nuñez GM, Rojo-Martinez G, Saez GT, Martín-Escudero JC. Plasma selenium levels and oxidative stress biomarkers: a gene–environment interaction population-based study. Free Radic Biol Med. 2014;74:229–36.
40. Reich HJ, Hondal RJ. Why nature chose selenium. ACS Chem Biol. 2016;11(4):821–41.
41. Fordyce FM. Selenium deficiency and toxicity in the environment. In: Essentials of medical geology. Amsterdam: Elsevier; 2013. p. 375–416.
42. Longchamp M, Angeli N, Castrec-Rouelle M. Selenium uptake in Zea mays supplied with selenate or selenite under hydroponic conditions. Plant and Soil. 2013;362(1):107–17.
43. Khanam A, Platel K. Bioaccessibility of selenium, selenomethionine and selenocysteine from foods and influence of heat processing on the same. Food Chem. 2016;194:1293–9.
44. Steinbrenner H, Sies H. Selenium homeostasis and antioxidant selenoproteins in brain: implications for disorders in the central nervous system. Arch Biochem Biophys. 2013;536 (2):152–7.
45. Pillai R, Uyehara-Lock JH, Bellinger FP. Selenium and selenoprotein function in brain disorders. IUBMB Life. 2014;66(4):229–39.
46. Hsueh YM, Su CT, Shiue HS, Chen WJ, Pu YS, Lin YC, Tsai CS, Huang CY. Levels of plasma selenium and urinary total arsenic interact to affect the risk for prostate cancer. Food Chem Toxicol. 2017;107:167–75.
47. Lyons MP, Papazyan TT, Surai PF. Selenium in food chain and animal nutrition: lessons from nature-review. Asian Australas J Anim Sci. 2007;20(7):1135–55.
48. Dennert G, Horneber M. Selenium for alleviating the side effects of chemotherapy, radiotherapy and surgery in cancer patients. Cochrane Database Syst Rev. 2006;3
49. Lippman SM, Klein EA, Goodman PJ, Lucia MS, Thompson IM, Ford LG, Parnes HL, Minasian LM, Gaziano JM, Hartline JA, Parsons JK. Effect of selenium and vitamin E on

risk of prostate cancer and other cancers: the Selenium and Vitamin E Cancer Prevention Trial (SELECT). JAMA. 2009;301(1):39–51.
50. Klein EA, Thompson IM, Tangen CM, Crowley JJ, Lucia MS, Goodman PJ, Minasian LM, Ford LG, Parnes HL, Gaziano JM, Karp DD. Vitamin E and the risk of prostate cancer: the Selenium and Vitamin E Cancer Prevention Trial (SELECT). JAMA. 2011;306(14):1549–56.
51. Combs GF, Lü J. Selenium as a cancer preventive agent. In: Hatfield DL, Berry MJ, Gladyshev VN, editors. Selenium. Berlin: Springer; 2006.
52. Rayman MP. The argument for increasing selenium intake. Proc Nutr Soc. 2002;61 (2):203–15.
53. Ramoutar RR, Brumaghim JL. Effects of inorganic selenium compounds on oxidative DNA damage. J Inorg Biochem. 2007;101(7):1028–35.
54. Battin EE, Perron NR, Brumaghim JL. The central role of metal coordination in selenium antioxidant activity. Inorg Chem. 2006;45(2):499–501.
55. Battin EE, Zimmerman MT, Ramoutar RR, Quarles CE, Brumaghim JL. Preventing metal-mediated oxidative DNA damage with selenium compounds. Metallomics. 2011;3(5):503–12.
56. Ramoutar R. Understanding the antioxidant mechanism of inorganic selenium, oxo-sulfur, and polyphenol compounds, and the biological implications of functionalized nanoparticles.
57. Guo J, He L, Li T, Yin J, Yin Y, Guan G. Antioxidant and anti-inflammatory effects of different zinc sources on diquat-induced oxidant stress in a piglet model. Biomed Res Int. 2020;21:2020.
58. Skalny AV, Rink L, Ajsuvakova OP, Aschner M, Gritsenko VA, Alekseenko SI, Svistunov AA, Petrakis D, Spandidos DA, Aaseth J, Tsatsakis A. Zinc and respiratory tract infections: Perspectives for COVID-19. Int J Mol Med. 2020;46(1):17–26.
59. Prasad AS. Zinc is an antioxidant and anti-inflammatory agent: its role in human health. Front Nutr. 2014;1:14.
60. Prasad AS. Lessons learned from experimental human model of zinc deficiency. J Immunol Res. 2020:1–12.
61. De la Vieja A, Santisteban P. Role of iodide metabolism in physiology and cancer. Endocr Relat Cancer. 2018;25(4):R225–45.
62. Aceves C, Mendieta I, Anguiano B, Delgado-González E. Molecular iodine has extrathyroidal effects as an antioxidant, differentiator, and immunomodulator. Int J Mol Sci. 2021;22(3):122.
63. Venturi S. Evolutionary significance of iodine. Curr Chem Biol. 2011;5:155–62.
64. Cann SA, Van Netten JP, van Netten C. Hypothesis: iodine, selenium and the development of breast cancer. Cancer Causes Control. 2000;11(2):121–7.
65. Smyth PP. Role of iodine in antioxidant defence in thyroid and breast disease. Biofactors. 2003;19(3-4):121–30.
66. Venturi S, Venturi M. Iodine in evolution of salivary glands and in oral health. Nutr Health. 2009;20(2):119–34.
67. Aceves C, Anguiano B, Delgado G. The extrathyronine actions of iodine as antioxidant, apoptotic, and differentiation factor in various tissues. Thyroid. 2013;23(8):938–46.
68. Juvenal JG, Thomasz L, Oglio R, Perona M, Pisarev AM, Rossich L, Salvarredi L. Thyroid: iodine beyond the thyronines. Curr Chem Biol. 2011;5(3):163–7.
69. Torremante PE, Rosner H. Antiproliferative effects of molecular iodine in cancers. Curr Chem Biol. 2011;5:168–76.
70. Bilal MY, Dambaeva S, Kwak-Kim J, Gilman-Sachs A, Beaman KD. A role for iodide and thyroglobulin in modulating the function of human immune cells. Front Immunol. 2017;8:1573.
71. Moore K, Thomas A, Harding KG. Iodine released from the wound dressing Iodosorb modulates the secretion of cytokines by human macrophages responding to bacterial lipopolysaccharide. Int J Biochem Cell Biol. 1997;29(1):163–71.
72. Kim SH, Lee JM, Kim SC, Park CB, Lee PC. Proposed cytotoxic mechanisms of the saffron carotenoids crocin and crocetin on cancer cell lines. Biochem Cell Biol. 2014;92(2):105–11.

73. Fiedor J, Burda K. Potential role of carotenoids as antioxidants in human health and disease. Nutrients. 2014;6(2):466–88.
74. Parker RS. Carotenoids in human blood and tissues. J Nutr. 1989;119(1):101–4.
75. Khachik F. Distribution and metabolism of dietary carotenoids in humans as a criterion for development of nutritional supplements. Pure Appl Chem. 2006;78(8):1551–7.
76. Beecher GR, Khachik F. Qualitative relationship of dietary and plasma carotenoids in human beings. Ann N Y Acad Sci. 1992;669(1):320–1.
77. Fiedor J, Fiedor L, Haeßner R, Scheer H. Cyclic endoperoxides of β-carotene, potential pro-oxidants, as products of chemical quenching of singlet oxygen. Biochim Biophys Acta. 2005;1709(1):1–4.
78. Edge R, Truscott TG. Properties of carotenoid radicals and excited states and their potential role in biological systems. Boca Raton, FL: CRC Press; 2010.
79. Cvetkovic D, Fiedor L, Fiedor J, Wiśniewska-Becker A, Markovic D. Molecular base for carotenoids antioxidant activity in model and biological systems: the health-related effects. In: Carotenoids: Food sources, production and health benefits. Hauppauge, NY: Nova Science Publisher; 2013. p. 93–126.
80. Johary A, Jain V, Misra S. Role of lycopene in the prevention of cancer. Int J Nutr Pharmacol Neurol Dis. 2012;2(3):167.
81. Milani A, Basirnejad M, Shahbazi S, Bolhassani A. Carotenoids: biochemistry, pharmacology and treatment. Br J Pharmacol. 2017;174(11):1290–324.
82. Tanaka T, Shnimizu M, Moriwaki H. Cancer chemoprevention by carotenoids. Molecules. 2012;17(3):3202–42.
83. Zare M, Norouzi Roshan Z, Assadpour E, Jafari SM. Improving the cancer prevention/ treatment role of carotenoids through various nano-delivery systems. Crit Rev Food Sci Nutr. 2021;61(3):522–34.
84. Gong X, Smith JR, Swanson HM, Rubin LP. Carotenoid lutein selectively inhibits breast cancer cell growth and potentiates the effect of chemotherapeutic agents through ROS-mediated mechanisms. Molecules. 2018;23(4):905.
85. Bekhechi C, Boti JB, Bekkara FA, Abdelouahid DE, Casanova J, Tomi F. Isothymol in Ajowan essential oil. Nat Prod Commun. 2010;5(7):1934578X1000500726.
86. Zarshenas MM, Moein M, Samani SM, Petramfar P. An overview on ajwain (Trachyspermum ammi) pharmacological effects; modern and traditional. J Nat Remedies. 2013;14(1):98–105.
87. Kamboj A, Saluja AK. Phytopharmacological review of Xanthium strumarium L.(Cocklebur). Int J Green Pharm. 2010;4(3).
88. Sharifi-Rad J, Hoseini-Alfatemi SM, Sharifi-Rad M, Sharifi-Rad M, Iriti M, Sharifi-Rad M, Sharifi-Rad R, Raeisi S. Phytochemical compositions and biological activities of essential oil from Xanthium strumarium L. Molecules. 2015;20(4):7034–47.
89. Mandala SC, Dharab AK, Kumara CKA, Maitic BC. Neuropharmacological activity of Xanthium strumarium Linn. extract. J Herbs Spices Med Plants. 2001;8:69–77.
90. Grossman S, Dovrat S, Gottlieb HE, Bergman M. Growth inhibitory activity of cucurbitacin glucosides isolated from Citrullus colocynthis on human breast cancer cells. Biochem Pharmacol. 2007;73(1):56–67.
91. Jayaraman R, Christina AJM. Evaluation of Citrullus colocynthis fruits on in vitro antioxidant activity and in vivo DEN/PB induced hepatotoxicity. Int J Appl Res Nat Prod. 2013;6(1):1–9.
92. Al-Snafi AE. Chemical constituents and pharmacological effects of Citrullus colocynthis-A review. IOSR Jf Pharm. 2016;6(3):57–67.
93. Zarei A, Changizi-Ashtiyani S, Taheri S, Ramezani M. A quick overview on some aspects of endocrinological and therapeutic effects of Berberis vulgaris L. Avicenna J Phytomed. 2015;5 (6):485.
94. Imenshahidi M, Hosseinzadeh H. Berberis vulgaris and berberine: an update review. Phytother Res. 2016;30(11):1745–64.
95. Rahimi-Madiseh M, Lorigoini Z, Zamani-Gharaghoshi H, Rafieian-Kopaei M. Berberis vulgaris: specifications and traditional uses. Iran J Basic Med Sci. 2017;20(5):569.

96. Moshiri M, Vahabzadeh M, Hosseinzadeh H. Clinical applications of saffron (Crocus sativus) and its constituents: a review. Drug Res. 2015;65(6):287–95.
97. Samarghandian S, Borji A. Anticarcinogenic effect of saffron (Crocus sativus L.) and its ingredients. Pharmacogn Res. 2014;6(2):99.
98. Patil DD, Mhaske DK, Wadhawa GC. Antibacterial and Antioxidant study of Ocimum basilicum Labiatae (sweet basil). J Adv Pharm Edu Res. 2011;2:104–12.
99. Marwat SK, Khan MS, Ghulam S, Anwar N, Mustafa G, Usman K. Phytochemical constituents and pharmacological activities of sweet Basil-Ocimum basilicum L.(Lamiaceae). Asian J Chem. 2011;23(9):3773.
100. da Silva Ramos R, Rodrigues AB, Farias AL, Simões RC, Pinheiro MT, Ferreira RM, Costa Barbosa LM, Picanço Souto RN, Fernandes JB, Santos LD, de Almeida SS. Chemical composition and in vitro antioxidant, cytotoxic, antimicrobial, and larvicidal activities of the essential oil of Mentha piperita L.(Lamiaceae). Sci World J. 2017; https://doi.org/10.1155/2017/4927214.
101. Pramila DM, Xavier R, Marimuthu K, Kathiresan S, Khoo ML, Senthilkumar M, Sathya K, Sreeramanan S. Phytochemical analysis and antimicrobial potential of methanolic leaf extract of peppermint (Mentha piperita: Lamiaceae). J Med Plant Res. 2012;6(2):331–5.
102. Seidavi AR, Laudadio V, Khazaei R, Puvača N, Selvaggi M, Tufarelli V. Feeding of black cumin (Nigella sativa L.) and its effects on poultry production and health. Worlds Poult Sci J. 2020;76(2):346–57.
103. Grauso L, de Falco B, Lanzotti V, Motti R. Stinging nettle, Urtica dioica L.: Botanical, phytochemical and pharmacological overview. Phytochem Rev. 2020:1–37.
104. Ahmed KM, Parsuraman S. Urtica dioica L (Urticaceae): a stinging nettle. Syst Rev Pharm. 2014;5(1):6.
105. Scherer R, Lemos MF, Lemos MF, Martinelli GC, Martins JD, da Silva AG. Antioxidant and antibacterial activities and composition of Brazilian spearmint (Mentha spicata L.). Ind Crop Prod. 2013;50:408–13.
106. Scherer R, Godoy HT. Antioxidant activity index (AAI) by 2,2-diphenyl-1- picrylhydrazyl method. Food Chem. 2009;112:654–8.
107. Bayan L, Koulivand PH, Gorji A. Garlic: a review of potential therapeutic effects. Avicenna J Phytomed. 2014;4(1):1.
108. Borkowska A, Knap N, Antosiewicz J. Diallyl trisulfide is more cytotoxic to prostate cancer cells PC-3 than to noncancerous epithelial cell line PNT1A: a possible role of p66Shc signaling axis. Nutr Cancer. 2013;65:711–7.
109. Capasso A. Antioxidant action and therapeutic efficacy of Allium sativum L. Molecules. 2013;18:690–700.
110. Kim SH, Choi KC. Anti-cancer effect and underlying mechanism(s) of kaempferol, a phytoestrogen, on the regulation of apoptosis in diverse cancer cell models. Toxic Res. 2013;29(4):229.
111. Kumar S, Pandey AK. Chemistry and biological activities of flavonoids: an overview. Sci World J. 2013;2013:162750.
112. Pareek S, Sagar NA, Sharma S, Kumar V. Onion (Allium cepa L.). Fruit Vegetable Phytochem Chem Human Health. 2017;2:1145–62.
113. Kim KH, Moon E, Kim SY, Choi SU, Lee JH, Lee KR. 4-Methylthio-butanyl derivatives from the seeds of Raphanus sativus and their biological evaluation on anti-inflammatory and antitumor activities. J Ethnopharmacol. 2014;151:503–8.
114. Banihani SA. Radish (Raphanus sativus) and diabetes. Nutrients. 2017;9(9):1014.
115. Amri E. The role of selected plant families with dietary Ethnomedicinal species used as anticancer. J Med Plants Stud. 2014;2(1):28–39.
116. Rahman M, Amina Khatun LL, Barkla BJ. Brassicaceae Mustards: Traditional and Agronomic Uses in Australia and New Zealand Mahmudur. Molecules. 2018;23:1–18.
117. Kidwai MK. Effect of Mancozeb on Mustard (Brassica juncea L.): an in-vitro study. Trop plant Res. 2017;4(1):55–61.

118. Pasko P, Zagrodzki P, Barton H, Chlopicka J, Gorinstein S. Effect of quinoa seeds (Chenopodium quinoa) in diet on some biochemical parameters and essential elements in blood of high fructose-fed rats. Plant Foods Hum Nutr. 2010a;65(4):333e338.
119. Pasko P, Barton H, Zagrodzki P, Izewska A, Krosniak M, Gawlik M, Gawlik M. Effect of diet supplemented with quinoa seeds on oxidative status in plasma and selected tissues of high fructose-fed rats. Plant Foods Hum Nutr. 2010;65(2):146e151.
120. Yao Y, Yang X, Shi Z, Ren G. Anti-inflammatory activity of saponins from quinoa (Chenopodium quinoa Willd.) seeds in lipopolysaccharide-stimulated RAW 264.7 macrophage cells. J Food Sci. 2014;79(5):H1018eH1023.
121. Bhadra P. An Overview of Ajwain (Trachyspermum ammi); 2020.
122. Sahoo JP, Behera L, Praveena J, Sawant S, Mishra A, Sharma SS, Ghosh L, Mishra AP, Sahoo AR, Pradhan P, Sahu S. The golden spice turmeric (Curcuma longa) and its feasible benefits in prospering human health—a review. Am J Plant Sci. 2021;12(03):455.
123. Süleyman K, Nesrin H, Veysel T, Ersin K, Uyan Y. Mineral content, essential oil components and biological activity of two mentha species (M. piperita L., M. spicata L). Turkish J Field Crops. 2010;15(2):148–53.
124. Srinivasan K. Cumin (Cuminum cyminum) and black cumin (Nigella sativa) seeds: traditional uses, chemical constituents, and nutraceutical effects. J Cereal Sci. 2018;2*(1):1–16.*
125. Navruz-Varli S, Sanlier N. Nutritional and health benefits of quinoa (Chenopodium quinoa Willd.). J Cereal Sci. 2016;1(69):371–6.
126. Shahrajabian MH, Sun W, Cheng Q. Chemical components and pharmacological benefits of Basil (Ocimum Basilicum): a review. Int J Food Prop. 2020;23(1):1961–70.
127. Mzabri I, Addi M, Berrichi A. Traditional and modern uses of saffron (Crocus sativus). Cosmetics. 2019;6(4):63.
128. Jesus F, Gonçalves AC, Alves G, Silva LR. Health benefits of Prunus avium plant parts: an unexplored source rich in phenolic compounds. Food Rev Intl. 2020;12:1–29.
129. Varvara M, Bozzo G, Celano G, Disanto C, Pagliarone CN, Celano GV. The use of ascorbic acid as a food additive: technical-legal issues. Ital J Food Saf. 2016;5(1):4313.
130. Carr AC, Rowe S. Factors affecting vitamin C status and prevalence of deficiency: a global health perspective. Nutrients. 2020;12(7):1963.
131. Jarosz M, Rychlik E, Stoś K, Wierzejska R, Wojtasik A, Charzewska J, Mojska H, Szponar L, Sajór I, Kłosiewicz-Latoszek L, Chwojnowska Z. Normy żywienia dla populacji Polski. Instytut Żywności i Żywienia; 2017.
132. Kaźmierczak-Barańska J, Boguszewska K, Adamus-Grabicka A, Karwowski BT. Two faces of vitamin C—antioxidative and pro-oxidative agent. Nutrients. 2020;12(5):1501.
133. Szarka A, Kapuy O, Lőrincz T, Bánhegyi G. Vitamin C and cell death. Antioxid Redox Signal. 2021;34(11):831–44.
134. Tóth SZ, Lőrincz T, Szarka A. Concentration does matter: the beneficial and potentially harmful effects of ascorbate in humans and plants. Antioxid Redox Signal. 2018;29 (15):1516–33.
135. Csala M, Szarka A, Margittai É, Mile V, Kardon T, Braun L, Mandl J, Bánhegyi G. Role of vitamin E in ascorbate-dependent protein thiol oxidation in rat liver endoplasmic reticulum. Arch Biochem Biophys. 2001;388(1):55–9.
136. Szarka A, Bánhegyi G, Asard H. The inter-relationship of ascorbate transport, metabolism and mitochondrial, plastidic respiration. Antioxid Redox Signal. 2013;19(9):1036–44.
137. Khallouki F, Owen RW, Akdad M, El Bouhali B, Silvente-Poirot S, Poirot M. Vitamin E: an overview. Mol Nutr. 2020:51–66.
138. Torquato P, Marinelli R, Bartolini D, Galli F. Vitamin E: nutritional aspects. In: Molecular nutrition; 2020. pp. 447-485.
139. Niki E. Role of vitamin E as a lipid-soluble peroxyl radical scavenger: in vitro and in vivo evidence. Free Radic Biol Med. 2014;66:3–12.
140. Jiang Q. Natural forms of vitamin E: metabolism, antioxidant, and anti-inflammatory activities and their role in disease prevention and therapy. Free Radic Biol Med. 2014;72:76–90.

141. Peh HY, Tan WD, Liao W, Wong WF. Vitamin E therapy beyond cancer: Tocopherol versus tocotrienol. Pharmacol Ther. 2016;162:152–69.
142. Poirot M, Silvente-Poirot S. Cholesterol-5, 6-epoxides: chemistry, biochemistry, metabolic fate and cancer. Biochimie. 2013;95(3):622–31.
143. Krishnaveni M, Mirunalini S. Chemopreventive efficacy of Phyllanthus emblica L.(amla) fruit extract on 7, 12-dimethylbenz (a) anthracene induced oral carcinogenesis–A dose–response study. Environ Toxicol Pharmacol. 2012;34(3):801–10.
144. Gaire BP, Subedi L. Phytochemistry, pharmacology and medicinal properties of Phyllanthus emblica Linn. Chin J Integr Med. 2014;9:1–8.
145. Pientaweeratch S, Panapisal V, Tansirikongkol A. Antioxidant, anti-collagenase and anti-elastase activities of Phyllanthus emblica, Manilkara zapota and silymarin: An in vitro comparative study for anti-aging applications. Pharm Biol. 2016;54(9):1865–72.
146. Srivastava R, Jyoti B, Pathak S, Wazir SS, Shukla A, Sajid Z. Aloe vera: The herbal magic wand. J Clin Den Res Edu. 2014;3
147. Sharrif Moghaddasi M, Res M. Aloe vera their chemicals composition and applications: A review. Int J Biol Med Res. 2011;2(1):466–71.
148. Joseph B, Raj SJ. Pharmacognostic and phytochemical properties of Aloe vera linn an overview. Int J Pharm Sci Rev Res. 2010;4(2):106.
149. Akbar S. Lactuca sativa L.(Asteraceae/Compositae). In: Handbook of 200 medicinal plants. Cham: Springer; 2020. p. 1067–75.
150. Noumedem JA, Djeussi DE, Hritcu L, Mihasan M, Kuete V. Lactuca sativa. In: Medicinal spices and vegetables from Africa. Cambridge, MA: Academic Press. 2017. pp. 437-449
151. Moharib SA, Maksoud NAE, Ragab HM, Mahmoud Shehata M. Anticancer activities of mushroom polysaccharides on chemically-induced colorectal cancer in rats. J Appl Pharm Sci. 2014;4(7):054–63.
152. Lepage C, Leger DY, Bertrand Y, Martin F, Beneytout JL, Liagre B. Diosgenin induces deathreceptor-5 through activation of p38 pathway and promotes TRAIL-induced apoptosis in colon cancer cells. Cancer Lett. 2011;301(2):193–202.
153. Agarwal M, Agarwal M, Jain SC. In vitro regulation of bioactive compounds in Trigonella species by mutagenic treatments. J Plant Sci. 2015;3:40–4.
154. Chaudhary S, Chaudhary PS, Chikara SK, Sharma MC, Iriti M. Review on Fenugreek (Trigonella foenum-graecum L.) and its important secondary metabolite diosgenin. Notulae Botanicae Horti Agrobotanici Cluj-Napoca. 2018;46(1):22–31.
155. De Sarker D, Saha MR, Saha S. Perspective of dietetic and antioxidant medicinal plants. Chennai: Notion Press; 2015.
156. Malla KJ, Kunwar RM, Jan HA, Bussmann RW, Paniagua-Zambrana NY. Boerhavia diffusa L. N yctaginaceae Ethnobotany of the Himalayas. 2020:1–6.
157. Apu AS, Liza MS, Jamaluddin AT, Howlader MA, Saha RK, Rizwan F, Nasrin N. Phytochemical screening and in vitro bioactivities of the extracts of aerial part of Boerhavia diffusa Linn. Asian Pac J Trop Biomed. 2012;2(9):673–82.
158. Murti K, Panchal MA, Lambole V. Pharmacological properties of Boerhaavia diffusa-a review. Int J Pharm Sci Rev Res. 2010;5(2):107–10.
159. Devanathan K. Abrus precatorius L. Fabaceae. Ethnobotany of the Mountain Regions of Southeast Asia; 2020. pp. 1-1.
160. Riaz G, Chopra R. A review on phytochemistry and therapeutic uses of Hibiscus sabdariffa L. Biomed Pharmacother. 2018;102:575–86.
161. Mossalam HH, Aty OAAE, Morgan EN, Youssaf SMS, Mackawy AMH. Biochemical and ultra structure studies of the antioxidant effect of aqueous extract of Hibiscus sabdariffa on the Nephrotoxicity Induced by organophosphorous pesticide (Malathion) on the adult albino rats. Life Sci J. 2011;8(5):561–74.
162. Lin HH, Chan KC, Sheu JY, Hsuan SW, Wang CJ, Cheng JH. Hibiscus sabdariffa leaf induces apoptosis of human prostate cancer cells in vitro and in vivo. Food Chem. 2012;132 (2):880–91.

163. Okhale SE, EM N. Abrus precatorius Linn (Fabaceae): phytochemistry, ethnomedicinal uses, ethnopharmacology and pharmacological activities. Int J Pharm Sci Res. 2016;1:37–43.
164. Sudhakar P, Thenmozhi V, Srivignesh S, Dhanalakshmi M. Colocasia esculenta (L.) Schott: Pharmacognostic and pharmacological review. J Pharmacogn Phytochem. 2020;9(4):1382–6.
165. Ranju Pal S, Ariharasivakumar G, Girhepunje K, Upadhyay A. In-vitro antioxidative activity of phenolic and flavonoid compounds extracted from seeds of Abrus Precatorius. Int J Pharm Pharm Sci. 2009;1(2):136–40.
166. Kundu N, Campbell P, Hampton B, Lin CY, Ma X, Ambulos N, et al. Antimetastatic activity isolated from Colocasia esculenta (taro). Anticancer Drugs. 2012;23(2):200–11.
167. Yadav M, Kushawaha DK, Chatterji S, Watal G. Assessment of antioxidant activity and phytochemical screening of Colocasia esculenta corm. Int J Pharm Sci Res. 2017;8 (4):1758–64.
168. Labban L. Medicinal and pharmacological properties of Turmeric (Curcuma longa): A review. Int J Pharm Biomed Sci. 2014;5(1):17–23.
169. Verma RK, Kumari P, Maurya RK, Kumar V, Verma RB, Singh RK. Medicinal properties of turmeric (Curcuma longa L.): a review. Int J Chem Stud. 2018;6(4):1354–7.
170. Barrajón-Catalán E, Fernández-Arroyo S, Saura D, Guillén E, Fernández-Gutiérrez A, Segura-Carretero A, Micol V. Cistaceae aqueous extracts containing ellagitannins show antioxidant and antimicrobial capacity, and cytotoxic activity against human cancer cells. Food Chem Toxicol. 2010;1:48.
171. Cordero-Herrera I, Martín MA, Bravo L, Goya L, Ramos S. Epicatechin gallate induces cell death via p53 activation and stimulation of p38 and JNK in human colon cancer SW480 cells. Nutr Cancer. 2013;65(5):718–28.
172. Granato D, Shahidi F, Wrolstad R, Kilmartin P, Melton LD, Hidalgo FJ, Miyashita K, van Camp J, Alasalvar C, Ismail AB, Elmore S. Antioxidant activity, total phenolics and flavonoids contents: Should we ban in vitro screening methods? Food Chem. 2018;264:471–5.
173. Del Rio D, Rodriguez-Mateos A, Spencer JP, Tognolini M, Borges G, Crozier A. Dietary (poly) phenolics in human health: structures, bioavailability, and evidence of protective effects against chronic diseases. Antioxid Redox Signal. 2013;18(14):1818–92.
174. Heleno SA, Martins A, Queiroz MJRP, Ferreira ICFR. Bioactivity of phenolic acids: metabolites versus parent compounds: a review. Food Chem. 2015;173:501–13.
175. Williamson G. The role of polyphenols in modern nutrition. Nutr Bull. 2017;42(3):226–35.
176. Rice-Evans CA, Miller NJ, Paganga G. Structure-Antioxidant activity relationships of flavonoids and pHenolic acids. Free Radic Biol Med. 1996;20:933–56.
177. Vuolo MM, Lima VS, Roberto M, Junior M. Phenolic compounds: structure, classification, and antioxidant power [Internet]. Bioactive Compounds.
178. Birt DF, Jeffery E. Flavonoids. Adv Nutr. 2013;4:576–7.
179. Huang WY, Cai YZ, Zhang Y. Natural phenolic compounds from medicinal herbs and dietary plants: potential use for cancer prevention. Nutr Cancer. 2009;62(1):1–20.
180. Xu D, Hu MJ, Wang YQ, Cui YL. Antioxidant activities of quercetin and its complexes for medicinal application. Molecules. 2019;24(6):1123.
181. Bubolsa GB, Viannac DR, Medina-Remónd A, Poserb GV, Lamuela-Raventosd RM, Eifler-Limab VL, Garcia SC. The antioxidant activity of coumarins and flavonoids. Mini-Rev Med Chem. 2013;13:318–34.
182. Boots AW, Haenen GR, Bast A. Health effects of quercetin: from antioxidant to nutraceutical. Eur J Pharmacol. 2008;585(2-3):325–37.
183. Nichols JA, Katiyar SK. Skin photoprotection by natural polyphenols: anti-inflammatory, antioxidant and DNA repair mechanisms. Arch Dermatol Res. 2010;302(2):71–83.
184. Li Y, Zhang T. Targeting cancer stem cells by curcumin and clinical applications. Cancer Lett. 2014;346(2):197–205.
185. Manikandan R, Beulaja M, Arulvasu C, Sellamuthu S, Dinesh D, Prabhu D, Babu G, Vaseeharan B, Prabhu NM. Synergistic anticancer activity of curcumin and catechin: An in vitro study using human cancer cell lines. Microsc Res Tech. 2012;75(2):112–6.

186. Ferrer JL, Austin MB, Stewart C, Noel JP. Structure and function of enzymes involved in the biosynthesis of phenylpropanoids. Plant Physiol Biochem. 2008;46:356–70.
187. Haslam E. Plant polyphenols: vegetable tannins revisited. CUP Archive; 1989.
188. Afzal S, Ahmad HI, Jabbar A, Tolba MM, AbouZid S, Irm N, Zulfiqar F, Iqbal MZ, Ahmad S, Aslam Z. Use of medicinal plants for respiratory diseases in Bahawalpur, Pakistan. BioMed Res Int. 2021;2021:5578914.
189. Sundaram R, Mitra SK. Antioxidant activity of ethyl acetate soluble fraction of Acacia arabica bark in rats. Indian J Pharm. 2007;39(1):33.
190. Rajvaidhya S, Nagori BP, Singh GK, Dubey BK, Desai P, Jain S. A review on Acacia Arabica-an Indian medicinal plant. Int J Pharm Sci Res. 2012;3(7):1995.
191. Baliga MS, Bhat HP, Baliga BR, Wilson R, Palatty PL. Phytochemistry, traditional uses and pharmacology of Eugenia jambolana Lam.(black plum): a review. Food Res Int. 2011;44 (7):1776–89.
192. Goyal PK, Verma P, Sharma P, Parmar J, Agarwal A. Evaluation of anticancer and anti-oxidative potential of Syzygium cumini against benzo[a]pyrene (BaP) induced gastric carcinogenesis in mice. Asian Pac J Cancer Prev. 2010;11:753–8.
193. Baliga MS. Anticancer, chemopreventive and radioprotective potential of black plum (Eugenia jambolana lam.). Asian Pac J Cancer Prev. 2011;12(1):3–15.
194. Jain S, Yadav PP, Gill V, Vasudeva N, Singla N. Terminalia arjuna a sacred medicinal plant: phytochemical and pharmacological profile. Phytochem Rev. 2009;8(2):491–502.
195. Amalraj A, Gopi S. Medicinal properties of Terminalia arjuna (Roxb.) Wight & Arn.: a review. J Tradit Complement Med. 2017;7(1):65–78.
196. Moulisha B, Kumar GA, Kanti HP. Anti-leishmanial and anti-cancer activities of a pentacyclic triterpenoid isolated from the leaves of Terminalia arjuna Combretaceae. Trop J Pharm Res. 2010;9(2).
197. Ardekani MR, Hajimahmoodi M, Oveisi MR, Sadeghi N, Jannat B, Ranjbar AM, Gholam N, Moridi T. Comparative antioxidant activity and total flavonoid content of Persian pomegranate (Punica granatum L.) cultivars. Iran J Pharm Res. 2011;10(3):519.
198. Kumari A, Dora J, Kumar A, Kumar A. Pomegranate (Punica granatum)—overview. Int J Pharm Chem Sci. 2012;1:1218–22.
199. Miguel MG, Neves MA, Antunes MD. Pomegranate (Punica granatum L.): A medicinal plant with myriad biological properties-A short review. J Med Plant Res. 2010;4(25):2836–47.
200. Kang NJ, Shin SH, Lee HJ, Lee KW. Polyphenols as small molecular inhibitors of signaling cascades in carcinogenesis. Pharmacol Ther. 2011;130(3):310–24.
201. Sporn MB. Perspectivesin cancer research carcinogenesis and cancer: different perspectives on the same disease1. Cancer Res. 1991;51:6215–8.
202. Gao S, Hu M. Bioavailability challenges associated with development of anti-cancer phenolics. Mini Rev Med Chem. 2010;10(6):550–67.
203. Visioli F, Lastra CA, Andres-Lacueva C, Aviram M, Calhau C, Cassano A, D'Archivio M, Faria A, Favé G, Fogliano V, Llorach R. Polyphenols and human health: a prospectus. Crit Rev Food Sci Nutr. 2011;51(6):524–46.
204. Sirerol JA, María LR, Mena S, Asensi MA, Estrela JM, Angel L. Ortega. Role of natural stillbenes in the prevention of cancer. Oxid Med Cell Longev. 2016;3128951:2016.
205. Cai YZ, Sun M, Xing J, Luo Q, Corke H. Structure–radical scavenging activity relationships of phenolic compounds from traditional Chinese medicinal plants. Life Sci. 2006;78 (25):2872–88.
206. Surveswaran S, Cai YZ, Corke H, Sun M. Systematic evaluation of natural phenolic antioxidants from 133 Indian medicinal plants. Food Chem. 2007;102(3):938–53.
207. De Fátima ND, De Souza MM, Neto RA, Golin V, Niero R, Yunes RA, Delle Monache F, Cechinel FV. Phytochemical analysis and analgesic properties of Curcuma zedoaria grown in Brazil. Phytomedicine. 2002;9(5):427–32.
208. Masuda T. Anti-inflammatory Antioxidants from Tropical Zingiberaceae plants: isolation and synthesis of new curcuminoids.

209. Guerrero S, Inostroza-Riquelme M, Contreras-Orellana P, Diaz-Garcia V, Lara P, Vivanco-Palma A, Cárdenas A, Miranda V, Robert P, Leyton L, Kogan MJ. Curcumin-loaded nanoemulsion: a new safe and effective formulation to prevent tumor reincidence and metastasis. Nanoscale. 2018;10(47):22612–22.
210. Zorofchian Moghadamtousi S, Abdul Kadir H, Hassandarvish P, Tajik H, Abubakar S, Zandi K. A review on antibacterial, antiviral, and antifungal activity of curcumin. Biomed Res Int. 2014;2014:186864.
211. Fritsche S, Wang X, Jung C. Recent advances in our understanding of tocopherol biosynthesis in plants: an overview of key genes, functions, and breeding of vitamin E improved crops. Antioxidants. 2017;6(4):99.
212. Llano S, Gómez S, Londoño J, Restrepo A. Antioxidant activity of curcuminoids. Phys Chem Chem Phys. 2019;21(7):3752–60.
213. Menon VP, Sudheer AR. Antioxidant and anti-inflammatory properties of curcumin. Adv Exp Med Biol. 2007;595:105–25.
214. Yousef JM, Saddiq AA. Some microbiological, biochemical and histological investigations on pendant coumarin thiocarbohydrazone and its Cobalt (II) complex in rats. Int J Microbiol Res. 2010;1:1–13.
215. Al-Amiery AA, Al-Majedy YK, Kadhum AA, Mohamad AB. Novel macromolecules derived from coumarin: synthesis and antioxidant activity. Sci Rep. 2015;5(1):1–7.
216. Egan D, O'kennedy R, Moran E, Cox D, Prosser E, Thornes RD. The pharmacology, metabolism, analysis, and applications of coumarin and coumarin-related compounds. Drug Metab Rev. 1990;22(5):503–29.
217. Završnik D, Muratović S, Makuc D, Plavec J, Cetina M, Nagl A, Clercq ED, Balzarini J, Mintas M. Benzylidene-bis-(4-hydroxycoumarin) and benzopyrano-coumarin derivatives: synthesis, 1H/13C-NMR conformational and X-ray crystal structure studies and in vitro antiviral activity evaluations. Molecules. 2011;16(7):6023–40.
218. Nasr T, Bondock S, Youns M. Anticancer activity of new coumarin substituted hydrazide–hydrazone derivatives. Eur J Med Chem. 2014;76:539–48.
219. Kostova I. Studying plant derived coumarins for their pharmacological and therapeutic properties as potential anticancer drugs. Expert Opin Drug Discovery. 2007;2(12):1605–18.
220. Goel A, Prasad AK, Parmar VS, Ghosh B, Saini N. Apoptogenic effect of 7, 8-diacetoxy-4-methylcoumarin and 7, 8-diacetoxy-4-methylthiocoumarin in human lung adenocarcinoma cell line: Role of NF-κB, Akt, ROS and MAP kinase pathway. Chem Biol Interact. 2009;179 (2-3):363–74.
221. Tanaka T, Sugiura H, Inaba R, Nishikawa A, Murakami A, Koshimizu K, Ohigashi H. Immunomodulatory action of citrus auraptene on macrophage functions and cytokine production of lymphocytes in female BALB/c mice. Carcinogenesis. 1999;20(8):1471–6.
222. Murakami A, Nakamura Y, Tanaka T, Kawabata K, Takahashi D, Koshimizu K, Ohigashi H. Suppression by citrus auraptene of phorbol ester-and endotoxin-induced inflammatory responses: role of attenuation of leukocyte activation. Carcinogenesis. 2000;21(10):1843–50.
223. Kostova I, Bhatia S, Grigorov P, Balkansky S, Parmar SV, Prasad KA, Saso L. Coumarins as antioxidants. Curr Med Chem. 2011;18(25):3929–51.
224. Higuchi M. Antioxidant properties of wheat bran against oxidative stress. In: Wheat and rice in disease prevention and health. Cambridge, MA: Academic Press; 2014. p. 181–99.
225. Wcislo G, Szarlej-Wcislo K. Colorectal cancer prevention by wheat consumption: a three-valued logic–true, false, or otherwise? In: Wheat and rice in disease prevention and health. Cambridge, MA: Academic Press; 2014. p. 91–111.
226. Cañete A, Armijo F, Del Valle MA, Tapia RA, Theoduloz C, Pessoa CD, Cantuarias L, Recabarren G. Biological activities and correlations tendency of electrochemical properties of some indolizino [1, 2-B] quinoline derivatives. J Chilean Chem Soc. 2012;57(2):1126–9.
227. Lu JJ, Bao JL, Wu GS, Xu WS, Huang MQ, Chen XP, Wang YT. Quinones derived from plant secondary metabolites as anti-cancer agents. Anti-Cancer Agents Med Chem. 2013;13 (3):456–63.

228. Taguchi C, Fukushima Y, Kishimoto Y, et al. Estimated dietary polyphenol intake and major food and beverage sources among elderly Japanese. Nutrients. 2015;7:10269–81. https://doi.org/10.3390/nu7125530.
229. Evans WC. Trease and evans pharmacognosy. 15th ed. Amsterdam: Elsevier; 2006.
230. Masoko P, Eloff JN. Screening of twenty-four South African Combretum and six Terminalia species (Combretaceae) for antioxidant activities. Afr J Tradit Complement Altern Med. 2007;4(2):231–9.
231. Jaberian H, Piri K, Nazari J. Phytochemical composition and in vitro antimicrobial and antioxidant activities of some medicinal plants. Food Chem. 2013;136(1):237–44.
232. Gunjan MC, Mahajan RT. Comparative antioxidant activity of twenty traditional Indian medicinal plants and its correlation with total flavonoid and phenolic content. Int J Pharm Sci Rev Res. 2015;30(1):105–11.
233. Gupta VK, Sharma SK. Plants as natural antioxidants. Nat Prod Rad. 2006;5(4):326–34.
234. Singh N, Mathur C, Sase NA, Rai S, Abraham J. Pharmaceutical properties of emblica officinalis and phyllanthus emblica extracts. RJPBCS. 2015;6(1):1007–16.
235. Ansari A, Shariar MSZ, Hassan MM, Das SR, Rokeya B, Haque MA, et al. Emblicaofficinalis improves glycemic status and oxidative stress in STZ induced type 2 diabetic model rats. Asian Pac J Trop Med. 2014:21–5.
236. Moses RS, Maheswari R. In-vitro antioxidant potential of Terminalia arjuna bark aqueous extract on sheep red blood cells. Int J Res Appl Chem. 2016;2(5):1–4.
237. Konda RGV, Eerike M, Raghuraman PL, Rajamanickam KM. Antioxidant and nephroprotective activities of aconitum heterophyllum root in glycerol induced acute renal failure in rats. J Clin Diagn Res. 2016;10(3):FF01–2.
238. Refahy LA, Saad AM. Characterization of chemical constituents, reducing power and anticancer activities of TerminaliabellericaRoxb. Acad J Cancer Res. 2014;7(2):117–25.
239. Assa JR, Widjanarko SB, Kusnadi J, Berhimpon S. Antioxidant potential of flesh, seed and mace of Myristicafragrans. IJCRGG. 2014;6(4):2460–8.
240. Talke P, Satyapal US, Mhajan DC, Nharwar V. Phytochemical analysis, in vitro antioxidant and antimicrobial activities of flower petals of Rosa damascene. Int J Pharmacogn Phytochem Res. 2015;7(2):246–50.
241. Sarwar S, Malik AH, Rahman MA, Rahman MZ, Rana MS. Antioxidant, cytotoxic and analgesic activities of the methanolic fruit extract of Terminaliachebula Retz. Int Curr Pharm J. 2013;3(1):219–22.
242. Rani AA, Jeeva S, Punitha SMJ. Antioxidant, anti-inflammatory, antiproliferative and apoptotic properties of Terminaliachebula (fruit) towards raw 264.7 and oral KB cell lines. IJAPSA. 2016;02(05):90–100.
243. Jana K, Ghosh A, Ghosh D. In vitro antioxidant potentiality of ethyl acetate fraction of seed of *Eugenia jambolana*. Asian J Pharm Clin Res. 2015;8(1):167–70.
244. Rao N, Sudhanshu MS, Menghani E. In vitro phytochemical screening, antioxidant & antimicrobial activity of the methanolic extract of Quercusinfectoria L. Int J Pharm Sci. 2013;5(2):273–7.
245. Rana RK, Patel RK. Antioxidant activity of bark of Myricanagi. Int J Pharm Sci Rev Res. 2014;28(1):99–101.
246. Chougule P, Pawar R, Limaye D, Joshi MY, Kadam V. In-vitro antioxidant activity of ethanolic extract of centaureabehen. J Appl Pharm Sci. 2012;02(04):106–10.
247. Kalaivani T, Methew L. Free radical scavenging activity from leaves of Acacia nilotica (L.) Wil. exDelile, an Indian medicinal tree. Food Chem Toxicol. 2010;298–305.

248. Teh SS, LianEe GC, Mah SH, Yong YK, Lim YM, Rahmani M, et al. In vitro cytotoxic, antioxidant, and antimicrobial activities of Mesuabeccariana (Baill.) Kosterm, Mesuaferrea Linn, and Mesuacongestiflora Extracts. Biomed Res Int. 2013;517072:1–9.
249. Keawsa-ard S, Kongtaweelert S. Antioxidant, antibacterial, anticancer activities and chemical constituents of the essential oil from mesuaferrea leaves. Chiang Mai J Sci. 2012;39 (3):455–63.
250. Chahar MK, Sanjaya Kumar DS, Lokesh T, Manohara KP. In-vivo antioxidant and immunomodulatory activity of mesuol isolated from Mesua ferrea L. seed oil. Int Immunopharmacol. 2012;13(4):386–91.
251. Garg S, Kameshwar S, Rajeev R, Pankaj A, Parshuram M. In-vivo Antioxidant activity and hepatoprotective effects of methanolic extracts of Mesuaferrea L. Int J Pharmatechnol Res. 2009;1:1692–6.

Polyphenols Targeting and Influencing Cellular Signaling During Progression and Treatment of Cancer

4

Sidharth Mehan, Saloni Rahi, Shubham Upadhayay, and Andleeb Khan

Abstract

Long-term dietary intake of natural polyphenols shows chemoprotective and anticancer activity through scavenging and removing free radicals. Polyphenols have been reported to influence and alter the initiation, promotion, and progression of cancer. The broad range of these polyphenol compounds' biological and pharmacological activities is well supported by numerous studies in metabolism regulation, microbiome interaction, and interference with primary cell signaling responsible for cancer development. A number of polyphenols from various dietary sources demonstrate the regulation of cancer-causing transcription factors, and polyphenols control signaling molecules and modulate cancer cell apoptosis, proliferation, invasion, and metastasis. Here, we focus on multiple cell signals that play a significant role in cancer progression and discuss the beneficial role of polyphenols in different cancer progression stages, including metastasis and apoptosis. In addition, we attempted to provide a more consistent and reliable relationship between how different polyphenols affect cancer signaling. To summarize, using polyphenols as nutraceuticals aids in the development of potential new drugs with a particular target pathway involved in cancer pathogenesis and medication production as a possible strategy in cancer treatment.

S. Mehan (✉) · S. Rahi · S. Upadhayay
Department of Pharmacology, Neuropharmacology Division, ISF College of Pharmacy, Moga, Punjab, India
e-mail: sidharthmehan@isfcp.org

A. Khan
Department of Pharmacology and Toxicology, College of Pharmacy, Jazan University, Jazan, Saudi Arabia

S. Tabrez, M. Imran Khan (eds.), *Polyphenols-based Nanotherapeutics for Cancer Management*, https://doi.org/10.1007/978-981-16-4935-6_4

Keywords

Polyphenols · Chemoprevention · Cancer · Cellular signaling · Metastasis · Tumorigenesis

Abbreviations

AGL	Apigenin 7-O-glucoside
AKT	Protein kinase B (PKB)
CaMK	Calmodulin-dependent protein kinase
CBR1	Human carbonyl reductase 1
EGCG	Epigallocatechin gallate
EGF	Epidermal growth factor
EGFR	Epidermal growth factor receptor
ERK	Extracellular signal-regulated kinases
GLI	Glioma-associated homolog
GLI-R	Glioma-associated homolog repressor
GSH	Glutathione
GST	Glutathione S-transferase
hGCCs	Human gastric cancer cells
IGF	Insulin-like growth factor
IGFR	Insulin-like growth factor receptor
JAK	Janus Tyrosine Kinase
JNK	c-Jun N-terminal kinase
MAPK	Mitogen-activated protein
MMP	Mitochondrial membrane potential
mTOR	Mechanistic target of rapamycin
NF-κB	Nuclear Factor kappa B
PARP	Poly ADP-ribose polymerase
PI3K	Phosphoinositide 3-kinases
PIP2	Phosphatidylinositol 4,5-bisphosphate
PIP3	Phosphatidylinositol 3,4,5-trisphosphate
PKc	Protein kinase C
PATCH-1	Patched-1
PTEN	Phosphatase and tensin homolog
ROS	Reactive Oxidative species
SHH	Sonic Hedgehog
SMO	Smoothened
STAT	Signal Transducer and Activator of Transcription
TNF-α	Tumor necrosis factor
TP53	Tumor protein P53
TRAIL	TNF-related apoptosis-inducing ligand
TSC	Tuberous sclerosis complex
VEGF	Vascular endothelial growth factor

4.1 Introduction

Recent developments in phytochemical-based preparations have played an essential role in treating various diseases related to cell growth, differentiation, and proliferation [1]. One such critically reviewed and widely studied class of phytochemicals is polyphenols. Polyphenols have a wide range of evidence demonstrating their beneficial effects on diseases caused by cell degeneration, deregulation, and abnormal differentiation, such as cancer tumorigenesis, neurodegenerative diseases, and a variety of other cell abnormalities [2]. Cancer, one of the most hotly discussed and prevalent diseases of the twenty-first century, has had no targeted treatment or cure to date [3]. Since the last few decades, many studies and clinical work have been performed on various phytocomponents related to cancer treatment. Polyphenols are among the most significant parts of clinical and preclinical research [4].

Polyphenols are secondary metabolites present in various medicinal plants and are an essential bioactive dietary compound [5]. Consumption of a rich polyphenol diet, such as fruits and vegetables, provides multiple health benefits [5]. Polyphenols are made up of several subclasses, including flavonoids and other phenolic compounds, all of which contribute to the protective mechanism against different diseases [6–8]. The primary polyphenol subclasses are flavonoids and non-flavonoids. Due to polyphenols' antioxidant properties, polyphenols' regular consumption (up to 1g) helps to minimize reactive oxidative species and pro-oxidants [9]. Besides, several studies in recent years have shown that polyphenols play a significant role in chemoprevention and cancer cell apoptosis [5, 10].

One of the major factors contributing to the development of cancer is the interrupted intracellular signaling network, which transmits aberrant signals that result in abnormal cellular activity [11–13]. In chemoprevention, targeting these deregulated intracellular signaling mechanisms may help by modulating one or more cell signaling pathways in a manner that inhibits the carcinogenic mechanism [14–16].

Several cell lines, animal models, and human epidemiological studies indicate that dietary polyphenols play a protective function against multiple forms of cancer. Dietary polyphenols by modulation and targeting several signaling pathways are opposed to the cells' carcinogenic nature [17]. Clinical studies also relate polyphenolic intake to cancer prevention, indicating a decreased risk of different types of cancer and reduced recurrence following intake of flavonoids or certain foods or beverages that are high in these phenolic compounds [18, 19]. Human trials, by contrast, have demonstrated no beneficial effects. Since carcinogenesis is a multistep process involving multiple cellular signaling pathways such as NF-κB, PI3K/Akt signaling, mTOR signaling, IGF (Insulin-like growth factor) pathway, and many more [20]. Minor deregulation of major signaling pathways leads to many alterations related to cell differentiation and proliferation [21]. Also, deregulated signaling contributes to the carcinogenic activity of the cells and leads to cancer. Intake of different dietary polyphenols modulates aberrant cell signaling to normalize and reverse cancer development [22, 23]. Many hypotheses often operate on the concept of polyphenols linked to the apoptotic signaling system for cancer cells. Polyphenols cause cell apoptosis through induction of cell cycle arrest in cancer cells [24]. Figure 4.1 *depicts the cellular signaling pathways involved in cancer progression, as well as polyphenols' involvement in chemoprevention by modulation of these pathways.*

There is currently a wide amount of knowledge available that supports polyphenols' biological role and anti-carcinogenic activity. So far, several researchers have provided information on the use of polyphenols in cancer care. However, to the best of our knowledge, there is still a limited number of studies on the use of polyphenols as an alternative therapy in cancer treatment. We searched for all of the details on polyphenol bioavailability or ADME (Absorption, Distribution, Metabolism, and Elimination). In that case, we will see that the concentration of polyphenols in food products and their consumption varies by individual. Since there are several polyphenols, determining which one is showing anticancer activity is difficult. In contrast, the associations of polyphenolic compounds ingested as dietary supplements with drug pharmacology should be studied. The "omics" technology can be used to investigate the pharmacological effects of polyphenols. Furthermore, using polyphenols as a nutraceutical is one of the most promising steps toward incorporating them into chemoprevention drug formulations. The profile of safety and toxicity must also be taken into account, especially in terms of bioavailability. In this chapter, we will discuss the function of polyphenol in chemoprevention and its impact on modulating various signaling pathways.

4.2 Polyphenols and Cancer Chemoprevention

4.2.1 Introduction of Dietary Polyphenols

Several cancers are linked to dietary nutrients and other constituents [25]. Polyphenols can be present in a variety of fruits, vegetables, nuts, and beverages. Dietary sources of polyphenols include green tea, almonds, and berries [26]. Polyphenols have been shown to have effective and pharmacological activities in preventing neurodegeneration, aging, tumorigenesis, and metabolic disorders such as diabetes [27]. Polyphenol has also been shown to control pathogenic, hypertensive, and cardiovascular infections [27]. Polyphenols are essentially polyhydroxyphenols, which are distinguished by a large number of phenolic units. These phenolic units are glycosides [28].

Polyphenols are usually categorized into different groups based on their structure, source, and therapeutic action [29]. They are known as phenolic acids, flavonoids, phenolic amides, and other polyphenols based on their chemical nature [30]. Flavonoids are one of the leading and largest polyphenols that are further subclassified as isoflavones, flavanols, and anthocyanidins. Phenolic acid is also subclassified as benzoic acids and cinnamic acid derivatives [30–33]. They also play a significant role in angiogenesis and tumorigenesis [2]. Polyphenols, which are found in a variety of foods, including vegetables and fruits, can be used in

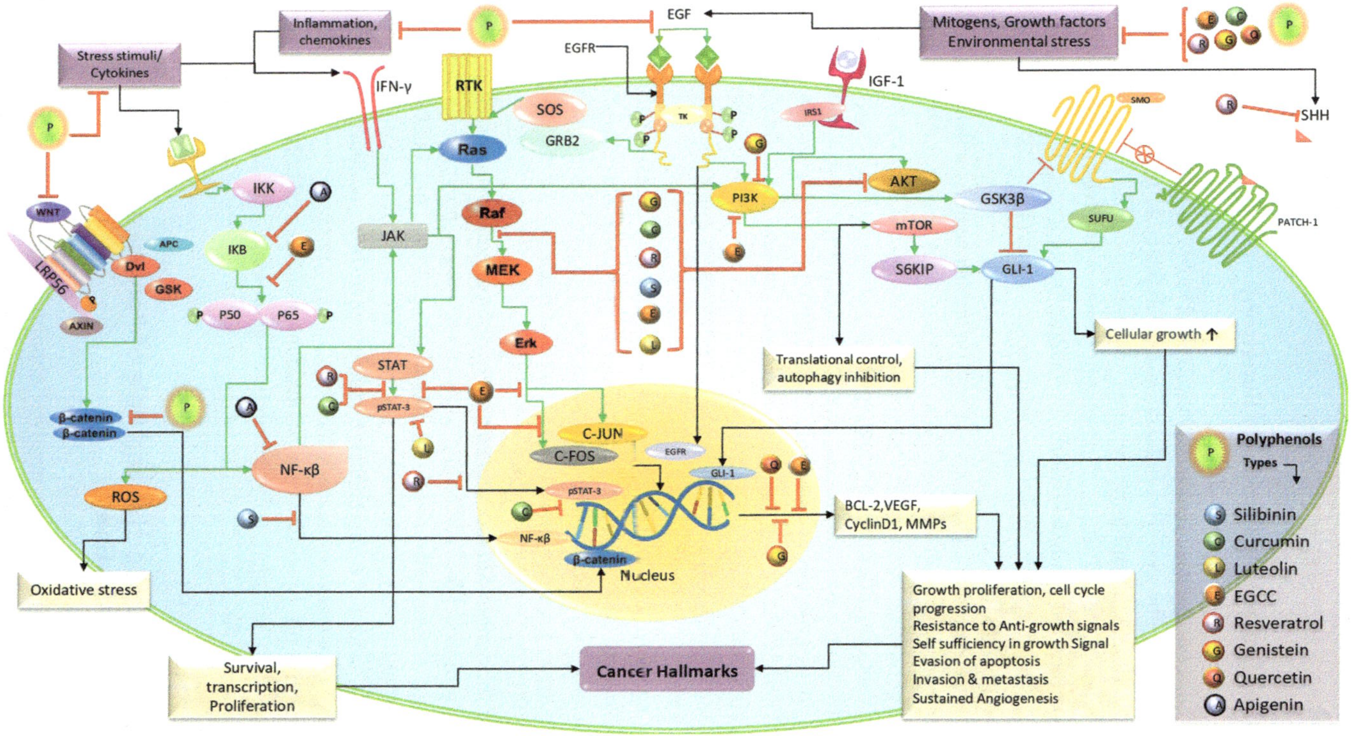

Fig. 4.1 Cellular signaling and polyphenols' involvement in chemoprevention. Cancer generation is a dynamic and multistage phenomenon involving various signals from cells and molecules. Polyphenols control cancer growth and metastases. This diagram shows the different cell signal transductions that play a significant role in cancer cells' state and condition and contribute to cancer development. Different polyphenols are targeted and mediate chemoprotective effects by modulating the cell signaling pathways involved in cancer growth, as well as increasing the potency of the chemotherapy agent in many types of cancer. (↓: downregulated/decrease; ↑: upregulated/increase; ⊥ inhibition)

chemoprevention and as therapeutic agents because they significantly control several signaling pathways and include cell cycle arrest and apoptosis [34].

4.2.2 How Dietary Polyphenols Function?

Various studies have shown that polyphenols interfere with multiple cell signaling mechanisms and pathways. The interaction of polyphenols, primarily flavonoids, appears to modulate the different signaling mechanisms [35]. This modulation, in some way, leads to the activation of transcription factors involved in gene expression [35]. Gene expression ultimately works by facilitating various cellular deregulation processes, such as cellular viability, inflammatory pathways, and the release of various other factors [36].

Polyphenols have various bioactive effects on human health, including anticancer activity; polyphenols affect the cell cycle, making them one of the most effective compounds in tumorigenesis [37]. Oxidative stress is one of the key factors behind multiple cell abnormalities [38]. Oxidative stress induces ROS (Reactive Oxidative species) activation, which further triggers many cellular pathways such as NF-κB [39], ERK (Extracellular signal-regulated kinases) [40], JNK (c-Jun N-terminal kinase) [41], PI3K/Akt [42], P38 [40], and many others; the regulation of these pathways affects transcription [43]. Transcription is the pathway responsible for activating, controlling, and releasing various mediators for inflammation and cellular oxidative stress.

Dietary polyphenols have an impact on ROS and play an essential role in free radical scavenging [44, 45]. Polyphenols also promote the activity of endogenous antioxidant enzymes thus inhibiting oxidant enzymes [46]. They have also been shown to play an important role in signaling and releasing the effects of different cytokines [47].

Phenolic substances can modulate a variety of biochemical processes induced by tumor cell promoters [48]. According to research, dietary polyphenols inhibit pre-malignant and cancer cell growth by inducing apoptosis and inhibit cell tumor growth by inhibiting cell cycle phases [48, 49]. The roles of these polyphenols are still unknown, and no comprehensive studies have been conducted to provide complete data on cancer suppression and chemoprevention by polyphenols. Various research includes information on the antioxidant properties of polyphenols. A few studies have also revealed polyphenol findings in other diseases affecting the glycemic process [50–52].

4.2.3 Current Perspective and Role of Polyphenols in Cancer Chemoprevention

Cancer is a disease group that involves abnormal cell growth and metabolism [53]. The primary mechanism underlying cancer growth is unbalanced and dysregulated cell proliferation and differentiation [54–56]. To date, no specific cause of disrupted cell growth and differentiation is identified, and all cancer prevention and treatment therapies include cell growth inhibitors with severe side effects [57].

Polyphenol can inhibit the cell cycle, making it one of the potential chemopreventive agents [58, 59]. High dietary consumption of fruits and vegetables is widely believed to help prevent cancer onset [60]. However, there is a degree of uncertainty in that some studies have not shown any reduction in cancer growth incidence due to the intake of fruit and vegetables [60]. Despite this, there is still a chance that certain fruits or vegetables or specific polyphenols found within them could have protective effects against cancer production [61].

Cancer is a complex and multistep process that involves multiple cells and molecular signaling [62]. The initiation method, in which the cell is exposed to the carcinogenic agent, is the most crucial step in cancer development [63]. Second, the process of promotion begins when cells replicate from their original state to pre-cancer cells [64]. In the final stage, tumor formation starts, which leads to uncontrolled cell development. These steps result in metastases and the formation of new blood vessels, a process known as angiogenesis. During cancer cell growth, signaling pathways such as cell proliferation and differentiation, as well as increased cellular oxidative stress, are activated [65].

Polyphenols in the diet play an important role in carcinogenesis by upregulating and downregulating major cell pathways involved in cancer progression [66, 67]. Polyphenols regulate cell proliferation, transduction, apoptosis, angiogenesis, and metastasis by modulating cell signaling [48]. The potential chemoprotective existence of polyphenols helps to prevent carcinogenic processes and signaling molecules [16]. One of the polyphenols in green tea, which is extensively researched in cancer polyphenol, with more than 700 reports claiming chemoprotective effects in the case of multiple cancers [68]. The main phytochemicals present in green tea are catechins in the form of ()-epigallocatechin-3-gallate (EGCG), ()-epicatechin-3-gallate, ()-epigallocatechin, and ()-epicatechin [66, 68]. These EGCGs are the most common and important defense mechanisms against skin, lung, breast, colon, liver, stomach, prostate, and other cancers [2, 5]. The EGCG study notes that polyphenols' protective effects include inhibition of genotoxic molecules and inhibition of mutagen activity. In addition to these polyphenols, the enzyme Cytochrome P450s is regulated [69]. Numerous studies have been performed to date concerning polyphenols as chemoprotective agents. However, the bioavailability and safety data for polyphenols for clinical use in cancer are still missing.

4.3 Involvement of Intracellular Molecular Signaling During Cancer Progression

4.3.1 EGFR-mediated Signal Transduction Pathway

The epidermal growth factor (EGF) receptor signaling is an important signaling pathway that is part of the complex mechanism that drives cancer progression [70, 71]. Combination therapies include anti-EGFR serving as a chemopreventive agent along with other anticancer therapies [72]. The EGF was described as a factor contributing to cellular growth by Nobel laureate Stanely Cohen [73]. EGFR is a family of receptor tyrosine kinases that is excessively expressed in cancer progression and responsible for activating various carcinogenic mediators in different types of cancers such as breast, lung, colon, esophageal many others [74, 75]. EGFR has shown a significant role in cell development, migration, proliferation, differentiation, and carcinogenic translation and transcription [76]. They also contribute to cancer survival and metastasis and have emerged as one of the most critical cancer research pathways [77].

Over-activation of EGFR activity is responsible for tumor cells' growth and involves various cellular activities that over-regulate normal proliferation and differentiation and cause apoptosis [78]. The EGFR family structurally consists of three major domains, including the cysteine-rich extracellular N-terminal ligand-binding domain, the hydrophobic transmembrane domain, and the intracellular domain C-terminal tyrosine kinase cytoplasm [79]. The intracellular domain is strongly conserved, and thus all binding has taken place in the extracellular domain, which also has four major sub-domains in it [80]. Sub-domains I and III are responsible for the open conformation and activation of sub-domains II and IV [80, 81]. This translocation allows sub-domains I and III to reveal the ligand-binding pocket to interact with the adjacent dimer arm to form the homodimer [81]. EGFR also promotes heterodimerization with a relative member receptor of the same family [82]. When EGFR homodimerizes or heterodimerizes, it initiates a variety of cellular signaling cascades and promotes complex signaling factors [82].

EGFR activation is caused by ligand-binding and receptor dimerization, promoting the phosphorylation of the tyrosine residue binding at the EGFR C-terminus [83]. This phosphorylation helps supply the effector proteins and the phosphotyrosine motif present in the receptor intracellular domain [83, 84]. As a result, this activation and the effector proteins promote the activation of the RAS-RAF-MEK-ERK pathway, P13K-AKT pathway, anti-apoptotic and (Signal Transducer and Activator of Transcription) STAT signaling [85]. All these activations signaling pathways contribute to cell proliferation, migration, survival, and adhesion along with angiogenesis [86]. These cellular processes are deregulated and over-activated in malignant cells triggered by mutations in associated genes [85, 86]. If activated, start signaling from the cell membrane, and all these signals are transmitted to the nucleus via cytoplasmic intermediates.

EGFR is present in the nucleus of nearly all cancer cells, including those from the breast, ovaries, cervix, skin, prostate, and esophagus [77]. In human cancers, EGFR signaling occurs through two distinct pathways. One is the conventional EGFR pathway, which is considered a significant transduction cascade involving PLC-c-CaMK/PKC, RAS-RAF-MEK-ERK, P13-AKT-GSK, and JAK-STAT [85, 87]. Many of these signaling pathways have been actively involved in the transduction of cellular growth factors via signal cascades' activation to particular cytoplasmic targets and the nucleus to engage in the genetic transcription [87] actively. Under the deregulated/over-regulated condition, these signaling mechanisms led to malignant development, increased spread and differentiation, tumor progression, apoptosis invasion, and cancer mediator resistance [76]. Another primary cascade of EGFR is novel direct transduction involving the translocation of the EGFR cell surface and the target gene's transcription [87]. More on EGFR nuclear accumulation has also been associated with tumor proliferation and cell survival [88].

4.3.2 RAS–RAF–MEK–ERK (MAPK ERK) Signaling Pathway

Overactivated EGFR promotes tumorigenic factors and decreases apoptosis pathways controlled by PI3k-AKT signaling [85]. MAPK (mitogen-activated protein kinase) is important for cell proliferation and survival [89]. This pathway involves the activation of various cascades, including RAF, MEK (MAP-ERK kinases), and ERK (Extracellular Signal-Regulated Kinases)[90]. In normal cells, the RAS activation, which further signals the RAF kinases' activation, facilitates the RAF's dimerization and development [91]. The RAF then activated further phosphorylates and activated the MEK's (1&2) [92].

MEK activation results in the phosphorylation of ERK 1 and ERK 2. ERK serves an essential role by actively promoting cellular effects such as nuclear gene transcription and cytosolic protein expression [91, 92]. Even minor changes in this signaling cascade facilitate tumor progression by inducing mutations in specific genes, such as RAS genes, kRAS, nRAS, and hRAS, as well as MEK1 mutations [93]. It also causes deletion of mutations and promotes the methylation of specific genes. These factors have an effect on tumor cell survival and the production of the cancer process [85].

4.3.3 PI3K–AKT–mTOR Pathway

PI3K (Phosphoinositide 3-kinase)/AKT (protein kinase B)/mTOR (mammalian target of rapamycin) pathway is another signaling system found to be deregulated in the event of cancer progression and human malignancies and various varieties of neoplasms [94]. The oncogenic activity of PI3K/AKT/mTOR is due to its role in cell progression, differentiation, and survival [95, 96]. The PI3K signal cascade is triggered after dimerization and activation of the EGFR [85]. It is also triggered by RTK activation, which activates the tyrosine kinase receptor on the cell membrane's surface. Ras and oncogenic proteins also play a role in PI3K activation [97]. When active, PI3k interacts with the other signaling cascades and is involved in a variety of processes, including mutation and gene involvement, as well as the activation of RAS isoforms [93].

Studies show that the PI3K/AKT/mTOR pathway is actively involved in cancer progression and results in the amplification of gene encoding components [99].

Besides, activation of PI3K/AKT/mTOR is also mutated in various cancers, including head and neck cancer, breast cancer, colon cancer, lung cancer, and ovarian cancer [95]. When activated, PIP3 (phosphatidylinositol 3,4,5-trisphosphate) is activated via PIP2 (phosphatidylinositol 4,5-diphosphate) phosphorylation. Under normal conditions, the PIP3 level is regulated by the PTEN (Phosphatase and tensin homolog), which is responsible for the dephosphorylation of the PIP3 and converts it back to PIP2, and triggers the negative feedback loop of the PI3K cascade [96, 98, 99].

Under normal circumstances, AKT phosphorylates the TSC2 (tuberous sclerosis complex 2) and inhibits the activity of the TSC1/TSC2 complex, and causes mTOR to be activated via RAS and spreads the signal [100, 101]. MTOR is available in two isoforms, i.e., mTORC1 and mTORC2, for which mTORC1 is responsible for protein synthesis and protein translation [102]. MTORC2 is primarily known to phosphorylate the AKT to its full activation [103, 104]. Genetic mutations and modifications disrupt the standard PI3K/AKT/mTOR signaling cascade, resulting in molecular changes contributing to cancer progression [105].

As most studies to date have shown, the modification, including PIK3CA mutations, overexpression of ER, HER2, etc., in a variety of cancers directly linked to PI3K/AKT/mTOR cascade signaling [106]. Together with the mTOR mutation, it causes mTOR-related signaling changes and leads to human malignancies, including cancer. Increased phosphorylation of mTOR and Akt signaling modulates cancer progression and influences cell proliferation/differentiation [98]. These causes, as well as the role of the PI3K/AKT/mTOR signaling cascade, make it an important signaling cascade for cancer research in order to establish successful treatment strategies for future use [94].

4.3.4 PLC-c-CaMK/PKC Signaling Pathway

Protein kinase C belongs to the family of phospholipid-dependent serine/threonine kinases that help in cellular functioning [107]. PKC (Protein kinase C) is categorized into three subfamilies of isozymes, i.e., conventional isozymes, novel or nonclassical isozymes, and atypical isozymes [107]. DAG (Diacylglycerol) is needed as the primary activator for the activation of PKCs and other activation cofactors such as phosphatidylserine and calcium [108]. PKC isozymes are responsible for multistep signal transduction, including growth hormones and ligand proteins, which respond to multiple stress/stimulus reactions.

In cancer progression, PKC isozymes function as a significant factor in cell proliferation, survival, and migration [109]. PKC isozymes also include various cellular signaling cascades in cellular apoptosis and angiogenesis along with cancer resistance [107, 109]. During the cancerous environment, PKC isozymes actively modulate cell signalings, such as RAS–RAF–MEK–ERK (MAPK ERK) or PI3K–AKT–mTOR in cell proliferation, differentiation, and survival [89]. Besides, activated PKCs help to inhibit the apoptosis cascade and anticancer factors such as Caspase and Bax. Activation of PKC isozymes and downregulation of apoptosis signaling cascades significantly impact cellular conditions [110].

In chronic lymphocytic leukemia, PKC acts as an antiapoptotic regulator, whereas in acute myeloid leukemia, it acts as a proapoptotic regulator [111]. It also involves the spread of cancer cells in the case of colon cancer and other cancers [112, 113]. PKCs are regarded as a critical signaling factor in cancer progression due to their role in the expression and spread of cancer factors.

4.3.5 JAK-STAT Pathway

STAT is a family transcription factor involving six prominent members, i.e., Stat-1, 2, 3, 4, 5a, 6b. STAT is one of the main signaling factors involved in various cancer progressions, including breast cancer and colon cancer [114, 115]. Deregulated EGFR and JAK pathways are linked with elevated STAT3 tumor activity [116]. This improper STAT3 signal transduction is most likely to increase cytokine levels, as well as have an impact on cell growth, proliferation, and differentiation [117, 118]. It directly activates the transcription of genes involved in cell proliferation in a cancerous environment such as c-Jun and C-Fos. It includes the cell cycle's progression and the downflow of apoptosis factors such as BCL-xl and Fas [119]. Besides, STAT helps in VEGF (Vascular endothelial growth factor) activation, one of the modulating factors for angiogenesis and tumor metastasis [120]. The role of STAT in oncogenesis, cancer, angiogenesis, and other cancer-promoting actors makes it one of the targeted import signaling mechanisms for cancer research [85].

STAT phosphorylation promotes STAT release from its receptor and induces dimerization into two distinct STAT molecules after receptor activation [121]. This dimer has been translocated into the nucleus, where it binds to the DNA fragment and causes gene expression. This binding to DNA expresses genes that are receptive to cytokines, such as interferons and interleukins, involved in cancer progression by linking to various receptors [118]. This binding phosphorylates the JAK and helps to form a dimer in association with another STAT molecule. This molecule is then translocated into the nucleus and further added to the DNA and promotes cell proliferation and differentiation via gene expression [117].

Studies show elevated levels of STAT 1, 3, and 5 in a variety of cancer cells. These proteins are actively involved in the signal transduction of hormones and cytokines. Above all, STAT protein regulates cell function, including organogenesis, fetal development, cellular apoptosis pathways, growth, immune function, and cell inflammation [122]. STAT is activated during tumor formation by several tyrosine kinases, including JAK and EGFR. JAK/STAT activation has a significant impact on cell proliferation, inflammation, angiogenesis, and metastasis, all of which contribute to cancer progression [123, 124].

4.3.6 IGF-mediated Pathway for Signal Transduction

IGF or IGFR (Insulin-like growth factor receptor) transduction is a transduction cascade strongly involved in cell growth and survival [125]. It also includes chemo-responses under particular conditions. IGF-I and IGF-II ligands bind to the receptors, i.e., IGFR-I and IGFR-II, which further promote the different signaling cascades and involve DNA synthesis and cell growth and survival [76, 126]. The abnormal activation or over-expression of IGF and IGFR is linked to the development of several forms of cancer. IGF/IGFR is linked to a number of cancers, including cancer cell survival and metastasis [127].

4.3.7 Nuclear Factor-B Signaling Pathway

NF-κB is a transcriptional factor responsible for regulating and expressing immune and growth genes [128]. It is a homo-or hetero-dimeric mixture of protein subunits, namely RelA, RelB, c-Rel, NF-κB1, and NF-κB2 [128, 129]. These subunits share the N-terminal Rel domain, mainly involved in DNA binding and dimerization [130]. In normal cells, NF-κB dimers are sequestered in the cytoplasm by I£B. Still, under stimulation from an external environment, they are rapidly translocated to the nucleus, promoting gene expression [131]. NF-κB is mediated either by phosphorylation of IκB members accompanied by proteasomal degradation or by the degradation of p100 and p105 to p52 and p50 [132]. Under normal circumstances, NF-κB is controlled by the control of IκB. NF-κB is highly activated in cancerous conditions and translocated to the nucleus to improve cell proliferation and survival, together with the deregulation of many other signaling pathways [133].

MiRNAs also play a significant role in affecting major components and proteins, such as TNF and other inflammatory cytokines responsible for regulating NF-κB [85]. Reduction in the expression level of the miR-9 aids in the promotion of the NF-κB expression and upregulation of the activities relevant to the NF-κB [134]. This leads to NF-B overexpression and activation, which affects cell proliferation and survival. NF-κB signaling is also implicated in angiogenesis, metastasis, and cellular invasion. Enabling NF-B mediates the upregulation of interleukins and VEGF expression, which serves as a cancer marker [135].

4.3.8 Wnt Pathway

Wnt signaling is a transduction pathway that involves several proteins and is activated by cell surface receptors. Wnt signaling follows either a canonical or a non-canonical signaling direction. The key differentiating factor that distinguishes between canonical and non-canonical pathways is β-catenin [136]. Both signaling pathways are triggered through the Wnt ligand receptor connection to the Frizzled (Fz) cell surface receptor [137]. This receptor binding transmits a signal to Dishevelled (Dsh), which is an intracellular protein. Numerous glycoproteins are involved in Wnt signaling and are responsible for key roles such as cell survival, proliferation, differentiation, migration, and other vital functions, including cell patterning and stem cell regeneration [85, 138].

Deregulated Wnt signaling causes an abrupt mutation in the genes, altering the role of the necessary proteins in signal transduction [139]. This abrupt signaling plays a role in cellular changes, including the development of cancer. Wnt signaling is altered in cancer and is actively involved in cancers such as breast cancer, hepatocellular carcinoma, lung cancer, and gastric cancer [140–143]. Increased level of β-catenin correlates with increased expression of cyclone D1 and is also observed in different melanomas [144]. Inhibition of β-catenin indicates it decreased abrupt cell proliferation, migration, and invasion and causes apoptosis signaling [145].

4.3.9 Sonic Hedgehog Signaling

SHH signaling stands for sonic hedgehog signaling, one of the main signaling pathways responsible for embryonic cell differentiation and proliferation [85, 146]. SHH signaling is responsible for embryonic limb and craniofacial development. SHH is a vital signaling mechanism that helps preserve tissue polarity [146]. In the absence of SHH ligand, PATCH-1 inhibits SMO and inhibits translocation to activate GLI-1(Glioma-associated homolog-1) [147]. PATCH-1-mediated inhibition of SMO is abolished in the presence of SHH ligand, and SMO is available to promote nuclear accumulation of GLI1 and trigger genetic transcription [148]. The rapid activation of SHH signaling is seen in many human cancers and is responsible for the promotion of oncogenic factors in cancer cells [149]. Abnormal SHH signaling has been linked to the development of many cancers, including basal cell carcinomas, medulloblastomas, and rhabdomyosarcomas [150].

Mutation in SMO and PATCH-1 is a major factor responsible for the deregulation of SHH signaling. Several studies have shown that endocrine and paracrine SHH deregulation is induced in various tumors and cancers [151]. SHH hyperactivation is involved in pancreatic, colorectal, prostate, and glioma cancers and is responsible for tumor angiogenesis, tumor cell proliferation, differentiation, and survival [152].

SHH transduction pathways are also helpful in the preservation of cancer stem cells (CSCs) in cancers such as chronic myeloid leukemia and breast cancer [153, 154]. The SHH pathway is inhibited, which reduces the distribution and regeneration of stem cells. SHH signaling's role in CSC maintenance has also been linked to metastatic progression in cancers such as pancreatic and colon-rectal cancers [155].

4.4 Anticarcinogenic Activity of Dietary Polyphenols by Modulating Various Signaling Pathways

4.4.1 Modulation of Cellular Signaling Associated with Cancer Through Polyphenols

Numerous studies to date have shown that a diet rich in polyphenols decreases the risk of various chronic diseases, including cancer. According to several researchers, the intake of a diet rich in polyphenols and other phenolic compounds has beneficial effects, including preventing various diseases by modulating different cellular signaling that is actively responsible for controlling inflammation and oxidative stress, apoptosis, and many more [156]. Polyphenols are the most abundant and diverse phytochemical group found in the majority of plant products, including vegetables and berries.

Polyphenols, as previously mentioned, are a major class of phytoconstituents with various roles, such as antioxidant, antiproliferative, and anti-inflammatory, all of which lead to the reduction of carcinogenic cell survival [157]. These widely distributed polyphenols function on various cell signaling pathways and reduce the production of numerous cytokines that are found to be responsible for cell inflammation and oxidative stress. Polyphenols, such as resveratrol and epigallocatechin gallate, are actively responsible for the direct control of cell signals transduction pathways, such as inflammatory cascades, cell proliferation signaling cascades, and other pathways responsible for cell abnormalities.

Resveratrol demonstrates anticarcinogenic activity through a signaling mechanism by upregulation of death receptors or TRAIL (TNF-related apoptosis-inducing ligand) by death receptor expression (TRAIL-R1/DR4 and TRAIL-R2/DR5). TRAIL has had further effects on the upregulation of Bax and inhibition of Bcl-2 [160]. Resveratrol Inhibit cell proliferation by activation of apoptosis in hepatocarcinogenesis [164]. Effects of cell proliferation reduction, colony formation failure. Curcumin Prevents Small Cell Lung Cancer [172]. EGCG inhibits cell proliferation and migration of pancreatic cancer cells by inducing apoptosis by interference with the STAT3 signaling pathway. EGCG has improved the therapeutic effects of gemcitabine and CP690550 on pancreatic cancer [173].

The apoptotic effect of luteolin was facilitated by mitogen-activated protein kinase stimulation. The authors confirm that luteolin induced apoptotic cell death by inducing antioxidant activity and activating MAPK signaling in colon cancer cells [193]. Silibinin decreased proliferation and increased delayed mutation apoptosis in TP53 (Tumor protein P53) cells. Silibinin toxicogenic activity on FRAP/mTOR, AKT2, FGFR3, DNMT1, and miR100 was dependent on the status of TP53 cells [190]. Apigenin 7-O-glucoside facilitates apoptotic cell death through PTEN/PI3K/AKT and inhibits cell proliferation in the cervical tumor cell HeLa [181].

Quercetin inhibited the progression of breast cancer by inhibiting mobility and glycolysis through mTOR-mediated autophagy activation. In MDA-MB-435 and Hs578t breast cancer cells, genistein prevents cell proliferation by activating apoptosis. Genistein inhibits miR-155 expression, which has anticancer properties in metastatic breast cancer [199]. Table 4.1 ***describes the research-based detailed evidence (preclinical and clinical studies) on polyphenols in cancer chemoprevention, including specific signaling)***

4.4.2 The Potential Therapeutic Effect of Dietary Chemopreventive Polyphenols on Cancer Cell Apoptosis

Some research has already looked into the idea of polyphenols being related to apoptotic cancer cell signaling mechanisms. Polyphenols trigger cell apoptosis in cancer cells by disrupting the cell cycle. Polyphenols have been shown in previous studies to have a therapeutic effect on apoptosis in cancer cells, and some therapeutically active polyphenols are used to prevent cancer cells.

Luteolin is a dietary flavone that suppresses the development of tumors in human colon cancer. Luteolin modulated DNA demethylation and complexity between p53 and Nrf2 (Nuclear factor erythroid 2-related factor 2) is associated with the apoptotic effects of luteolin [194]. Kang et al. show that luteolin triggered the MAPK signaling pathway mediated apoptotic effects. Luteolin activates apoptosis in human colon cancer cells by inducing antioxidant activity by triggering MAPK signaling. Leutin has a possible therapeutic effect on colon cancer [193]. Another polyphenol is Apigenin 7-O-glucoside (AGL), which induces cell apoptosis through the PTEN/PI3K/ACT pathway. AGL can facilitate the release of cytochrome c by controlling the Bcl-2 family proteins and instead cause caspase 9/3 to enhance cell apoptosis. AGL shows potential therapeutic activity against cervical cancer [181].

Casticin, a flavonoid extract from Vitex rotundifolia, induced G0/G1 arrest and mitochondrial-related apoptosis by Bcl-2 expression and upregulating Bax, cleaved caspase-9, cleaved caspase-3, and cleaved poly ADP-ribose polymerase expression. Casticin significantly disrupted the dose- and time-dependent proliferation of gallbladder cancer cells [216]. Resveratrol has a potent chemopreventive effect on DENA-initiated hepatocarcinogenesis by controlling cell proliferation and apoptosis activation [164]. The ability of resveratrol to suppress tumor growth, the therapeutic potential of TRAIL, suggests that resveratrol alone or in conjunction with TRAIL can be used to treat prostate cancer [160]. Cardamonin greatly strengthened 5-FU chemosensitivity in GC cells by blocking the Wnt/β-catenin signaling pathway. The addition of cardamonin and 5-FU resulted in apoptosis and inhibition of the cell cycle in BGC-823/5-FU cells and downregulate expression levels of P-glycoprotein, β-catenin, and TCF4 [219]. The author previously studied bavachin-induced cell death mechanisms in choriocarcinoma cells. Bavachin increased 3/7 caspase activation in JEG3 and JAR cells by 2.6 and 3.4-fold, respectively. By interfering with the STAT3 signaling pathway, EGCG inhibits pancreatic cancer cell growth and promotes apoptosis [173].

Pterostilbene (PTER) was found in blueberries. Preclinical results suggest that PTER is an inexpensive, specific, and therapeutically safe natural product that can be tested for prostate cancer. Pterostilbene inhibits MTA1 signaling by enhanced p53 acetylation, the high apoptotic index for prostate cancer [161]. Chrysin induced

Table 4.1 Research-based detailed evidence (preclinical and clinical studies) on polyphenols in cancer chemoprevention

S. no.	Cancer type	Target/factor involvement	Study type	Dose, route, and duration	Action	Key finding	References
1.	*Resveratrol*						
	Squamous cell carcinoma	• Apoptosis-related factors, • p53, ERK	In vivo	10, 20, 40μg i.p. for 14 days	• ⊥ and upgrades p53 protein • mRNA expression and ↓ SVV protein • ↑Tumor cell apoptosis.	• Xenograft volume↓ • Free radical scavenging Incidence↓ • Number of tumors per mouse↓	[158]
	Breast cancer	• p21Waf1/Cip1	In vivo	40 mg/kg/day orally for 30 days	• Increase the level of P21 • ⊥ LP-BER	• Tumor volume↓	[159]
	Prostate cancer	• VEGF, VEGFR2 • FOXO (Forkhead box O) transcription factors	In vivo	30 mg/kg/day Thrice/week for 6 weeks	• ↑apoptosis-inducing potential of TRAIL in PC-3 • ↑ caspase-3 activity and apoptosis	• Tumor volume↓ • Apoptosis↑ • Cell proliferation↓ • Number of blood vessels↓	[160]
		• MTA1 signaling	In vivo	50 mg/kg/day i.p. daily 14 days after implantation for 6 weeks	• Anti-inflammatory • Regulation of multiple and diverse molecular targets • Cell cycle arrest and apoptosis • ⊥ Angiogenesis	• Tumor growth↓ • Progression, local invasion↓ • metastasis↓ • Angiogenesis↓ • Apoptosis↑	[161]
	Lung Cancer	• Apoptosis signaling cascades	In vivo	15, 30, or 60 mg/kg i.v. daily for 15 days	• Alter ROS-dependent apoptosis pathway	• Tumor volume↓	[162]

	Colon cancer	• Apoptosis pathway	In vivo	45µg/kg/day orally for 60 days	• Alters cell cycle profiles • Induces apoptosis • ⊥ the growth of colon adenocarcinoma	• Colon adenomas number ↓ • Dysplasia occurrence↓	[163]
	Liver Cancer (Hepatocellular carcinoma)	• Glutathione (GSH) activity • glutathione S-transferase (GST)-induced DNA damage	In vivo	50, 100, 300 mg/kg for 20 weeks	• ⊥ of cell proliferation • Cardiotonic	• Tumor growth↓ • Apoptosis↑, Bcl2↓; Bax↑ • Cell proliferation↓	[164]
	Colorectal cancer	• Inflammatory signaling cascades	Clinical trial	0.5–5.0 g for 29 days	• ⊥ Proliferation of preneoplastic or malignant cells • Ameliorated formation of aberrant crypt foci and/or adenocarcinoma	• Reduction of Ki-67 levels in cancerous and normal tissue by 5 and 7%, respectively.	[165]
	Benign prostate hyperplasia	• Circulating Androgen Precursors	Clinical trial	150 mg or 1000 mg, daily for 4 months	• ⊥ 17, 20 lyase activity of the CYP17A1 enzyme in human adrenocortical carcinoma cells • ↓ androgen receptor expression (genetic and protein level)	• ↓serum levels of androgens • No changes in prostate tumor growth.	[166]

(continued)

Table 4.1 (continued)

S. no.	Cancer type	Target/factor involvement	Study type	Dose, route, and duration	Action	Key finding	References
2.	*Curcumin*						
	Prostate cancer	• Free radicals • Glutathione S-transferases • Glutathione peroxidase • Superoxide dismutases	Pilot Clinical Trial	3 g of curcumin (as 6, 500 mg capsules, 2 capsules with each meal)	• ↓ Deleterious effects induced by ionizing radiation • ↑ Antioxidant status, ↓ lipid peroxidation • ↑ Glutathione S-transferases	• ↓ severity of radiotherapy-related urinary symptoms, which are of the most common side effects of radiation therapy	[50]
	Solid tumors	• Plasma free radical • Pro-inflammatory transcription factors • Kinases	RCT	500 mg, three times a day for 60 days	• ⊥ Carcinogenesis • Block of signal transduction pathways associated with the development of cancer • Functional and genomic ⊥ of enzymes generating ROS and inflammatory lipids	• Curcumin reduced side effects seen after the radiotherapy	[167]
	Advanced and metastatic breast cancer	• Vascular endothelial growth factor • Tumor markers	Phase trial study	500–600 mg for 16 months	• Antioxidant and antiproliferative activities • ⊥ Tumor initiation and promotion against carcinogenesis	• ↓ concentration of the CEA marker tumor.	[51]
	Colorectal cancer	• Chemokine ligand 1 (CXCL1)	Randomized Phase Trial	2 g per day for 291 days	• ↓ Aberrant crypt foci • ↓Inflammatory mediators • ↓Cellular	• Curcumin was safe and tolerable in patients with	[168]

					proliferation • ↓Angiogenesis • ↓ metastatic spread • ↑Cell cycle arrest and apoptosis	metastatic colorectal cancer	
		• HCT-8/5-Fu cells • Erythroid 2-related factor (Nrf2)	In vivo	10μM		• Curcumin enhances the chemosensitivity • Down regulates the expression ratio of Bax/Bcl-2 • Repressed the mRNA and protein expression levels of Nrf2	[169]
		• SIRT1	Preclinical study	Dose range	• ↓Xenograft tumor growth • ⊥ Migration and growth of HCT-116 cells	• Facilitates proteasomal degradation of oncogenic SIRT1 • Covalent modification of SIRT1 at the cysteine 67 residue	[170]
	Human gastric cancer	• Human gastric cancer cells (hGCCs	In vitro	10μM, 20μM	• ⊥ Proliferation, Colony Formation, and Migration of hGCCs • ↑ROS levels and triggers mitochondrial damage, DNA damage, and apoptosis of hGCCs	• Prooxidative effects of curcumin facilitate oxidative stress, ↑ DNA damage, ↑ DNA demethylation of hGCCs	[171]
	Small cell lung cancer	• JAK/STAT pathway	In vitro	15μmol/L for 24, 48, 72 h	• Proliferation inhibition in human small cell lung cancer	• ⊥ STAT3 phosphorylation • ↓ STAT3	[172]

(continued)

Table 4.1 (continued)

S. no.	Cancer type	Target/factor involvement	Study type	Dose, route, and duration	Action	Key finding	References
					cells (NCI-H446 and NCI-1688)	downstream gene expression	
3.	*Epigallocatechin-3-gallate (EGCG)*						
	Human Pancreatic Cancer	• JAK1, JAK2, JAK3 • STAT3	In vitro	0, 20, 40, 60 mM for 48 h	• ↓Cancer progression in human pancreatic cells (AsPC-1 and PANC-1), breast cancer (T47D), head and neck cancer (YCU-H861)	• ⊥ viability, invasion, and migration • ↑apoptosis in pancreatic cancer cells. • ⊥ STAT3 • ↓ STAT3-target genes.	[173]
	Prostate cancer	• PC-3ML cells	In vitro, In vivo	228 mg/kg or 200μmol/L	• ⊥ Mitochondrial membrane potential • ↑ Vesiculation of mitochondria • ↑ Elevated poly (ADP-ribose) polymerase (PARP) cleavage • ↑ apoptosis	• ↓ fibroblast growth • ↓ tumor cell viability • ⊥ expression of genes essential for invasion and metastases	[174]
		• Twist /VE-Cadherin/AKT Pathway	Preclinical	10, 20, and 40μM	• ⊥ Twist/VE-cadherin/AKT	• ↓ the nuclear localization of twist • ⊥ and suppress VM formation	[175]
	Neuroblastoma	• SH-SY5Y • SK-N-BE2	Preclinical	50 μM	• control growth of human malignant neuroblastoma	• ↓cell survival • ↓expression of VEGFR-2	[176]

					SH-SY5Y and SK-N-BE2 cells	• ⊥ cell migration • ↑ cell cycle arrest	
	Bladder urothelial carcinoma	• Glucose-Regulated Protein (GRP) 78	Preclinical	10, 20, 33.3, and 40μM	• Binds to GRP78 and ⊥ its function • ↑apoptosis in NTUB1 and T24 cells	• ↓ ER chaperone GRP78 • ⊥ GRP78	[177]
	Breast cancer	• GRP78 • JNK	in vivo, in vitro	30 mg/kg, i.p	• ↑ 4T1 cells apoptosis • ⊥ Tumor growth	• ↑ JNK phosphorylation and cell death	[178]
	Hepatocellular carcinoma	• Human carbonyl reductase 1 (CBR1)	Preclinical	0.08, 0.16, 0.32, 0.63, 1.25, 2.5, and 5lM	• Chemopreventive • Anticarcinogenic	• ⊥ CBR1 activity • ⊥ CBR1-mediated tumor resistance to DNR (daunorubicin)	[179]
4.	*Apigenin*						
	Colon cancer	• STAT3	Clinical	0, 5, 15, and 50μM	• ↑Cleavage of PARP • ↑apoptosis	• ↓ Bcl-xL and Mcl-1 • ⊥ STAT3	[180]
	Cervical cancer	• PTEN/PI3K/AKT pathway		47.26μM at 48 h	• ↑ Cell apoptosis • ↑Cell cycle arrest • ↑ Mitochondrial • ↑ Death receptor	• ⊥ Hela cell migration • ↓MMP2/9	[181]
	Triple-negative breast cancer	• hnRNPA2 (Heterogeneous ribonuclear protein A2/B1)	In vivo	50μM	• Regulate the expression of DNR-selective efflux transporters.	• Regulates expression of ABCC4 and ABCG2	[182]
	Ovarian cancer	• SKOV3/DDP	In vitro	50μM	• ↓ Mitochondrial transmembrane potential • ↑ Ratios of cleaved caspase-3/caspase-3 and Bax/Bcl-2	• ↓ Apoptosis • ⊥ Transcription and translation of Mcl-1 in SKOV3 and SKOV3/DDP	[183]

(continued)

Table 4.1 (continued)

S. no.	Cancer type	Target/factor involvement	Study type	Dose, route, and duration	Action	Key finding	References
	Breast Cancer	• Akt/FOXM1	Preclinical	10μM	• ⊥ Growth of BC cells • ⊥ Growth xenograft tumors in hormone receptor-positive BC • ⊥Expression of mucin 1 C-terminal subunit oncoprotein	• ⊥ Expression of FOXM1 • ↓ Proliferation of MCF-7/Akt cells	[184]
5.	*Silibinin*						
	Breast cancer	• MDA-MB-231 • Mitochondrial fusion	Preclinical	30–90μM	• ↑ Expression of epithelial marker, E-cadherin • ↓ Expression of mesenchymal markers, N-cadherin and vimentin	• ⊥ Epithelial to mesenchymal transition (EMT) of MDA-MB-231 • ↓ Migration and invasion of the MDA-MB-231 breast cancer cells	[185]
		• hTERT and cyclin D1 genes		10–150μM	• ⊥ Cell proliferation	• ⊥ growth of T47D cells • ⊥ hTERT and Cyclin D1 genes	[186]
		• STAT3 • ERK		50–600μM	• ↑ BAX • ↓ Survivin, Bcl2	• ↓ STAT3 • ↓ERK • ↓survivin in MDAMB435 cells	[187]
	Lung Cancer	• hTERT gene	In vitro, In vivo	5–150μM	• ↓ Progression, angiogenesis, and tumor growth	• ⊥ growth of A549 • ⊥ hTERT gene expression	[188]
	Ovarian cancer		Preclinical				[189]

		• P53 • P21 • β-actin		50μM, 100μM, 200μM	• Affect apoptotic genes	• ⊥ Inhibits cell proliferation in SKOV-3 cells	
	Urinary bladder tumors (urothelial cell carcinoma)	• PI3K/AKT/FRAP-mTOR pathway	Preclinical	100, 115, 130, 150, 200, and 250μM for 48 h	• ⊥ Cell proliferation • ↑ DNA damage of cancer cells	• ↓ FRAP/mTOR • ↓FGFR3 • ↓DNMT1 • ↓AKT2 genes and miR100	[190]
6.	*Luteolin*						
	Breast cancer	• Estrogen receptor (ER) • Progesterone receptor (PR) • Human epidermal growth factor receptor (HER2/neu)	In vivo, In vitro	10 or 20 mg/kg, i.p.	• Disrupt the growth and migration of TNBC cells	• ↓ TNBC cell viability • ⊥ metastasis into lung	[191]
		• T47-D and BT-474 cells • VEGF	In vitro, In vivo	20 mg/kg, i.p. and 1–100μM	• ⊥ Angiogenesis • Restricts conversion of breast cancer cells → stem cell-like cells	• ⊥ Progestin-dependent human breast cancer tumor growth • ⊥ Stem cell-like phenotype in human breast cancer cells	[192]
	Colon cancer	• JNK and p38 MAPK	Preclinical	50μg/ml	• ↓ Mitochondrial membrane action potential • ↑ Mitochondrial Ca2+ level • ↑ Bax, ↓ Bcl-2, ↑release of cytochrome c	• ↑Apoptosis • ↑MAPK signaling	[193]

(continued)

Table 4.1 (continued)

S. no.	Cancer type	Target/factor involvement	Study type	Dose, route, and duration	Action	Key finding	References
		• Nrf2 • p53	Preclinical	30µM	• ↑Apoptosis • ↑ DNA demethylation	• ↑ Nrf2 transcription • ↑Interaction between Nrf2 and p53	[194]
	Colorectal cancer	• miR-384/ pleiotrophin	In vitro, In vivo	100 mg/kg every 2 days for 30 days	• ⊥ Cells migration and invasion • ⊥ Metastasis	• Chemoprotective nature of luteolin is partially mediated by miR-384/PTN axis	[195]
	Ovarian cancer	Mitochondrial membrane potential • MMP2 • MMP9	In vitro	5, 10, 15µg/ml 50 mg/kg	• ⊥ Cellular proliferation and migration	• ⊥ Expression of MMPs • ⊥ Metastasis	[196]
7.	*Genistein*						
	Prostate Cancer	• ZEB1	In vitro	40µM daily for 7 days	• Alters the expression of various miRNA	• Demethylation of specific CpG sites in its promoter • ↑miR-200c expression in PCa cells	[197]
		• sFRP1 • Smad4	In vitro and in vivo	25µM for 4 days	• Anti-invasion • Anti-proliferation • Pro-apoptotic • Modulate cell cycle	• ↑ miRNA-1260b expression • ↑ expression of sFRP1 and Smad4 • ↓ H3K9-me2, H3K9-me3 and H3K27-me3 level	[198]
	Breast cancer	• FOXO3, PTEN, casein kinase, and p27	Preclinical	10, 25, and 50µM	• Cell cycle arrest • Apoptosis	• ↓ miR-155	[199]
		• Hep2	Preclinical	100µM			[200]

	Human Laryngeal cancer				• Alter cellular miRNA expression	• ↑Hep2 cell apoptosis • ↑miR-1469 expression	
	Kidney cancer	• HOX transcript antisense RNA (HOTAIR)	Preclinical	10 and 25μM	• ↓Cell proliferation and migration	• ↓ EED levels in PRC2 • ⊥ HOTAIR/PRC2 interaction	[201]
	Cervical cancer	• DNA methyltransferases (DNMTs) • Histone deacetylases (HDACs)	Preclinical	15μM for 24, 48, 72, and 96 h	• Regulates cell growth by ⊥ tyrosine kinase, angiogenesis • Antioxidant	• ↓expression and enzymatic activity of DNMTs and HDACs	[52]
	Colorectal cancer	• MCL1, KDR, and APP	Preclinical in vivo	20, 40, 80 mg/kg	• Antioxidation • Cyto-protection • Anti-neoplastic	• ↓MCL1, KDR, and APP positive cells	[202]
8.	*Quercetin*						
	Gastric cancer	• GSK-3β/β-catenin	In vitro, In vivo	6.25–100μM, 20 mg/kg BW	• Reduced cell viability • Increase apoptosis • Modulate angiogenesis-associated and EMT-related factors.	• Ameliorate p-GSK-3βSer9 and β-catenin protein expression levels • ↓ tumor VEGF-R and VEGF-A • ↓COX-2 gene expression	[203]
	Breast Cancer	• Akt-mTOR	In vitro, In vivo	0–100μM 50 g/kg BW	• ↑ Autophagy, • ↓ Migration rate and ↓ MMP-2, MMP-9 • ↓ Glucose uptake, lactate production	• ↑AKT, mTOR, and p70-S6K • ↓VEGF, PKM2, and p-AKT level	[204]
	Ovarian cancer	• p-STAT3	In vivo	80 mg/kg twice a week	• ↑ Protective autophagy		[205]

(continued)

Table 4.1 (continued)

S. no.	Cancer type	Target/factor involvement	Study type	Dose, route, and duration	Action	Key finding	References
					• ↑ Apoptosis • ↑ ER stress •	• Activate p-STAT3/ Bcl2 axis •	
		• Apoptosis • Intrinsic pathway • PA-1 cells	In vitro	0–200μM for 24 h	• ↓ Viability • ↑ Apoptosis • ↓ Bcl-2 and Bcl-xL • ↑ caspase-3, caspase-p, Bid, Bad, Bax, cytochrome c	• ⊥ Growth of PA-1 cells • Modulate intrinsic apoptotic pathway	[206]
	Colon cancer	• ERK	In vitro	15μM	• Induction of autophagy	• ↑ERK phosphorylation and activation	[207]
	Prostate cancer	• hnRNPA1	In vivo	0, 2.5, 5, 10, 20, or 50μM	• Antagonizes androgen receptor signaling • Desensitizes enzalutamide-resistant prostate cancer cells	• ↓ hnRNPA1 expression • ↓ Expression of AR-V7	[208]
9.	*Chalcones*						
	Breast cancer	• p53	In vitro	Dose range	• ↑ apoptosis • Antiproliferative • ↑ p53 expression in ER-positive cells (MCF-7 line	• ↑ p53 protein expression • No effect on Sp1 protein expression	[209]
		• Microtubule cytoskeleton	Preclinical	Dose range	• Prolong mitotic arrest at the spindle assembly checkpoint (SAC)	• Target colchicine-binding pocket and kill MDR1- and	[210]

						MRP1-overexpressing tumor cells	
	Human urinary bladder, cervical, and breast cancer	• Topoisomerase IIα	In silico, in vitro	–	• Topoisomerase inhibition	• Inhibitory activity against hTopoIIa-ATPase • Interact with ATP-binding pocket residue	[211]
10.	*Chrysin/5,7-Dihydroxyflavone*						
	Skin cancer	• Apoptosis signaling cascades	In vitro	50μg/mL	• Promote apoptotic death, act via caspase • Nuclear fragmentation and cell cycle arrest	• ⊥ Human epidermoid carcinoma (A431) cells	[58]
	Lung cancer	• Apoptosis signaling cascades	In vitro, In vivo	Dose range (500, 250, 125, 62.5, 31.25, and 15.62 mg/kg), i. p.	• Induce cytotoxicity	• ↑ Cell growth arrest • ↑Apoptosis and ER stress • ⊥ The activation of signal transducer and ↑ transcription 3	[212]
	Prostate cancer	• PI3K-AKT • MAPK • ERK1/2	In vitro	Dose range (0, 5, 10, 20, 50, and 100μM)	• Initiates cell death • ↑ Mitochondrial-mediated apoptosis • ↑ ER stress and regulation of signaling pathways	• ↓ PI3K-AKT, P70S6K, S6 and P90RSK proteins • ↑ MAPK • ↑ ERK1/2 and • P38 proteins	[213]
	Gastric cancer	• miR-22 • miR-34a • miR-126	In vitro	Dose range (0–160μM)	• Anti-inflammatory • Antioxidant • ↑ apoptosis	• ↑ Expression of miR-22, miR-34a, and miR-126 gene	[214]
	Ovarian cancer	• MAPK and PI3K/AKT pathways	In vitro		• Stimulate apoptosis • Cause mitochondrial	• ↓ Proliferation of ES2 and OV90 cells	[215]

(continued)

Table 4.1 (continued)

S. no.	Cancer type	Target/factor involvement	Study type	Dose, route, and duration	Action	Key finding	References
				Dose range (5, 10, 20, 50, and 100μM)	dysfunction, ROS generation, • ↓ Intracellular Ca^{2+} concentration	• ↓ PCNA protein expression • ↑MAPK and PI3K/AKT	
11.	*Casticin*						
	Gallbladder cancer	• p27 • cyclinD1 • Protein kinase B	In vitro, In vivo	0.1, 0.5, 1, 4, 7μM for 24, 48, or 72 h	• ↑ Bax, cleaved caspase-3, cleaved caspase-9, and cleaved poly ADP-ribose polymerase expression • ↓ Bcl-2 expression	• ↑ G0/G1 arrest • ↑ Mitochondrial-related apoptosis • ↑ p27 • ↓ CyclinD1/cyclin-dependent kinase4 and phosphorylated protein kinase B	[216]
	Prostate cancer	• Ras/Akt/NF-κB	In vitro	Dose range (0, 1.25, 2.5, 5, 10, 20, 40, and 50 μM)	• ↓ Cell mobility, suppressed cell migration and invasion, and reduced cell gelatinolytic activities	• ↓ Metastatic effect • ↓ Viable cell number • ⊥ Migration, invasion, and adhesion • ↓ Matrix metalloproteinases activity on human prostate DU 145 cells • ↓GRB2, SOS-1, Ras, MEK-1, p-ERK1/2, and p-JNK1/2	[217]
	Bladder cancer	• p-ATM • p-ATR • BRCA1	In vitro	Dose range (0, 0.5, 1, 2.5, 5, and 10μM)	• ↓ Viability of cells and ↑ DNA damage	• ↓ Expression of p-ATM, p-ATR, MDC1, and MGMT	[112]

		• MDC1 • MGMT				levels • ↑ p-ATR and MGMT levels • ↑ p-p53, p-H2A.X, and PARP levels. • Affect translocation of DNA-PKcs and p-p53	
	Oral cancer	• Mitochondria-dependent pathways	In vitro	Dose range (0, 0.25, 0.5, 1, 2.5, and 5μM)	• ↑ Cell morphological changes, DNA condensation, and damage • ↓ The total viable cells	• ↑ G2/M phase arrest in SCC-4 cells • ↑ ROS and Ca21 productions • ↑ caspase-3, -8, and -9 activities in SCC-4 cells	[218]
	Lung cancer	• p-H2A.X, PARPp, H2A.X, MDC1, DNA-PKcs, MGMT, p-ATM, p-ATR, and BRCA1	In vitro	Dose range (0, 10, 20, 30, 40, and 50μM)	• ↓ Cell number through DNA damage and condensation • ↑ Expressions and nuclear translocation of p-H2AX in A549 cells	• ↑ PARPp, H2A.X, MDC1, DNA-PKcs, and MGMT at different intervals • ↑ p-ATM, p-ATR, and BRCA1 at 6–24 h treatment but ↓ the same at 24–48 h treatment • ↓p-p53 at 6–24 h but ↑ at 48 h	[113]

(continued)

Table 4.1 (continued)

S. no.	Cancer type	Target/factor involvement	Study type	Dose, route, and duration	Action	Key finding	References
12.	*Cardamonin*						
	Breast cancer	• mTOR/p70S6K	In vitro In vivo	5, 10, 20, and 40 μM 3 mg/kg	• Repress mTOR/p70S6K pathway	• ⊥ Expression of HIF-1α at mRNA and protein levels • ↑ Mitochondrial oxidative phosphorylation • ↑ Induced reactive oxygen species (ROS) accumulation • ⊥ Nrf2-dependent ROS scavenging system	[59]
	Gastric cancer	• Wnt/β-catenin	In vivo In vitro	0, 5, 10, and 20μM 25 mg/kg	• ↑ Chemosensitivity of 5-FU in GC cells via suppression of Wnt/β-catenin signaling pathway	• ↑ Apoptosis and cell cycle arrest of BGC-823/5-FU • ↓ Expression levels of P-glycoprotein, β-catenin, and TCF4 • Disrupt formation of β-catenin/TCF4 complex	[140]
	Lung cancer	• PI3K/Akt/mTOR	In vitro, In vivo	Dose range (0, 5, 10, 20, and 40μmol/l) 5.0 mg/kg	• ↑ Apoptosis, activate caspase-3, upregulate Bax, downregulate Bcl-2. • Suppress cell	• Arrested cells in G2/M phase • ⊥ expression levels of cyclin D1/CDK4 • Reduce PI3K-Akt-mTOR	[219]

					migration and invasion	phosphorylation • Retard tumor growth	
	Ovarian Cancer	• mTOR pathway • Anti-apoptotic proteins	In vitro	20 µM	• ⊥ proliferation • Suppress expression of anti-apoptotic proteins	• ↓ expression of B cell lymphoma-2, X-linked inhibitor of apoptosis protein and Survivin • Activate mTOR	[220]
	Colorectal cancer	• NF-kB signaling • MicroRNA expression	In vivo In vitro	10 mg/kg, 10, 20µM	• ⊥ Tumor incidence, tumor multiplicity, Ki-67, and β-catenin positive cells • Regulate replication stress and chromosomal stability	• ↓ NF-κB translocation • Restore RNF20 expression • Restore Mex3 C expression • ↑ p38 and JNK	
13.	*Formononetin*						
	Gastric cancer	• AKT/mTOR • Wnt/β-Catenin	In vitro In vivo	Dose range (0.1µM, 0.4µM, 0.8µM, 1µM, 2.5µM, and 3µM)	• Act on Wnt/β-Catenin and AKT/mTOR pathways • Promote cellular growth and proliferation	• ⊥ Migration against SGC7901 tumor cells	[141]
	Bladder cancer	• PTEN, p-Akt	In vitro	50, 100, 200µM	• ↑Apoptosis and lower invasiveness	• ⊥ The proliferation of T24 cells • ↓ miR-21 expression • ↑ PTEN and ↓ p-Akt	[222]
	Breast cancer	• p-ERK1/2	In vitro	40µM and 80µM	• Antioxidant • Antitumor • ⊥ Proliferation of	• ⊥ Proliferation and ↑ Apoptosis in MCF-7 cells • ↓ bcl-2 mRNA	[223]

(continued)

Table 4.1 (continued)

S. no.	Cancer type	Target/factor involvement	Study type	Dose, route, and duration	Action	Key finding	References
					ER-positive human breast cancer	expression • ↓ protein expression of bcl-2 • ↓ p-ERK1/2	
	Cervical cancer	• HIF-1α and VEGF	In vivo	10 mg/kg	• ↑Apoptosis • Antitumor effect	• ⊥ Expression levels of HIF-1α and VEGF • ↓ mRNA levels of HIF-1α and VEGF	[224]
	Lung cancer	• EGFR-Akt-Mcl-1	In vitro In vivo	0–10 μM 10 mg/kg	• Antitumor effect • ↓ Tumor growth	• Suppress EGFR signaling • ↓ The protein level of Mcl-1	[225]
14	*Ascochlorin*						
	Brain tumors (glioblastomas)	• FAK • JAK-STAT	In vitro	1, 5, 10, 25, 50μM for 24 h	• ⊥ Cell migration • Invade U373MG and A172 cancer cells	• ⊥ MMP-9 expression and MMP-2 gelatinolytic action • ⊥ JAK2/STAT3 phosphorylation • ⊥ nuclear translocation of STAT3	[226]
	Tumor growth	• ERK /c-Myc	In vitro	10 μM	• Induce G1 arrest • ⊥ Tumor growth	• Repression of ERK phosphorylation and c-Myc expression • ↓ c-Myc protein expression	[227]
15.	*Bergamottin*						
		• STAT3	In vitro	100μM			[228]

	Multiple myeloma				• ↑ Substantial apoptosis at sub-G1 stage	• ↓ Expression of STAT3-regulated gene factors like COX-2, VEGF, cyclin D1, survivin, IAP-1, Bcl-2, and Bcl-xl	
	Colon cancer	• Ras/Raf/ERK	In vivo	15, 30, and 60 mg/kg	• Antiproliferative • ↑Apoptosis • Cell cycle arrest	• Block Raf/MEK/ERK signaling cascade.	[229]
	Pancreatic cancer	• Akt/mTOR • PANC-1	Preclinical	6.25, 12.5, 25 μM	• Antitumor effect	• ↑ Apoptosis, cell cycle arrest, and ⊥ of cell migration and invasion. • ⊥ PANC-1 cell migration and colony formation • ⊥ Akt/mTOR	[230]
16.	*Capillarisin*						
	Tumors	• STAT3 • *SHP*-1 and *SHP*-2 tyrosine phosphatases	Preclinical *study*	Not mentioned	• ↓ Growth and *metastasis in human* multiple myeloma cells • ↑ Apoptosis • ↓ Expression level of various STAT3-regulated proteins	• ⊥ STAT3 activation *at tyrosine 705 and its* phosphorylation • ⊥ Activation of JAK1, JAK2, and c-Src kinase •	[231]
	Prostate cancer	• STAT3 or IL-6-inducible STAT3	In vitro	10, 50, 100, 200μmol/L	• Cell cycle arrest at the G0/G1 phase • block migration and invasion of DU145 cells	• ⊥ Androgen-independent DU145 and androgen-dependent LNCaP cell growth	[232]

(continued)

Table 4.1 (continued)

S. no.	Cancer type	Target/factor involvement	Study type	Dose, route, and duration	Action	Key finding	References
						• ↑ p21 and p27 • ↓ expression of cyclin D1, cyclin A, and cyclin B • ↓ protein expression of survivin, MMP-2, and MMP-9 • ⊥ protein levels of phospho-STAT3 but not STAT3	
17.	*Bavachin*						
	Multiple myeloma	• NF-κB • STAT3	Preclinical study	10μM	• ↑cytotoxicity in multiple myeloma cell line • ↑ apoptosis • ⊥ NF-κB, expression levels of Bcl-2	• ⊥ STAT3 activation and Phosphorylation	[233]
	Placental choriocarcinoma	• Placental mitochondria factors	In vitro	12μM	• ↑ apoptosis and caspase activation • ↑ calcium overload and ER stress activation	• Suppress placental choriocarcinoma cells • ↑ MMP depolarization and mitochondrial dysfunction • ↓ ETC complexes lead to ↓ OXPHOS and glycolytic capacity in choriocarcinoma cells	[234]

(↓: downregulated/decrease; ↑: upregulated/increase; ⊥ inhibition) apoptosis and suppressed cells during the sub-G1 phase of the cell cycle and decreased proliferation in both prostate cancer cells. Chrysin inactivated the PI3K/AKT pathway and stimulated the ERK1/2 MAPK and P38 MAPK pathways, which led to the apoptosis of DU145 and PC-3 cells. Chrysin has the potential to be a therapeutic agent for human prostate cancer cells [213]. Basic chalcones 11 and 17 were antiproliferative agents that inhibited the growth of human breast cancer cells by activating the intestinal apoptotic pathway. Chalcones induced apoptosis in ER-positive cells by increasing p53 expression (MCF-7 line).

4.5 Conclusion and Future Perspectives

Based on the evidence provided in this study, the conclusion is that polyphenols play an important role in carcinogenesis by upregulating and downregulating various cancer-related mechanistic pathways. Apoptosis is induced by dietary polyphenols, which prevent the production of premalignant and cancer cells and suppress tumor growth by stopping cell cycle phases, cytokine levels, and cellular oxidative stress. Polyphenols derived from natural products are currently at the forefront of drug research and development due to the potential for many of these compounds to interfere with cancer development at different stages.

The positive effects of polyphenols have been reported and published in numerous in vitro and animal studies. While several polyphenols are shown to have beneficial effects on various signaling pathways, further research is needed to validate polyphenols' anticancer mechanisms. In addition, more research must be performed on the therapeutic effect of dietary polyphenols on cancer risk in relation to the anticancer function of multiple polyphenols and their mechanisms of action. Furthermore, promising new drugs with a specific target pathway involved in cancer pathogenesis and dosage can be engineered using polyphenols as a good replacement and supplementary resource in cancer care and potential future sources for drug development and research.

Acknowledgments The authors express their gratitude to Chairman, Mr. Parveen Garg and Director, Dr. G. D. Gupta, ISF College of Pharmacy, Moga (Punjab), India, for their great vision and support.

Disclosure of Potential Conflicts of Interest The authors declare that they have no competing interests.

Authors' Contributions All data were generated in-house, and no paper mill was used. All authors agree to be accountable for all aspects of work, ensuring integrity and accuracy.

References

1. Forni C, Facchiano F, Bartoli M, Pieretti S, Facchiano A, D'Arcangelo D, Norelli S, Valle G, Nisini R, Beninati S, Tabolacci C. Beneficial role of phytochemicals on oxidative stress and age-related diseases. Biomed Res Int. 2019;2019:8748253.
2. Piwowarczyk L, Stawny M, Mlynarczyk DT, Muszalska-Kolos I, Goslinski T, Jelińska A. Role of curcumin and (−)-epigallocatechin-3-O-gallate in bladder cancer treatment: a review. Cancer. 2020;12(7):1801.
3. Williams SA, Anderson WC, Santaguida MT, Dylla SJ. Patient-derived xenografts, the cancer stem cell paradigm, and cancer pathobiology in the 21st century. Lab Invest. 2013;93 (9):970–82.
4. Lall RK, Syed DN, Adhami VM, Khan MI, Mukhtar H. Dietary polyphenols in prevention and treatment of prostate cancer. Int J Mol Sci. 2015;16(2):3350–76.
5. Khan N, Afaq F, Saleem M, Ahmad N, Mukhtar H. Targeting multiple signaling pathways by green tea polyphenol (−)-epigallocatechin-3-gallate. Cancer Res. 2006;66(5):2500–5.
6. Cartea ME, Francisco M, Soengas P, Velasco P. Phenolic compounds in Brassica vegetables. Molecules. 2011;16(1):251–80.
7. Arfaoui L. Dietary plant polyphenols: effects of food processing on their content and bioavailability. Molecules (Basel, Switzerland). 2021;26(10):2959. https://doi.org/10.3390/molecules26102959.
8. Pandey KB, Rizvi SI. Plant polyphenols as dietary antioxidants in human health and disease. Oxid Med Cell Longev. 2009;2(5):270–8.
9. Tresserra-Rimbau A, Lamuela-Raventos RM, Moreno JJ. Polyphenols, food and pharma. Current knowledge and directions for future research. Biochem Pharmacol. 2018;156:186–95.
10. Miyata Y, Shida Y, Hakariya T, Sakai H. Anti-cancer effects of green tea polyphenols against prostate cancer. Molecules. 2019;24(1):193.
11. Nakada M, Kita D, Watanabe T, Hayashi Y, Teng L, Pyko IV, Hamada JI. Aberrant signaling pathways in glioma. Cancer. 2011;3(3):3242–78.
12. Syed V. TGF-β Signaling in Cancer. J Cell Biochem. 2016;117(6):1279–87.
13. Sedgwick AE, D'Souza-Schorey C. Wnt signaling in cell motility and invasion: drawing parallels between development and cancer. Cancer. 2016;8(9):80.
14. Millimouno FM, Dong J, Yang L, Li J, Li X. Targeting apoptosis pathways in cancer and perspectives with natural compounds from mother nature. Cancer Prev Res. 2014;7 (11):1081–107.
15. Singh BN, Shankar S, Srivastava RK. Green tea catechin, epigallocatechin-3-gallate (EGCG): mechanisms, perspectives and clinical applications. Biochem Pharmacol. 2011;82 (12):1807–21.
16. Kang NJ, Shin SH, Lee HJ, Lee KW. Polyphenols as small molecular inhibitors of signaling cascades in carcinogenesis. Pharmacol Ther. 2011;130(3):310–24.
17. Neergheen VS, Bahorun T, Taylor EW, Jen LS, Aruoma OI. Targeting specific cell signaling transduction pathways by dietary and medicinal phytochemicals in cancer chemoprevention. Toxicology. 2010;278(2):229–41.
18. Aguilera Y, Martin-Cabrejas MA, de Mejia EG. Phenolic compounds in fruits and beverages consumed as part of the mediterranean diet: their role in prevention of chronic diseases. Phytochem Rev. 2016;15(3):405–23.
19. Durazzo A, Lucarini M, Souto EB, Cicala C, Caiazzo E, Izzo AA, Novellino E, Santini A. Polyphenols: A concise overview on the chemistry, occurrence, and human health. Phytother Res. 2019;33(9):2221–43.
20. Rajput M, Dwivedi L, Sabarwal A, Singh RP. The biology of aging and cancer: a complex association. In: Models, molecules and mechanisms in biogerontology. Singapore: Springer; 2020. p. 465–97.
21. Duronio RJ, Xiong Y. Signaling pathways that control cell proliferation. Cold Spring Harb Perspect Biol. 2013;5(3):a008904.

22. Kedhari Sundaram M, Raina R, Afroze N, Bajbouj K, Hamad M, Haque S, Hussain A. Quercetin modulates signaling pathways and induces apoptosis in cervical cancer cells. Biosci Rep. 2019;30:39(8).
23. Li Y, Go VL, Sarkar FH. The role of nutraceuticals in pancreatic cancer prevention and therapy: targeting cellular signaling, miRNAs and epigenome. Pancreas. 2015;44(1):1.
24. Szliszka E, Krol W. The role of dietary polyphenols in tumor necrosis factor-related apoptosis inducing ligand (TRAIL)-induced apoptosis for cancer chemoprevention. Eur J Cancer Prev. 2011;20(1):63–9.
25. Ramos S. Cancer chemoprevention and chemotherapy: Dietary polyphenols and signalling pathways. Mol Nutr Food Res. 2008;52(5):507–26.
26. Alam MN, Almoyad M, Huq F. Polyphenols in colorectal cancer: current state of knowledge including clinical trials and molecular mechanism of action. Biomed Res Int. 2018;2018:4154185.
27. Li AN, Li S, Zhang YJ, Xu XR, Chen YM, Li HB. Resources and biological activities of natural polyphenols. Nutrients. 2014;6(12):6020–47.
28. Zhang H, Tsao R. Dietary polyphenols, oxidative stress and antioxidant and anti-inflammatory effects. Curr Opin Food Sci. 2016;8:33–42.
29. Otles S, Nakilcioglu E. Determination of phenolic compounds (gallic, caffeic, ferulic, and p-coumaric acids). Flow Inj Anal of Food Addit. 2015;1:393.
30. Tsao R. Chemistry and biochemistry of dietary polyphenols. Nutrients. 2010;2(12):1231–46.
31. Singla RK, Dubey AK, Garg A, Sharma RK, Fiorino M, Ameen SM, Haddad MA, Al-Hiary M. Natural polyphenols: chemical classification, definition of classes, subcategories, and structures. J AOAC Int. 2019;102(5):1397–400.
32. Kumar N, Goel N. Phenolic acids: natural versatile molecules with promising therapeutic applications. Biotechnol Rep. 2019;24:e00370.
33. Alan M, Aslanipour B. Anticancer properties of some effective phytochemicals. Drug development for cancer and diabetes: a path to 2030. London: Apple Academic Press; 2020. p. 59.
34. Kapinova A, Kubatka P, Golubnitschaja O, Kello M, Zubor P, Solar P, Pec M. Dietary phytochemicals in breast cancer research: anticancer effects and potential utility for effective chemoprevention. Environ Health Prev Med. 2018;23(1):1–8.
35. Wahle KW, Brown I, Rotondo D, Heys SD. Plant phenolics in the prevention and treatment of cancer. Bio-Farms for Nutraceuticals. 2010:36–51.
36. Multhoff G, Molls M, Radons J. Chronic inflammation in cancer development. Front Immunol. 2012;2:98.
37. Fantini M, Benvenuto M, Masuelli L, Frajese GV, Tresoldi I, Modesti A, Bei R. In vitro and in vivo antitumoral effects of combinations of polyphenols, or polyphenols and anticancer drugs: perspectives on cancer treatment. Int J Mol Sci. 2015;16(5):9236–82.
38. Sosa V, Moliné T, Somoza R, Paciucci R, Kondoh H, LLeonart ME. Oxidative stress and cancer: an overview. Ageing Res Rev. 2013;12(1):376–90.
39. Gloire G, Legrand-Poels S, Piette J. NF-κB activation by reactive oxygen species: fifteen years later. Biochem Pharmacol. 2006;72(11):1493–505.
40. McCubrey JA, LaHair MM, Franklin RA. Reactive oxygen species-induced activation of the MAP kinase signaling pathways. Antioxid Redox Signal. 2006;8(9-10):1775–89.
41. Lo YY, Wong JM, Cruz TF. Reactive oxygen species mediate cytokine activation of c-Jun NH2-terminal kinases. J Biol Chem. 1996;271(26):15703–7.
42. Clerkin JS, Naughton R, Quiney C, Cotter TG. Mechanisms of ROS modulated cell survival during carcinogenesis. Cancer Lett. 2008;266(1):30–6.
43. Reuter S, Gupta SC, Chaturvedi MM, Aggarwal BB. Oxidative stress, inflammation, and cancer: how are they linked? Free Radic Biol Med. 2010;49(11):1603–16.
44. Lobo V, Patil A, Phatak A, Chandra N. Free radicals, antioxidants and functional foods: Impact on human health. Pharmacogn Rev. 2010;4(8):118.

45. Gupta RK, Patel AK, Shah N, Choudhary AK, Jha UK, Yadav UC, Gupta PK, Pakuwal U. Oxidative stress and antioxidants in disease and cancer: a review. Asian Pac J Cancer Prev. 2014;15(11):4405–9.
46. Rodrigo R, Miranda A, Vergara L. Modulation of endogenous antioxidant system by wine polyphenols in human disease. Clin Chim Acta. 2011;412(5-6):410–24.
47. Chiva-Blanch G, Urpi-Sarda M, Llorach R, Rotches-Ribalta M, Guillen M, Casas R, Arranz S, Valderas-Martinez P, Portoles O, Corella D, Tinahones F. Differential effects of polyphenols and alcohol of red wine on the expression of adhesion molecules and inflammatory cytokines related to atherosclerosis: a randomized clinical trial. Am J Clin Nutr. 2012;95(2):326–34.
48. Lewandowska H, Kalinowska M, Lewandowski W, Stępkowski TM, Brzoska K. The role of natural polyphenols in cell signaling and cytoprotection against cancer development. J Nutr Biochem. 2016;32:1–9.
49. Niedzwiecki A, Roomi MW, Kalinovsky T, Rath M. Anticancer efficacy of polyphenols and their combinations. Nutrients. 2016;8(9):552.
50. Molana SH. A pilot clinical trial of radioprotective effects of curcumin supplementation in patients with prostate cancer. J Cancer Sci Ther. 2013;5(10):320–4.
51. Bayet-Robert M, Kwiatowski F, Leheurteur M, Gachon F, Planchat E, Abrial C, Mouret-Reynier MA, Durando X, Barthomeuf C, Chollet P. Phase I dose escalation trial of docetaxel plus curcumin in patients with advanced and metastatic breast cancer. Cancer Biol Ther. 2010;9(1):8–14.
52. Sundaram MK, Ansari MZ, Al Mutery A, Ashraf M, Nasab R, Rai S, Rais N, Hussain A. Genistein induces alterations of epigenetic modulatory signatures in human cervical cancer cells. Anticancer Agents Med Chem. 2018;18(3):412–21.
53. Seyfried TN, Flores RE, Poff AM, D'Agostino DP. Cancer as a metabolic disease: implications for novel therapeutics. Carcinogenesis. 2014;35(3):515–27.
54. Dimri M, Satyanarayana A. Molecular signaling pathways and therapeutic targets in hepatocellular carcinoma. Cancer. 2020;12(2):491.
55. Wu WK, Cho CH, Lee CW, Fan D, Wu K, Yu J, Sung JJ. Dysregulation of cellular signaling in gastric cancer. Cancer Lett. 2010;295(2):144–53.
56. Hirschey MD, DeBerardinis RJ, Diehl AM, Drew JE, Frezza C, Green MF, Jones LW, Ko YH, Le A, Lea MA, Locasale JW. Dysregulated metabolism contributes to oncogenesis. In: Seminars in cancer biology, vol. 35. Cambridge, MA: Academic Press; 2015. p. S129–50.
57. Wang H, Oo Khor T, Shu L, Su ZY, Fuentes F, Lee JH, Tony Kong AN. Plants vs. cancer: a review on natural phytochemicals in preventing and treating cancers and their druggability. Anticancer Agents Med Chem. 2012;12(10):1281–305.
58. Boothapandi M, Ravichandran R. Antiproliferative activity of chrysin (5, 7-dihydroxyflavone) from Indigofera tinctoria on human epidermoid carcinoma (A431) cells. Eur J Integr Med. 2018;24:71–8.
59. Jin J, Qiu S, Wang P, Liang X, Huang F, Wu H, Zhang B, Zhang W, Tian X, Xu R, Shi H, Wu X. Cardamonin inhibits breast cancer growth by repressing HIF-1α-dependent metabolic reprogramming. J Exp Clin Cancer Res: CR. 2019;38(1):377. https://doi.org/10.1186/s13046-019-1351-4.
60. MollakhaliliMeybodi N, Mortazavian AM, BahadoriMonfared A, Sohrabvandi S, AghaeiMeybodi F. Phytochemicals in cancer prevention: a review of the evidence. Iran J Cancer Prev. 2017;10(1):e7219.
61. Upadhyay S, Dixit M. Role of polyphenols and other phytochemicals on molecular signaling. Oxid Med Cell Longev. 2015;2015:504253.
62. Khan AQ, Ahmed EI, Elareer NR, Junejo K, Steinhoff M, Uddin S. Role of miRNA-regulated cancer stem cells in the pathogenesis of human malignancies. Cell. 2019;8(8):840.
63. Barcellos-Hoff MH, Lyden D, Wang TC. The evolution of the cancer niche during multistage carcinogenesis. Nat Rev Cancer. 2013;13(7):511–8.
64. Basu AK. DNA damage, mutagenesis and cancer. Int J Mol Sci. 2018;19(4):970.

65. Rajabi M, Mousa SA. The role of angiogenesis in cancer treatment. Biomedicine. 2017;5 (2):34.
66. Khan N, Mukhtar H. Modulation of signaling pathways in prostate cancer by green tea polyphenols. Biochem Pharmacol. 2013;85(5):667–72.
67. Khan H, Reale M, Ullah H, Sureda A, Tejada S, Wang Y, Zhang ZJ, Xiao J. Anti-cancer effects of polyphenols via targeting p53 signaling pathway: updates and future directions. Biotechnol Adv. 2020;38:107385.
68. Du GJ, Zhang Z, Wen XD, Yu C, Calway T, Yuan CS, Wang CZ. Epigallocatechin Gallate (EGCG) is the most effective cancer chemopreventive polyphenol in green tea. Nutrients. 2012;4(11):1679–91.
69. Cao J, Han J, Xiao H, Qiao J, Han M. Effect of tea polyphenol compounds on anticancer drugs in terms of anti-tumor activity, toxicology, and pharmacokinetics. Nutrients. 2016;8(12):762.
70. Sigismund S, Avanzato D, Lanzetti L. Emerging functions of the EGFR in cancer. Mol Oncol. 2018;12(1):3–20.
71. Pandey MK, Gupta SC, Nabavizadeh A, Aggarwal BB. (2017) Regulation of cell signaling pathways by dietary agents for cancer prevention and treatment. In: Seminars in cancer biology. 46 Academic Press, Cambridge, MA, pp 158-181.
72. Howe LR, Brown PH. Targeting the HER/EGFR/ErbB family to prevent breast cancer. Cancer Prev Res. 2011;4(8):1149–57.
73. Carpenter G, Coffey R. Stanley Cohen (1922–2020). Science. 2020;367(6484):1307.
74. Hsu JL, Hung MC. The role of HER2, EGFR, and other receptor tyrosine kinases in breast cancer. Cancer Metastasis Rev. 2016;35(4):575–88.
75. Yewale C, Baradia D, Vhora I, Patil S, Misra A. Epidermal growth factor receptor targeting in cancer: a review of trends and strategies. Biomaterials. 2013;34(34):8690–707.
76. Isali I, Al-Sadawi MA, Qureshi A, Khalifa AO, Agrawal MK, Shukla S. Growth factors involve in cellular proliferation, differentiation and migration during prostate cancer metastasis. Int J Cell Biol Physiol. 2019;2(1–2):1.
77. Seshacharyulu P, Ponnusamy MP, Haridas D, Jain M, Ganti AK, Batra SK. Targeting the EGFR signaling pathway in cancer therapy. Expert Opin Ther Targets. 2012;16(1):15–31.
78. Lichtenberger BM, Tan PK, Niederleithner H, Ferrara N, Petzelbauer P, Sibilia M. Autocrine VEGF signaling synergizes with EGFR in tumor cells to promote epithelial cancer development. Cell. 2010;140(2):268–79.
79. Lu C, Mi LZ, Grey MJ, Zhu J, Graef E, Yokoyama S, Springer TA. Structural evidence for loose linkage between ligand binding and kinase activation in the epidermal growth factor receptor. Mol Cell Biol. 2010;30(22):5432–43.
80. Lemmon MA, Schlessinger J, Ferguson KM. The EGFR family: not so prototypical receptor tyrosine kinases. Cold Spring Harb Perspect Biol. 2014;6(4):a020768.
81. Sheng Q, Liu J. The therapeutic potential of targeting the EGFR family in epithelial ovarian cancer. Br J Cancer. 2011;104(8):1241–5.
82. Kovacs E, Zorn JA, Huang Y, Barros T, Kuriyan J. A structural perspective on the regulation of the epidermal growth factor receptor. Annu Rev Biochem. 2015;84:739–64.
83. Purba ER, Saita EI, Maruyama IN. Activation of the EGF receptor by ligand binding and oncogenic mutations: the "rotation model". Cell. 2017;6(2):13.
84. Tsai CJ, Nussinov R. Emerging allosteric mechanism of EGFR activation in physiological and pathological contexts. Biophys J. 2019;117(1):5–13.
85. Nisar S, Hashem S, Macha MA, Yadav SK, Muralitharan S, Therachiyil L, Sageena G, Al-Naemi H, Haris M, Bhat AA. Exploring dysregulated signaling pathways in cancer. Curr Pharm Des. 2020;26(4):429–45.
86. Zhao X, Guan JL. Focal adhesion kinase and its signaling pathways in cell migration and angiogenesis. Adv Drug Deliv Rev. 2011;63(8):610–5.
87. Villaseñor R, Nonaka H, Del Conte-Zerial P, Kalaidzidis Y, Zerial M. Regulation of EGFR signal transduction by analogue-to-digital conversion in endosomes. Elife. 2015;4:e06156.

88. Dittmann K, Mayer C, Rodemann HP. Nuclear EGFR as novel therapeutic target. Strahlenther Onkol. 2010;186(1):1–6.
89. Aksamitiene E, Kiyatkin A, Kholodenko BN. Cross-talk between mitogenic Ras/MAPK and survival PI3K/Akt pathways: a fine balance. Biochem Soc Trans. 2012;40(1):139–46.
90. Sun J, Nan G. The extracellular signal-regulated kinase 1/2 pathway in neurological diseases: a potential therapeutic target. Int J Mol Med. 2017;39(6):1338–46.
91. Santarpia L, Lippman SM, El-Naggar AK. Targeting the MAPK–RAS–RAF signaling pathway in cancer therapy. Expert Opin Ther Targets. 2012;16(1):103–19.
92. Steelman LS, Chappell WH, Abrams SL, Kempf CR, Long J, Laidler P, Mijatovic S, Maksimovic-Ivanic D, Stivala F, Mazzarino MC, Donia M. Roles of the Raf/MEK/ERK and PI3K/PTEN/Akt/mTOR pathways in controlling growth and sensitivity to therapy-implications for cancer and aging. Aging (Albany NY). 2011;3(3):192.
93. De Luca A, Maiello MR, D'Alessio A, Pergameno M, Normanno N. The RAS/RAF/MEK/ERK and the PI3K/AKT signalling pathways: role in cancer pathogenesis and implications for therapeutic approaches. Exp Opin Ther Targets. 2012;16(sup2):S17–27.
94. Guimarães IS, Tessarollo NG, Lyra-Junior P, dos Santos DZ, Zampier RC, de Oliveira LF, Siqueira KV, Silva IV, Rangel LB. Targeting the PI3K/AKT/mTOR pathway in cancer cells. Updates on Cancer Treatment 2015 Oct 28.
95. Khan KH, Yap TA, Yan L, Cunningham D. Targeting the PI3K-AKT-mTOR signaling network in cancer. Chin J Cancer, 2013;32(5):253–65. https://doi.org/10.5732/cjc.013.10057
96. Edlind MP, Hsieh AC. PI3K-AKT-mTOR signaling in prostate cancer progression and androgen deprivation therapy resistance. Asian J Androl. 2014;16(3):378.
97. Jason SL, Cui W. Proliferation, survival and metabolism: the role of PI3K/AKT/mTOR signalling in pluripotency and cell fate determination. Development. 2016;143(17):3050–60.
98. Fransecky L, Mochmann LH, Baldus CD. Outlook on PI3K/AKT/mTOR inhibition in acute leukemia. Mol Cell Ther. 2015;3(1):1–7.
99. Shull AY, Latham-Schwark A, Ramasamy P, Leskoske K, Oroian D, Birtwistle MR, Buckhaults PJ. Novel somatic mutations to PI3K pathway genes in metastatic melanoma. PLoS One. 2012;7(8):e43369.
100. Chen M, Lu J, Wei W, Lv Y, Zhang X, Yao Y, Wang L, Ling T, Zou X. Effects of proton pump inhibitors on reversing multidrug resistance via downregulating V-ATPases/PI3K/Akt/mTOR/HIF-1α signaling pathway through TSC1/2 complex and Rheb in human gastric adenocarcinoma cells in vitro and in vivo. OncoTargets Ther. 2018;11:6705.
101. Keppler-Noreuil KM, Parker VE, Darling TN, Martinez-Agosto JA. Somatic overgrowth disorders of the PI3K/AKT/mTOR pathway & therapeutic strategies. Am J Med Genet C Semi Med Genet. 2016;172(4):402–21.
102. Jhanwar-Uniyal M, Wainwright JV, Mohan AL, Tobias ME, Murali R, Gandhi CD, Schmidt MH. Diverse signaling mechanisms of mTOR complexes: mTORC1 and mTORC2 in forming a formidable relationship. Adv Biol Regul. 2019;72:51–62.
103. Xia P, Xu XY. PI3K/Akt/mTOR signaling pathway in cancer stem cells: from basic research to clinical application. Am J Cancer Res. 2015;5(5):1602.
104. Jhanwar-Uniyal M, Amin AG, Cooper JB, Das K, Schmidt MH, Murali R. Discrete signaling mechanisms of mTORC1 and mTORC2: Connected yet apart in cellular and molecular aspects. Adv Biol Regul. 2017;64:39–48.
105. Houédé N, Pourquier P. Targeting the genetic alterations of the PI3K–AKT–mTOR pathway: Its potential use in the treatment of bladder cancers. Pharmacol Ther. 2015;145:1–8.
106. Araki K, Miyoshi Y. Mechanism of resistance to endocrine therapy in breast cancer: the important role of PI3K/Akt/mTOR in estrogen receptor-positive, HER2-negative breast cancer. Breast Cancer. 2018;25(4):392–401.
107. Kang JH. Protein kinase C (PKC) isozymes and cancer. New J Sci. 2014;2014:231418.
108. Mérida I, Arranz-Nicolás J, Rodríguez-Rodríguez C, Ávila-Flores A. Diacylglycerol kinase control of protein kinase C. Biochem J. 2019;476(8):1205–19.

109. Kazanietz MG, editor. Protein Kinase C in cancer signaling and therapy. Singapore: Springer; 2010.
110. Zhao M, Xia L, Chen GQ. Protein kinase cδ in apoptosis: a brief overview. Arch Iumimmunol Ther Exp. 2012;60(5):361–72.
111. Di Marcantonio D, Martinez E, Sidoli S, Vadaketh J, Nieborowska-Skorska M, Gupta A, Meadows JM, Ferraro F, Masselli E, Challen GA, Milsom MD. Protein kinase C epsilon is a key regulator of mitochondrial redox homeostasis in acute myeloid leukemia. Clin Cancer Res. 2018;24(3):608–18.
112. Huang AC, Cheng YD, Huang LH, Hsiao YT, Peng SF, Lu KW, Lien JC, Yang JL, Lin TS, Chung JG. Casticin induces DNA damage and impairs DNA repair in human bladder cancer TSGH-8301 cells. Anticancer Res. 2019;39(4):1839–47.
113. Cheng ZY, Hsiao YT, Huang YP, Peng SF, Huang WW, Liu KC, Hsia TC, Way TD, Chung JG. Casticin induces DNA damage and affects DNA repair associated protein expression in human lung cancer A549 cells (Running Title: Casticin induces DNA damage in lung cancer cells). Molecules. 2020;25(2):341.
114. Groner B, von Manstein V. Jak Stat signaling and cancer: opportunities, benefits and side effects of targeted inhibition. Mol Cell Endocrinol. 2017;451:1–4.
115. Slattery ML, Lundgreen A, Kadlubar SA, Bondurant KL, Wolff RK. JAK/STAT/SOCS-signaling pathway and colon and rectal cancer. Mol Carcinog. 2013;52(2):155–66.
116. Steelman LS, Chappell WH, Akula SM, Abrams SL, Cocco L, Manzoli L, Ratti S, Martelli AM, Montalto G, Cervello M, Libra M. Therapeutic resistance in breast cancer cells can result from deregulated EGFR signaling. Adv Biol Regul. 2020;28:100758.
117. Jang YN, Baik EJ. JAK-STAT pathway and myogenic differentiation. Jak-stat. 2013;2(2): e23282.
118. Vainchenker W, Constantinescu SN. JAK/STAT signaling in hematological malignancies. Oncogene. 2013;32(21):2601–13.
119. Bournazou E, Bromberg J. Targeting the tumor microenvironment: JAK-STAT3 signaling. Jak-Stat. 2013;2(2):e23828.
120. Sansone P, Bromberg J. Targeting the interleukin-6/Jak/stat pathway in human malignancies. J Clin Oncol. 2012;30(9):1005.
121. Mohr A, Chatain N, Domoszlai T, Rinis N, Sommerauer M, Vogt M, Müller-Newen G. Dynamics and non-canonical aspects of JAK/STAT signalling. Eur J Cell Biol. 2012;91 (6–7):524–32.
122. Loh CY, Arya A, Naema AF, Wong WF, Sethi G, Looi CY. Signal transducer and activator of transcription (STATs) proteins in cancer and inflammation: functions and therapeutic implication. Front Oncol. 2019;9:48.
123. Siveen KS, Sikka S, Surana R, Dai X, Zhang J, Kumar AP, Tan BK, Sethi G, Bishayee A. Targeting the STAT3 signaling pathway in cancer: role of synthetic and natural inhibitors. Biochim Biophys Acta. 2014;1845(2):136–54.
124. Bose S, Banerjee S, Mondal A, Chakraborty U, Pumarol J, Croley CR, Bishayee A. Targeting the JAK/STAT signaling pathway using phytocompounds for cancer prevention and therapy. Cell. 2020;9(6):1451.
125. Yao X, Sun S, Zhou X, Guo W, Zhang L. IGF-binding protein 2 is a candidate target of therapeutic potential in cancer. Tumor Biol. 2016;37(2):1451–9.
126. Gallagher EJ, LeRoith D. Minireview: IGF, insulin, and cancer. Endocrinology. 2011;152 (7):2546–51.
127. Kudo M. Signaling pathway/molecular targets and new targeted agents under development in hepatocellular carcinoma. World J Gastroenterol: WJG. 2012;18(42):6005.
128. DiDonato JA, Mercurio F, Karin M. NF-κB and the link between inflammation and cancer. Immunol Rev. 2012;246(1):379–400.
129. Perkins ND. The diverse and complex roles of NF-κB subunits in cancer. Nat Rev Cancer. 2012;12(2):121–32.

130. Serasanambati M, Chilakapati SR. Function of nuclear factor kappa B (NF-kB) in human diseases-a review. South Indian J Biol Sci. 2016;2(4):368–87.
131. Xia L, Tan S, Zhou Y, Lin J, Wang H, Oyang L, Tian Y, Liu L, Su M, Wang H, Cao D. Role of the NFκB-signaling pathway in cancer. OncoTargets Ther. 2018;11:2063.
132. Hoesel B, Schmid JA. The complexity of NF-κB signaling in inflammation and cancer. Mol Cancer. 2013;12(1):1–5.
133. Tyagi N, Bhardwaj A, Singh AP, McClellan S, Carter JE, Singh S. p-21 activated kinase 4 promotes proliferation and survival of pancreatic cancer cells through AKT-and ERK-dependent activation of NF-κB pathway. Oncotarget. 2014;5(18):8778.
134. Wan HY, Guo LM, Liu T, Liu M, Li X, Tang H. Regulation of the transcription factor NF-κB1 by microRNA-9 in human gastric adenocarcinoma. Mol Cancer. 2010;9(1):16.
135. Dmitrieva OS, Shilovskiy IP, Khaitov MR, Grivennikov SI. Interleukins 1 and 6 as main mediators of inflammation and cancer. Biochemistry (Mosc). 2016;81(2):80–90.
136. Rao TP, Kühl M. An updated overview on Wnt signaling pathways: a prelude for more. Circ Res. 2010;106(12):1798–806.
137. MacDonald BT, He X. Frizzled and LRP5/6 receptors for Wnt/β-catenin signaling. Cold Spring Harb Perspect Biol. 2012;4(12):a007880.
138. Wang J, Sinha T, Wynshaw-Boris A. Wnt signaling in mammalian development: lessons from mouse genetics. Cold Spring Harb Perspect Biol. 2012;4(5):a007963.
139. Sheikh A, Niazi AK, Ahmed MZ, Iqbal B, Anwer SM, Khan HH. The role of Wnt signaling pathway in carcinogenesis and implications for anticancer therapeutics. Hereditary Cancer Clin Pract. 2014;12(1):13.
140. Hou G, Yuan X, Li Y, Hou G, Liu X. Cardamonin, a natural chalcone, reduces 5-fluorouracil resistance of gastric cancer cells through targeting Wnt/β-catenin signal pathway. Invest New Drugs. 2020;38(2):329–39.
141. Yao JN, Zhang XX, Zhang YZ, Li JH, Zhao DY, Gao B, Zhou HN, Gao SL, Zhang LF. Discovery and anticancer evaluation of a formononetin derivative against gastric cancer SGC7901 cells. Invest New Drugs. 2019;37(6):1300–8.
142. Pohl SG, Brook N, Agostino M, Arfuso F, Kumar AP, Dharmarajan A. Wnt signaling in triple-negative breast cancer. Oncogenesis. 2017;6(4):e310.
143. Yang J, Chen J, He J, Li J, Shi J, Cho WC, Liu X. Wnt signaling as potential therapeutic target in lung cancer. Expert Opin Ther Targets. 2016;20(8):999–1015.
144. Damsky WE, Curley DP, Santhanakrishnan M, Rosenbaum LE, Platt JT, Rothberg BE, Taketo MM, Dankort D, Rimm DL, McMahon M, Bosenberg M. β-catenin signaling controls metastasis in Braf-activated Pten-deficient melanomas. Cancer Cell. 2011;20(6):741–54.
145. Sinnberg T, Menzel M, Ewerth D, Sauer B, Schwarz M, Schaller M, Garbe C, Schittek B. β-Catenin signaling increases during melanoma progression and promotes tumor cell survival and chemoresistance. PLoS One. 2011;6(8):e23429.
146. Rimkus TK, Carpenter RL, Qasem S, Chan M, Lo HW. Targeting the sonic hedgehog signaling pathway: review of smoothened and GLI inhibitors. Cancer. 2016;8(2):22.
147. Carballo GB, Honorato JR, de Lopes GP. A highlight on Sonic hedgehog pathway. Cell Commun Signal. 2018;16(1):1–5.
148. Choudhry Z, Rikani AA, Choudhry AM, Tariq S, Zakaria F, Asghar MW, Sarfraz MK, Haider K, Shafiq AA, Mobassarah NJ. Sonic hedgehog signalling pathway: a complex network. Ann Neurosci. 2014;21(1):28.
149. Seto M, Ohta M, Asaoka Y, Ikenoue T, Tada M, Miyabayashi K, Mohri D, Tanaka Y, Ijichi H, Tateishi K, Kanai F. Regulation of the hedgehog signaling by the mitogen-activated protein kinase cascade in gastric cancer. Mol Carcinog. 2009;48(8):703–12.
150. Carpenter RL, Paw I, Zhu H, Sirkisoon S, Xing F, Watabe K, Debinski W, Lo HW. The gain-of-function GLI1 transcription factor TGLI1 enhances expression of VEGF-C and TEM7 to promote glioblastoma angiogenesis. Oncotarget. 2015;6(26):22653.
151. Farooqi AA, Pinheiro M, Granja A, Farabegoli F, Reis S, Attar R, Sabitaliyevich UY, Xu B, Ahmad A. EGCG mediated targeting of deregulated signaling pathways and non-coding

RNAs in different cancers: Focus on JAK/STAT, Wnt/β-Catenin, TGF/SMAD, NOTCH, SHH/GLI, and TRAIL mediated signaling pathways. Cancer. 2020;12(4):951.
152. Hanna A, Shevde LA. Hedgehog signaling: modulation of cancer properties and tumor microenvironment. Mol Cancer. 2016;15(1):1–4.
153. Su W, Meng F, Huang L, Zheng M, Liu W, Sun H. Sonic hedgehog maintains survival and growth of chronic myeloid leukemia progenitor cells through β-catenin signaling. Exp Hematol. 2012;40(5):418–27.
154. Cui W, Wang LH, Wen YY, Song M, Li BL, Chen XL, Xu M, An SX, Zhao J, Lu YY, Mi XY. Expression and regulation mechanisms of Sonic Hedgehog in breast cancer. Cancer Sci. 2010;101(4):927–33.
155. Rasheed ZA, Yang J, Wang Q, Kowalski J, Freed I, Murter C, Hong SM, Koorstra JB, Rajeshkumar NV, He X, Goggins M. Prognostic significance of tumorigenic cells with mesenchymal features in pancreatic adenocarcinoma. J Natl Cancer Inst. 2010;102(5):340–51.
156. Maraldi T, Vauzour D, Angeloni C. Dietary polyphenols and their effects on cell biochemistry and pathophysiology. Oxid Med Cell Longev. 2014;2014:576363.
157. Alissa EM, Ferns GA. Functional foods and nutraceuticals in the primary prevention of cardiovascular diseases. J Nutr Metabol. 2012;2012:569486.
158. Hao Y, Huang W, Liao M, Zhu Y, Liu H, Hao C, Liu G, Zhang G, Feng H, Ning X, Li H. The inhibition of resveratrol to human skin squamous cell carcinoma A431 xenografts in nude mice. Fitoterapia. 2013;86:84–91.
159. Mohapatra P, Satapathy SR, Das D, Siddharth S, Choudhuri T, Kundu CN. Resveratrol mediated cell death in cigarette smoke transformed breast epithelial cells is through induction of p21Waf1/Cip1 and inhibition of long patch base excision repair pathway. Toxicol Appl Pharmacol. 2014;275(3):221–31.
160. Ganapathy S, Chen Q, Singh KP, Shankar S, Srivastava RK. Resveratrol enhances antitumor activity of TRAIL in prostate cancer xenografts through activation of FOXO transcription factor. PLoS One. 2010;5(12):e15627.
161. Li K, Dias SJ, Rimando AM, Dhar S, Mizuno CS, Penman AD, Lewin JR, Levenson AS. Pterostilbene acts through metastasis-associated protein 1 to inhibit tumor growth, progression and metastasis in prostate cancer. PLoS One. 2013;8(3):e57542.
162. Yin HT, Tian QZ, Guan L, Zhou Y, Huang XE, Zhang H. In vitro and in vivo evaluation of the antitumor efficiency of resveratrol against lung cancer. Asian Pac J Cancer Prev. 2013;14(3):1703–6.
163. Huderson AC, Myers JN, Niaz MS, Washington MK, Ramesh A. Chemoprevention of benzo (a) pyrene-induced colon polyps in ApcMin mice by resveratrol. J Nutr Biochem. 2013;24(4):713–24.
164. Bishayee A, Dhir N. Resveratrol-mediated chemoprevention of diethylnitrosamine-initiated hepatocarcinogenesis: inhibition of cell proliferation and induction of apoptosis. Chem Biol Interact. 2009;179(2-3):131–44.
165. Patel KR, Brown VA, Jones DJ, Britton RG, Hemingway D, Miller AS, West KP, Booth TD, Perloff M, Crowell JA, Brenner DE. Clinical pharmacology of resveratrol and its metabolites in colorectal cancer patients. Cancer Res. 2010;70(19):7392–9.
166. Kjær TN, Ornstrup MJ, Poulsen MM, Jørgensen JO, Hougaard DM, Cohen AS, Neghabat S, Richelsen B, Pedersen SB. Resveratrol reduces the levels of circulating androgen precursors but has no effect on, testosterone, dihydrotestosterone, PSA levels or prostate volume. A 4-month randomised trial in middle-aged men. Prostate. 2015;75(12):1255–63.
167. Belcaro G, Hosoi M, Pellegrini L, Appendino G, Ippolito E, Ricci A, Ledda A, Dugall M, Cesarone MR, Maione C, Ciammaichella G. A controlled study of a lecithinized delivery system of curcumin (Meriva®) to alleviate the adverse effects of cancer treatment. Phytother Res. 2014;28(3):444–50.
168. Howells LM, Iwuji CO, Irving GR, Barber S, Walter H, Sidat Z, Griffin-Teall N, Singh R, Foreman N, Patel SR, Morgan B. Curcumin combined with FOLFOX chemotherapy is safe

and tolerable in patients with metastatic colorectal cancer in a randomized phase IIa trial. J Nutr. 2019;149(7):1133–9.
169. Zhang C, He LJ, Ye HZ, Liu DF, Zhu YB, Miao DD, Zhang SP, Chen YY, Jia YW, Shen J, Liu XP. Nrf2 is a key factor in the reversal effect of curcumin on multidrug resistance in the HCT-8/5-Fu human colorectal cancer cell line. Mol Med Rep. 2018;18(6):5409–16.
170. Lee YH, Song NY, Suh J, Kim DH, Kim W, Ann J, Lee J, Baek JH, Na HK, Surh YJ. Curcumin suppresses oncogenicity of human colon cancer cells by covalently modifying the cysteine 67 residue of SIRT1. Cancer Lett. 2018;431:219–29.
171. Tong R, Wu X, Liu Y, Liu Y, Zhou J, Jiang X, Zhang L, He X, Ma L. Curcumin-induced DNA Demethylation in human gastric Cancer cells is mediated by the DNA-damage response pathway. Oxid Med Cell Longev. 2020;2020:2543504.
172. Yang CL, Liu YY, Ma YG, Xue YX, Liu DG, Ren Y, Liu XB, Li Y, Li Z. Curcumin blocks small cell lung cancer cells migration, invasion, angiogenesis, cell cycle and neoplasia through Janus kinase-STAT3 signalling pathway. PLoS One. 2012;7(5):e37960.
173. Tang SN, Fu J, Shankar S, Srivastava RK. EGCG enhances the therapeutic potential of gemcitabine and CP690550 by inhibiting STAT3 signaling pathway in human pancreatic cancer. PLoS One. 2012;7(2):e31067.
174. Stearns ME, Amatangelo MD, Varma D, Sell C, Goodyear SM. Combination therapy with epigallocatechin-3-gallate and doxorubicin in human prostate tumor modeling studies: inhibition of metastatic tumor growth in severe combined immunodeficiency mice. Am J Pathol. 2010;177(6):3169–79.
175. Yeo C, Han DS, Lee HJ, Lee EO. Epigallocatechin-3-gallate suppresses vasculogenic mimicry through inhibiting the twist/VE-cadherin/AKT pathway in human prostate cancer PC-3 cells. Int J Mol Sci. 2020;21(2):439.
176. Mohan N, Karmakar S, Banik NL, Ray SK. SU5416 and EGCG work synergistically and inhibit angiogenic and survival factors and induce cell cycle arrest to promote apoptosis in human malignant neuroblastoma SH-SY5Y and SK-N-BE2 cells. Neurochem Res. 2011;36 (8):1383–96.
177. Huang KH, Kuo KL, Chen SC, Weng TI, Chuang YT, Tsai YC, Pu YS, Chiang CK, Liu SH. Down-regulation of glucose-regulated protein (GRP) 78 potentiates cytotoxic effect of celecoxib in human urothelial carcinoma cells. PLoS One. 2012;7(3):e33615.
178. Luo T, Wang J, Yin Y, Hua H, Jing J, Sun X, Li M, Zhang Y, Jiang Y. (-)-Epigallocatechin gallate sensitizes breast cancer cells to paclitaxel in a murine model of breast carcinoma. Breast Cancer Res. 2010;12(1):R8.
179. Huang W, Ding L, Huang Q, Hu H, Liu S, Yang X, Hu X, Dang Y, Shen S, Li J, Ji X. Carbonyl reductase 1 as a novel target of (−)-epigallocatechin gallate against hepatocellular carcinoma. Hepatology. 2010;52(2):703–14.
180. Maeda Y, Takahashi H, Nakai N, Yanagita T, Ando N, Okubo T, Saito K, Shiga K, Hirokawa T, Hara M, Ishiguro H. Apigenin induces apoptosis by suppressing Bcl-xl and Mcl-1 simultaneously via signal transducer and activator of transcription 3 signaling in colon cancer. Int J Oncol. 2018;52(5):1661–73.
181. Liu MM, Ma RH, Ni ZJ, Thakur K, Cespedes-Acuña CL, Jiang L, Wei ZJ. Apigenin 7-O-glucoside promotes cell apoptosis through the PTEN/PI3K/AKT pathway and inhibits cell migration in cervical cancer Hela cells. Food Chem Toxicol. 2020;146:111843.
182. Sudhakaran M, Parra MR, Stoub H, Gallo KA, Doseff AI. Apigenin by targeting hnRNPA2 sensitizes triple-negative breast cancer spheroids to doxorubicin-induced apoptosis and regulates expression of ABCC4 and ABCG2 drug efflux transporters. Biochem Pharmacol. 2020;182:114259.
183. Qi Y, Ding Z, Yao Y, Ren F, Yin M, Yang S, Chen A. Apigenin induces apoptosis and counteracts cisplatin-induced chemoresistance via Mcl-1 in ovarian cancer cells. Exp Ther Med. 2020;20(2):1329–36.

184. Pham TH, Page YL, Percevault F, Ferrière F, Flouriot G, Pakdel F. Apigenin, a partial antagonist of the estrogen receptor (ER), inhibits ER-positive breast cancer cell proliferation through Akt/FOXM1 signaling. Int J Mol Sci. 2021;22(1):470.
185. Si L, Fu J, Liu W, Hayashi T, Nie Y, Mizuno K, Hattori S, Fujisaki H, Onodera S, Ikejima T. Silibinin inhibits migration and invasion of breast cancer MDA-MB-231 cells through induction of mitochondrial fusion. Mol Cell Biochem. 2020;463(1-2):189–201.
186. Maasomi ZJ, Soltanahmadi YP, Dadashpour M, Alipour S, Abolhasani S, Zarghami N. Synergistic anticancer effects of silibinin and chrysin in T47D breast cancer cells. Asian Pac J Cancer Prev. 2017;18(5):1283.
187. Molavi O, Narimani F, Asiaee F, Sharifi S, Tarhriz V, Shayanfar A, Hejazi M, Lai R. Silibinin sensitizes chemo-resistant breast cancer cells to chemotherapy. Pharm Biol. 2017;55 (1):729–39.
188. Amirsaadat S, Pilehvar-Soltanahmadi Y, Zarghami F, Alipour S, Ebrahimnezhad Z, Zarghami N. Silibinin-loaded magnetic nanoparticles inhibit hTERT gene expression and proliferation of lung cancer cells. Artif Cells Nanomed Biotechnol. 2017;45(8):1649–56.
189. Pashaei-Asl F, Pashaei-Asl R, Khodadadi K, Akbarzadeh A, Ebrahimie E, Pashaiasl M. Enhancement of anticancer activity by silibinin and paclitaxel combination on the ovarian cancer. Artif Cells Nanomed Biotechnol. 2018;46(7):1483–7.
190. de Oliveira DT, Sávio AL, de Castro Marcondes JP, Barros TM, Barbosa LC, Salvadori DM, da Silva GN. Cytotoxic and toxicogenomic effects of silibinin in bladder cancer cells with different TP53 status. J Biosci. 2017;42(1):91–101.
191. Cook MT, Liang Y, Besch-Williford C, Hyder SM. Luteolin inhibits lung metastasis, cell migration, and viability of triple-negative breast cancer cells. Breast Cancer Targets Ther. 2017;9:9.
192. Cook MT, Liang Y, Besch-Williford C, Goyette S, Mafuvadze B, Hyder SM. Luteolin inhibits progestin-dependent angiogenesis, stem cell-like characteristics, and growth of human breast cancer xenografts. Springerplus. 2015;4(1):444.
193. Kang KA, Piao MJ, Ryu YS, Hyun YJ, Park JE, Shilnikova K, Zhen AX, Kang HK, Koh YS, Jeong YJ, Hyun JW. Luteolin induces apoptotic cell death via antioxidant activity in human colon cancer cells. Int J Oncol. 2017;51(4):1169–78.
194. Kang KA, Piao MJ, Hyun YJ, Zhen AX, Cho SJ, Ahn MJ, Yi JM, Hyun JW. Luteolin promotes apoptotic cell death via upregulation of Nrf2 expression by DNA demethylase and the interaction of Nrf2 with p53 in human colon cancer cells. Exp Mol Med. 2019;51(4):1–4.
195. Yao Y, Rao C, Zheng G, Wang S. Luteolin suppresses colorectal cancer cell metastasis via regulation of the miR-384/pleiotrophin axis. Oncol Rep. 2019;42(1):131–41.
196. Liu H, Zeng Z, Wang S, Li T, Mastriani E, Li QH, Bao HX, Zhou YJ, Wang X, Liu Y, Liu W. Main components of pomegranate, ellagic acid and luteolin, inhibit metastasis of ovarian cancer by down-regulating MMP2 and MMP9. Cancer Biol Ther. 2017;18(12):990–9.
197. Lynch SM, O'Neill KM, McKenna MM, Walsh CP, McKenna DJ. Regulation of miR-200c and miR-141 by methylation in prostate cancer. Prostate. 2016;76(13):1146–59.
198. Hirata H, Hinoda Y, Shahryari V, Deng G, Tanaka Y, Tabatabai ZL, Dahiya R. Genistein downregulates onco-miR-1260b and upregulates sFRP1 and Smad4 via demethylation and histone modification in prostate cancer cells. Br J Cancer. 2014;110(6):1645–54.
199. De La Parra C, Castillo-Pichardo L, Cruz-Collazo A, Cubano L, Redis R, Calin GA, Dharmawardhane S. Soy isoflavone genistein-mediated downregulation of miR-155 contributes to the anticancer effects of genistein. Nutr Cancer. 2016;68(1):154–64.
200. Ma CH, Zhang YX, Tang LH, Yang XJ, Cui WM, Han CC, Ji WY. MicroRNA-1469, a p53-responsive microRNA promotes Genistein induced apoptosis by targeting Mcl1 in human laryngeal cancer cells. Biomed Pharmacother. 2018;106:665–71.
201. Imai-Sumida M, Dasgupta P, Kulkarni P, Shiina M, Hashimoto Y, Shahryari V, Majid S, Tanaka Y, Dahiya R, Yamamura S. Genistein represses HOTAIR/chromatin remodeling pathways to suppress kidney cancer. Cell Physiol Biochem. 2020;54(1):53.

202. Zhang L, Zhang J, Gong Y, Lv L. Systematic and experimental investigations of the anti-colorectal cancer mediated by genistein. Biofactors. 2020;46(6):974–82.
203. Lei CS, Hou YC, Pai MH, Lin MT, Yeh SL. Effects of quercetin combined with anticancer drugs on metastasis-associated factors of gastric cancer cells: in vitro and in vivo studies. J Nutr Biochem. 2018;51:105–13.
204. Jia L, Huang S, Yin X, Zan Y, Guo Y, Han L. Quercetin suppresses the mobility of breast cancer by suppressing glycolysis through Akt-mTOR pathway mediated autophagy induction. Life Sci. 2018;208:123–30.
205. Liu Y, Gong W, Yang ZY, Zhou XS, Gong C, Zhang TR, Wei X, Ma D, Ye F, Gao QL. Quercetin induces protective autophagy and apoptosis through ER stress via the p-STAT3/Bcl-2 axis in ovarian cancer. Apoptosis. 2017;22(4):544–57.
206. Teekaraman D, Elayapillai SP, Viswanathan MP, Jagadeesan A. Quercetin inhibits human metastatic ovarian cancer cell growth and modulates components of the intrinsic apoptotic pathway in PA-1 cell line. Chem Biol Interact. 2019;300:91–100.
207. Zhao Y, Fan D, Zheng ZP, Li ET, Chen F, Cheng KW, Wang M. 8-C-(E-phenylethenyl) quercetin from onion/beef soup induces autophagic cell death in colon cancer cells through ERK activation. Mol Nutr Food Res. 2017;61(2):1600437.
208. Tummala R, Lou W, Gao AC, Nadiminty N. Quercetin targets hnRNPA1 to overcome enzalutamide resistance in prostate cancer cells. Mol Cancer Ther. 2017;16(12):2770–9.
209. Dos Santos MB, Bertholin Anselmo D, de Oliveira JG, Jardim-Perassi BV, Alves Monteiro D, Silva G, Gomes E, Lucia Fachin A, Marins M, de Campos Zuccari DA, Octavio RL. Antiproliferative activity and p53 upregulation effects of chalcones on human breast cancer cells. J Enzyme Inhib Med Chem. 2019;34(1):1093–9.
210. Lindamulage IK, Vu HY, Karthikeyan C, Knockleby J, Lee YF, Trivedi P, Lee H. Novel quinolone chalcones targeting colchicine-binding pocket kill multidrug-resistant cancer cells by inhibiting tubulin activity and MRP1 function. Sci Rep. 2017;7(1):1–3.
211. Sangpheak K, Mueller M, Darai N, Wolschann P, Suwattanasophon C, Ruga R, Chavasiri W, Seetaha S, Choowongkomon K, Kungwan N, Rungnim C. Computational screening of chalcones acting against topoisomerase IIα and their cytotoxicity towards cancer cell lines. J Enzyme Inhib Med Chem. 2019;34(1):134–43.
212. Lakshmi S, Suresh S, Rahul BS, Saikant R, Maya V, Gopi M, Padmaja G, Remani P. In vitro and in vivo studies of 5, 7-dihydroxy flavones isolated from Alpinia galanga (L.) against human lung cancer and ascetic lymphoma. Med Chem Res. 2019;28(1):39–51.
213. Ryu S, Lim W, Bazer FW, Song G. Chrysin induces death of prostate cancer cells by inducing ROS and ER stress. J Cell Physiol. 2017;232(12):3786–97.
214. Mohammadian F, Abhari A, Dariushnejad H, Nikanfar A, Pilehvar-Soltanahmadi Y, Zarghami N. Effects of chrysin-PLGA-PEG nanoparticles on proliferation and gene expression of miRNAs in gastric cancer cell line. Ira J Cancer Prev. 2016;9(4):3786–97.
215. Lim W, Ryu S, Bazer FW, Kim SM, Song G. Chrysin attenuates progression of ovarian cancer cells by regulating signaling cascades and mitochondrial dysfunction. J Cell Physiol. 2018;233 (4):3129–40.
216. Song XL, Zhang YJ, Wang XF, Zhang WJ, Wang Z, Zhang F, Zhang YJ, Lu JH, Mei JW, Hu YP, Chen L. Casticin induces apoptosis and G0/G1 cell cycle arrest in gallbladder cancer cells. Cancer Cell Int. 2017;17(1):9.
217. Lin CC, Chen KB, Tsai CH, Tsai FJ, Huang CY, Tang CH, Yang JS, Hsu YM, Peng SF, Chung JG. Casticin inhibits human prostate cancer DU 145 cell migration and invasion via Ras/Akt/NF-κB signaling pathways. J Food Biochem. 2019;43(7):e12902.
218. Chou GL, Peng SF, Liao CL, Ho HC, Lu KW, Lien JC, Fan MJ, La KC, Chung JG. Casticin impairs cell growth and induces cell apoptosis via cell cycle arrest in human oral cancer SCC-4 cells. Environ Toxicol. 2018;33(2):127–41.
219. Zhou X, Zhou R, Li Q, Jie X, Hong J, Zong Y, Dong X, Zhang S, Li Z, Wu G. Cardamonin inhibits the proliferation and metastasis of non-small-cell lung cancer cells by suppressing the PI3K/Akt/mTOR pathway. Anticancer Drugs. 2019;30(3):241–50.

220. Niu P, Shi D, Zhang S, Zhu Y, Zhou J. Cardamonin enhances the anti-proliferative effect of cisplatin on ovarian cancer. Oncol Lett. 2018;15(3):3991–7.
221. James S, Aparna JS, Paul AM, Lankadasari MB, Mohammed S, Binu VS, Santhoshkumar TR, Reshmi G, Harikumar KB. Cardamonin inhibits colonic neoplasia through modulation of MicroRNA expression. Sci Rep. 2017;7(1):1–6.
222. Wu Y, Zhang X, Li Z, Yan H, Qin J, Li T. Formononetin inhibits human bladder cancer cell proliferation and invasiveness via regulation of miR-21 and PTEN. Food Funct. 2017;8(3):1061–6.
223. Xin M, Wang Y, Ren Q, Guo Y. Formononetin and metformin act synergistically to inhibit growth of MCF-7 breast cancer cells in vitro. Biomed Pharmacother. 2019;109:2084–9.
224. Zhang Y, Chen C, Zhang J. Effects and significance of formononetin on expression levels of HIF-1α and VEGF in mouse cervical cancer tissue. Oncol Lett. 2019;18(3):2248–53.
225. Yu X, Gao F, Li W, Zhou L, Liu W, Li M. Formononetin inhibits tumor growth by suppression of EGFR-Akt-Mcl-1 axis in non-small cell lung cancer. J Exp Clin Cancer Res. 2020;39:1–7.
226. Cho HJ, Park JH, Nam JH, Chang YC, Park B, Hoe HS. Ascochlorin suppresses MMP-2-mediated migration and invasion by targeting FAK and JAK-STAT signaling cascades. J Cell Biochem. 2018;119(1):300–13.
227. Jeong YJ, Hoe HS, Cho HJ, Park KK, Kim DD, Kim CH, Magae J, Kang DW, Lee SR, Chang YC. Suppression of c-Myc enhances p21WAF1/CIP1-mediated G1 cell cycle arrest through the modulation of ERK phosphorylation by ascochlorin. J Cell Biochem. 2018;119(2):2036–47.
228. Kim SM, Lee JH, Sethi G, Kim C, Baek SH, Nam D, Chung WS, Kim SH, Shim BS, Ahn KS. Bergamottin, a natural furanocoumarin obtained from grapefruit juice induces chemosensitization and apoptosis through the inhibition of STAT3 signaling pathway in tumor cells. Cancer Lett. 2014;354(1):153–63.
229. Zhang H, Yang S, Lin T. Bergamottin exerts anticancer effects on human colon cancer cells via induction of apoptosis, G2/M cell cycle arrest and deactivation of the Ras/Raf/ERK signalling pathway. Arch Med Sci. 2019;15(1) https://doi.org/10.5114/aoms.2019.86226.
230. Sun S, Phrutivorapongkul A, Dibwe DF, Balachandran C, Awale S. Chemical constituents of Thai citrus hystrix and their antiausterity activity against the PANC-1 human pancreatic cancer cell line. J Nat Prod. 2018;81(8):1877–83.
231. Lee JH, Chiang SY, Nam D, Chung WS, Lee J, Na YS, Sethi G, Ahn KS. Capillarisin inhibits constitutive and inducible STAT3 activation through induction of SHP-1 and SHP-2 tyrosine phosphatases. Cancer Lett. 2014;345(1):140–8.
232. Tsui KH, Chang YL, Yang PS, Hou CP, Lin YH, Lin BW, Feng TH, Juang HH. The inhibitory effects of capillarisin on cell proliferation and invasion of prostate carcinoma cells. Cell Prolif. 2018;51(2):e12429.
233. Takeda T, Tsubaki M, Tomonari Y, Kawashima K, Itoh T, Imano M, Satou T, Nishida S. Bavachin induces the apoptosis of multiple myeloma cell lines by inhibiting the activation of nuclear factor kappa B and signal transducer and activator of transcription 3. Biomed Pharmacother. 2018;100:486–94.
234. Lee JY, Lim W, Song G. Bavachin suppresses human placental choriocarcinoma cells by targeting electron transport chain complexes and mitochondrial dysfunction. Free Radic Biol Med. 2020;156:26–35.

Polyphenols as Modulators of Oxidative Stress in Cancer Disease

5

Ekta Yadav, Pankajkumar Yadav, Mohammad A. Kamal, and Amita Verma

Abstract

Epidemiologic reports have revealed that cancer is a major health risk and considered a leading cause of increasing death rates all over the world. High oxidative stress can mediate chronic diseases such as onset of cancer because of damaging effects on vital molecules, DNA mutation, cell proliferation, and genome modification. Among bioactive phytoconstituents, dietary polyphenols are widely distributed in fruits, vegetables, spices, etc., having strong antioxidant activity and believed to act extensively as chemopreventive agents causing interference with carcinogenesis. Anticancer effect of polyphenols is induced via regulation of antioxidant enzymatic activity, apoptosis induction by downregulation of various signaling pathways, and cell cycle arrest by initiating cell senescence associated with oxidative stress. Several polyphenols are demonstrated to act directly by affecting epigenetic process via modulating level of oxidative stress and reactive oxygen species (ROS) generation. Additionally, prooxidant mechanism of polyphenols impedes the metabolic process of cancer stem cells as well as self-renewal signaling pathways. Polyphenols can be suggested as a beneficial anticancer tool in a combinational protocol with a standard chemotherapeutic agent resulting in significantly fewer side effects.

Pankajkumar Yadav and Amita Verma contributed equally to this work.

E. Yadav · A. Verma
Bioorganic and Medicinal Chemistry Research Laboratory, Department of Pharmaceutical Sciences, Sam Higginbottom University of Agriculture, Technology and Sciences, Prayagraj, India

P. Yadav (✉)
Pharmaceutics Laboratory, Department of Pharmaceutical Sciences, Sam Higginbottom University of Agriculture, Technology and Sciences, Prayagraj, India

M. A. Kamal
King Fahd Medical Research Center, King Abdulaziz University, Jeddah, Saudi Arabia

S. Tabrez, M. Imran Khan (eds.), *Polyphenols-based Nanotherapeutics for Cancer Management*, https://doi.org/10.1007/978-981-16-4935-6_5

Keywords

Polyphenols · oxidative stress · Anticancer · Reactive oxygen species · Antioxidant

5.1 Introduction

Life expectancy, mortality rate as well as economic standards of people is greatly affected by health challenges globally. Over the years, cancer has emerged as an epidemiologically evidenced health risk, which granted global pressures with more than 14 million new cases approximately and 8 million deaths yearly [1]. Cancer, a multistage process described by three phases primarily, i.e., initiation, promotion, and progression [2]. Oxidative stress contributes to all three stages of cancer. During the first stage (initiation stage), over-generated reactive oxygen species (ROS) may lead to damaging effects on DNA molecules by causing gene mutations along with morphological changes in DNA. Whereas during the promotion phase (under the influence of ROS), aberrant gene expression, interference with cellular communication, and modulation of second messenger system occur which promotes cell proliferation or reduction in apoptotic process of an early-stage cell population. Oxidative stress may also actively contribute to the cancer progression stage by forming critical DNA modification to the initiated cell growth [3].

Many epidemiological reports suggested that a rapid increase in the rate of mortality is attributed to frequent tumor recurrence, which is believed to be arising in response to chemo or radiotherapy-induced cell resistance [4]. Additionally, despite the availability of advanced diagnostic methods, cancer is usually diagnosed in a later stage in most cases. Nevertheless, nowadays smart drugs with promisingly improved anticancer effects have been introduced, which especially targets the pathologically responsible signaling pathways [5, 6]. Thus, it is a strict need of time to develop a potential alternative approach for the effective management and treatment of cancer. Over the past few decades, a plant-based diet, including vegetables and fruits comprising polyphenols, is consumed all over the world which increases interest to understand its chemical and biological nature along with beneficial effects on human health [7]. The literature revealed various experimental models, such as cellular, molecular, and transgenic animal models, which explored the relevant underlying mechanism of action concerning polyphenols. The ability of polyphenols to scavenge the endogenously produced free radicals, radiation, and even xenobiotics are considered as potential bioactivity which contributes to the treatment of a variety of cancers in animal models as well as humans [8, 9]. Polyphenols have chemotherapeutic property, as they owe redox activities, which directly targets ROS and oxidative stress [10].

Over the recent years, several reports have evidenced that ROS is implicated as a strong bridge between cancer and chronic inflammation. Even tumor promoters are

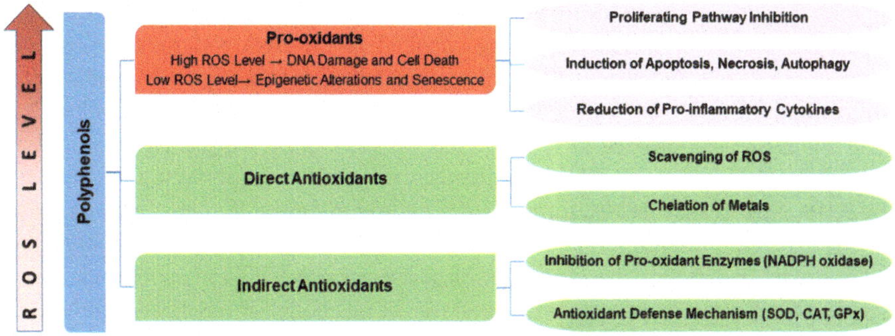

Fig. 5.1 Role of polyphenols in cancer cells through prooxidant and antioxidant mechanisms attributed to different cellular ROS level

characterized by the ability to accelerate and activate inflammatory cells for the production of ROS [11, 12]. Certain antioxidants are evidenced to possess significant potential to inhibit tumor promotion in animal models [3].

However, the anticancer activity of polyphenols is not fully credited to their antioxidant action and it has been suggested that the prooxidant capacity of polyphenols is widely attributed to its antitumor activity by following both direct and indirect mechanisms. They act by initiating DNA damage and consequently cellular death. Direct mechanism of prooxidant activity promotes the generation of some redox chemical species, e.g., aroxyl radical and metal cation complex, in a favorable environment of high pH and increased amount of transition metals [13, 14]. Whereas, the indirect mechanism involves the interaction of polyphenols with specific cellular pathways, such as NADPH (reduced form of nicotinamide adenine dinucleotide phosphate) oxidase (NOX), via activation of intracellular ROS production [10] (Fig. 5.1).

It has been evident that elevation in the level of copper within cancer cells activates the prooxidant mechanism in the redox-active microenvironment. Copper, assembled by a metal chelating agent, is a crucial chromatin redox-active metal ion linked with DNA bases [15]. Pathological reports have suggested a significant increase in copper level in cells, serum, and tissue samples of patients who suffered from cancer [16]. As cancer cells show aberrant redox hemostasis, it was advised that these polyphenols may selectively get involved in cancer cells' behavior attributed to their redox status [17].

5.1.1 Major Risk Factors of ROS Generation

5.1.1.1 Endogenous Factors of ROS Generation

Mitochondrial oxidative phosphorylation, peroxisomes, metabolism by cytochrome P450, and activation of inflammatory cell response are several important endogenous risk factors responsible for the generation of ROS. About 4–5% of molecular oxygen majorly gets converted to superoxides in response to oxidative metabolism in mitochondria. Superoxide dismutase act on the generated superoxides gives rise to hydrogen peroxide, which ultimately changed to the hydroxyl radical [18]. Past studies have revealed a potential connection between tumorigenesis and level of mitochondrial ROS as cancer cells have identified with high ROS induced by mitochondria as compared to normal cells. In addition, various inflammatory cells such as neutrophils, macrophages, and eosinophils also contribute to the generation of ROS. Superoxide anion, nitric oxide, hydrogen peroxide, and nitric oxide are ROS, which are produced by macrophage activation. Peroxisomes are also responsible organelle towards the formation of hydrogen peroxide and superoxide anions by acyl-CoA oxidase and xanthine oxidase. In rat model, it has been reported that from normally utilized oxygen about 35% of total hydrogen peroxide in liver is associated with peroxisomes. Moreover, different external chemical sources including halogenated solvents, phthalate esters, and hypolipidemic drugs are known to increase the level of hydrogen peroxide via an elevation in the concentration of peroxisomes, which are associated with the development of tumors in liver. Therefore, it advises a promising connection between liver tumorigenesis and ROS generation by peroxisome proliferation [19].

5.1.1.2 Exogenous Sources of ROS

Exogenous sources involving different chemical and physical agents induced cancer by involving the activation of oxidative stress-mediated pathways in mammals. Ionizing radiation plays a vital role as a carcinogen that adversely affects every phase of cancer [20]. Moreover, Ionizing radiation cause DNA damaging effects due to ROS generation from water radiolysis, which further results in mutation of genes and carcinogenesis effects. ROS formation by nongenotoxic carcinogens, which are non-DNA reactive in nature mediated by way of directly acting on different metabolized intermediates or by stimulating the responsible endogenous factors of ROS. Even exposure to some xenobiotics such as barbiturates, chlorinated compounds, metal ions, phorbol esters, and peroxisome proliferating compounds are also considered as producers of oxidative stress as well as cancer. Antineoplastic agents including adriamycin and cisplatin induce DNA damage and cell death via generating high levels of ROS. Human beings are continuously exposed to other exogenous factors such as tobacco smoking, air pollution, pesticides as well as ultraviolet rays that prominently cause oxidative stress [19, 21].

5.2 Role of Oxidative Stress in Cancer

5.2.1 ROS-Mediated Cellular Transformation Mechanisms

Oxidative stress is one of the major events among others to cause the favorable environment to initiate tumor onset, progression, and further survival of tumor cells by mediating cellular signal transduction pathways [22]. Tumor cells are characterized by their enhanced efficiency towards cell survival rate compared to normal cells. These signaling pathways participate in inter or intracellular communication and are essential for tumor cell survival and cell fate. Additionally, chronic inflammation leads to preneoplastic condition via stimulation of dysfunctional and damaging processes by the production of a huge amount of ROS leading to further immune cell activation [23, 24]. Overcoming of the endogenous antioxidant response occurs if the cellular ROS is overproduced and it can cause irretrievable oxidative damage to vital cellular components such as nucleic acids, lipids, and proteins leading to dysregulation of oncogenes and tumor suppressor genes. Therefore, the process of oxidative stress and chronic inflammation are closely associated with each other, and negligence to control these major processes could initiate carcinogenesis in response to cellular modulation at the genetic/epigenetic level [25]. Moreover, oxidative stress is also observed to affect several important signaling pathways linked with the process of cell proliferation including epidermal growth factor receptor signaling pathway (EGFR) along with chief signaling proteins, i.e., mitogen-activated protein kinase (MAPK), extracellular signal-regulated kinase 1/2 (ERK1/2), nuclear factor erythroid 2-related factor 2 (NRF2), reticular activating system (Ras)/rapidly accelerated fibrosarcoma (Raf), phosphatidylinositol 3-kinase (PI3K), protein kinase C, and phospholipase C [26, 27]. Furthermore, ROS modifies tumor protein p53 suppressor gene expression, which plays a key role in apoptosis. These reports advocate that oxidative stress is a key factor in the onset and further progression of a tumor through gene expression alterations, cell proliferation, and apoptosis [28, 29]. On one side of the coin, ROS is attributed to carcinogenesis, whereas, on the other side, extreme amounts of ROS may contribute to inhibition of proliferation of cancer cells, apoptotic damage to cancer cells, or its necrosis by acting as a strong cellular toxicant. Under the influence of high oxidative stress, malignant cells are more susceptible to the damaging effects of ROS [30]. Several studies explored that patients suffering from cancer show an elevated level of oxidative stress and decreased level of antioxidant status during pretreatment of cancer [31]. Thus, assessment of tissue redox condition has great potential for cancer diagnosis and this could be significantly beneficial to rectify the appropriate approach for patient treatment. The conventional method for oncology therapeutics primarily relies on the mechanism of ROS overproduction persuaded apoptosis in cancer cells. However, in long run, this strategy proved to exhibit serious and inevitable toxic side effects towards surrounding normal tissues. A less sturdy state of ROS status along with a steady level of decreasing equivalents occurs within normal cells rather than cancerous cells [32]. Therefore, based on the regulation of the redox-signaling pathway, a new effective therapeutic tool can be designed by assessing the redox status of normal as well as cancer cells.

Antioxidant agents are evidenced to minimize the adverse reaction that occurs with cancer treatment therapy, i.e., neurotoxicity, weight loss, stomatitis, and asthenia [33]. A significant decrease in dose-dependent toxic effects by antioxidants may allow more patients to successfully complete prescribed chemotherapy or radiotherapy to demonstrate a better and convincing therapeutic index. Moreover, antioxidants also play a promising role as a chemopreventive agent. Various reported studies evidenced that people who consume the polyphenolic type of

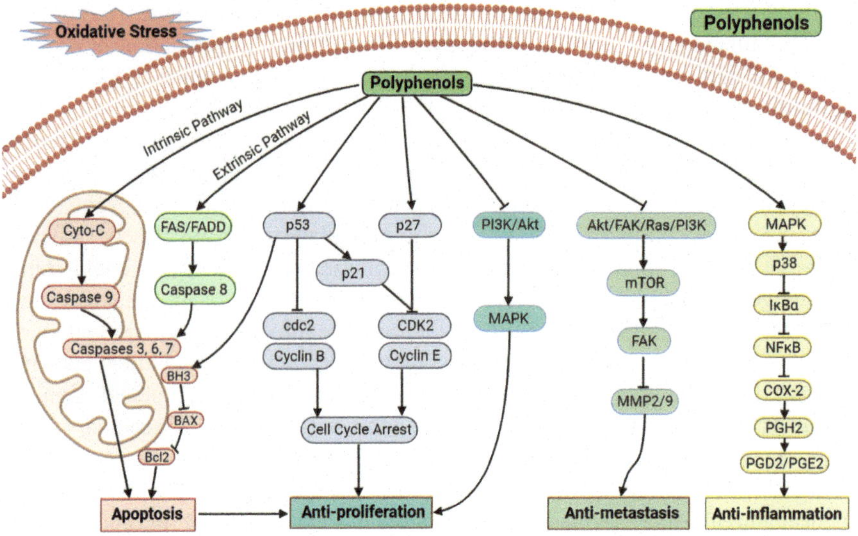

Akt, serine specific protein kinase; BAX, Bcl2-associated X protein; Bcl, B-cell lymphoma; BH3, Bcl-2 homology domain 3; Caspase, cysteine-aspartic protease; cdc, cell division cycle; CDK, cyclin-dependent kinase; COX, cyclooxygenase; Cyto-C, cytochrome complex; FADD, Fas-associated protein with death domain; FAK, focal adhesion kinase; FAS, receptor protein of the TNF receptor family; IκBα, nuclear factor of kappa light polypeptide gene enhancer; MAPK, mitogen-activated protein kinase; MMP, matrix metalloproteinase; mTOR, mechanistic target of rapamycin; NFκB, nuclear factor kappa B; PGD2, prostaglandin D2; PGE2, prostaglandin E2; PGH2, prostaglandin H2; PI3K, phosphoinositide 3-kinase; Ras, reticular activating system

Fig. 5.2 Schematic representation of different signaling pathways followed by polyphenols for activation of apoptosis, anti-proliferation, anti-metastasis, and anti-inflammation in cancer cells. (Left to right) Cellular apoptosis caused by inhibition of Bax and Bcl-2 as well as by actuating Caspase signaling pathway via increasing Cytochrome C which ultimately leads to anti-proliferation. Anti-proliferation induced via PI3K/Akt pathway inhibition by arresting cell cycle division by increasing p53, p21, and p27. Anti-metastasis occurs due to suppression of Akt/FAK/Ras/PI3K pathway through regulation of MMP 2/9 level. Anti-inflammation activity initiated by modulating MAPK pathway via reduction in p38 and COX-2 expression

antioxidant-rich food such as vegetables, fruits, and other related food may bear a significantly lesser probability of cancer incidence. The Mediterranean diet habit has a beneficial effect on cancer prevention and it is majorly occupied with antioxidants. Therefore, it is capable of modulating the progression of the inflammatory process, proliferation, apoptosis, cell cycle, and expression of various related genes [34, 35] (Fig. 5.2).

It has been reported that inflammatory cytokines, as well as cells, have the potential to onset and further perpetuate various cancers including liver, lung, breast, stomach, colon, and skin. About 20 % of cancer is induced in response to chronic inflammation or persistent infection [36]. Several pathways implicated in a tumor are associated with chronic inflammation have been documented. The onset of the inflammatory microenvironment leads to increase in levels of cytokines, prostaglandins, nuclear factor kappa B (NF-κB), and microRNAs (miRNAs) that influences various cellular process including cell proliferation, cell senescence, cellular death, DNA methylation, angiogenesis along with DNA mutation rate [37]. Presence of interleukin 6 (IL-6) cytokine is observed in various cancers, which accounts for tumor initiation and metastasis by modulating the NF-κB and signal transducer and activator of transcription protein (STAT3) signaling pathways [38]. Protein kinase B (Akt) and ATP-binding cassette protein (ARRB1) pathways are involved in the instigation of hepatocellular carcinoma in partial liver resection-associated inflammation. Tumor necrosis factor-α (TNF-α) is observed to promote spontaneous mammary cancer in rodents [39].

Cyclooxygenase-2 (COX-2) derived proinflammatory lipid prostaglandin E_2 (PGE2) and its receptors are known to exhibit a vital role in tumor progression through the proliferation of tumor cells, immunosuppression, and angiogenesis. Numerous human solid tumors samples from various organs such as stomach, breast, and colon were observed with a high level of PGE2. Additionally, thromboxane A2 (TxA2) is another COX-2 derived prostaglandin that is reported to be involved in process of oncogenesis by affecting angiogenesis. Incidence of colon carcinogenesis-associated tumor was prominently increased with PGE2 in rat model [40]. Therefore, based on past reports, it is established that various inflammatory cells and biomolecules may contribute to tumorigenesis and tumoral growth.

5.2.1.1 Oxidative Stress Biomarkers in Cancer Diagnosis

Measurement of free radicals and level of oxidative stress is commonly performed with the estimation of free radicals reaction products along with their biomolecules in terms of biomarkers. Oxidative stress biomarkers impart clinical relevance for diagnosis of disease, pathological condition, status, and type of cancer by evaluating tissue or fluid sample of patients.

It is believed that ROS mainly targets PUFA (polyunsaturated fatty acids) which exists within the cell membrane, susceptible to be oxidized as a result of lipid peroxidation. Further different metabolites including 4-hydroxynoneal, malondialdehyde, and acrolein generated by lipid peroxidation induce inhibition of enzyme as well as receptor alterations via binding and functional modification to protein leads to cell injury. Various reports suggested elevated level of malondialdehyde (oxidative stress biomarker) is observed in various types of cancer [41]. ROS is also responsible for DNA damage. Hydroxyl radicals (OH-) are highly unstable and a strong oxidizing agent which has the ability to react with most organic or inorganic cellular components such as DNA, lipids, proteins, amino acids, and sugars at a high rate. Hydrogen abstraction, addition, and electron transfer are key chemical reactions induced by hydroxyl radicals. These radicals target DNA and modify the deoxyribose by causing cross-linking [41].

Thymine glycol and 8-hydroxydeoxy guanosine (8-OHdG) are formed as a product of DNA damage. An oxidized form of guanine, i.e., 8-OHdG, is known as a chief oxidative DNA damage metabolite that causes transmutations such as C:C and G:C from A:T and T:A due to its potential to base pair with adenine and cytosine. Increase in 8-OHdG level was observed in various types of human tumors, i.e., high-grade glioma, than neighboring healthy tissue or even from low-grade glioma. Numerous reports suggested a strong link between oxidative stress and tumor onset and progression. Accumulation of 8-OHdG in salivary cell DNA was reported in patients with squamous cell carcinoma of head and neck attributed to a notable imbalance in their redox system. Its concentration was elevated in the case of breast tumor cells, too. Consequently, 8-OHdG is considered a significant tumor marker for clinical diagnosis [21, 42].

Glutathione is a major antioxidant as well as reducing agent present in the body in two different forms; one is resuscitated and oxidized, i.e., GSH and GSSG, respectively. Since an increased level of the reduced form of glutathione is observed in a healthy person thus elevated level of cellular GSSG and reduced level of GSH can be utilized as an oxidative stress marker. Various reports also exhibited a reduction in blood GSH status in breast cancer patients [41].

5.2.2 ROS-Mediated Epigenetic Modification in Cancer

Conventional epigenetic changes such as DNA methylation and histone alterations disrupt the availability of DNA transcription factors or may cause reorganization of chromatin structure and ultimately particular gene expression gets affected. It has been suggested that noncoding RNAs in general and specific miRNAs modulated gene expressions are closely associated with epigenetic alterations [43]. At the post-transcription stage, miRNAs can negatively control their concerned genes expression and after binding with their specific mRNAs, it attenuates the stability or even translation process. Moreover, epigenetic modifications are considered pathophysiological characteristics of cancer [44]. Besides acquired genetic alterations, epigenetic modifications of gene expression also play a major role in the onset and progression of cancer [45]. In cancerous cells, gene silencing occurs as a result of excessive hypermethylation of specific areas of tumor suppressor genes and this results in blockade of essential gene expression [46]. Oxidative stress and inflammation cause modulated epigenetic expression of cytokines, oncogenes as well as tumor suppressor genes, leading to chronic inflammation-mediated carcinogenesis [12, 47]. Even significantly reduced methylation of DNA molecules leads to global chromosomal instability, mutations, and ultimately carcinogenesis [48]. A new therapeutic approach could be an emphasis on epigenomes to reverse the epigenetic alteration linked with cancer or to maintain the regular gene expressions as these epigenetic damaging starts in the early stage of cancer [49].

5.2.2.1 Modern Techniques for Detection of ROS-Mediated DNA Damage

Since the endogenous and exogenous stimuli target the DNA molecules in eukaryotic cells to induce DNA lesions such as genomic instability, DNA helix breakage by altering the base, loss of genetic information by breaking the DNA double-strand, and accounts for various diseases, including cancer. DNA damage can be evaluated by utilizing different available modern strategies such as molecular, fluorescence, chemiluminescence, and analytical.

Molecular Approach

Polymerase Chain Reaction (PCR) and Agarose Gel Electrophoresis

PCR and agarose gel electrophoresis can be used to detect DNA lesions and breakage on the basis of reduction in the molecular weight of a single DNA strand. PCR is considered an effective and most common technique to estimate ROS-mediated DNA damage. In this technique, the amplification process of DNA molecule is arrested at the point of damage by preventing the *Taq* polymerase progression, which further quantitatively reduces the PCR product and produces DNA templates devoid of *Taq* obstructed lesions. PCR is an easy and consistent process in which precise replication of a specific DNA segment is performed and then agarose gel is employed to resolve an array of DNA fragments (50–50,000 bp) based on the percentage of agarose. Whereas quantification of the damaging effects on DNA strands is analyzed with quantitative PCR (qPCR) along with the kinetics study, concerned with the removal of mitochondrial DNA damage in human beings [50]. Damaging effect to the mitochondrial DNA in hydrogen peroxide treated *Schizosaccharomyces pombe* cells is reported to measure with this PCR technique. Various parameters need to be considered in qPCR such as quantification of DNA as well as amplified product, high-molecular-weight DNA, qPCR specific conditions, and estimation of DNA lesion frequency. Therefore, based on previous reports, detection of DNA damage with gene-specificity and repairing can be efficiently performed with PCR [51].

Additionally, UV-associated photoproducts of DNA, including cyclobutane pyrimidine dimers and 6-4 photoproducts distribution, can be detected with Ligation-mediated PCR. This technique has high sensitivity as it analyzes even a single DNA photoproduct at a very low UV range of 10–20 J/m^2 and in vivo DNA interactions with proteins [52].

Immuno-coupled PCR assay is especially used to couple the product of nucleic acid amplification with an antibody and further, in the enzyme-linked immunosorbent assay (ELISA) a biotinylated DNA attached with an antigen-antibody complex reinstates the detection enzyme. Gene thymine dimer generation is measured by this methodology and has been accounted directly proportional to the global concentration of human genomic DNA exposed to UV radiations. As compared to typical PCR and qPCR, PCR-based short interspersed DNA element (SINE) mediated assay is extremely sensitive towards detection of UV-B as well as xenobiotics induced DNA lesions, including cisplatin, by involving the faster amplification of extended DNA segments at the site of the genome transcription [53].

Fluorescence Strategies

Comet Assay

The comet assay is a highly efficient method to assess DNA adducts either single or double-stranded in eukaryotes. This technique is one of the easy and simple benchmark assays also called as single-cell gel electrophoresis [54]. Along with detecting the DNA lesions, it is also capable to analyze oxidized bases, pyrimidine dimers associated with UV, and alkylation abrasion through the development of lesion-specified endonucleases [55]. This assay is based on the identification of intact DNA as a comet head in the form of spherical mass whereas the strand breaks surrounded by DNA surge out like a tail from the head. In general, comet assay is performed with DNA immobilization by implanting in agarose followed by a lysis process with detergent and a high amount of salt. The restricted resolution power (10–800 kb) is considered as a limitation of comet assay when performed with standard conditions [56]. Other versions of comet assays are also available to detect DNA damage such as by using lesion-specific enzymes, alkaline and neutral single-cell gel electrophoresis.

Alkaline Single-cell Gel Electrophoresis

This variant of comet assay causes alkaline denaturation around the point of DNA breakage and extends the tails of comet. However, sensitivity and preciseness is the limitation of this technique as compared to a method including lesion-specific enzymes [57].

Neutral Single-cell Gel Electrophoresis

In this assay, alkaline treatment is initially utilized and after restoring in the neutral condition, the gel electrophoresis process is executed in a neutral or mild alkaline environment. This method is also considered less sensitive as compared to others [50].

Utilization of Lesion-specific Enzyme Technique

The lesion-specific enzymes technique has the ability to assess different types of DNA damage such as pyrimidine dimers or oxidized bases [58]. Briefly, these enzymes cause the formation of apyrimidic or apurinic region by removing the afflicting base. Whereas, impairments like 8-oxo-7,8-dihydroguanine and ring opened-purines are detected by formamidopyrimidine DNA glycosylases and endonucleases which specifically identify the oxidized pyrimidines [54].

Halo Assay

In this assay, a supercoiled DNA is created by embedding propidium iodide (PI) into the DNA helix followed by a lysis process in which the halos are generated from the particular cell's nucleoids and subjected to determine the chromatin damage. The "halo" diameter is considered as directly proportional with PI level and is represented in terms of supercoils either relaxed or rewound at a low and high PI, correspondingly. The advantage of this assay is the detection of DNA lesions in single-cell without using radioactive precursors labeling [59].

DNA Breakage Detection (DBD): Fluorescence In Situ Hybridization (FISH) Assay

The FISH technique deals with multiple target progression simultaneously, imaging of live cells and fast quantitative estimation. It allows detecting various aberrations at genetic, chromosomal, and genomic levels linked with various diseases. Consequently, it has clinical significance in tracing gene modifications in cancer patients.

Whereas, a variant of this FISH technique, i.e., DBD FISH is capable to analyze as well as quantify the single and double-strand DNA abrasion at the genomic level or with a single-cell's specific DNA sequence. Clinically, it has been utilized to diagnose the status of cervical cancer development based on quantification of DNA breakage within the genomic area, which is susceptible to destabilization [50].

Radioimmunoassay (RIA)

In this assay, synthesis of the marked antigen is performed either with a radiolabel or without any labeling and further coupled with a particular antibody. RIA technique is based on the assessment of antigens amount by using specific antibodies [60]. Additionally, this assay may be used to estimate the DNA abrasion including cyclobutane dimers in DNA and level of 6-4 photoproducts [59].

Chemiluminescence Tools

Enzyme-linked Immunosorbent Assay (ELISA)

ELISA is a frequently used immunological technique for the detection and quantification of damaging effects on DNA [61]. Briefly, it is performed with an unknown amount of antigen attached to a surface exposed to an unknown concentration of antibody to instigate the binding of the antibody with the antigen. After adding a suitable substrate, quantification of antibodies associated with an enzyme is carried out [59, 61].

Immunohistochemical Assay

Immunohistochemical assay is subjected to utilize proteases and RNase pretreated fixed cells. This method arrests the cross-reaction with DNA by removing proteins and RNA [61]. An immunohistochemical assay offers more precise screening and analysis of certain metabolites impairments for instance ALK gene within non-small-cell cancer of the lung [62].

Immunological Assay

This assay determines the existence of oxidative DNA by using the immunoslot-blot method and detection with chemiluminescence followed by conjugation of secondary antibodies with alkaline phosphatase enzymes and radioactive iodine [63]. This assay is limited in terms of the occurrence of antibodies' cross-reaction with normal DNA bases.

Analytical Strategies

High Performance Liquid Chromatography (HPLC) Electrospray Tandem Mass Spectrometry (MS)

Oxidative DNA damage due to oxidative stress and UV light absorption by nucleic acids is considered as one of the major causative factors for the promotion of carcinogenesis. The advancement in HPLC technique by coupling tandem MS along with an electrospray ionization mode represents an accurate and highly precise assay to estimate the oxidative damage to DNA bases as well as dimeric pyrimidine photoproducts associated with UV. With this technique, modified genomic DNA nucleobases can be easily identified and quantified during the early phase of the base excision repair [64]. Thus, HPLC-MS technique may act as a beneficial tool for the detection of single-stranded lesions as these are associated with proteins of the base excision repair pathway [65]. It has been reported that quantification of various oxidized nucleosides such as 8-oxo-7,8-dihydro-2'-deoxyadenosine, 8-oxo-7,8-dihydro-2'-deoxyguanosine, 5-formyl-2'-deoxyuridine, 5-hydroxymethyl-2'--deoxyuridine, and 5-hydroxy-2'-deoxyuridine can be performed with cellular DNA exposed to γ-rays [66]. Estimation of type of DNA lesion along with Tandem DNA lesions, i.e., dinucleoside monophosphates, also gives information about the exact site and extent of DNA damage [66, 67]. Since this technique offers high accuracy and is a preferred method, it has some limitations as it is expensive and requires skilled human resources to observe the oxidized base formation even at a low level in cellular DNA [66].

Gas Chromatography-mass Spectrometry (GC-MS) Technique

GC-MS has the ability to analyze different products of DNA adduction including heterocyclic bases as well as sugar moiety. Basically, gas chromatography aids in the detection of complex samples, while MS offers structural elucidation in terms of biological or chemical analysis. It detects a single DNA lesion within multiple DNA lesions or nucleobases linked with chemical or enzyme degradation of the nucleic acids with high sensitivity. In general, this technique involves DNA hydrolysis followed by derivatization and separation of hydrolysates by using gas chromatography, which is further detected and quantified with MS [50].

Electrochemical Methods

Electrochemical methods have been established for analyzing DNA damage induced by ROS and DNA modification on the basis of DNA-mediated charge transport. These techniques can observe numerous types of base damage products as well as discrepancies within base pairs [68]. Additionally, development of a sensor to estimate the single base mutations and duplex DNA base lesions has been hypothesized with respect to charge sensitivity against DNA film transport [69]. Other electrochemical methods such as electrocatalysis are novel methods to identify lesions even at a low level hence can be used as an early diagnostic approach. It is recommended as a sensitive, precise, selective, and economic method for DNA damage detection, but it is unable to rapidly distinguish thymidine dimer-related lesions without associating with the DNA double helix distortion [59].

5.3 Bioactive Polyphenols in Cancer Treatment

5.3.1 Epigenetic and Antioxidant Approach

Numerous epidemiological reports have advised that cellular damage induced by overproduced ROS (superoxide, hydrogen peroxide, and hydroxyl free radicals) is recognized as a basic causative factor of cancer as well as age-associated diseases [70]. Therefore, despite the availability of standard cancer treatment methods, reduction of oxidative stress by regular utilization of antioxidant molecules is implied as a quintessential strategy for cancer treatment or prevention [71]. Experimental evidence based on animal and human studies have focused on antioxidant effect of dietary polyphenol molecules [72–74]. Polyphenols could be a beneficial tool in cancer prevention as well as associated mortality [75]. Besides the antioxidant potential to prevent oxidative damage, polyphenols also exhibit beneficial activities through restructuring of chromatin and other epigenetic remodeling [76]. Polyphenols, in terms of chemoprevention, can act as a reversible modulator in epigenetic pathways, concerned with tumorigenesis, resulting in activation or silencing of gene expression [77]. Various polyphenols [apigenin, epigallocatechin-3-gallate (EGCG), luteolin, delphinidin] directly activate or block the epigenetic enzymes [histone acetyltransferase (HAT), DNA methyltransferase (DNMT), and histone deacetylases (HDAC) [78]], regulate the expression of NF-κB and remodulate the chromatin structure. Past reports have revealed that several polyphenols including curcumin, sulforaphane, and resveratrol exhibits antitumor potential via histone protection from deacetylation during epigenetic alterations. Polyphenols such as EGCG, curcumin, and genistein prevent acetylation of histone proteins [79]. Resveratrol, lycopene, EGCG, curcumin, and genistein dietary polyphenols act by inhibiting the methylation process of DNA molecules via DNMT activity modulation [80].

Cancer cells are mainly characterized by the presence of some distinguished features in response to cumulative epigenetic modification of multiple genes along with their related cell signaling pathways. Some pathways are closely connected to the process of inflammation [81]. Furthermore, tumor cells allow immune cell infiltration; thus, the anti-inflammation approach might affect the therapy of cancer [82]. Modulation of epigenetic cofactor including inflammatory cascades associated with cancer with minimum toxicity by polyphenols is well-established [83]. Most polyphenols act as strong anti-inflammatory agents due to their ability to persuade HDAC enzyme activity [84]. Whereas some polyphenols have the ability to regulate the activity of HDAC as well as HAT, may be due to interconnection of responsible mechanism. Polyphenol, such as curcumin, a potential free radical scavenger, downregulates the oxidative damage possibly by both mechanisms of acetylation and deacetylation modulation [85]. It has been reported that oxidative stress ultimately leads to the acceleration of proinflammatory mediators via inhibition of HDAC and stimulation of HAT intrinsic enzyme activity, which is involved with NF-κB pathway [86].

Luteolin act as a chemopreventive polyphenol that modulates ROS-mediated specific signal transduction pathways as well as enzymes related to DNA replication. Elangovan et al. reported 1% luteolin-containing diet exhibited a significant decrease in fibrosarcoma rate in mice model by alleviating the enhanced concentrations of lipid peroxides and cytochrome P450 [87]. Luteolin is believed to be engaged with various possible mechanisms such as reduction in oxidative stress by ROS level regulation, NF-kB and activator protein-1 (AP-1) hypofunction, topoisomerases (I, II) inhibition, downregulation of PI3K, signal transducer and activator of transcription protein 3 (STAT3), insulin-like growth factor I receptor (IGF1R), as well as human epidermal growth factor receptor 2 (HER2), and p53 stabilization to wield chemopreventive activity [88].

Tea is widely consumed and the second most prevalent beverage worldwide. Green, black, and oolong tea is rich in polyphenols. Tea polyphenols are reported to have photo-protective activity against DNA damages induced by UV rays, which directly or indirectly cause the onset of inflammation, oxidative stress, and alteration in cell signaling pathways as well as epigenetic modifications [89]. The most popular tea polyphenols are green tea polyphenols with EGCG, an abundant (50–88%) component present in green tea [71]. Polyphenols in green tea possess strong antioxidant potential, which contributes to anti-inflammatory and cancer prevention effects. It has been reported that treatment with green tea polyphenol at a dose level of 0.05% in the form of sole source of drinking fluid results in an average increase (5–7%) in mean survival time along with a reduction in tumor load (25–39%) in mice with mammary adenocarcinoma via significant reduction in malondialdehyde–DNA adduct [90]. In cultured cells, EGCG has been reported to hamper some key transduction signaling pathways and responsible to activate several redox-sensitive transcription factors including NF-κB and AP-1 [91]. Moreover, in the mouse skin model, EGCG inhibits the DNA binding of NF-κB and cAMP response element-binding protein (CREB) mediated by 12-O-tetradecanoylphorbol 13-acetate [92]. During in vitro study, EGCG inhibits the process of carcinogenesis by acting on several signal transduction pathways such as PI3K/Akt, Janus kinase/signal transducer and activator of transcription protein (JAK/STAT), Wnt, MAPK, and Notch [93]. Additionally, EGCG blocks phosphorylation of MAPK induced by oxidative stress in human fibrosarcoma HT1080 cells as well as breast cancer cell line T47D and skin cells [88]. EGCG is also able to prevent cisplatin, a cancer chemotherapeutic agent, induced side effects specifically nephrotoxicity induced by oxidative stress. Cisplatin is known to cause mitochondrial oxidative stress in the kidney and disturb the activity of antioxidant enzymes. EGCG may be utilized as a promising adjunct to cisplatin chemotherapy [94]. Moreover, these polyphenols are extensively beneficial from epigenetic side. EGCG treatment modulated methylation level of DNA molecules and remodeling of chromatin protein in human prostate cancer cell line as well as decreased the Class I HDACs activity [95]. Among all green tea polyphenols, EGCG promisingly blocks HAT activity while rest of the polyphenol derivatives including epicatechin, catechin, and epigallocatechin exerted less effect on HAT inhibition. EGCG also prevents the coupling of p300/CREB binding protein (CBP) with the IL-6 gene promoter area and accelerated HDAC3 level, which plays a major role in HATs and histone deacetylases equilibrium during NF-κB associated inflammatory signaling pathway [96]. For the treatment of skin cancer, EGCG exhibited beneficial effects by regulating the DNA methylation process along with histone alteration and tumor suppressor genes p16INK4a and p21 (CIP1/WAF1) regulation [97]. Combinational therapy of polyphenols demonstrated the possible synergistic chemopreventive approach. For instance, a DNA methyltransferase inhibitor (dietary green tea polyphenols) and a histone deacetylase inhibitor (sulforaphane) in breast cancer cell lines caused an epigenetic modification of muted tumor suppressor genes such as p21 (CIP1/WAF1) and Klotho via chromatin activation [98]. Past studies have revealed that treatment of different human cancer cell lines with EGCG regulates the hypermethylation of p15, p16INK4a, MGMT, hMLH1, and RARβ genes in time as well as dose-dependent manner [99, 100]. Epigenetic silencing in various human cancers is basically characterized by abnormal and accelerated methylation of Wnt inhibitory factor-1 (WIF-1). EGCG potential to promote WIF-1 is attributed to increased demethylation in lung cancer cell lines [101]. Polyphenols exist in tea and coffee act via demethylation in cell lines concerned with human breast cancer. Likewise, caffeic acid and chlorogenic acid exhibited dose-dependent effect on DNMT1 inhibition [102]. Caffeic acid exhibits anticancer and antimetastatic effects by controlling the phase of tumor promotion through inhibition of inflammatory responses and oxidative stress events via reducing the expression level of COX-2 and NF-κB [103, 104]. Black tea has been reported as an anti-tumorigenic in the lung and liver [105]. Theaflavin present in black tea modulates the signal transduction pathway linked with PI3K, which affects inflammation, proliferation, and apoptosis in mice [106]. In multiple myeloma human cells, theaflavins showed antitumor activity by preventing chymotrypsin-like activity against tumor proteasome [107]. Past reports demonstrated that polyphenols, chlorogenic and caffeic acids present in coffee beans and other plant sources, have shown a strong antioxidant effect in vitro as well as in vivo. Furthermore, chlorogenic acid is observed as an anticancer agent by inhibiting the DNA damage by modulating the NF-κB pathway associated with ROS. An interesting study has explored a reciprocal relationship between regular coffee intake with the risk of endometrial, liver, breast, and colon cancer onset. It showed daily consumption of at least one cup of coffee reduced the risk of cancer associated with the upper gastrointestinal tract by 49% in the Japanese population [108].

Over the recent years, apigenin has gained attention due to its therapeutic point of view such as potential anticancer effect with low toxicity than other flavonoids having structural similarities [109]. It acts through restraining ornithine decarboxylase as well as cell growth and inhibits the tumor growth via modulation of different signaling pathways such as PI3K/Akt, MAPK, and B-cell lymphoma (Bcl)-2-associated X protein (Bax)/Bcl-2 ratio [110–113]. It has also been suggested that treatment of malignant cells with apigenin causes a blockage of G2/M and G0/G1 phase arrest by affecting the activity of p34 (cdc2) kinase along with stabilization of p53 protein [114]. Apigenin exhibited doxorubicin sensitivity reversal effect against hepatocellular carcinoma BEL-7402 and BEL-7402/ADM cells, which were resistant to doxorubicin at a dose level of 10 μM. This effect is associated with a reduction in expression of nuclear factor erythroid 2-related factor 2 (NRF2) mRNA as well as protein via attenuating PI3K/Akt pathway. Interestingly, in BEL-7402 xenografts, the combinational approach of apigenin and doxorubicin showed a synergistic effect on the reduction of tumor growth along with cellular proliferation rate and increase in apoptosis [115].

Vegetables belonging to the cruciferous family including broccoli, cabbage, cauliflower, and kale are highly rich in bioactive polyphenol, i.e., sulforaphane, has the ability to persuade the expression of various enzymes such as detoxification enzymes (phase II) through stimulation of cytoplasmic NRF2 and murine hepatocytes associated glutathione transferase [116, 117]. Under oxidative stress conditions, NRF2 promotes the expression of different antioxidant enzymes after binding with an antioxidant responsive element in the nucleus [118]. Sulforaphane significantly reduced the tumor size and promoted the process of apoptosis in xenograft murine when administered orally. Anticancer effect of sulforaphane exerted through various mechanisms including a reduction in oxidative stress caused by NRF2 linked pathways and inhibition of HDAC activity explored in colon cancer cell line HCT116 dose-dependently [119]. Histones acetylation was found affected in prostate, ileum, and colon of C57BL/6J mice whose food was supplemented with sulforaphane for 10 weeks [120]. Furthermore, two bioactive metabolites generated from sulforaphane [sulforaphane-*N*-acetylcysteine and sulforaphane-cysteine], in response to the mercapturic acid pathway, also showed the effective inhibition of HDAC [121].

Curcumin, a well-known polyphenol, is widely utilized for its broad-spectrum beneficial effects such as antioxidant and anti-inflammation contributed to various diseases including cancer [122]. Curcumin has been explored as a long-term chemopreventive agent by accelerating the level of antioxidant enzymes attributed to activation of NRF2 signaling pathway, promoting effect on tumor suppressor p53, and regulation of various inflammatory mediators (TGF-β and COX2) in mice with liver lymphoma. Curcumin is also reported to affect the activity of HAT and HDAC enzymes through histones modulation [123]. Numerous reports based on in vitro studies on different cancer cell lines have suggested that curcumin reduced the activity of p300/CBP HAT which particularly curbs acetylation of histone as well as nonhistone protein, i.e., p53 [124]. Additionally, in hepatoma-cultured cells, curcumin significantly reduced the level of histone acetylation by inhibiting the HAT activity without affecting HDAC [125]. Curcumin reserved the p300/CBP-related HAT activity along with various classes of HDACs when explored in hematopoietic cell lines, which restrict the cell proliferation and initiates apoptosis [85]. Antitumor effect exerted by curcumin via regulation of miRNA level in cancer cells. For instance, curcumin has demonstrated to reduce the level of expression of protein Bcl-2 attributed to antiapoptosis in breast cancer cell line MCF7 through ameliorating effect on miRNA-15a as well as miRNA-16 [126]. Intake of dietary curcumin (2%) alone and combination of curcumin (1%) and PEITC have been found effective in high-grade carcinoma and cause apoptosis by modulating the Akt signaling pathway in mice prostate model with transgenic adenocarcinoma

[127]. Numerous reports have reported that curcumin can inhibit cell cycle progression, tumor growth, and angiogenesis along with apoptosis induction in ovarian cancer at a dose level of 500 mg/kg in vivo [128]. Curcumin acts as a chemopreventive agent by targeting various mechanisms including NF-κB pathway inhibition, increase in Apo2L/TNF-related apoptosis-inducing ligand (TRAIL) induced apoptosis [129], regulation of Akt and p38 MAPK pathway which further results in the introduction of G2/M cell cycle arrest and apoptosis [130] and affecting different enzymes associated with drug metabolism [131]. Curcumin slowed down the tumor formation against HER-2 positive breast cancer in mice [132]. When curcumin was administered with other established polyphenols, such as EGCG, it was effective in oral cancer [133] and breast cancer (with genistein) [134] via TRAIL in lymph node carcinoma of the prostate (LNCaP) cells [135].

An important polyphenol, i.e., resveratrol, occurs in various types of fruit berries like blueberries, cranberries, raspberries as well as in nuts, red grapes, and wine. It exhibits a strong anti-inflammatory, antioxidant effect and influences the metabolic process of glucose directly or indirectly contributing to anticancer activity [136]. Furthermore, it regulates cellular growth, angiogenesis, cell apoptosis, and metastasis processes of a tumor by affecting responsible signaling pathways [137]. Cancer cells are characterized by a high level of oxidative stress along with glycolytic flux. Therefore, resveratrol can reduce the level of intracellular ROS as well as glycolytic metabolism of cancer cells. It generates the inactive chromatin molecules in response to stimulation of protein deacetylase sirtuin (SIRT) 1 and modifies the gene transcriptional process [138]. Whereas, considering the other side, p300/CBP HAT is activated by resveratrol, which is involved in the production of the active form of chromatin [139]. Additionally, Tili et al. demonstrated that resveratrol causes various epigenetic modifications and participates in the activation of tumor suppressor miRNAs during the oncogenesis process [140]. The cytoprotective effect of resveratrol has been suggested against paclitaxel-induced cytotoxicity in breast cancer cell lines such as MDA-MB-231, MDA-MB-435s, and SKBR-3, except MCF-7 cell lines [141]. Daily and high utilization of freeze-dried black raspberries act as a chemopreventive agent in Barrett's esophagus, a premalignant esophageal condition characterized by oxidative stress-induced metaplastic columnar-lined epithelium estimated in urine [142] due to significant reduction in oxidative stress level and tumor incidence [143].

At the onset of breast cancer, different hallmark epigenetic alterations are observed such as alleviation in the level of SIRT expression attributed to tumor suppressor gene. In vitro as well as in vivo experimental studies revealed that resveratrol has the potential to inhibit the expression of survivin in response to elevate the BRCA1 expression with an accelerating effect on SIRT1 expression. Therefore, resveratrol therapy can be utilized as targeted drug therapy for the treatment of breast cancer associated with Breast cancer type 1 susceptibility protein (BRCA1) [144]. Resveratrol and curcumin possess significant chemopreventive effects in mice induced with lung carcinogenesis by regulating enzymes associated with drug metabolism as well as antioxidant activity when utilized in combination therapy [145].

Isoflavones such as genistein and daidzein have similar chemopreventive effect as estrogens against different types of cancers particularly in breast cancer and prostate cancer induced by hormones in human [146]. Genistein is capable to compete with both natural estrogen receptors [estrogen receptor alpha (ERα) and the estrogen receptor beta (ERβ)]. Ratio of ERα/ERβ is considered as a predictive indicator for breast cancer and the status of ERα expression could hint at the existence of malignant tumors. ERα/ERβ ratio is majorly affected by genistein treatment in addition to regulation of enzymatic antioxidant status, oxidative stress, function of mitochondria, and SIRT in human breast cancer cell lines [147, 148]. It was also found to modulate gene transcription by affecting DNA methylation and histone alteration like epigenetic modification incidence. Regarding human esophageal squamous carcinoma cell line, genistein acts by regulating the hypermethylation of DNA molecules and reactivation of methylated silenced genes such as tumor suppressor gene p16INK4a [149]. Under the influence of renal carcinoma, B-cell translocation gene 3 (BTG3) and tumor suppressor gene is inhibited in response to an increase in 5'-cytosine-phosphate-guanine-3' (CpG) methylation. This was significantly upregulated by genistein administration by causing demethylation of CpG, DNMT reduction, and modifications of active histone [150]. Additionally, genistein can influence at miRNAs level as it accelerates the expression of miRNA-1296 along with S phase cells accumulation and reduces the target of miRNA-1296, i.e., mini chromosome maintenance gene (MCM-2) in prostate cancer cells [151].

A dietary polyphenol, i.e., quercetin, occurs in various vegetables and citrus fruits which reduce intracellular oxidative stress by scavenging the ROS. Past reports of in vitro head and neck tumor model suggest that quercetin caused reduction of aldehyde dehydrogenase (ALDH) 1 level, and inhibited head and neck cancer associated spheres induced stemness expression [152]. Whereas in pancreatic cancer it works by inhibition of β-catenin [153]. Quercetin also inhibits HDAC and DNMT1 activity leading to activation of SIRT1 deacetylase, which ultimately results in cell cycle arrest, and apoptosis by p53-linked mechanism and retard the growth of the tumor as well as angiogenesis [154]. Quercetin and genistein have an enzyme inhibitory effect on protein tyrosine kinase concerned with cell proliferation [155].

Antitumor potential of ellagic acid was exhibited by affecting the cellular pathways like deactivation of PI3K/Akt, which resulted in regulation of Bcl-2 family proteins [156]. Supplementation of ellagic acid modulates the expression of Bax and caspase-3 caused an acceleration in cytochrome concentration and ultimately cell death. Study explored with in vitro and in vivo tumor models concluded the chemopreventive effect of proanthocyanidins via targeting at various molecular levels. In different cancer cells, oleuropein inhibited the cell cycle and induced apoptosis [157]. Oleuropein and hydroxytyrosol have also been reported to downregulate the HER2/neu receptor overexpression induced by Herceptin in breast cancer [158].

Polyphenolic rich fraction extracted from artichoke showed significant cytotoxic and apoptosis induction effects in colorectal cancer cells by modulating the expression of Bax gene as well as p21CIP1/WAF1 cell cycle inhibition [159]. It is also found effective against different human cell lines including hepatoma cell line [160]. On human breast cancer cell line, it induced the process of apoptosis dose-dependently without affecting the normal breast epithelial cell line. Moreover, artichoke causes epigenetic modification including reduction in DNA hypermethylation and enhances the level of lysine acetylation [161]. Interestingly, artichoke polyphenols exhibit prooxidant effect on breast cancer cells [162], while in normal hepatocytes it acts through antioxidant mechanism [160].

5.3.2 Therapy-Induced Senescence Approach

Cytotoxicity is the basic approach for cancer treatment therapy. As this therapeutic strategy may cause the death of a cell in neoplastic tissues but the frequent incidence of therapy resistance or induction of advanced stage of primary as well as metastatic tumors has been observed in various types of cancers. Therefore, against such case, a promising alternative approach, i.e., induction of cytostasis, has been utilized which inhibits the ability of cells to proliferate without causing the death of the cancerous cell [163]. This cancer treatment strategy provides minimal or no side effects associated with chemoprevention in cancer patients along with an equal or extended survival rate. It may represent a more pragmatic and targeted therapeutic approach for the management or treatment of some chronic cancer types. For induction of cytostasis, a potential therapeutic tool such as therapy-induced senescence (TIS) persuades a complete and irreversible arrest of cell growth with different anatomical and biochemical properties [164]. It mainly affects morphologically with flat, extended characters and accelerates β-galactosidase enzyme activity linked with senescence in tissues as well as cultured cells [165]. With the conventional approach of cytotoxic drugs, the apoptotic process continuously progresses but regarding senescent cells, they have the ability to endure permanently [166]. Tumor suppressor genes such as retinoblastoma protein (Rb) and p53 are considered essential genes possessing promising inhibitory effects on tumor cell growth. It has been reported that cells having active p53 and Rb genes are, more susceptible to stress conditions and oncogenic behavior, responsible to activate senescence [167]. However, tumor cells devoid of active Rb, p53, and several other tumor suppressive proteins greatly respond to TIS, and it is accounted as an important therapeutic approach. For instance, doxorubicin accelerated senescence in more than 50% of cells without affecting Rb and p53 genes in cancer cell lines deficit to these characteristic tumor suppressor genes [168].

The underlying mechanism, i.e., cells affected by senescence or cell death, can be defined by p53 and Rb mutual function [169, 170]. As of now, the specific role of these tumor suppressor proteins in response to senescence activity is quite intricate and not even known to its complete level. Along with p53 and Rb, several other overexpressed genes involved with cell cycle such as p16INK4a, p27, cyclin-dependent kinase inhibitors (CDKI), and p21CIP1/WAF1 [171, 172] play a vital role in process of senescence by promoting the senescent status in cancer cell lines. It is noticed that a reduced level of p21CIP1/WAF1 expression delays the cell cycle arrest associated with senescence, while its overexpressed state causes rapid initiation of cell cycle arrest influenced by senescence [173]. Likewise, p16INK4a regulates Rb phosphorylation via reducing CDK4 and CDK6 activation [174]. The p16INK4a is attributed to Rb functional activity, its hypophosphorylated state, which leads to inhibit various genes regulated by E2F transcription factors participating in the arrest of G1 cell cycle. Various reports have suggested the importance of both, p53/p21 and Rb/p16, pathways in significant promotion of cell senescence in two ways; the first is caused by the shortening of telomere and damaging effects on DNA, and another one is associated with stress-induced premature senescence (SIPS) [175, 176].

Development of novel cancer therapeutic tool with a combination approach by using induction of prosenescence with well-established treatment therapy could be worthwhile. This combination of neoadjuvant with adjuvant protocol has a beneficial role in various neoplasias treatment, such as prostate, colon, and breast cancer, and it is found to enhance the survival rate in patients or disease-free survival [177]. A conventional treatment approach could be provided in combination with prosenescence therapy before the process of surgery to lessen the tumor mass within a neoadjuvant protocol. Furthermore, natural compounds, particularly polyphenols, may be utilized as senescence-inducing moieties in a combinational approach along with radiotherapy but due to some physiological limitations, such as age or severe stage of the disease, they are not suitable for surgical therapy [178, 179]. Such type of treatment is believed to act by introducing senescence where it causes the inhibition of tumoral growth and clears senescent cells by stimulating the immune system. This ultimately contributes to diminishing the mass of the tumor. Both factors, senescence and apoptosis contribute to p53; therefore, a synergistic effect on cancer cells could be observed with the combination of prosenescence protocol along with conventional radiotherapeutic or chemotherapeutic approach, which directs induction of senescent and apoptotic cell death.

Various prosenescence agents are gaining attention and clinically explored to assess their potential for cancer management. Nowadays, natural compounds involved epigenetically in senescence control are mainly focused to develop beneficial prosenescence tools in cancer therapy [180]. Most polyphenols present in fruit and vegetables are proved as anticancer via inhibiting the cellular growth majorly by inducing premature senescence associated with ROS. A natural compound extracted from ginseng, i.e., 20(S)-ginsenoside Rg3, produced senescence-linked cell growth arrest at subapoptosis level and elevated ROS in human glioma cells [181]. Additionally, bisdemethoxycurcumin naturally derived from curcumin was reported to curb cell proliferation via induction of oxidative stress-related senescence in human breast cancers [182]. Similarly, phenethyl isothiocyanate also exhibited cellular apoptosis along with tumor senescence [183]. Artichoke extract rich in polyphenols at high doses has the ability to act as a chemopreventive agent explored in human breast cancer cell line MDA-MB231 through apoptosis and restricting its invasion potential [184]. Artichoke extract administration at sublethal dose stimulates premature senescence by following epigenetic and ROS-mediated pathways to suppress cell growth in human breast cancer. Since artichoke polyphenols possess a strong antioxidant effect, an elevated concentration of ROS has been observed as a responsible key stimulus for the induction of senescence with chronic administration of artichoke extract. These reports demonstrated the essential contribution of ROS in cancer cells as a precursor for causing prooxidant damage induced by polyphenols. The key role of ROS was substantiated with attenuation of the potential effect of artichoke extract on MDA-MB231 cell line by antioxidant N-acetyl cysteine. Additionally, artichoke extract exhibited a prooxidant effect in breast cancer cells, [161] whereas in normal hepatocytes it showed antioxidant activity [185]. As numerous tumor cells are characterized by the occurrence of an aberrant redox system, artichoke extract may act via selectively restricting the cellular growth of tumor without or with minor toxic effects on normal cells attributed to their redox system status.

Resveratrol was also found to be effective in chemoprevention through the onset of premature type of senescence in lung cancer cells when treated at a low dose. Increased damage to DNA double strands as well as over generation of ROS in response to increased expression of NAPDH oxidase-5 is known to correspond with the antitumor effect of resveratrol [186]. Another study reported that resveratrol cause inhibition of gastric cancer cell growth and further promote apoptosis at a high dose, while at low dose it induced senescence instead of apoptotic response by arresting cell growth at G1 phase. In vivo model, i.e., a nude mice xenograft also supported the inhibitory activity of resveratrol on gastric cancer cells. Additionally, resveratrol was observed to be a gastric cancer progression inhibitory agent and it significantly reduced Ki67-positive cells within the tumor sample of nude mice [187]. With the treatment of resveratrol, a similar type of response was estimated in vitro as well by causing an alteration in regulators engaged with the cell cycle and triggering the senescence-associated pathways. The ability of various tumor cells to get affected by senescence at a low dose and chronic administration with resveratrol, and undergo apoptosis mechanism after providing high doses of resveratrol was corroborated with C6 rat glioma cell lines. Furthermore, it has been investigated that resveratrol and quercetin given chronically at subapoptotic doses can produce cell growth arrest associated with senescence. Based on the results, this combinational therapy can be utilized as a beneficial tool for the treatment of glioma cell tumors [188].

5.4 Contribution of Polyphenols in Targeting Cancer Stem Cells (CSCs)

5.4.1 Effect of Polyphenols on CSCs Self-renewal Regulation

Over recent years, many reports confirmed the presence of CSCs in many solid as well as nonsolid tumors associated with colon, head, breast, brain, neck, leukemia, etc. [189]. CSCs are attributed to tumor recurrence and therapy-resistant tumors [190]; consequently targeting CSCs for novel therapeutic approaches is gaining attention [191]. Although, CSCs are distinct cancer cells having a comparatively low level of ROS because of high concentration of ROS scavenging molecules. They respond more competently towards DNA repair and on the process of glycolysis and autophagy [192]. Numerous CSCs targeting approaches have been suggested which includes (1) inhibition of self-renewal potential along with other pathways related to chemoresistance, (2) induction of cell differentiation ability [193], (3) targeting several molecular markers on their cellular surface [194], (4) inhibiting the glycolysis by affecting their energy metabolism [195], by targeting cell organelle including mitochondria [196], and (e) constructing novel strategies for complete inhibition of cancer stemness based on miRNA [197]. It has been estimated that CSCs might stay in a special microenvironment characterized by the presence of hypoxia-like conditions [198], a peri-tumor acidic pH [199], oxidative stress [22], and chronic inflammation [200] in almost every type of tumor. Therefore, considering the situation, many scientists have advised that cancer disease can be treated by involving one of the two mechanisms; one is by CSCs metabolism arrest or the second is by disturbing the adjoining cancer cell environment [201].

Design of a novel anticancer tool depends on carefully targeting the CSCs. To fulfill this objective, natural compounds having anticancer potential might exhibit a relevant beneficial role. Various organic natural polyphenolic compounds are addressed in numerous reports as CSCs' regulating substances.

5.4.2 Effect of Polyphenols on CSCs Metabolism

Polyphenols are reported to possess the ability to influence the pathways (Wnt/β-catenin, Hedgehog, and Notch) associated with the self-renewal of CSCs [202]. Particularly, isothiocyanates exhibited a beneficial effect in preventing human tumors [203]. It follows different mechanisms to inhibit signaling pathways, i.e., NF-κB and STAT3, related to oncogenesis via regulation of apoptosis process, epithelial-mesenchymal transition, stimulation of enzymatic detoxification of carcinogens, and inhibition of cell proliferation as well as CSCs self-regeneration [204].

Sulforaphane, mostly present in plants of the cruciferous family, has been identified as CSCs targeting agent in different cancers by involving various pathways such as NF-κB, Hedgehog, and Wnt/ β-catenin regulation along with transitional induction of epithelial mesenchyma [205]. Therefore, keeping these properties in mind, some preclinical studies recommended sulforaphane along with chemotherapy as an ancillary agent [206]. Sulforaphane was found to have reducing properties on cancer cell growth against human breast cancer cells due to alleviating the level of ALDH positive cells as well as mammospheres detected during in vitro study [207]. Additionally, in vitro and in vivo models revealed sulforaphane is responsible to inhibit cell proliferation in pancreatic CSCs via stimulation of the Hedgehog pathway responsible for the self-renewal of CSCs [208].

Quercetin was also observed to be beneficial in pancreatic CSCs studies by decreasing ALDH1, inducing apoptosis and reducing epithelial–mesenchymal transition proteins expression in vitro [209]. In vivo studies also exhibited that treatment with quercetin reduced cell proliferation and decreased gene expression of angiogenesis and stemness, which caused arrest of xenografts associated with CSCs [210]. Reports suggested the combination therapy of various polyphenolic compounds to design a potent synergistic tool for cancer treatment as sulforaphane and quercetin exhibited improved effects when given in combination [211]. Regular utilization of soy foods, rich in isoflavones, has reduced the risk of mammary tumors and controlled breast cancer-related adiposity along with bodyweight in animal as well as human models [212, 213]. Culture medium rich with genistein isoflavone treated adipocytes-like condition exhibits a reduced level of mammospheres formation in human MCF-7 breast cancer cells [214].

Curcumin extracted from *Curcuma longa* has an anti-inflammatory effect against acute pancreatitis and targeted pancreatic CSCs [215] by affecting mitogen-activated protein kinase signaling pathway [216]. Combination approach of curcumin with different well-known chemoprotective agents including oxaliplatin against colorectal cancer cell lines [217], gemcitabine in a pancreatic cancer orthotopic model, paclitaxel against bladder cancer has been observed as potentially synergistic. One more report suggested that curcumin with metformin imparted a promising anticancer effect via CSC mechanism in oral squamous cell carcinoma [218].

5.4.3 Effect of Polyphenols on CSCs Metabolism

Hyperglycolitic metabolism is the characteristic property of CSCs [219] and they have decreased level of mitochondrial respiration in tumor mass than other cells [220]. Therefore, impairment in the metabolic process either by blocking glycolysis or by forced mitochondrial metabolism of CSCs and their oxidative phosphorylation could be an important possibility to thwart CSCs [221]. A number of polyphenols are known to contribute to the regulation of cancer metabolism. For instance, genistein has been reported to modulate the pentose phosphate pathway without affecting fatty acids synthesis in pancreatic adenocarcinoma cells [222]. Furthermore, in human breast cancer cells, EGCG was observed to stimulate AMP-activated protein kinase (AMPK) which is essential for cellular energy level regulation, protein synthesis, cell cycle as well as cell viability [223]. AMPK activation primarily causes inhibition of cell proliferation, increased level of CDK inhibitor p21CIP1/WAF1 whereas decreased the level of rapamycin pathway associated with targeting and arrest of CSCs growth [224]. Additionally, olive oil polyphenols possess anticancer activity by alleviating the level of gene expression partakes in CSCs self-renewal and aerobic glycolysis (Warburg effect) [225]. Since a high level of oxidative stress is observed in CSCs with enhanced glycolytic activity, they are more prone to additional damaging effect induced by prooxidant polyphenols as compared to normal cells [226]. One more report based on polyphenol, i.e., curcumin, exhibited chemopreventive effect by inducing cell death via accelerated ROS formation and cell apoptosis, and degraded potential of the mitochondrial membrane in different cancer models [227, 228].

It has been demonstrated that CSCs lay within specific locations particularly at the site of inflammation, oxidative stress, and low level of oxygen along with low pH [3]. Therefore, polyphenols are suggested to target the concerned signaling pathways supporting tumor microenvironmental characteristics. Regarding these features, pterostilbene extracted from berries (blueberries) exhibited an anticancer effect by targeting hypoxia. In vitro studies revealed that upon a coculture process of breast cancer cell lines (MCF-7 and MDA-MB231) and tumor-promoted malignant metastasis showed significantly populated CSCs with increased formation of mammospheres through modulation of β-catenin, Twist1, hypoxia-inducible factor 1α, and NF-κB pathways. Rate of CSC formation was promisingly decreased with the incorporation of pterostilbene into the cell culture medium. In vivo experiments further exhibited the beneficial antitumor effects of these polyphenols by inhibition of various key processes such as tumorigenesis as well as metastasis [229, 230].

5.4.4 Effect of Polyphenols on Proinflammatory Signaling Pathways

Neoplastic niche is majorly characterized by the existence of chronic inflammation [231]; therefore, most polyphenols play a vital therapeutic role in counteracting chronic inflammation responsible for initiating various diseases like cancer [232]. Natural phenolic and flavonoid compounds that exist in vegetables and fruits are suggested to act as anti-inflammatory by suppressing NF-κB pathway, contributing in different pathological processes including cell transformation, inflammation, proliferation, metastasis, and angiogenesis of tumor cells [233]. Carotenoids showed anti-inflammatory and anticancer effects by downregulating the NF-κB signaling pathway [234]. Glucosinolates, present in Brassicaceae family reported to possess a significant protective effect against inflammation and tumor in a murine model with inflammation-induced colon cancer [235].

5.4.5 Effect of Polyphenols in Regulation of Peritumoral pH

An acidic environment is the distinct feature of CSCs' extracellular surroundings induced by aerobic glycolysis [236]. In vivo animal studies demonstrated that utilization of sodium bicarbonate neutralizes acidic cancer pH and thereby it arrest tumor growth as well as cancer cell invasion [237]. Moreover, the consumption of vegetables and fruits diet, rich in potassium, along with less intake of animal proteins might be a promising tool to counterbalance cancer-induced acidosis.

Various polyphenols including resveratrol and genistein also contributed to neutralizing the acidic pH and they can be used as a potent therapeutic and chemopreventive strategy by causing damaging effects on CSC metabolism or by enforced oxidative phosphorylation of tumor cells. Besides, other bioactive phytocompounds have also been advised to elevate the cellular pH level by influencing the activity of the proton pump and ultimately induction of cell apoptosis [238]. Some important polyphenolic anticancer agents are listed in Table 5.1.

5.5 Polyphenols in Anticancer Clinical Trials

Preclinical studies of various polyphenols including curcumin, resveratrol, EGCG, lycopene, quercetin, and sulforaphane have proved the effectiveness against different cancers; therefore, clinical trials of some of these compounds are presently in progress.

Curcumin is widely reported as a potential chemopreventive and chemotherapeutic agent in different types of cancer cells. Curcumin has been observed safe, nontoxic, and tolerable in Phase I clinical trials administered even at a high dose of 8 g/day but it showed poor bioavailability in humans. Even after the curcumin bioavailability issue, clinical trials have exhibited efficacy towards prostate cancer, breast cancer, and hematological malignancies [274] when given either alone or in combination as an anticancer agent. Pastorelli et al. reported curcumin Meriva® (2000 mg/day) enhances the efficacy of gemcitabine to the local or advanced metastatic pancreatic cancer patients without exerting any toxic effects [275]. Presently, determination of curcumin (300 mg/i.v./day) efficacy in combination with Paclitaxel (80 mg/m^2 BS; i.v.) administered once weekly for consecutive 12 weeks in patients with advanced and metastatic breast cancer is in progress by using randomized, double-blind, and placebo-controlled phase 2/3 trial (NCT03072992). Additionally, curcumin is registered on clinicaltrials.gov with other 18 actively ongoing clinical trials associated with cancer.

EGCG also proved safe by clinical data when administered in patients with high-grade prostatic intraepithelial neoplasia and/or atypical small acinar proliferation at a dose level of 200 mg/day. Polyphenon E, a polyphenol-rich formulation majorly containing EGCG (1200 mg/day), was observed to cause a reduction in proliferation process, apoptosis and accumulation of EGCG in cancer tissue during a pilot study of randomized, presurgical placebo-controlled phase II in bladder cancer. One more report exhibited the significantly enhanced efficacy of EGCG along with indole-3-carbinol against patients with advanced ovarian cancer [274]. Recently, chemoprotective activity detection of Teavigo™ (contain 94% EGCG) at a dose level of 450 mg/PO/day in colorectal cancer patients is ongoing with randomized, early phase I trial (NCT03072992).

Chen et al. suggested the decrease in prostate cancer risk is attributed to lycopene consumption observed in persons ingesting a high concentration of lycopene [276]. In contrast, intake of multisupplement with high dose lycopene (35 mg), green tea catechins (600 mg), and selenium (55 μg) for 6 months induced an insignificant reduction in the level of prostate-specific antigen (PSA). Whereas elevation in prostate cancer incidence (accounted with re-biopsy) as well as miRNAs expression observed with a randomized, double-blinded, and controlled trial in multifocal high-grade prostatic intraepithelial neoplasia and/or atypical small acinar proliferation patient [277]. While Beynon et al. observed a metabolomic study with

Table 5.1 List of polyphenolic anticancer agents

Source	Polyphenols	Cancer type	Anticancer mechanism	References
Kiwi, cherry, plum, apple, pear, and coffee	Caffeic acid	Human colon cancer cells	PI3K/Akt and AMPK signaling pathways modulation	[239]
		Human breast cancer cell line	Apoptosis	[239]
		Human cervical cancer	Apoptosis/prooxidant	[239]
Coffee and berries	Chlorogenic acid	Human hepatocellular carcinoma cell line	Matrix metalloproteinase-2 and -9 suppression	[240]
		Breast cancer cell lines	DNA methylation	[102]
Red wine, purple cabbage, berries, and grapes	Delphinidin	Prostate cancer	Suppress NF-κB pathway to induce apoptosis and cell cycle arrest	[241]
		Breast cancer	Apoptosis, prevention of angiogenesis	[242]
Green tea, black tea, and white tea	Epigallocatechin gallate (EGCG)	Skin cancer cell line	Histone alteration and DNA methylation	[97]
		Hepatocellular carcinoma	miRNAs modulation /apoptosis	[243]
		Non-small-cell lung cancer cells	miRNAs/MAPK signaling modulation	[244]
		Promyelocytic leukemia cells	Regulation of DNMT1, HDAC1, HDAC2	[245]
		Melanoma cancer cells	ROS-dependent apoptosis	[246]
		Breast cancer stem cells	Mammosphere formation inhibition	[194]
Onions, kale, teas, berries, andapples	Quercetin	Human leukemia cell lines	Promotes apoptosis	[247]
		Breast cancer cell lines	ROS-dependent apoptosis and cell cycle arrest	[248]
		Prostate cancer	Apoptosis	[249]
Citrus fruits, oranges, and grapefruits	Hesperetin	Prostate cancer cells	Apoptosis mediated by NF-κB pathway	[250]

		Gastric tumor cells	Mitochondria-mediated apoptosis through ROS accumulation	[251]
		Breast cancer cells	Promote ROS, apoptosis signal-regulating kinase 1/c-Jun N-terminal kinase activation pathways and induce growth inhibition through mitochondria-mediated apoptosis	[252]
	Naringenin	Prostate cancer	Oxidative stress	[253]
		Placental choriocarcinoma	Oxidative stress	[254]
		Pancreatic cancer cells	Oxidative stress and apoptosis	[255]
Club moss, celery, andparsley	Apigenin	Prostate cancer	Apoptosis and cell cycle arrest via suppressing the HDAC activity during hyperacetylation of histone	[256]
		Colon cancer (human)	Apoptotic effect by suppression of antiapoptotic proteins Bcl-xL and myeloid leukemia cell differentiation protein-1	[257]
		Hepatocarcinoma	Apoptosis	[257]
		Colorectal cancer cells	Oxidative stress-induced senescence	[257]
Soybeans, fava beans, and psoralen	Genistein	Lung cancer	*Inhibition of cell proliferation and migration* of H446 cell by the induction of cycle arrest at G2/M-stages and apoptosis	[258]
		Prostate cancer cells and esophageal cell carcinoma	Histone modification as well as DNA methylation	[149]
		Renal carcinoma cell line	Histone modification as well as DNA methylation	[259]
		Breast cancer cell lines	Oxidative stress modulation	[147]
Cranberries, red grapes, nuts, and blueberries	Resveratrol	Colon cancer cell lines	miRNAs modulation	[140]
		Gastric cancer cell lines	SIRT/senescence	[187]
		Lung cancer cell lines	ROS/senescence	[260]

(continued)

Table 5.1 (continued)

Source	Polyphenols	Cancer type	Anticancer mechanism	References
Turmeric	Curcumin	Pancreatic cancer	Inhibition of NF-κB-regulated gene products and apoptosis	[261]
		Lung cancer	Inhibition of STAT3 pathway as well as matrix metalloproteinases and vascular endothelial growth factor modulation	[262]
		Breast cancer	miRNAs modulation	[126]
		Human acute monocytic leukemia	Apoptosis	[263]
Soybeans and soy foods	Daidzein	Breast cancer cell lines	Apoptosis	[264]
		Human hepatic cancer cells	Apoptosis	[265]
Vegetables of cruciferous family	Phenethylisothiocyanate	Prostate cancer cell lines	Histone modification and DNA methylation	[266]
		Human oral squamous carcinoma	Mitochondria-mediated apoptotic cell death	[267]
		Human gastric cancer cells	Inhibition of NF-κB and MAPK	[268]
Celery, parsley, broccoli, onion leaves, carrots, peppers, cabbages, and apple skin	Luteolin	Hepatocellular cancer cells	Apoptosis	[269]
		Colon cancer cells	Apoptosis	[270]
		Liver cancer mice model	Redox homeostasis	[271]
Tomato	Lycopene	Breast cancer cells	Methylation of DNA	[80]
Blueberries	Pterostilbene	Breast cancer stem cells	Modulation of NF-κB/miRNA-488 circuit	[272]
Vegetables of cruciferous family	Sulforaphane	Colon cancer cells	HDAC inhibition	[121]
		Breast cancer stem cells		[207]

			Alteration in Wnt/β-catenin self-renewal pathway	
		Pancreatic cancer stem cells	Activation of Hedgehog pathway	[273]
		Human cervical cancer cell lines	DNA methylation and apoptosis	[119]

lycopene (15 mg) provided with green tea catechins containing EGCG (600 mg) for 6 months caused a decrease in circulating pyruvate level in individuals with elevated PSA without prostate cancer. The link between pyruvate level and prostate cancer is suggested in a report performed with Mendelian randomization analysis [278]. Due to the lack of solid and homogeneous clinical data, the conclusions drawn can be conflicting or ambiguous. However, assessment of lycopene (20 mg/PO/day) efficacy for the reduction of skin toxicity against metastasis colorectal carcinoma patients administered with panitumumab is currently in progress with a double-blind, placebo-controlled phase II trial (NCT03167268).

It has been noticed that consumption of pulverized muscadine grape skin extract having 4000 mg resveratrol increased the PSA doubling time (PSADT) up to 3–5 months by interrupting the incidence of recurrence as compared to placebo [279]. Recently, a clinical trial has been completed on the effectiveness of resveratrol (2.5 g/p.o./twice/day) in low-grade gastrointestinal neuroendocrine tumors via Notch-1 signaling but no data is available based on this clinical trial yet (NCT01476592).

A double-blinded, randomized, placebo-controlled trial on SFN has been performed with 78 patients having elevated levels of PSA after radical prostatectomy. It showed SFN oral treatment (60 mg/day) for consecutive 6 months induced significant acceleration in PSADT without any adverse effect than a placebo group. While after 2 months of SFN administration, PSA slope was observed as unaltered. In another study of single-arm trial, various parameters including safety, efficacy, pharmacokinetics as well as pharmacodynamics of broccoli sprout extracts rich in SFN at a dose level of 200 μM/day provided for 20 weeks were performed by using 20 patients with PSA recurrent prostate cancer. Though the primary end result was not attained, it has been observed that there was a significant elevation in PSADT with on-treatment as compared to pretreatment PSADT (6.1 months pretreatment vs. 9.6 months) [280]. Presently, chemopreventive efficacy of Avmacol (sulforaphane) tablets administration twice a day (120 μM/p.o.) is going on with a double-blind, placebo-controlled phase II trial in former smokers highly prone to develop lung cancer (NCT03232138).

5.6 Conclusion

All over the world, the scientific community is facing challenges towards the treatment and prevention of cancer. Though there are numerous conventional chemotherapeutic medicines available in the market, due to inevitable toxic effects, less bioefficacy, and high cost, there is a strict need to explore natural compounds such as polyphenols for the treatment of cancer. Cancer cells bear a condition of oxidative stress due to high-level ROS than physiological cells and different regulating pathways to manage their concerned redox status. Since ROS plays a vital role in tumorigenesis, utilizing antioxidant agents, especially dietary polyphenols, serves a good strategy in the reduction of oncogenesis or chemoprevention. While in another case, overproduced ROS is responsible to cause cytotoxicity in cancer cells and

Table 5.2 List of ongoing anticancer clinical trials on different natural polyphenols

S. no.	Clinical trial reference no.	Polyphenol	Cancer type	Analysis
1	NCTO1912820[a]	Quercetin	Prostate cancer	Accumulation of EGCG, ECG, quercetin along with their methylated metabolites in prostate tissue as well as plasma. COMT, MRP1, and DNMT1 enzymatic expression. Inter-individually genotype variation in COMT.
2	NCTO3232138[a]	Sulforaphane	Lung cancer development associated with smoking	Bronchial dysplasia index, apoptosis marker, such as caspase-3 and TUNEL, cell proliferation marker Ki-67
3	NCTO3072992[a]	Curcumin	Advanced and metastatic breast cancer	Combination safety, progression-free survival, disease progression duration, treatment failure duration
4	NCTO2891538[a]	Epigallocatechin	Colorectal cancer	Alteration in methylation pattern than baseline
5	NCTO1476592[a]	Resveratrol	Low-grade GI Neuroendocrine tumors	Activation of Notch1 and toxicity

[a]Clinical trial reference number at www.clinicaltrials.govt

ultimately cell death. Literature suggested that consideration of redox status of tumor cells is an important factor for the selection of polyphenols as a potent anticancer treatment therapy. Polyphenols regulate epigenetic alterations in tumorigenesis at the gene level via intracellular modulation of ROS concentration and inflammation. Under pathological conditions, natural polyphenols (Table 5.2) display potent anti-oxidant activity whereas prooxidant-like activity has been exhibited in typical conditions leading to activation of apoptosis along with inhibition of inflammatory and cell proliferative processes. Bioactive polyphenols are known to persuade a complex balance between cell proliferation, apoptosis, and senescence; therefore, they can be utilized, from the therapeutic point of view, as a new antitumor tool with advanced bioefficacy, bioavailability along with no or minimum side effects as compared to conventional anticancer therapy (Fig. 5.3). It has been demonstrated that the anatomy and physiology of chromatin are greatly endorsed by DNA methylation and post-translational histone modifications in the epigenomic cascade. Several polyphenols alter the inflammatory process by affecting enzymes associated with the epigenetic modification that might dither the tumor. Therefore, it is necessary for polyphenol anti-inflammatory therapies to intensely explore their anticancer potency in terms of epigenetic regulators. However, it has been noticed that the

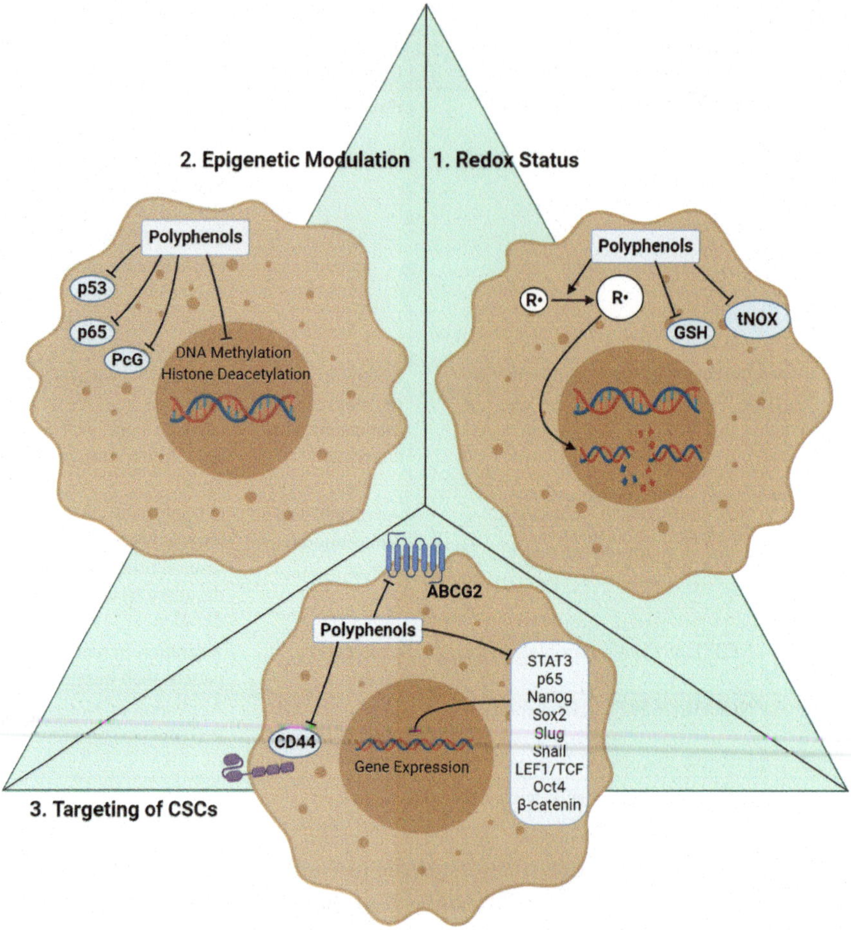

Fig. 5.3 Different molecular targets of polyphenols induced anticancer activity. (*1*) Redox status: ↑ generation of free radical, ↓ tNox activity, ↓ GSH concentration; (*2*) Epigenetic modulation: DNA methylation activity (↓ DNMT1, ↓ HDAC), transcriptional regulation (↓ in p53 and p65 level) and polycomb proteins, (*3*) Targeting of CSCs: ↓ transcriptional factors associated with CSCs, ↓ drug carriers (ABCG2), ↓ CSCs receptor (CD44)

antitumor approach by utilizing polyphenol as DNMT and HAT/HDAC modulators suffers from few limitations including nonselectivity. A combinational synergistic approach of polyphenol nonselective epigenetic treatment along with specific standard therapies at a low dose can be utilized as an alternative. Further, polyphenols are responsible to maintain the concentration of miRNAs, responsible to act directly on specific enzymes linked with epigenetic modification, and regulate the epigenome landscape. They play a vital role in harmonizing ROS homeostasis within tumor cells. Combination therapy of polyphenols with the conventional chemotherapeutic drug might be a potential tool to conquer drug resistance and a better alternative to cancer patients.

References

1. Rizeq B, Gupta I, Ilesanmi J, AlSafran M, Rahman MDM, Ouhtit A. The power of phytochemicals combination in cancer chemoprevention. J Cancer. 2020;11:4521–33.
2. Pitot HC. The molecular biology of carcinogenesis. Cancer. 1993;72:962–70.
3. Reuter S, Gupta SC, Chaturvedi MM, Aggarwal BB. Oxidative stress, inflammation, and cancer: how are they linked? Free Radic Biol Med. 2010;49:1603–16.
4. Kawasaki BT, Hurt EM, Mistree T, Farrar WL. Targeting cancer stem cells with phytochemicals. Mol Interv. 2008;8:174–84.
5. Stepanic V, Gasparovic A, Troselj K, Amic D, Zarkovic N. Selected attributes of polyphenols in targeting oxidative stress in cancer. Curr Top Med Chem. 2015;15:496–509.
6. Pignatti F, Jonsson B, Blumenthal G, Justice R. Assessment of benefits and risks in development of targeted therapies for cancer - The view of regulatory authorities. Mol Oncol. 2015;9:1034–41.
7. Maraldi T. Natural compounds as modulators of NADPH oxidases. Oxid Med Cell Longev. 2013;2013:271602.
8. Kurutas EB. The importance of antioxidants which play the role in cellular response against oxidative/nitrosative stress: Current state. Nutr J. 2016;15:71.
9. Kalaiselvan I, Samuthirapandi M, Govindaraju A, Sheeja Malar D, Kasi PD. Olive oil and its phenolic compounds (hydroxytyrosol and tyrosol) ameliorated TCDD-induced hepatotoxicity in rats via inhibition of oxidative stress and apoptosis. Pharm Biol. 2016;54:338–46.
10. León-González AJ, Auger C, Schini-Kerth VB. Pro-oxidant activity of polyphenols and its implication on cancer chemoprevention and chemotherapy. Biochem Pharmacol. 2015;98:371–80.
11. Mittal M, Siddiqui MR, Tran K, Reddy SP, Malik AB. Reactive oxygen species in inflammation and tissue injury. Antioxidants Redox Signal. 2014;20:1126–67.
12. Aggarwal V, Tuli HS, Varol A, Thakral F, Yerer MB, Sak K, et al. Role of reactive oxygen species in cancer progression: molecular mechanisms and recent advancements. Biomolecules. 2019;9:735.
13. Vittorio O, Curcio M, Cojoc M, Goya GF, Hampel S, Iemma F, et al. Polyphenols delivery by polymeric materials: challenges in cancer treatment. Drug Deliv. 2017;24:162–80.
14. Park E-J, M. Pezzuto J. Flavonoids in cancer prevention. Anticancer Agents Med Chem. 2012;12:836–51.
15. Zubair H, Khan HY, Sohail A, Azim S, Ullah MF, Ahmad A, et al. Redox cycling of endogenous copper by thymoquinone leads to ROS-mediated DNA breakage and consequent cell death: Putative anticancer mechanism of antioxidants. Cell Death Dis. 2013;4:e660.
16. Margalioth EJ, Schenker JG, Chevion M. Copper and zinc levels in normal and malignant tissues. Cancer. 1983;52:868–72.
17. Khan HY, Zubair H, Faisal M, Ullah MF, Farhan M, Sarkar FH, et al. Plant polyphenol induced cell death in human cancer cells involves mobilization of intracellular copper ions and reactive oxygen species generation: a mechanism for cancer chemopreventive action. Mol Nutr Food Res. 2014;58:437–46.
18. Betteridge DJ. What is oxidative stress? Metabolism. 2000;49:3–8.
19. Klaunig JE, Wang Z. Oxidative stress in carcinogenesis. Curr Opin Toxicol. 2018;7:116–21.
20. Little MP, Heidenreich WF, Moolgavkar SH, Schöllnberger H, Thomas DC. Systems biological and mechanistic modelling of radiation-induced cancer. Radiat Environ Biophys. 2008;47:39–47.

21. Klaunig JE, Kamendulis LM, Hocevar BA. Oxidative stress and oxidative damage in carcinogenesis. Toxicol Pathol. 2010;38:96–109.
22. Sosa V, Moliné T, Somoza R, Paciucci R, Kondoh H, LLeonart ME. Oxidative stress and cancer: an overview. Ageing Res Rev. 2013;12:376–90.
23. Guina T, Biasi F, Calfapietra S, Nano M, Poli G. Inflammatory and redox reactions in colorectal carcinogenesis. Ann N Y Acad Sci. 2015;1340:95–103.
24. Thapa D, Ghosh R. Chronic inflammatory mediators enhance prostate cancer development and progression. Biochem Pharmacol. 2015;94:53–62.
25. Murata M, Thanan R, Ma N, Kawanishi S. Role of nitrative and oxidative DNA damage in inflammation-related carcinogenesis. J Biomed Biotechnol. 2012;2012:623019.
26. Huo L, Li CW, Huang TH, Lam YC, Xia W, Tu C, et al. Activation of keap1/nrf2 signaling pathway by nuclear epidermal growth factor receptor in cancer cells. Am J Transl Res. 2014;6:649–63.
27. Korbecki J, Baranowska-Bosiacka I, Gutowska I, Chlubek D. The effect of reactive oxygen species on the synthesis of prostanoids from arachidonic acid. J Physiol Pharmacol. 2013;64:409–21.
28. Wiemer EAC. Stressed tumor cell, chemosensitized cancer. Nat Med. 2011;17:1552–4.
29. Barrera G. Oxidative stress and lipid peroxidation products in cancer progression and therapy. ISRN Oncol. 2012;2012:137289.
30. Brigelius-Flohé R, Kipp A. Glutathione peroxidases in different stages of carcinogenesis. Biochim Biophys Acta. 1790;2009:1555–68.
31. Malik UU, Siddiqui IA, Hashim Z, Zarina S. Measurement of serum paraoxonase activity and MDA concentrations in patients suffering with oral squamous cell carcinoma. Clin Chim Acta. 2014;430:38–42.
32. Spencer CM, Faulds D. Paclitaxel: a review of its pharmacodynamic and pharmacokinetic properties and therapeutic potential in the treatment of cancer. Drugs. 1994;48:794–847.
33. Bekaii-Saab T, Kim R, Kim TW, O'Connor JM, Strickler JH, Malka D, et al. Third- or later-line therapy for metastatic colorectal cancer: reviewing best practice. Clin. Colorectal Cancer. 2019;18:e117–29.
34. Mentella MC, Scaldaferri F, Ricci C, Gasbarrini A, Miggiano GAD. Cancer and mediterranean diet: a review. Nutrients. 2019;11:2059.
35. Schwingshackl L, Schwedhelm C, Galbete C, Hoffmann G. Adherence to mediterranean diet and risk of cancer: an updated systematic review and meta-analysis. Nutrients. 2017;9:1063.
36. Wang K, Karin M. Tumor-elicited inflammation and colorectal cancer. Adv Cancer Res. 2015;128:173–96.
37. Schetter AJ, Heegaard NHH, Harris CC. Inflammation and cancer: interweaving microRNA, free radical, cytokine and p53 pathways. Carcinogenesis. 2009;31:37–49.
38. Dmitrieva OS, Shilovskiy IP, Khaitov MR, Grivennikov SI. Interleukins 1 and 6 as main mediators of inflammation and cancer. Biochem. 2016;81:166–78.
39. Munn LL. Cancer and inflammation. Wiley Interdiscip Rev Syst Biol Med. 2017;9:e1370.
40. Wang D, Dubois RN. Prostaglandins and cancer. Gut. 2006;55:115–22.
41. Nourazarian AR, Kangari P, Salmaninejad A. Roles of oxidative stress in the development and progression of breast cancer. Asian Pacific J Cancer Prev. 2014;15:4745–51.
42. Sies H. What is oxidative stress? J Japan Med Assoc. 2000;45:1–8.
43. Supic G, Jagodic M, Magic Z. Epigenetics: a new link between nutrition and cancer. Nutr Cancer. 2013;65:781–92.
44. Sandoval J, Esteller M. Cancer epigenomics: beyond genomics. Curr Opin Genet Dev. 2012;22:50–5.
45. Baxter E, Windloch K, Gannon F, Lee JS. Epigenetic regulation in cancer progression. Cell Biosci. 2014;4:45.
46. Wajed SA, Laird PW, DeMeester TR. DNA methylation: an alternative pathway to cancer. Ann Surg. 2001;234:10–20.

47. Shanmugam MK, Sethi G. Role of epigenetics in inflammation-associated diseases. Subcell Biochem. 2013;61:627–57.
48. Cheung HH, Lee TL, Rennert OM, Chan WY. DNA methylation of cancer genome. Birth Defects Res C Embryo Today Rev. 2009;87:335–50.
49. Olzscha H, Sheikh S, La Thangue NB. Deacetylation of chromatin and gene expression regulation: a new target for epigenetic therapy. Crit Rev Oncog. 2015;20:1–17.
50. Figueroa-González G, Pérez-Plasencia C. Strategies for the evaluation of DNA damage and repair mechanisms in cancer. Oncol Lett. 2017;13:3982–8.
51. Van Houten B, Cheng S, Chen Y. Measuring gene-specific nucleotide excision repair in human cells using quantitative amplification of long targets from nanogram quantities of DNA. Mutat Res. 2000;460:81–94.
52. Strauss EC, Orkin SH. Guanine-adenine ligation-mediated PCR in vivo footprinting. Methods. 1997;11:164–70.
53. Wang G, Hallberg LM, Englander EW. Rapid SINE-mediated detection of cisplatin:DNA adduct formation in vitro and in vivo in blood. Mutat Res. 1999;434:67–74.
54. Collins AR. Measuring oxidative damage to DNA and its repair with the comet assay. Biochim Biophys Acta. 1840;2014:794–800.
55. Collins AR, Azqueta A. DNA repair as a biomarker in human biomonitoring studies; further applications of the comet assay. Mutat Res. 2012;736:122–9.
56. Glei M, Hovhannisyan G, Pool-Zobel BL. Use of Comet-FISH in the study of DNA damage and repair: review. Mutat Res. 2009;681:33–43.
57. Collins AR. The comet assay for DNA damage and repair: principles, applications, and limitations. Mol Biotechnol. 2004;26:249–61.
58. Collins AR, Azqueta A. single-cell gel electrophoresis combined with lesion-specific enzymes to measure oxidative damage to DNA. In: Conn PM, editor. Methods in cell biology. Cambridge, MA: Academic Press; 2012. p. 69–92.
59. Kumari S, Rastogi R, Singh K, Singh S, Sinha R. DNA damage: detection strategies. Excli J. 2008;7:44–62.
60. Berton TR, Mitchell DL. Quantification of DNA photoproducts in mammalian cell DNA using radioimmunoassay. Methods Mol Biol. 2012;920:177–87.
61. Santella RM. Immunological methods for detection of carcinogen-DNA damage in humans. Cancer Epidemiol Biomarkers Prev. 1999;8:733–9.
62. Yatabe Y. ALK FISH and IHC: You cannot have one without the other. J Thorac Oncol. 2015;10:548–50.
63. Kriste AG, Martincigh BS, Salter LF. A sensitive immunoassay technique for thymine dimer quantitation in UV-irradiated DNA. J Photochem Photobiol A Chem. 1996;93:185–92.
64. Mullins EA, Rubinson EH, Pereira KN, Calcutt MW, Christov PP, Eichman BF. An HPLC-tandem mass spectrometry method for simultaneous detection of alkylated base excision repair products. Methods. 2013;64:59–66.
65. Caldecott KW. DNA single-strand break repair. Exp Cell Res. 2014;329:2–8.
66. Cadet J, Douki T, Frelon S, Sauvaigo S, Pouget JP, Ravanat JL. Assessment of oxidative base damage to isolated and cellular DNA by HPLC-MS/MS measurement. Free Radic Biol Med. 2002;33:441–9.
67. Pouget JP, Douki T, Richard MJ, Cadet J. DNA damage induced in cells by γ and UVA radiation as measured by HPLC/GC-MS and HPLC-EC and comet assay. Chem Res Toxicol. 2000;13:541–9.
68. Fojta M, Daňhel A, Havran L, Vyskočil V. Recent progress in electrochemical sensors and assays for DNA damage and repair. Trends Anal Chem. 2016;79:160–7.
69. Boon EM, Ceres DM, Drummond TG, Hill MG, Barton JK. Mutation detection by electrocatalysis at DNA-modified electrodes. Nat Biotechnol. 2000;18:1096–100.
70. Hail N, Cortes M, Drake EN, Spallholz JE. Cancer chemoprevention: a radical perspective. Free Radic Biol Med. 2008;45:97–110.

71. Lambert JD, Elias RJ. The antioxidant and pro-oxidant activities of green tea polyphenols: a role in cancer prevention. Arch Biochem Biophys. 2010;501:65–72.
72. Yadav E, Singh D, Yadav P, Verma A. Attenuation of dermal wounds via downregulating oxidative stress and inflammatory markers by protocatechuic acid rich n-butanol fraction of Trianthema portulacastrum Linn. in wistar albino rats. Biomed Pharmacother. 2017;96:86–97.
73. Yadav E, Singh D, Yadav P, Verma A. Ameliorative effect of biofabricated ZnO nanoparticles of: Trianthema portulacastrum Linn. on dermal wounds via removal of oxidative stress and inflammation. RSC Adv. 2018;8:21621–35.
74. Yadav E, Singh D, Debnath B, Rathee P, Yadav P, Verma A. Molecular docking and cognitive impairment attenuating effect of phenolic compound rich fraction of trianthema portulacastrum in scopolamine induced Alzheimer's disease like condition. Neurochem Res. 2019;44:1665–77.
75. Dai J, Mumper RJ. Plant phenolics: Extraction, analysis and their antioxidant and anticancer properties. Molecules. 2010;15:7313–52.
76. Rahman I, Chung S. Dietary polyphenols, deacetylases and chromatin remodeling in inflammation. J Nutrigenet Nutrigenomics. 2010;3:220–30.
77. Yang P, He X, Malhotra A. Epigenetic targets of polyphenols in cancer. J Environ Pathol Toxicol Oncol. 2014;33:159–65.
78. Gerhauser C. Cancer chemoprevention and nutri-epigenetics: state of the art and future challenges. In: Pezzuto JM, Suh N, editors. Natural products in cancer prevention and therapy. Topics in current chemistry. Berlin: Springer; 2012. p. 73–132.
79. Hardy TM, Tollefsbol TO. Epigenetic diet: impact on the epigenome and cancer. Epigenomics. 2011;3:503–18.
80. Shankar S, Kumar D, Srivastava RK. Epigenetic modifications by dietary phytochemicals: implications for personalized nutrition. Pharmacol Ther. 2013;138:1–17.
81. Baylin SB, Jones PA. Epigenetic determinants of cancer. Cold Spring Harb Perspect Biol. 2016;8:a019505.
82. Gonzalez H, Hagerling C, Werb Z. Roles of the immune system in cancer: From tumor initiation to metastatic progression. Genes Dev. 2018;32:1267–84.
83. Vanden BW. Epigenetic impact of dietary polyphenols in cancer chemoprevention: lifelong remodeling of our epigenomes. Pharmacol Res. 2012;65:565–76.
84. Biswas S, Rahman I. Modulation of steroid activity in chronic inflammation: a novel anti-inflammatory role for curcumin. Mol Nutr Food Res. 2008;52:987–94.
85. Hassan FU, Rehman MSU, Khan MS, Ali MA, Javed A, Nawaz A, et al. Curcumin as an alternative epigenetic modulator: mechanism of action and potential effects. Front Genet. 2019;10:514.
86. Rahman I. Dietary polyphenols mediated regulation of oxidative stress and chromatin remodeling in inflammation. Nutr Rev. 2008;66:S42–5.
87. Elangovan V, Sekar N, Govindasamy S. Chemopreventive potential of dietary bioflavonoids against 20-methylcholanthrene-induced tumorigenesis. Cancer Lett. 1994;87:107–13.
88. Tabrez S, Priyadarshini M, Urooj M, Shakil S, Ashraf GM, Khan MS, et al. Cancer chemoprevention by polyphenols and their potential application as nanomedicine. J Environ Sci Heal C Environ Carcinog Ecotoxicol Rev. 2013;31:67–98.
89. Camouse MM, Domingo DS, Swain FR, Conrad EP, Matsui MS, Maes D, et al. Topical application of green and white tea extracts provides protection from solar-simulated ultraviolet light in human skin. Exp Dermatol. 2009;18:522–6.
90. Kaur S, Greaves P, Cooke DN, Edwards R, Steward WP, Gescher AJ, et al. Breast cancer prevention by green tea catechins and black tea theaflavins in the C3(1) SV40 T,t antigen transgenic mouse model is accompanied by increased apoptosis and a decrease in oxidative DNA adducts. J Agric Food Chem. 2007;55:3378–85.
91. Sahnoun Z, Jamoussi K, Mounir ZK. Free radicals: fundamental notions and methods of exploration. Thérapie (Paris). 1997;52:251–70.

92. Kundu JK, Surh YJ. Epigallocatechin Gallate inhibits phorbol ester-induced activation of NF-κB and CREB in mouse skin role of p38 MAPK. Ann N Y Acad Sci. 2007;1095:504–12.
93. Singh BN, Shankar S, Srivastava RK. Green tea catechin, epigallocatechin-3-gallate (EGCG): mechanisms, perspectives and clinical applications. Biochem Pharmacol. 2011;82:1807–21.
94. Pan H, Chen J, Shen K, Wang X, Wang P, Fu G, et al. Mitochondrial modulation by epigallocatechin 3-gallate ameliorates cisplatin induced renal injury through decreasing oxidative/nitrative stress, inflammation and NF-kB in mice. PLoS One. 2015;10:e0124775.
95. Thakur VS, Gupta K, Gupta S. Green tea polyphenols causes cell cycle arrest and apoptosis in prostate cancer cells by suppressing class I histone deacetylases. Carcinogenesis. 2012;33:377–84.
96. Choi KC, Myung GJ, Lee YH, Joo CY, Seung HK, Kang HB, et al. Epigallocatechin-3-gallate, a histone acetyltransferase inhibitor, inhibits EBV-induced B lymphocyte transformation via suppression of RelA acetylation. Cancer Res. 2009;69:583–92.
97. Nandakumar V, Vaid M, Katiyar SK. (-)-Epigallocatechin-3-gallate reactivates silenced tumor suppressor genes, Cip1/p21 and p16INK4a, by reducing DNA methylation and increasing histones acetylation in human skin cancer cells. Carcinogenesis. 2011;32:537–44.
98. Sinha S, Shukla S, Khan S, Tollefsbol TO, Meeran SM. Epigenetic reactivation of p21CIP1/WAF1 and KLOTHO by a combination of bioactive dietary supplements is partially ER-α-dependent in ERα-negative human breast cancer cells. Mol Cell Endocrinol. 2015;406:102–14.
99. Fang MZ, Wang Y, Ai N, Hou Z, Sun Y, Lu H, et al. Tea polyphenol (-)-epigallocatechin-3-gallate inhibits DNA methyltransferase and reactivates methylation-silenced genes in cancer cell lines. Cancer Res. 2003;63:7563–70.
100. Berner C, Aumüller E, Gnauck A, Nestelberger M, Just A, Haslberger AG. Epigenetic control of estrogen receptor expression and tumor suppressor genes is modulated by bioactive food compounds. Ann Nutr Metab. 2011;57:183–9.
101. Henning SM, Wang P, Carpenter CL, Heber D. Epigenetic effects of green tea polyphenols in cancer. Epigenomics. 2013;5:729–41.
102. Lee WJ, Zhu BT. Inhibition of DNA methylation by caffeic acid and chlorogenic acid, two common catechol-containing coffee polyphenols. Carcinogenesis. 2006;27:269–77.
103. Michaluart P, Masferrer JL, Carothers AM, Subbaramaiah K, Zweifel BS, Koboldt C, et al. Inhibitory effects of caffeic acid phenethyl ester on the activity and expression of cyclooxygenase-2 in human oral epithelial cells and in a rat model of inflammation. Cancer Res. 1999;59:2347–52.
104. Ozturk G, Ginis Z, Akyol S, Erden G, Gurel A, Akyol O. The anticancer mechanism of caffeic acid phenethyl ester (CAPE): review of melanomas, lung and prostate cancers. Eur Rev Med Pharmacol Sci. 2012;16:2064–8.
105. Mukhtar H, Ahmad N. Tea polyphenols: prevention of cancer and optimizing health. Am J Clin Nutr. 2000;71:1698S–702S.
106. Kumar G, Dange P, Kailaje V, Vaidya MM, Ramchandani AG, Maru GB. Polymeric black tea polyphenols modulate the localization and activity of 12-O-tetradecanoylphorbol-13-acetate-mediated kinases in mouse skin: Mechanisms of their anti-tumor-promoting action. Free Radic Biol Med. 2012;53:1358–70.
107. Mujtaba T, Dou QP. Black tea polyphenols inhibit tumor proteasome activity. In Vivo (Brooklyn). 2012;26:197–202.
108. Gorzynik-Debicka M, Przychodzen P, Cappello F, Kuban-Jankowska A, Gammazza AM, Knap N, et al. Potential health benefits of olive oil and plant polyphenols. Int J Mol Sci. 2018;19:686.
109. Wang M, Firrman J, Liu LS, Yam K. A review on flavonoid apigenin: dietary intake, ADME, antimicrobial effects, and interactions with human gut microbiota. Biomed Res Int. 2019;2019:7010467.
110. Tong X, Pelling J. Targeting the PI3K/Akt/mTOR axis by apigenin for cancer prevention. Anticancer Agents Med Chem. 2013;13:971–8.

111. Woo JS, Choo GS, Yoo ES, Kim SH, Lee JH, Han SH, et al. Apigenin induces apoptosis by regulating Akt and MAPK pathways in human melanoma cell A375SM. Mol Med Rep. 2020;22:4877–89.
112. Shukla S, Gupta S. Apigenin-induced cell cycle arrest is mediated by modulation of MAPK, PI3K-Akt, and loss of cyclin D1 associated retinoblastoma dephosphorylation in human prostate cancer cells. Cell Cycle. 2007;6:1102–14.
113. Lepley DM, Pelling JC. Induction of p21/WAF1 and G1 cell-cycle arrest by the chemopreventive agent apigenin. Mol Carcinog. 1997;19:74–82.
114. Choi EJ, Kim GH. Apigenin causes G2/M arrest associated with the modulation of p21Cip1 and Cdc2 and activates p53-dependent apoptosis pathway in human breast cancer SK-BR-3 cells. J Nutr Biochem. 2009;20:285–90.
115. Gao AM, Zhang XY, Ke ZP. Apigenin sensitizes BEL-7402/ADM cells to doxorubicin through inhibiting miR-101/Nrf2 pathway. Oncotarget. 2017;8:82085–91.
116. Fan P, Zhang Y, Liu L, Zhao Z, Yin Y, Xiao X, et al. Continuous exposure of pancreatic cancer cells to dietary bioactive agents does not induce drug resistance unlike chemotherapy. Cell Death Dis. 2016;7:e3346.
117. Hwang ES, Jeffery EH. Induction of quinone reductase by sulforaphane and sulforaphane N-acetylcysteine conjugate in murine hepatoma cells. J Med Food. 2005;8:198–203.
118. Volonte D, Liu Z, Musille PM, Stoppani E, Wakabayashi N, Di YP, et al. Inhibition of nuclear factor-erythroid 2-related factor (Nrf2) by caveolin-1 promotes stress-induced premature senescence. Mol Biol Cell. 2013;24:1852–62.
119. Su X, Jiang X, Meng L, Dong X, Shen Y, Xin Y. Anticancer activity of sulforaphane: The epigenetic mechanisms and the Nrf2 signaling pathway. Oxid Med Cell Longev. 2018;2018:5438179.
120. Shannon J, Ho E, Naik A, Troxell M, Cox A, Maxcy C, et al. Sulforaphane supplementation in women newly diagnosed with DCIS: a biomarker study. J Clin Oncol. 2010;28:TPS143.
121. Myzak MC, Karplus PA, Chung FL, Dashwood RH. A novel mechanism of chemoprotection by sulforaphane: Inhibition of histone deacetylase. Cancer Res. 2004;64:5767–74.
122. Galiniak S, Biesiadecki M, Czubat B, Bartusik-Aebisher D. Anti-glycation activity of curcumin. Postep Hig Med Dosw. 2019;73:182–8.
123. Zammataro M, Sortino MA, Parenti C, Gereau RW, Chiechio S. HDAC and HAT inhibitors differently affect analgesia mediated by group II metabotropic glutamate receptors. Mol Pain. 2014;10:68.
124. Balasubramanyam K, Varier RA, Altaf M, Swaminathan V, Siddappa NB, Ranga U, et al. Curcumin, a novel p300/CREB-binding protein-specific inhibitor of acetyltransferase, represses the acetylation of histone/nonhistone proteins and histone acetyltransferase-dependent chromatin transcription. J Biol Chem. 2004;279:51163–71.
125. Kang J, Chen J, Shi Y, Jia J, Zhang Y. Curcumin-induced histone hypoacetylation: the role of reactive oxygen species. Biochem Pharmacol. 2005;69:1205–13.
126. Yang J, Cao Y, Sun J, Zhang Y. Curcumin reduces the expression of Bcl-2 by upregulating miR-15a and miR-16 in MCF-7 cells. Med Oncol. 2010;27:1114–8.
127. Barve A, Khor TO, Hao X, Keum YS, Yang CS, Reddy B, et al. Murine prostate cancer inhibition by dietary phytochemicals - curcumin and phenyethylisothiocyanate. Pharm Res. 2008;25:2181–9.
128. Yallapu MM, Maher DM, Sundram V, Bell MC, Jaggi M, Chauhan SC. Curcumin induces chemo/radio-sensitization in ovarian cancer cells and curcumin nanoparticles inhibit ovarian cancer cell growth. J Ovarian Res. 2010;3:11.
129. Wahl H, Tan L, Griffith K, Choi M, Liu JR. Curcumin enhances Apo2L/TRAIL-induced apoptosis in chemoresistant ovarian cancer cells. Gynecol Oncol. 2007;105:104–12.
130. Camacho-Barquero L, Villegas I, Sánchez-Calvo JM, Talero E, Sánchez-Fidalgo S, Motilva V, et al. Curcumin, a Curcuma longa constituent, acts on MAPK p38 pathway modulating COX-2 and iNOS expression in chronic experimental colitis. Int Immunopharmacol. 2007;7:333–42.

131. Moon YJ, Wang X, Morris ME. Dietary flavonoids: Effects on xenobiotic and carcinogen metabolism. Toxicol In Vitro. 2006;20:187–210.
132. Grill AE, Shahani K, Koniar B, Panyam J. Chemopreventive efficacy of curcumin-loaded PLGA microparticles in a transgenic mouse model of HER-2-positive breast cancer. Drug Deliv Transl Res. 2018;8:329–41.
133. Feitelson MA, Arzumanyan A, Kulathinal RJ, Blain SW, Holcombe RF, Mahajna J, et al. Sustained proliferation in cancer: Mechanisms and novel therapeutic targets. Semin Cancer Biol. 2015;35:S25–54.
134. Liu D, Chen Z. The effect of curcumin on breast cancer cells. J Breast Cancer. 2013;16:133–7.
135. Mukhopadhyay A, Bueso-Ramos C, Chatterjee D, Pantazis P, Aggarwal BB. Curcumin downregulates cell survival mechanisms in human prostate cancer cell lines. Oncogene. 2001;20:7597–609.
136. Savouret JF, Quesne M. Resveratrol and cancer: a review. Biomed Pharmacother. 2002;56:84–7.
137. Srivastava RK, Unterman TG, Shankar S. FOXO transcription factors and VEGF neutralizing antibody enhance antiangiogenic effects of resveratrol. Mol Cell Biochem. 2010;337:201–12.
138. Jung KH, Lee JH, Quach CHT, Paik JY, Oh H, Park JW, et al. Resveratrol suppresses cancer cell glucose uptake by targeting reactive oxygen species-mediated hypoxia-inducible factor-1α activation. J Nucl Med. 2013;54:2161–7.
139. He H, Yu FX, Sun C, Luo Y. CBP/p300 and SIRT1 are involved in transcriptional regulation of S-Phase specific histone genes. PLoS One. 2011;6:e22088.
140. Tili E, Michaille JJ, Alder H, Volinia S, Delmas D, Latruffe N, et al. Resveratrol modulates the levels of microRNAs targeting genes encoding tumor-suppressors and effectors of TGFβ signaling pathway in SW480 cells. Biochem Pharmacol. Biochem Pharmacol. 2010;80:2057–65.
141. Fukui M, Yamabe N, Zhu BT. Resveratrol attenuates the anticancer efficacy of paclitaxel in human breast cancer cells in vitro and in vivo. Eur J Cancer. 2010;46:1882–91.
142. Wang KK, Sampliner RE. Updated guidelines 2008 for the diagnosis, surveillance and therapy of Barrett's esophagus. Am J Gastroenterol. 2008;103:788–97.
143. Kresty LA, Frankel WL, Hammond CD, Baird ME, Mele JM, Stoner GD, et al. Transitioning from preclinical to clinical chemopreventive assessments of lyophilized black raspberries: interim results show berries modulate markers of oxidative stress in Barrett's esophagus patients. Nutr Cancer. 2006;54:148–56.
144. Wang RH, Zheng Y, Kim HS, Xu X, Cao L, Luhasen T, et al. Interplay among BRCA1, SIRT1, and survivin during BRCA1-associated tumorigenesis. Mol Cell. 2008;32:11–20.
145. Liu Y, Wu YM, Yu Y, Cao CS, Zhang JH, Li K, et al. Curcumin and resveratrol in combination modulate drug-metabolizing enzymes as well as antioxidant indices during lung carcinogenesis in mice. Hum Exp Toxicol. 2015;34:620–7.
146. Ziaei S, Halaby R. Dietary isoflavones and breast cancer risk. Medicines. 2017;4:18.
147. Nadal-Serrano M, Pons DG, Sastre-Serra J, Blanquer-Rossellò MM, Roca P, Oliver J. Genistein modulates oxidative stress in breast cancer cell lines according to ERa/ERβ ratio: effects on mitochondrial functionality, sirtuins, uncoupling protein 2 and antioxidant enzymes. Int J Biochem Cell Biol. 2013;45:2045–51.
148. Zhou Y, Liu X. The role of estrogen receptor beta in breast cancer. Biomark Res. 2020;8:39.
149. Fang MZ, Chen D, Sun Y, Jin Z, Christman JK, Yang CS. Reversal of hypermethylation and reactivation of p16INK4a, RARβ, and MGMT genes by genistein and other isoflavones from soy. Clin Cancer Res. 2005;11:7033–41.
150. Pudenz M, Roth K, Gerhauser C. Impact of soy isoflavones on the epigenome in cancer prevention. Nutrients. 2014;6:4218–72.
151. Bosutti A, Zanconati F, Grassi G, Dapas B, Passamonti S, Scaggiante B. Epigenetic and miRNAs dysregulation in prostate cancer: the role of nutraceuticals. Anticancer Agents Med Chem. 2016;16:1385–402.

152. Chang WW, Hu FW, Yu CC, Wang HH, Feng HP, Lan C, et al. Quercetin in elimination of tumor initiating stem-like and mesenchymal transformation property in head and neck cancer. Head Neck. 2013;35:413–9.
153. Cao C, Sun L, Mo W, Sun L, Luo J, Yang Z, et al. Quercetin mediates β-catenin in pancreatic cancer stem-like cells. Pancreas. 2015;44:1334–9.
154. Nosrati N, Bakovic M, Paliyath G. Molecular mechanisms and pathways as targets for cancer prevention and progression with dietary compounds. Int J Mol Sci. 2017;18:2050.
155. Huang YT, Hwang JJ, Lee PP, Ke FC, Huang JH, Huang CJ, et al. Effects of luteolin and quercetin, inhibitors of tyrosine kinase, on cell growth and metastasis-associated properties in A431 cells overexpressing epidermal growth factor receptor. Br J Pharmacol. 1999;128:999–1010.
156. Ou HC, Lee WJ, Da Lee S, Huang CY, Chiu TH, Tsai KL, et al. Ellagic acid protects endothelial cells from oxidized low-density lipoprotein-induced apoptosis by modulating the PI3K/Akt/eNOS pathway. Toxicol Appl Pharmacol. 2010;248:134–43.
157. Shamshoum H, Vlavcheski F, Tsiani E. Anticancer effects of oleuropein. BioFactors. 2017;43:517–28.
158. Han J, Talorete TPN, Yamada P, Isoda H. Anti-proliferative and apoptotic effects of oleuropein and hydroxytyrosol on human breast cancer MCF-7 cells. Cytotechnology. 2009;59:45–53.
159. Simsek EN, Uysal T. In vitro investigation of cytotoxic and apoptotic effects of Cynara L. species in colorectal cancer cells. Asian Pacific J Cancer Prev. 2013;14:6791–5.
160. Miccadei S, Di Venere D, Cardinali A, Romano F, Durazzo A, Foddai MS, et al. Antioxidative and apoptotic properties of polyphenolic extracts from edible part of artichoke (Cynara scolymus L.) on cultured rat hepatocytes and on human hepatoma cells. Nutr Cancer. 2008;60:276–83.
161. Mileo AM, Di Venere D, Abbruzzese C, Miccadei S. Long term exposure to polyphenols of artichoke (cynara scolymus L.) Exerts induction of senescence driven growth arrest in the MDA-MB231 human breast cancer cell line. Oxid Med Cell Longev. 2015;2015:363827.
162. Al-Radadi NS. Artichoke (Cynara scolymus L.,) mediated rapid analysis of silver nanoparticles and their utilisation on the cancer cell treatments. J Comput Theor Nanosci. 2018;15:1818–29.
163. Cairney CJ, Bilsland AE, Evans TRJ, Roffey J, Bennett DC, Narita M, et al. Cancer cell senescence: a new frontier in drug development. Drug Discov Today. 2012;17:269–76.
164. Ewald JA, Desotelle JA, Wilding G, Jarrard DF. Therapy-induced senescence in cancer. J Natl Cancer Inst. 2010;102:1536–46.
165. Naylor RM, Baker DJ, Van Deursen JM. Senescent cells: a novel therapeutic target for aging and age-related diseases. Clin Pharmacol Ther. 2013;93:105–16.
166. Childs BG, Gluscevic M, Baker DJ, Laberge RM, Marquess D, Dananberg J, et al. Senescent cells: an emerging target for diseases of ageing. Nat Rev Drug Discov. 2017;16:718–35.
167. Guo X, Ngo B, Modrek A, Lee W-H. Targeting tumor suppressor networks for cancer therapeutics. Curr Drug Targets. 2014;15:2–16.
168. Lai D, Visser-Grieve S, Yang X. Tumour suppressor genes in chemotherapeutic drug response. Biosci Rep. 2012;32:361–74.
169. Qian Y, Chen X. Senescence regulation by the p53 protein family. Methods Mol Biol. 2013;965:37–61.
170. Larsson LG. Oncogene- and tumor suppressor gene-mediated suppression of cellular senescence. Semin Cancer Biol. 2011;21:367–76.
171. Lan L, Holland JD, Qi J, Grosskopf S, Rademann J, Vogel R, et al. Shp2 signaling suppresses senescence in Py MT -induced mammary gland cancer in mice. EMBO J. 2015;34:2383.
172. Law ME, Corsino PE, Narayan S, Law BK. Cyclin-dependent kinase inhibitors as anticancer therapeutics. Mol Pharmacol. 2015;88:846–52.

173. Al Bitar S, Gali-Muhtasib H. The role of the cyclin dependent kinase inhibitor p21cip1/waf1 in targeting cancer: molecular mechanisms and novel therapeutics. Cancers (Basel). 2019;11:1475.
174. Haferkamp S, Becker TM, Scurr LL, Kefford RF, Rizos H. p16INK4a-induced senescence is disabled by melanoma-associated mutations. Aging Cell. 2008;7:733–45.
175. Mijit M, Caracciolo V, Melillo A, Amicarelli F, Giordano A. Role of p53 in the regulation of cellular senescence. Biomolecules. 2020;10:420.
176. Herbig U, Jobling WA, Chen BPC, Chen DJ, Sedivy JM. Telomere shortening triggers senescence of human cells through a pathway involving ATM, p53, and p21CIP1, but not p16INK4a. Mol Cell. 2004;14:501–13.
177. Kim R, Osaki A, Tanabe K, Toge T. Neoadjuvant chemotherapy for local advanced breast cancer with stage IIIB. Oncol Rep. 2004;11:1265–72.
178. Yeo EJ, Hwang YC, Kang CM, Kim IH, Kim DI, Parka JS, et al. Senescence-like changes induced by hydroxyurea in human diploid fibroblasts. Exp Gerontol. 2000;35:553–71.
179. Chang BD, Xuan Y, Broude EV, Zhu H, Schott B, Fang J, et al. Role of p53 and p21(waf1/cip1) in senescence-like terminal proliferation arrest induced in human tumor cells by chemotherapeutic drugs. Oncogene. 1999;18:4808–18.
180. Zhang Y, Yang JM. The impact of cellular senescence in cancer therapy: is it true or not? Acta Pharmacol Sin. 2011;32:1199–207.
181. Sin S, Kim SY, Kim SS. Chronic treatment with ginsenoside Rg3 induces Akt-dependent senescence in human glioma cells. Int J Oncol. 2012;41:1669–74.
182. Li YB, Gao JL, Zhong ZF, Hoi PM, Lee SMY, Wang YT. Bisdemethoxycurcumin suppresses MCF-7 cells proliferation by inducing ROS accumulation and modulating senescence-related pathways. Pharmacol Rep. 2013;65:700–9.
183. Roy N, Elangovan I, Kopanja D, Bagchi S, Raychaudhuri P. Tumor regression by phenethyl isothiocyanate involves DDB2. Cancer Biol Ther. 2013;14:108–16.
184. Mileo AM, Di Venere D, Linsalata V, Fraioli R, Miccadei S. Artichoke polyphenols induce apoptosis and decrease the invasive potential of the human breast cancer cell line MDA MB231. J Cell Physiol. 2012;227:3301–9.
185. Salekzamani S, Ebrahimi-Mameghani M, Rezazadeh K. The antioxidant activity of artichoke (Cynara scolymus): a systematic review and meta-analysis of animal studies. Phyther Res. 2019;33:55–71.
186. Luo H, Yang A, Schulte BA, Wargovich MJ, Wang GY. Resveratrol induces premature senescence in lung cancer cells via ROS-mediated DNA damage. PLoS One. 2013;8:e60065.
187. Yang Q, Wang B, Zang W, Wang X, Liu Z, Li W, et al. Resveratrol inhibits the growth of gastric cancer by inducing G1 phase arrest and senescence in a Sirt1-dependent manner. PLoS One. 2013;8:e70627.
188. Zamin LL, Filippi-Chiela EC, Dillenburg-Pilla P, Horn F, Salbego C, Lenz G. Resveratrol and quercetin cooperate to induce senescence-like growth arrest in C6 rat glioma cells. Cancer Sci. 2009;100:1655–62.
189. Cho RW, Clarke MF. Recent advances in cancer stem cells. Curr Opin Genet Dev. 2008;18:48–53.
190. Ye J, Wu D, Wu P, Chen Z, Huang J. The cancer stem cell niche: cross talk between cancer stem cells and their microenvironment. Tumor Biol. 2014;35:3945–51.
191. Maccalli C, De Maria R. Cancer stem cells: perspectives for therapeutic targeting. Cancer Immunol Immunother. 2015;64:91–7.
192. Cojoc M, Mäbert K, Muders MH, Dubrovska A. A role for cancer stem cells in therapy resistance: cellular and molecular mechanisms. Semin Cancer Biol. 2015;31:16–27.
193. Yang L, Shi P, Zhao G, Xu J, Peng W, Zhang J, et al. Targeting cancer stem cell pathways for cancer therapy. Signal Transduct Target Ther. 2020;5:8.
194. Chen K, Huang YH, Chen JL. Understanding and targeting cancer stem cells: therapeutic implications and challenges. Acta Pharmacol Sin. 2013;34:732–40.

195. Takebe N, Harris PJ, Warren RQ, Ivy SP. Targeting cancer stem cells by inhibiting Wnt, Notch, and Hedgehog pathways. Nat Rev Clin Oncol. 2011;8:97–106.
196. Song IS. Mitochondria as therapeutic targets for cancer stem cells. World J Stem Cells. 2015;7:418.
197. Ramos EK, Hoffmann AD, Gerson SL, Liu H. New opportunities and challenges to defeat cancer stem cells. Trends Cancer. 2017;3:780–96.
198. Hill RP, Marie-Egyptienne DT, Hedley DW. Cancer stem cells, hypoxia and metastasis. Semin Radiat Oncol. 2009;19:106–11.
199. Neri D, Supuran CT. Interfering with pH regulation in tumours as a therapeutic strategy. Nat Rev Drug Discov. 2011;10:767–77.
200. Landskron G, De La Fuente M, Thuwajit P, Thuwajit C, Hermoso MA. Chronic inflammation and cytokines in the tumor microenvironment. J Immunol Res. 2014;2014:149185.
201. Zhang G, Yang P, Guo P, Miele L, Sarkar FH, Wang Z, et al. Unraveling the mystery of cancer metabolism in the genesis of tumor-initiating cells and development of cancer. Biochim Biophys Acta. 1836;2013:49–59.
202. Takebe N, Miele L, Harris PJ, Jeong W, Bando H, Kahn M, et al. Targeting Notch, Hedgehog, and Wnt pathways in cancer stem cells: clinical update. Nat Rev Clin Oncol. 2015;12:445–64.
203. Bao Y, Wang W, Zhou Z, Sun C. Benefits and risks of the hormetic effects of dietary isothiocyanates on cancer prevention. PLoS One. 2014;9:e114764.
204. Zhang Y. Cancer-preventive isothiocyanates: measurement of human exposure and mechanism of action. Mutat Res. 2004;555:173–90.
205. Naujokat C, McKee DL. The "Big Five" phytochemicals targeting cancer stem cells: curcumin, EGCG, sulforaphane, resveratrol and genistein. Curr Med Chem. 2020;27:1.
206. Bayat Mokhtari R, Baluch N, Homayouni TS, Morgatskaya E, Kumar S, Kazemi P, et al. The role of Sulforaphane in cancer chemoprevention and health benefits: a mini-review. J Cell Commun Signal. 2018;12:91–101.
207. Li Y, Zhang T, Korkaya H, Liu S, Lee HF, Newman B, et al. Sulforaphane, a dietary component of broccoli/broccoli sprouts, inhibits breast cancer stem cells. Clin Cancer Res. 2010;16:2580–90.
208. Rodova M, Fu J, Watkins DN, Srivastava RK, Shankar S. Sonic Hedgehog signaling inhibition provides opportunities for targeted therapy by sulforaphane in regulating pancreatic cancer stem cell self-renewal. PLoS One. 2012;7:e46083.
209. Thyagarajan A, Forino AS, Konger RL, Sahu RP. Dietary polyphenols in cancer chemoprevention: implications in pancreatic cancer. Antioxidants. 2020;9:1–20.
210. Zhou W, Kallifatidis G, Baumann B, Rausch V, Mattern J, Gladkich J, et al. Dietary polyphenol quercetin targets pancreatic cancer stem cells. Int J Oncol. 2010;37:551–61.
211. Brito A, Ribeiro M, Abrantes A, Pires A, Teixo R, Tralhao J, et al. Quercetin in cancer treatment, alone or in combination with conventional therapeutics? Curr Med Chem. 2015;22:3025–39.
212. He FJ, Chen JQ. Consumption of soybean, soy foods, soy isoflavones and breast cancer incidence: differences between Chinese women and women in Western countries and possible mechanisms. Food Sci Hum Wellness. 2013;2:146–61.
213. Messina M. Soy and health update: evaluation of the clinical and epidemiologic literature. Nutrients. 2016;8:754.
214. Montales MTE, Rahal OM, Nakatani H, Matsuda T, Simmen RCM. Repression of mammary adipogenesis by genistein limits mammosphere formation of human MCF-7 cells. J Endocrinol. 2013;218:135–49.
215. Subramaniam D, Kaushik G, Dandawate P, Anant S. Targeting cancer stem cells for chemoprevention of pancreatic cancer. Curr Med Chem. 2017;25:2585–94.
216. Wang Y, Bu C, Wu K, Wang R, Wang J. Curcumin protects the pancreas from acute pancreatitis via the mitogen-activated protein kinase signaling pathway. Mol Med Rep. 2019;20:3027–34.

217. Howells LM, Moiseeva EP, Neal CP, Foreman BE, Andreadi CK, Sun YY, et al. Predicting the physiological relevance of in vitro cancer preventive activities of phytochemicals. Acta Pharmacol Sin. 2007;28:1274–304.
218. Siddappa G, Kulsum S, Ravindra DR, Kumar VV, Raju N, Raghavan N, et al. Curcumin and metformin-mediated chemoprevention of oral cancer is associated with inhibition of cancer stem cells. Mol Carcinog. 2017;56:2446–60.
219. Sancho P, Barneda D, Heeschen C. Hallmarks of cancer stem cell metabolism. Br J Cancer. 2016;114:1305–12.
220. Viale A, Corti D, Draetta GF. Tumors and mitochondrial respiration: a neglected connection. Cancer Res. 2015;75:3685–6.
221. De Francesco EM, Sotgia F, Lisanti MP. Cancer stem cells (CSCs): metabolic strategies for their identification and eradication. Biochem J. 2018;475:1611–34.
222. Boros LG, Bassilian S, Lim S, Lee WNP. Genistein inhibits nonoxidative ribose synthesis in MIA pancreatic adenocarcinoma cells: a new mechanism of controlling tumor growth. Pancreas. 2001;22:1–7.
223. Zhao H, Orhan YC, Zha X, Esencan E, Chatterton RT, Bulun SE. AMP-activated protein kinase and energy balance in breast cancer. Am J Transl Res. 2017;9:197–213.
224. Manu KA, Cao PHA, Chai TF, Casey PJ, Wang M. P21Cip1/Waf1 coordinate autophagy, proliferation and apoptosis in response to metabolic stress. Cancers (Basel). 2019;11:1112.
225. Fabiani R, Vella N, Rosignoli P. Epigenetic modifications induced by olive oil and its phenolic compounds: a systematic review. Molecules. 2021;26:273.
226. Tanveer S, Fathi E, Guy F. Towards new anticancer strategies by targeting cancer stem cells with phytochemical compounds. In: Shostak S, editor. Cancer stem cells – the cutting edge. London: IntechOpen; 2011. p. 431–56.
227. Lee W-H, Loo C-Y, Bebawy M, Luk F, Mason R, Rohanizadeh R. Curcumin and its derivatives: their application in neuropharmacology and neuroscience in the 21st century. Curr Neuropharmacol. 2013;11:338–78.
228. Yang CL, Ma YG, Xue YX, Liu YY, Xie H, Qiu GR. Curcumin induces small cell lung cancer NCI-H446 cell apoptosis via the reactive oxygen species-mediated mitochondrial pathway and not the cell death receptor pathway. DNA Cell Biol. 2012;31:139–50.
229. Shin HJ, Han JM, Choi YS, Jung HJ. Pterostilbene suppresses both cancer cells and cancer stem-like cells in cervical cancer with superior bioavailability to resveratrol. Molecules. 2020;25:228.
230. McCormack D, McFadden D. A review of pterostilbene antioxidant activity and disease modification. Oxid Med Cell Longev. 2013;2013:575482.
231. Coussens LM, Werb Z. Inflammation and cancer. Nature. 2002;420:860–7.
232. Pandey KB, Rizvi SI. Plant polyphenols as dietary antioxidants in human health and disease. Oxid Med Cell Longev. 2009;2:270–8.
233. Prasad S, Phromnoi K, Yadav VR, Chaturvedi MM, Aggarwal BB. Targeting inflammatory pathways by flavonoids for prevention and treatment of cancer. Planta Med. 2010;76:1044–63.
234. Koklesova L, Liskova A, Samec M, Buhrmann C, Samuel SM, Varghese E, et al. Carotenoids in cancer apoptosis—the road from bench to bedside and back. Cancers (Basel). 2020;12:2425.
235. Soundararajan P, Kim JS. Anti-carcinogenic glucosinolates in cruciferous vegetables and their antagonistic effects on prevention of cancers. Molecules. 2018;23:2983.
236. Yadav UP, Singh T, Kumar P, Sharma P, Kaur H, Sharma S, et al. Metabolic adaptations in cancer stem cells. Front Oncol. 2020;10:1010.
237. Robey IF, Baggett BK, Kirkpatrick ND, Roe DJ, Dosescu J, Sloane BF, et al. Bicarbonate increases tumor pH and inhibits spontaneous metastases. Cancer Res. 2009;69:2260–8.
238. Shamim U, Hanif S, Albanyan A, Beck FWJ, Bao B, Wang Z, et al. Resveratrol-induced apoptosis is enhanced in low pH environments associated with cancer. J Cell Physiol. 2012;227:1493–500.

239. Sharma A, Kaur M, Katnoria JK, Nagpal AK. Polyphenols in food: cancer prevention and apoptosis induction. Curr Med Chem. 2017;25:4740–57.
240. Yan Y, Liu N, Hou N, Dong L, Li J. Chlorogenic acid inhibits hepatocellular carcinoma in vitro and in vivo. J Nutr Biochem. 2017;46:68–73.
241. Bin Hafeez B, Asim M, Siddiqui IA, Adhami VM, Murtaza I, Delphinidin MH. a dietary anthocyanidin in pigmented fruits and vegetables: a new weapon to blunt prostate cancer growth. Cell Cycle. 2008;7:3320–6.
242. Liu W, Xu J, Wu S, Liu Y, Yu X, Chen J, et al. Selective anti-proliferation of HER2-positive breast cancer cells by anthocyanins identified by high-throughput screening. PLoS One. 2013;8:e81586.
243. Tsang WP, Kwok TT. Epigallocatechin gallate up-regulation of miR-16 and induction of apoptosis in human cancer cells. J Nutr Biochem. 2010;21:140–6.
244. Bhardwaj V, Mandal AKA. Next-generation sequencing reveals the role of epigallocatechin-3-gallate in regulating putative novel and known microRNAs which target the MAPK pathway in non-small-cell lung cancer A549 cells. Molecules. 2019;24:368.
245. Borutinskaitė V, Virkšaitė A, Gudelytė G, Navakauskienė R. Green tea polyphenol EGCG causes anti-cancerous epigenetic modulations in acute promyelocytic leukemia cells. Leuk Lymphoma. 2018;59:469–78.
246. Xie J, Yun JP, Yang YN, Hua F, Zhang XW, Lin H, et al. A novel ECG analog 4-(S)-(2,4,6-trimethylthiobenzyl)-epigallocatechin gallate selectively induces apoptosis of B16-F10 melanoma via activation of autophagy and ROS. Sci Rep. 2017;7:42194.
247. Russo M, Spagnuolo C, Tedesco I, Bilotto S, Russo GL. The flavonoid quercetin in disease prevention and therapy: facts and fancies. Biochem Pharmacol. 2012;83:6–15.
248. Wu Q, Needs PW, Lu Y, Kroon PA, Ren D, Yang X. Different antitumor effects of quercetin, quercetin-3′-sulfate and quercetin-3-glucuronide in human breast cancer MCF-7 cells. Food Funct. 2018;9:1736–46.
249. Ward AB, Mir H, Kapur N, Gales DN, Carriere PP, Singh S. Quercetin inhibits prostate cancer by attenuating cell survival and inhibiting anti-apoptotic pathways. World J Surg Oncol. 2018;16:108.
250. Sambantham S, Radha M, Paramasivam A, Anandan B, Malathi R, Chandra SR, et al. Molecular mechanism underlying hesperetin-induced apoptosis by in silico analysis and in prostate cancer PC-3 cells. Asian Pac J Cancer Prev. 2013;14:4347–52.
251. Zhang J, Wu D, Vikash SJ, Wang J, Yi J, et al. Hesperetin induces the apoptosis of gastric cancer cells via activating mitochondrial pathway by increasing reactive oxygen species. Dig Dis Sci. 2015;60:2985–95.
252. Palit S, Kar S, Sharma G, Das PK. Hesperetin induces apoptosis in breast carcinoma by triggering accumulation of ROS and activation of ASK1/JNK pathway. J Cell Physiol. 2015;230:1729–39.
253. Lim W, Park S, Bazer FW, Song G. Naringenin-induced apoptotic cell death in prostate cancer cells is mediated via the PI3K/AKT and MAPK signaling pathways. J Cell Biochem. 2017;118:1118–31.
254. Park S, Lim W, Bazer FW, Song G. Naringenin suppresses growth of human placental choriocarcinoma via reactive oxygen species-mediated P38 and JNK MAPK pathways. Phytomedicine. 2018;50:238–46.
255. Park HJ, Choi YJ, Lee JH, Nam MJ. Naringenin causes ASK1-induced apoptosis via reactive oxygen species in human pancreatic cancer cells. Food Chem Toxicol. 2017;99:1–8.
256. Pandey M, Kaur P, Shukla S, Abbas A, Fu P, Gupta S. Plant flavone apigenin inhibits HDAC and remodels chromatin to induce growth arrest and apoptosis in human prostate cancer cells: In vitro and in vivo study. Mol Carcinog. 2012;51:952–62.
257. Dei Cas M, Ghidoni R. Cancer prevention and therapy with polyphenols: sphingolipid-mediated mechanisms. Nutrients. 2018;10:940.
258. Tian T, Li J, Li B, Wang Y, Li M, Ma D, et al. Genistein exhibits anti-cancer effects via down-regulating FoxM1 in H446 small-cell lung cancer cells. Tumor Biol. 2014;35:4137–45.

259. Majid S, Dar AA, Ahmad AE, Hirata H, Kawakami K, Shahryari V, et al. BTG3 tumor suppressor gene promoter demethylation, histone modification and cell cycle arrest by genistein in renal cancer. Carcinogenesis. 2009;30:662–70.
260. Luo H, Wang L, Schulte BA, Yang A, Tang S, Wang GY. Resveratrol enhances ionizing radiation-induced premature senescence in lung cancer cells. Int J Oncol. 2013;43:1999–2006.
261. Kunnumakkara AB, Guha S, Krishnan S, Diagaradjane P, Gelovani J, Aggarwal BB. Curcumin potentiates antitumor activity of gemcitabine in an orthotopic model of pancreatic cancer through suppression of proliferation, angiogenesis, and inhibition of nuclear factor-κB-regulated gene products. Cancer Res. 2007;67:3853–61.
262. Alexandrow MG, Song LJ, Altiok S, Gray J, Haura EB, Kumar NB. Curcumin: a novel Stat3 pathway inhibitor for chemoprevention of lung cancer. Eur J Cancer Prev. 2012;21:407–12.
263. Yang CW, Chang CL, Lee HC, Chi CW, Pan JP, Yang WC. Curcumin induces the apoptosis of human monocytic leukemia THP-1 cells via the activation of JNK/ERK Pathways. BMC Complem Altern Med. 2012;12:22.
264. Stocco B, Toledo KA, Fumagalli HF, Bianchini FJ, Fortes VS, Fonseca MJV, et al. Biotransformed soybean extract induces cell death of estrogen-dependent breast cancer cells by modulation of apoptotic proteins. Nutr Cancer. 2015;67:612–9.
265. Park HJ, Jeon YK, You DH, Nam MJ. Daidzein causes cytochrome c-mediated apoptosis via the Bcl-2 family in human hepatic cancer cells. Food Chem Toxicol. 2013;60:542–9.
266. Wang LG, Beklemisheva A, Liu XM, Ferrari AC, Feng J, Chiao JW. Dual action on promoter demethylation and chromatin by an isothiocyanate restored GSTP1 silenced in prostate cancer. Mol Carcinog. 2007;46:24–31.
267. Chen PY, Lin KC, Lin JP, Tang NY, Yang JS, Lu KW, et al. Phenethyl isothiocyanate (PEITC) inhibits the growth of human oral squamous carcinoma hsc-3 cells through g(0)/g (1) phase arrest and mitochondria-mediated apoptotic cell death. Evid Based Complem Altern Med. 2012;2012:718320.
268. Ho CC, Lai KC, Hsu SC, Kuo CL, Ma CY, Lin ML, et al. Benzyl isothiocyanate (BITC) inhibits migration and invasion of human gastric cancer AGS cells via suppressing ERK signal pathways. Hum Exp Toxicol. 2011;30:296–306.
269. Im E, Yeo C, Lee EO. Luteolin induces caspase-dependent apoptosis via inhibiting the AKT/osteopontin pathway in human hepatocellular carcinoma SK-Hep-1 cells. Life Sci. 2018;209:259–66.
270. Kang KA, Piao MJ, Ryu YS, Hyun YJ, Park JE, Shilnikova K, et al. Luteolin induces apoptotic cell death via antioxidant activity in human colon cancer cells. Int J Oncol. 2017;51:1169–78.
271. Zhang Q, Yang J, Wang J. Modulatory effect of luteolin on redox homeostasis and inflammatory cytokines in a mouse model of liver cancer. Oncol Lett. 2016;12:4767–72.
272. Mak KK, Wu ATH, Lee WH, Chang TC, Chiou JF, Wang LS, et al. Pterostilbene, a bioactive component of blueberries, suppresses the generation of breast cancer stem cells within tumor microenvironment and metastasis via modulating NF-κB/microRNA 448 circuit. Mol Nutr Food Res. 2013;57:1123–34.
273. Li Y, Zhang T. Targeting cancer stem cells with sulforaphane, a dietary component from broccoli and broccoli sprouts. Future Oncol. 2013;9:1097–103.
274. Choudhari AS, Mandave PC, Deshpande M, Ranjekar P, Prakash O. Phytochemicals in cancer treatment: From preclinical studies to clinical practice. Front Pharmacol. 2020;10:1614.
275. Pastorelli D, Fabricio ASC, Giovanis P, D'Ippolito S, Fiduccia P, Soldà C, et al. Phytosome complex of curcumin as complementary therapy of advanced pancreatic cancer improves safety and efficacy of gemcitabine: Results of a prospective phase II trial. Pharmacol Res. 2018;132:72–9.
276. Chen J, Song Y, Zhang L. Lycopene/tomato consumption and the risk of prostate cancer: a systematic review and meta-analysis of prospective studies. J Nutr Sci Vitaminol (Tokyo). 2013;59:213–23.

277. Gontero P, Marra G, Soria F, Oderda M, Zitella A, Baratta F, et al. A randomized double-blind placebo controlled phase I-II study on clinical and molecular effects of dietary supplements in men with precancerous prostatic lesions. Chemoprevention or "chemopromotion"? Prostate. 2015;75:1177–86.
278. Beynon RA, Richmond RC, Santos Ferreira DL, Ness AR, May M, Smith GD, et al. Investigating the effects of lycopene and green tea on the metabolome of men at risk of prostate cancer: The ProDiet randomised controlled trial. Int J Cancer. 2019;144:1918–28.
279. Paller CJ, Rudek MA, Zhou XC, Wagner WD, Hudson TS, Anders N, et al. A phase I study of muscadine grape skin extract in men with biochemically recurrent prostate cancer: Safety, tolerability, and dose determination. Prostate. 2015;75:1518–25.
280. Alumkal JJ, Slottke R, Schwartzman J, Cherala G, Munar M, Graff JN, et al. A phase II study of sulforaphane-rich broccoli sprout extracts in men with recurrent prostate cancer. Invest New Drugs. 2015;33:480–9.

Epigenetic Basis of Polyphenols in Cancer Prevention and Therapy

6

Mohammed Kaleem, Mahmoud Alhosin, Kabiruddin Khan, Wasim Ahmad, Salman Hosawi, Suza Mohammad Nur, Hani Choudhry, Mazin Abdulaziz Zamzami, Fahad A. Al-Abbasi, and MD Noushad Javed

Abstract

The dynamic landscapes of epigenetic patterns implicate in genetic expression, post-translational modifications as well as transcribing multivariate signals into the specific program. These patterns play an important roles in DNA methylation, histone modification, long noncoding RNA (lncRNA), and microRNA (miRNA) interference to alter the functions of tumor suppressor genes (TSGs) and oncogenes, followed by modulation in structures, functioning and assembling of normal cells, prior to transformed into cancerous cells. Additionally, scaffolds of natural polyphenols and their metabolites, owing to diverse, unique structural conformations and topography, significantly intervene above-mentioned altered epigenetic mechanisms of cancers.

This chapter aims to discuss recent findings in developmental cancer biology, followed by establishing dynamic roles and delineated mechanisms of polyphenols targeting various epigenetic landscape, their parameters, immunogenic responses, signaling pathways, and physiological barriers in cancerous cells. The challenges and evidence for the perspective of polyphenols would

M. Kaleem · M. Alhosin · S. Hosawi · S. M. Nur · H. Choudhry · M. A. Zamzami · F. A. Al-Abbasi
Department of Biochemistry, Faculty of Science, Centre for Artificial intelligence in Precision Medicines, King Abdulaziz University, Jeddah, Saudi Arabia
e-mail: mkaleem0002@stu.kau.edu.sa; malhaseen@kau.edu.sa; shosawi@kau.edu.sa; hchoudhry@kau.edu.sa; mzamzami@kau.edu.sa

K. Khan
Department of Pharmaceutical Technology, Jadavpur University, Kolkata, India

W. Ahmad
Department of Kuliyate Tib, National Institute of Unani Medicine, Bengaluru, India

M. N. Javed (✉)
Department of Biotechnology, Jamia Millia Islamia, New Delhi, India

S. Tabrez, M. Imran Khan (eds.), *Polyphenols-based Nanotherapeutics for Cancer Management*, https://doi.org/10.1007/978-981-16-4935-6_6

integrate advanced understanding for developing various dietary products to prevent and treat different cancers.

Keywords

Polyphenols · lncRNA and miRNA · Epigenetic · Cancer · Tumor · DNA methylation · Histone modification

6.1 Introduction

Cancer is an uncontrolled division of healthy cells, which can be affected via genetic disorders, epigenetic aberrations, and deregulation in post-translational modifications [1, 2]. Tumor suppressor genes (TSGs) and Oncogenes are influenced by genetic alterations and epigenetic changes that comprise DNA methylation, histone modification, long noncoding RNA, and microRNA (miRNA) interference that belong to post-translational modification [3]. Additionally, epigenetic alterations can be triggered by regular intake of dietary and environmental factors [4]. As a result, epigenetic aberrations and genetic disorders generally induce tumorigenesis [5]. Globally, there are around 18.1 million new cases of cancer diagnosed in the year 2018, while mortality rates increased to 9.6 million as compared to 2008, which was nearly 7.6 million cancer-related deaths [6]. In 2030, there would be an estimated increase of 23.6 million new cases of cancer, according to American Cancer Society statistics.

Epigenetics is reversible heritable modifications in the expression of a gene that takes place without modifying DNA in sequence, but alterations that are suitably potent to control gene expression dynamics [7]. DNA methylation and histone modifications are the significant contributors to cancer epigenetics machinery, which may trigger changes in expression of a gene but no alteration in DNA sequence [8–10]. In contrast to genetic alteration processes, such as mutations and deletions, which are often challenging to reverse back; however, epigenetics abnormalities are often considered as facile reversible one [11]. Epigenetic gene arrangements have critical roles in various biological processes such as genetic imprinting, X-chromosome inactivation, and embryonic development. Three crucial and distinctive complex mechanisms are well-known to be part of the "epigenome," which comprises DNA methylation, histone modifications, and post-transcriptional gene regulation by noncoding microRNAs (miRNAs) [12]. These methods influence DNA folding, transcript stability, nucleosome positioning, chromatin compaction, and complete nuclear organization of the genetic material (Fig. 6.1). Concomitantly and synergistically, they govern whether a gene is downregulated or upregulated, along with the effectiveness and tissue selectivity towards the gene expression. Interference of the epigenome causes the progression of the disease. Thus, disease sensitivity is a consequence of a complicated association between one's genetic

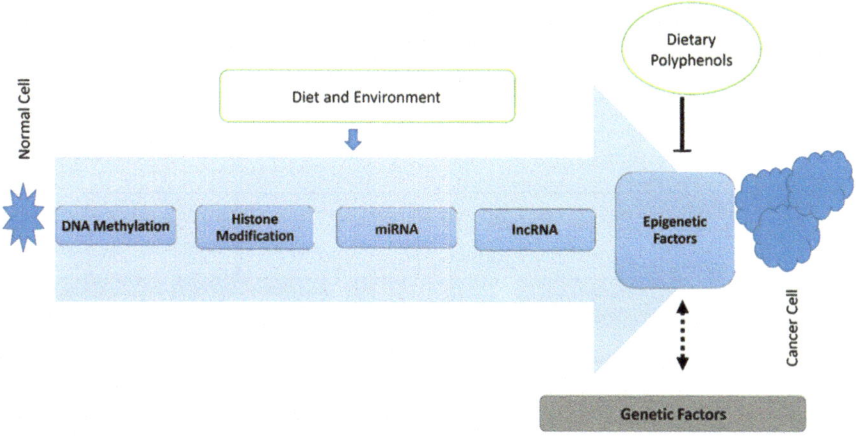

Fig. 6.1 Epigenetic mechanism in tumorigenesis

characteristics and epigenetic markers imprinted on one's genome by exogenous and endogenous attributes [13].

Tumorigenesis is a chronic inflammatory disease in which epigenetic and genetic characteristics change leading to tumor progression [14]. Epigenetic alterations, including histone modifications, microRNAs, noncoding RNA, and DNA methylation, in inflammatory disorders are affected by various factors; mainly by dietary and environmental attributes [15]. However, nutritional polyphenols are most likely influenced by these epigenetic changes, which correspondingly contribute towards their chemopreventive potential [13].

6.2 Polyphenols

Polyphenols are the most important factors of a human diet which primarily consists of phytochemicals [16]. In Fig. 6.2, polyphenols are divided into five different categories, such as phenolic acid, flavonoids, curcuminoids, stilbenes, as well as lignans [17], while flavonoids are subclassified into flavanols, flavones, flavanones, anthocyanins as well as isoflavones.

Polyphenols have been classified into flavonoids, stilbenoids, and phenolic acid; on the other hand, flavonoids are subcategorized into flavonols, flavanones, flavanols, flavones, isoflavones, and anthocyanins [17, 18].

6.3 Polyphenols for Tumor Prevention and Therapeutics

Several findings validated that animal or plant-based natural products (e.g., polyphenols) are used to inhibit and manage many diseases, including cardiac disorders, pathogenic infections, hyperglycemia, neuronal disorders, cancer, as

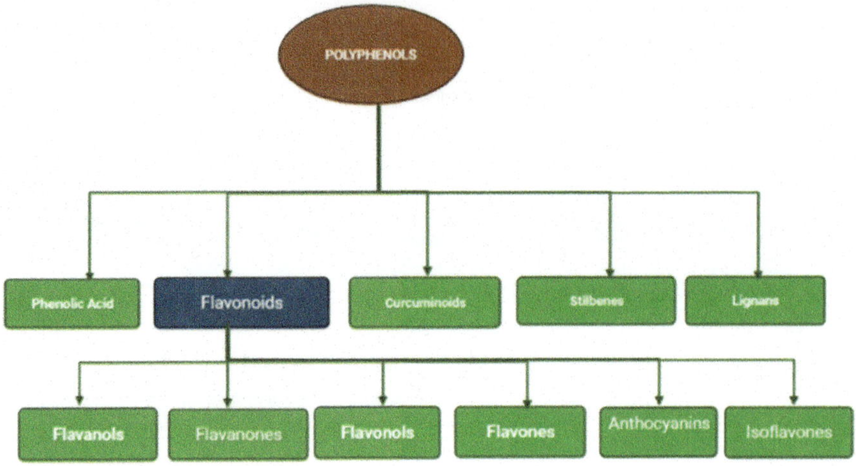

Fig. 6.2 The classifications of plant polyphenols

well as asthma [19, 20]. Tens of thousands of different polyphenols, isolated from plants, reported anti-carcinogenic characteristics, tumor growth suppressor, anti-proliferative, anti-inflammatory, anti-angiogenesis, apoptosis inducer, as well as anti-metastasis properties [21, 22]. Furthermore, these compounds can be utilized, such as bioactive molecules, to make innovative chemopreventive agents that show the most effective target organ with the least infectivity [18, 23]. Noteworthy, here role of nanotechnology-based delivery systems has emerged as a potential tool to combat such challenges, especially in viral infections and malignancy [24]. Among these nanoparticles, polymeric systems such as encapsulated [25] or polyelectric complexes [26]; metallic nanoparticles such as gold [27] and silver colloids [28]; lipid nanoformulations [29], bicontinuous carriers, such as limicubes [30] and cubosomes [31], as well as vesicular systems are most investigated delivery systems for such type of therapeutics, preferably being fabricated with experimental architects of factorial design tools [32] for optimal performances [33].

Multiple reports have shown that various nutraceuticals significantly regulate gene expression by targeting various factors/constituents of the epigenetic types of machinery [34]. Through the continuous improvement in the standard of living adaptations, it is essential to identify novel compounds, which can be most likely utilized as a hindrance of disease, and to discover novel molecules that could be anticancerous and shows better efficacy against malignancy [35]. These natural products are either derived from plants [36], microbial [37], and marine species [38] or designed in some nature mimicking systems hence called bioinspired [39] or biomimetic systems [40]. These polyphenols can commonly show anticancerous activities and effectiveness in many other disorders, including hyperglycemia [41], cardiovascular diseases [42], liver diseases [43], asthma [44], neurodegenerative disorders [45], neurodevelopmental [46]; osteoporosis [47], anemia [48], bulimia

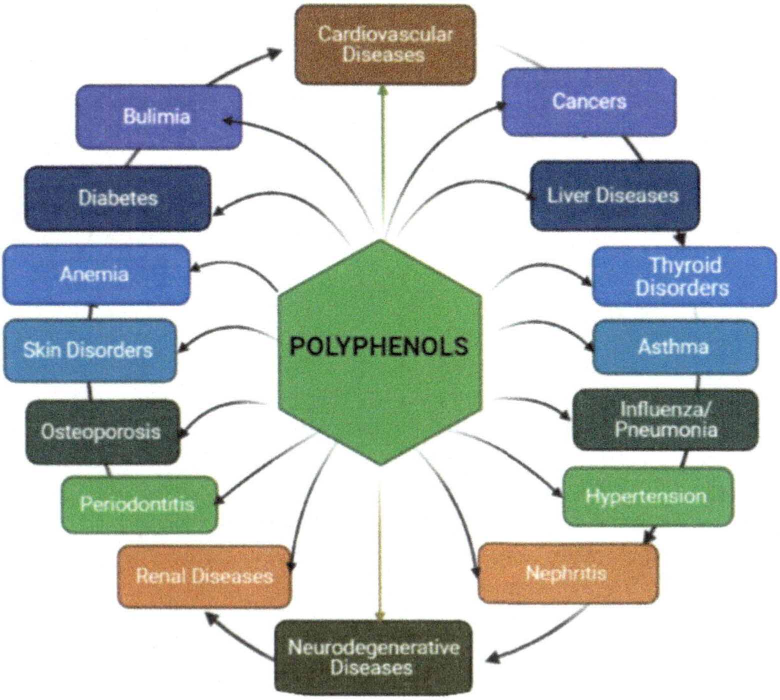

Fig. 6.3 Polyphenols have a beneficial effect on the health system

[18], influenza/ pneumonia [49], renal and thyroid disorders [50, 51], nephritis [52], periodontitis [53], hypertension [52], and skin disorders [55] (Fig. 6.3).

Polyphenols are mainly implicated with several mechanisms, via associations with numerous cellular constituents, including enzymes, carbohydrates, and protein to control gene expression and cancerous signaling pathways [23, 56]. Briefly, these plant-derived polyphenols regulate cancer pathways by preventing cell proliferation of cancer, tumoral mass reduction, and tumor regression.

Polyphenols are mainly found in vegetables, beverages, fruits, and spices. These products are chemopreventive against devastating diseases, including neurodegenerative diseases, cancer, diabetes, osteoporosis, liver, and cardiovascular diseases (CVDs) [18].

6.4 Role of Epigenetics in Cancer

6.4.1 DNA Methylation

Predominantly in cytosine, followed by guanine, a novel covalent bond with methyl group forms methylated CpG. Whereas human CpG islands domain is short cDNA sequences of more than 200 base-pair lengths, bearing very high frequency of CpG sites (observed-to-expected ratio > 60%), high GC frequency (>0.5), and interspersed; along with repeating units of centromeric repeats, retrotransposon elements, Recombinant DNA (rDNA) so these are significantly different from normal patterns of the genome [57, 58]. Subsequently, in small CpG enriched DNA stretches, methylation of the pyrimidine ring in cytosines at 5th carbon form 5-methylcytosine. CpG islands are preferably situated at 5′ gene end as well as covering around 0.6 fractions of human gene promoters [59]. Both methylations are also reported in several non-CpG domains namely, CpA, CpT, as well as CpC [60]. Differential types of methylated regions in CpG and non-CpG may decide the fate or regulation of genes, i.e., their silencing or activation hence may critically involve in pathological conditions of various diseases. In other words, the status of DNA methylation controls gene expression. Although both methylated CpG and non-CpG methylation are reported in complete genome accumulation of non-CpG methylation is very specific and limited, depending upon the type of cells, i.e., as pluripotent stem cells, oocytes, neurons, and glial cells [18].

Cancer is a major disorder owing to modification in enzymatic activities of DNA methyltransferases (DNMTs), leading to numerous diseases as well. DNMTs act on S-adenosyl-methionine to catalyze CH3 (methyl) domain relocation to cytosine. In mammals, DNMT family may be subdivided into five categories, i.e., 1, 2, 3a, 3b, and 3L subtypes [61]. In cell division, DNMT-1 maintains a pattern of DNA methylation with DNA replications [62]. While, DNMT-3a and DNMT-3b enzymes actively control de-novo DNA methyltransferase processes, essentially by integrating a CH_3 domain to cytosine, critical for differentiation [18, 63]. During tumorigenesis, CpGs hypermethylation process is reported at 5′ end in tumor-accompanied genes along with inactivation of many cancer-suppressor genes, despite hypomethylation of any single gene or its small subdivisions as reported in several tumors [64]. For example, among cyclin-dependent kinase inhibitors, $p16^{INK4a}$ (CDKN2A) is critical for tumor suppressor genes because differentially hypermethylated in cancer. Events of tumor suppressor gene hypermethylation, for example, H and E subtypes of cadherins, also induce metastasis and cancer proliferation [65]. Also, there is a closed relationship established between the inactivated gene that encodes cyclin-dependent kinase inhibitors, as well as progression in malignancy. Many hypermethylation events of DNA (genes) with repairing functionalities play a critical and direct role in epigenetics to mutate and alter tumor progression [66].

Subsequently, global DNA hypomethylation arrangement is a widespread cause in many carcinogenic processes [67, 68]. The recent findings have shown that the regulation of carcinogenesis is due to the combined impact of both DNA hypomethylation as well as hypermethylation sequences, while hypomethylation has an important key role in carcinogenic tissue in contrast with the normal tissue [69, 70]. The absence of satellite DNA methylation serves significant purposes in tumoral progression. For example, differential states of STAR-1 hypomethylation (satellite DNA sequence), a cluster with highly repetitive and tandem DNA sequences, contribute to both high frequencies of DNA rearrangements and chromosomal instability in more than 60% of breast tumorigenesis

[71]. Hypomethylation of satellite 2 (Sat2) in centromeric and juxtacentromeric (centromere-adjacent) in chromosome 1 served the role of independent biomarkers of poor prognosis in ovarian cancer and their elevated stages classify tumoral grade. Although, satellite DNA hypermethylation, as well as 15 5′ gene domain, are implicated in ovarian tumors changes in satellite DNA methylation are independent of gene region. Similarly, loci *CDH-13* (at 16q24) as well as *RNR-1* (at 13p12) hypermethylation is closely correlated to decreased Sat2 hypomethylation [72]. Subsequently, hypomethylation of chromatin helicase of DNA binding protein 3 gene promoter domain favors upregulated positive regulator of tumor cell proliferation (P cadherin) to impart invasiveness as well as metastasis in breast and colorectal tumors [73]. Noteworthy, DNA methylation significantly affects the progression of different cancers, and exploring the status of DNA methylation is crucial in all tumors and their staging [74].

Furthermore, APC gene silencing has been noted in several tumors, including colorectal, breast, prostate, as well as lung malignancy. APC serves an antagonist role in Wnt signaling pathway, effectively implicated in migratory functions as well as adhesiveness of cells. Briefly; WNT/β-catenin pathway majorly controls cell proliferation as well as survivals of many types of cancers. It also controls the members in the WNT pathway, which includes WNT inhibitory factor 1 (WIF1), secreted frizzled-related proteins (sFRPs), WNTs, and DDKs (Dickkopf) through epigenetic modifications [75]. Several other gene silencing events were duly illustrated in breast tumors, for example, BRCA1 silencing, causing DNA repair double-stranded breaks as well as transcriptional events [64]. Many FDA-approved drugs, for example, Doxorubicin, Cisplatin, Vorinostat, Decitabine, Azacitidine, as well as Paclitaxel revealed a promising approach in tumor treatment, through DNMTs targets [76].

6.4.2 Histone Modifications

Briefly, histones are groups of a soluble protein implicated in DNA wrapping on a structural bead unit of ~146 bp length but with a fixed distance intervals, i.e., nucleosomes [77]. Typically, a nucleosome involves linker histones type H-1 (main component) which establishes attachment with outer nucleosomal periphery to serve a linkage from one nucleosome to another nearby nucleosome. While, compared to H-1, core histones of nucleosome, i.e., 2A/2B, 3, and 4 variants of H; establish more favorable bonding with DNA [78, 79]. Histone modifications which are mainly reported at the globular N-terminus region that obtrudes outside from H-3 and H-4, susceptible to several chemical alterations with threonine, lysine, and serine. Thus, histone modifications are potently implicated in carcinogenesis as well as cancer development [80, 81].

Similarly, post-translational modifications (PTM) which frequently result in charge-mediated alterations in nucleosome are another critical component in epigenome assembly, leading to histone modifications and significantly altering gene expressions. Histones in relation to PTMs further support several processes and methods of cells, via chromatin changes to significantly influence gene expression, related to carcinogenesis as well as cancer development [81]. These PTMs are reversible as well as unrestricted towards lysine-arginine methylation, lysine ubiquitination, lysine acetylation, and serine-threonine phosphorylation [80]. Histone modifications also occur due to the action of several catalytic enzymes, including histone methyltransferases (HMTs), histone acetyltransferases (HATs), histone demethylases (HDMs), and histone deacetylases (HDACs). These mediated histone modifications can bring about cancer commencement and development via triggering genome-wide changes [82]. HATs actively participate in histone acetylation, accountable for regulating many cellular methods, including DNA repair, transcription, gene silencing, cell differentiation, and apoptosis [83]. HDAC enzymes reverse HAT enzyme actions via affecting many methods, including cell growth, signal transduction, and apoptosis [84]. These catalytic methods imbalance histone acetylation leading to tumor development. HDMs and HMTs also work as an inducement for histone modifications. HMTs have been implicated through chromatin-dependent transcriptional activation and repression in DNA methylation [85]. As a result of these stimulant methods, particular genes inside DNA involved with histone can either be stimulated or deactivated [86]. Among several kinds, EZH2, HMTs, and G9a are very important histone methyltransferases, because of their ability to histone H-3 methylation at lysine 27 (H-3: K27). While methylation of both lysine 9 histone H-3 (H-3:K9) as well as H-3:K27 help to enhance heterochromatin implicated in gene silencing and facilitate tumor development [87]. Various dietary polyphenols potentially regulate histone modifications to inhibit tumors thereby serving a purpose in treatments [88].

6.4.3 microRNAs

microRNAs (miRNAs) also play a significant role in epigenetic modulation. miRNAs can carry out RNA splicing associated with gain in functions, and miRNAs significantly facilitate post-translational gene modulations. miRNAs, 20–22 nucleotides long, are small single-stranded noncoding RNAs that control gene expression through post-translational silencing of the target genes [89]. miRNAs regulate several biological methods, including cell differentiation, cell proliferation, and apoptosis. As a result of their essential role in the physiology of cells, expression level changes are directly associated with disease development. The recent findings have demonstrated a direct relationship between miRNAs modifications and tumor ([90, 91]. MicroRNA expression can be monitored through various mechanisms, including single nucleotide polymorphisms (SNPs), chromosomal abnormalities, mutations in the primary transcripts, for example, *miR-15a* and *miR-16-1* [92], changed activity of many transcription factors, for instance, *miR-17-92* cluster, and alterations in the *miR-34* family because of activation of *p53*. These mechanisms can be related to various categories of tumors, including breast, bladder, and lung cancer [93, 94]. However, hypermethylation of *miR-9-1* in breast cancer occurs, whereas *miR-34c* and *miR-34b* groups are hypermethylated in colorectal cancer [95]. Aberrant methylation of *miR-148a*, miR-*9*, *miR-34b*, and *miR-34c* are frequently related to metastasis. Besides, methylation of *miR-9*, *miR-148a*, and *miR-34b/c* are directly associated with malignancy [96]. Similarly, these deviations, histone acetylation, and promoter methylation can also control expression of microRNA in various cancers [97].

6.4.4 lncRNA

lncRNAs, more than 200 nucleotides longer, are a category of non-translated RNAs [98] and have a crucial role in different biological methods implicated in cell progression and growth [99]. Numerous current studies showed their role in the epigenetic complex by altering chromatin remodeling enzymes and influencing gene expression arrangement, such as lncRNA TARID (TCF21 antisense RNA inducing demethylation) controls GADD45A (growth arrest and DNA-damage-inducible, alpha), which works as a regulator in the DNA methylation process by stimulating tumor suppressor transcription factor 21 (TCF21) via promoter demethylation [100]. A different class of lncRNA HOX transcript antisense RNA (HOTAIR) associates with Polycomb Repressive Complex 2 (PRC2) as well as mediating epigenetic silencing of the homeobox D cluster (HOXD) locus by causing its H3 lysine 27 trimethylation (H3K27me3) [101]. lncRNAs also control another joining method. For instance, the natural antisense transcript (NAT) of zinc finger E-box binding homeobox 2 ZEB2 inhibits intertwining of ZEB2 mRNA by interrelating with an intronic 5′ splice site and safeguards as anticancer cell metastasis [102]. Little lncRNAs work as oncogenes, whereas another group works as the tumor suppressor [103] such as TGF-β activated lncRNA (lncRNA-ATB) mediates epithelial to mesenchymal transition (EMT) and metastasis in hepatocellular carcinoma [104]. Interconnection of NF-κB with lncRNA (NKILA) works as a framework and triggers tumorigenic NF-κB pathway by impeding IκB phosphorylation [105]. Current findings report exhibited the tumor-suppressive nature of lncRNAs [106]. Here, the binding of PTENP1, a pseudogene for tumor suppressor PTEN to the miRNAs, inhibits PTEN activity by binding to 3′ untranslated region (UTR) of PTEN mRNA. These lncRNAs are identified as competitive endogenous RNA (ceRNA) for sequestration of miRNAs or target mimics for miRNA. Consequently, it is promising to investigate more about the lncRNAs function, which plays a significant role in clinical regulation of tumors [107]. A summary of the epigenetic changes during cancer development is demonstrated in Fig. 6.4.

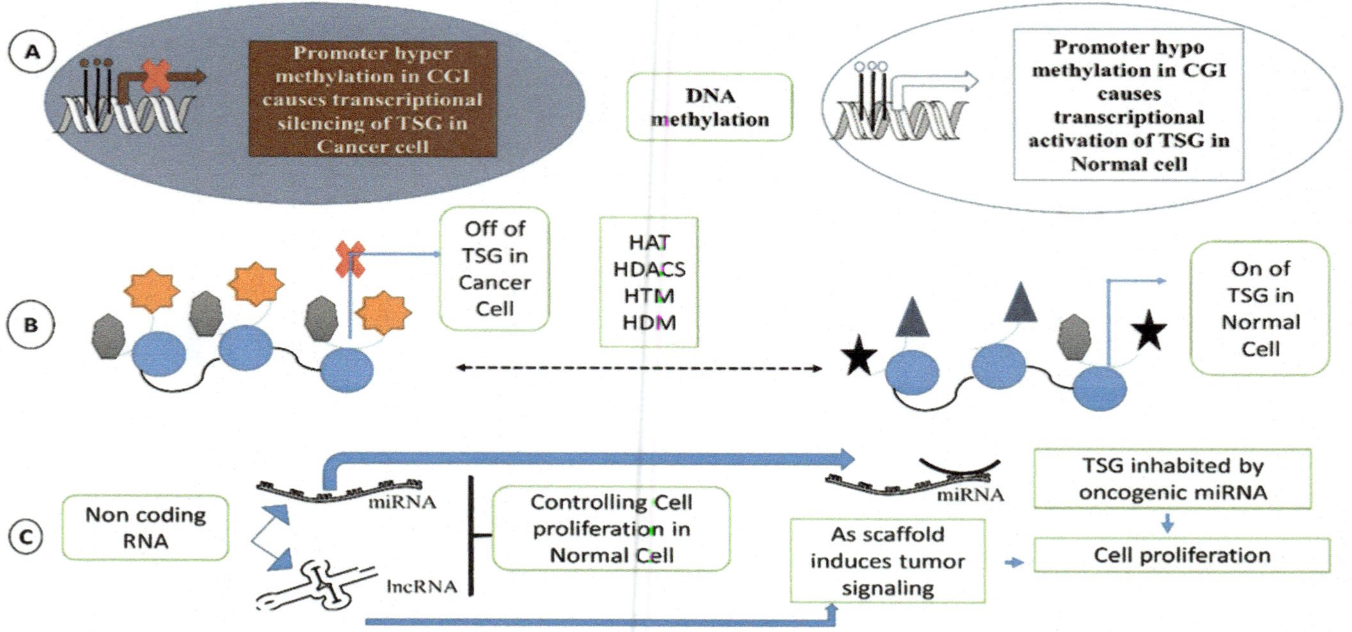

Fig. 6.4 Pictorial depiction of various epigenetic modifications during cancer progression. (**a**) DNA methylation mediated epigenetic modification interplays between normal cells and cancer cells through hypo or hypermethylation. When hypomethylation takes place in CpG Island (CGI) of tumor suppressor genes promoters' region it stimulates transcriptional activation of tumor suppressor genes (TSG). In contrast, cancer cells acquire hypermethylation which in turn causes transcription of TSG expression. (**b**) The histone tails become modified either by acetylation or by methylation at divergent positions. Based on this, it exerts divergent transcriptional output in normal cells and cancer cells. H3K4 methylation (star shaped) and acetylation (triangle shaped) fascinate transcription factor binding hence remarks the active gene expression in normal cells. In contrast, H3K9 (grey color) and H3K27 (orange triangles) methylation make compact chromatin structure hence remarks transcriptional suppression in cancer cells. (**c**) Noncoding RNA like miRNA and lncRNA differentially regulate gene expression in such a way that, noncoding RNA-mediated gene expression halts the cell proliferation in normal cells. In contrast, it inhibited the tumor suppressor gene expression and induces the tumorigenic signaling pathways, which in turn stimulates cell proliferation [107]

6.5 Polyphenols Inhibit Cancer Cell Proliferation Via Epigenetic Alterations

The uncontrollable proliferation converts normal cells into cancerous cells with the involvement of factors to control cell cycle progression and escape checkpoint. The cyclins (cyclin-dependent kinases (CDKs) and their inhibitors (CDKIs) regulate four (G1, S, G2, and M) phases of the cell cycle, acting as co-activators of CDK activities and trigger the cell cycle progression through making complexes of cyclin-CDK. Several reports indicate the involvement of polyphenols in regulating the arrest of the cell cycle, which leads to cancer through pathways involving upstream signaling. Some CDKIs examples involved in arresting cell cycle (at G1 stage) are p15INK4B, p21CIP1, and $p16^{INK4a}$. They do this (CDK4/6 inhibition) by creating complexes of CDKI-CDK4/6 [5].

6.5.1 Curcumin

The curcumin found in the rhizomes of Curcuma longa, belongs to the family Zingiberaceae putatively used for chemoprevention in several cancer types [108–110]. The chemoprevention is mainly by arresting cancerous cell growth in the G1 phase, primarily by expressing a high level of $p21^{CIP1}$ protein, reduction of miR-208 protein (responsible for the translation of $p21^{CIP}1$), and also restoring the levels of protein $p15^{INK4B}$ through downregulation/suppression in methylation state of a promoter [111, 112]. Additionally, cyclin D1 and CDK4/6 expression are inhibited by curcumin through miR-34a induction that acts on mRNA of these proteins, mainly colorectal cancerous cells [113]. The expression of $p21^{CIP1}$ and $p16^{INK4A}$ proteins are enhanced by genistein, GTPs (green tea polyphenols), and EGCG (epigallocatechin-3-gallate) through various (epigenetic) mechanisms in cancer [114, 115].

6.5.2 Genistein

Genistein represents isoflavone (bioactive) obtain from extracts of soybean. It induces expression of proteins like $p21^{CIP1}$ and $p16^{INK4A}$ mainly by an increase of transcriptional activators deployment, modification at H3K4me3, H4, and acetyl-H3, as well as by reducing repressor binding, altering chromatin H3K27me3 and H3K9me3, and lastly by enhancing $p21^{CIP1}$ and $p16^{INK4a}$ levels in cancerous or precancerous breast cells [116]. The EGCG represents another potent suppressor of HDACs and DNMTs [117]. The expression of $p16^{INK4a}$ leads to arresting G-1 stage of the cell cycle with EGCG treatment for further enhancing the methylation role of $p16^{INK4a}$, being identified by methylation-specific PCR (MSP) analysis [118]. The EGCG represents the primary active constituents from GTPs, which reduces cyclin (D1, D2) through induction of $p21^{CIP1}$, CDKIs, p53, and $p21^{CIP1}$, which is due to suppression of HDAC response and expression of HAT response that leads to relaxation of chromatin [114, 119]. The GTPs, when combined with sulforaphane (non-polyphenolic chemical obtained from vegetables), produce a synergistic effect in arresting the cell cycle at the G2/M phase along with induction of KLOTHO and $p21^{CIP1}$. The induction of KLOTHO and $p21^{CIP1}$ through GTPs sulforaphane combination changes the methylation pattern of DNA and modification of histone, which results in binding of MeCP2 to the former [115, 120]. This evidence suggests the strategy of applying combination therapy (a mixture of more than one biofunctional compound) for assessing antitumor efficacy. The demethylation of novel protocadherin 17 (TSG PCDH17, at promoter region) through genistein induces the arrest of gastric cancer cells in the G2/M phase [121]. Moreover, genistein enhances miR-34a expression, a tumor suppressor, suppressing the oncogenic HOX transcript antisense RNA (HOTAIR) expression, leading to cancer growth induction in prostate cells [122].

The Kras is an oncogene that is overexpressed and mutated in several types of cancers and is believed to play an essential role in uncontrolled proliferation, leading to malignancy [123]. Sulforaphane, GTPs, and Quercetin enhance miR-let-7 expression, suppresses, and controls Kras miRNA expression [124]. Orally administered Resveratrol significantly prevents colorectal cancer growth by inducing miR-96 and regulating Kras protein expression and Kras-related downstream signaling molecules [125].

The Isoliquiritigenin and Genistein of a licorice root extract (dietary chalcones) induce repressors of the WNT pathway through its expression mainly by producing miR-1260b and suppressing DNMT1 activity [126, 127]. The targeting effects of miR-1260b on WNT repressors such as sFRP1, SAMD4, and DDK2 were also reported by researchers. Additionally, there is a significant suppression of miR-1620b, which is expressed in renal tumor cell [126]. Isoliquiritigenin also stops breast tumor growth by suppressing DNMT1 expression, upregulating hypomethylation of WIF1 promoter and protein expression [127].

6.6 Polyphenols Induce Cell Death in Cancer Via Epigenetic Alterations

Sometimes, requirement of newer cells (cell population) is strictly being controlled by modulating rates of cell division processes. Alternatively, sometimes requirement of existing cells is no longer desirable so in these cells, programming of intracellular death is activated to induce cell suicidal events hence called programmed cell death (PCD) process. Inducing programmed cell death (PCD) in cancer cells represents an effective strategy for treating cancer [128]. Molecules that control apoptosis are type I PCD, while type II PCD molecules favor autophagy. To be more precise, apoptosis is regulated by caspases and Bcl-2, while autophagy is controlled by autophagy-related genes (ATGs) and microtubule-associated protein 1, also called light chain 3 (LC3). Curcumin's ability to manage several epigenetic modifications is responsible for its potential antitumor property. Additionally, treatment of curcumin led to induction of miR-7 and miR-181b and subsequently inhibited BCL-2 (anti-apoptotic protein). Moreover, curcumin also upregulates miR-215 and miR-192-5p thus acting on X-linked inhibitor (XIAP, responsible for apoptosis), leading to apoptosis [129–131]. Additionally, curcumin brings about induction of miR-29b, which inhibits expression of DNMT3b and increases the promoter methylation loss primarily in PTEN (pro-apoptotic protein) [132]. Curcumin has been demonstrated to possess inhibitory activity against HDAC, which leads to induction of apoptosis and DAN double-stranded breaks [133]. Several recent reports indicate the regulation of oncogenes and/or TSGs through epigenetic modifications. Apoptosis is induced by resveratrol and genistein through enhancing the level of miR-21 and miR-574-3p, which acts on mesoderm development candidate 1 (MESDC1 oncogenes) and also performs as a repressor of repeat flightless-interacting protein 1, which are leucine-rich (LRRFIP1) and NF-κB, respectively [134, 135]. The other mechanism with which resveratrol activates apoptosis is through miR-137 induction, leading to HMT EZH2 inhibition, a decrease in H3K27 me3, and reactivating CLU NGFR TSGs [136].

Autophagy is a leading mechanism responsible for anticancer activity. So far, several studies claim the role of polyphenols as an antitumor entity through induction of autophagic pathway by epigenetic mechanisms. The induction of novel TSG PCDH17 through genistein is mainly achieved by promoters by attaining methylation [121]. The PCDH17 induced autophagy is demonstrated in several in vivo and in vitro models [137]. The PCDH17 could be a suitable site for polyphenols responsible for their autophagic response achieved through epigenetic mechanisms [5].

6.7 Polyphenols Decrease Metastasis of Cancer Through the Regulation of Epigenetic Alterations

Tumor metastasis is the leading cause of most death caused by various types of cancers like breast, prostate, lung, and colorectal cancers. Metastasis in the early stage constitutes degradation and remodeling of extracellular matrix through matrix metalloproteinases (MMPs). Moreover, the tissue responsible for inhibiting matrix metalloproteinases (TIMPs) are crucial MMPs regulators [5].

The role of resveratrol in controlling the growth of cancer and its other beneficial properties in humans is well-known. The resveratrol's role on metastasis is mainly by miR-328 binding on MMP-2 mRNA and also by inhibiting MMP-2 translation (in cases of human osteosarcomas) [138]. Resveratrol hinders forkhead box protein C2 (FOXC2), representing metastasis-related oncoprotein and mesenchymal-epithelial transition (MET) by decreasing expression of miR-520h. The miR-520h targets PP2A/C mRNA leading to inhibition of Akt/NF-κB, which represents a transcriptional cascade [139]. Indirect inhibition of MMP3 and MMP1 expression by curcumin through induction of miR-181b expression. The MiR-181b-induced cancer proliferation/metastasis is through targeting 3′-UTR of CXCL-2 and chemokine (C-X-C motif) ligand)-1 (CXCL). Curcumin induces miR-181b expression, which leads to sufficient reduction of MMP-3 and MMP-1 protein levels [129]. Additionally, Deb et al. discovered that DNA methylation has no role in the regulation of TIMP-3, largely because TIMP-3 promoter was traced as unmethylated in MDA-MB-231 and MCF-7 cell lines of breast cancer. The induction of TIMP-3 expression by GTPs and EGCG is through suppression of HMT, HDAC2, EZH2, and HDAC8 protein expression that ends in reducing H3K27me3 level and increase in the level of H3K9/18 acetylation (on TIMP-3 promoter) [140] (Table 6.1).

6.8 Epigenetic Therapy

Epigenetic therapy is synonymous with applications of drugs to improve epigenetic defects also represents a treatment class that is a novel and innovative therapeutic method for treating or reducing cancer. This therapy represents an efficient and more advantageous treatment targeted in treating epigenetic defects, which, unlike genetic defects, is reversible [143]. These drugs also hold significant use in preventing several diseases and chemoprevention [144]. Furthermore, epigenetic drugs, either in combination or alone, can perform better than the conventional anticancer drugs, where later are found to be more toxic [145]. It is known that epigenetic alterations support a wide variety of human diseases thus enhancing the current prospect of epigenetic therapy which would be likely expanded in years to come.

The existing epigenetic drugs are designed to target inhibition of HDACs and DNMTs expression. Despite this, other available drugs exist which controls gene expression having potential targets which are still not discovered. The current epigenetic drugs under evaluation can be grouped into two broad categories (1) impede DNMTs and (2) impede HDACs. The two most commonly found DNMT inhibitors (nucleoside inhibitors) are 5-aza-2-deoxycytidine (5-Aza-CdR, or Decitabine) and 5-azacytidine (5-Aza-CR, or Vidaza), and are widely studied for their epigenetic effect [146]. Procainamide, EGCG, and procaine represent non-nucleoside inhibitors, having proved potential for reducing DNMT activity in many clinical and experimental studies [147]. As far as HDAC inhibitors are concerned, some compounds showing observable responses include trichostatin A (TSA), Valproic acid, Suberoylanilide hydroxamic acid (SAHA), and Phenylbutyrate [148, 149]. Most of the discussed drugs are currently under trial (preclinical/clinical). These trials are mainly involved in disease-related hematological malignancies and solid tumors [144, 150].

Despite promising evidence shown by the epigenetic drugs in cancer treatments, it also possesses several shortcomings. Among the major limitations including the inhibition of both HDAC and DNMT can trigger oncogenes present (largely due to nonspecific nature), leading to the proliferation of cancer cells [151]. Additionally, epigenetic states are reversible and can revert to their original state since DNA methylation patterns are reversible [152]. Poor specificity and high toxicity make the current synthetic epigenetic medications less valuable, so trends are emerging towards developing more specific and safer epigenetic therapeutical and chemopreventive drugs. The existing data (both experimental and epidemiological)

Table 6.1 Polyphenols show potential anticancer therapeutic effects via epigenetic alterations

Polyphenol	Target genes	Mechanism of action	Biological function	References
Curcumin	DNA miRNA miRNA miRNA miRNA miRNA, DNA Histone miRNA	Induce $p21^{CIP1}$ expression through repressing miR-208. Bring back the $p^{15INK4B}$ through reducing promoter methylation. Inhibit CDK4/6 and cyclin D1 expression via miR-34a. Downregulate BCL-2 via miR-7. Downregulate BCL-2 by miR-181b. Prevent XIAP expression through miR-215 and miR-192-5p. Increase PTEN expression and mediated DNTB3b inhibition by induction of miR-29b. Increase the level of DNA double-strand finding by inhibiting HDAC activity. Downregulate MMP 1 and 3, and mediated CXCL-1 and -2 through induction of miR-181b	Cell cycle arrest, Apoptosis Apoptosis	[111] [112] [113] [130] [129] [132] [133] [129]
Genistein	Histone	Upregulate $p21^{CIP1}$ and $p16^{INK4a}$ expression via alteration of histone methylation and acetylation.	Cell cycle arrest, Apoptosis	[116] [121] [122] [126] [134], [137], [121]
	DNA	Induce TSG Protocadherin 17 (PCDH17) expression-mediated promoter demethylation.		
	miRNA	Downregulate oncogenic HOTAIR via upregulating tumor suppressor miR-34a.		
	miRNA	Suppress Wnt pathway via inhibiting expressionmiR-1620b		
	miRNA	Upregulates miR-574-3p through targeting mesoderm development candidate 1		
	DNA	Upregulates PCDH17-mediated downregulation of PCDH17 promoter methylation		
Epigallocatechin-gallate (EGCG)	DNA	Reactivate expression of $p16^{INK4a}$ via decreasing promoter methylation	Cell cycle arrest, Apoptosis	[118] [140]
	Histone	Induce TIMP-3 via alteration of histone pattern at TIMP-3 promoter		

(continued)

Table 6.1 (continued)

Polyphenol	Target genes	Mechanism of action	Biological function	References
Isoliquiritigenin		Increase expression of inhibitory WNT pathway by preventing DNMT1 activity through promoter demethylation		[127]
Quercetin		Upregulate miR-let-7 via inhibiting Kras expression	Apoptosis	([124], [141])
GTPs (green tea polyphenols)	DNA	Upregulate p21^{CIP1}, p16^{INK4a}, and p53 expression due to HDAC activity reduction and enhancement of HAT activity	Cell cycle arrest, Apoptosis	[114] [119] [124] [140]
	Histone	Upregulate p21^{CIP1} via downregulation of the acetylated histone H3 at promoter range		
	DNA	Upregulate the miR-let-7 via decreasing the expression of Kras		
	Histone	Induce TIMP-3 through alteration of histone pattern at TIMP-3 promoter		
Resveratrol	miRNA	Upregulate miR-96 and inhibits tumorigenesis via decreasing the expression of Kras	Apoptosis	[125] [135, 142] [136] [138] [139]
	miRNA	Decrease miR-21 expression and mediated NF-κB activity through targeting LRRFIP1		
	miRNA, Histone	Induce upregulation of miR-137-mediated reduction of EZH2 and H3K27me3 via reactivation of tumor suppressor genes CLU and NGFR		
	miRNA	Inhibit MMP-2 expression through induction of miR-328		
	miRNA	Indirect inhibition of MET through induction of miR-520 h		
Combinatorial effect of Green tea with sulforaphane	DNA, Histone	Induce p21^{CIP1} and KLOTHO expression synergistically via alteration in arrangements of DNA methylation histone modification level	Cell cycle arrest at G2/M	[115]

provides us with evidence that plant polyphenols (dietary) carry significant anticancer properties and are involved in the treatment of several cancer types wherein the effect is measured through epigenetic machinery modulation within the cancer cells [13].

6.9 Polyphenols and DNA Methylation

6.9.1 Tea Polyphenols (Epigallocatechin-3-gallate (EGCG)

The intake of tea has several beneficial effects on health systems. Tea polyphenols include epigallocatechin (EGC), epicatechin-gallate (ECG), epicatechin (EC), and epigallocatechin-gallate (EGCG) [153]. Among all, EGCG consist of more than 50% of the total polyphenol, which is amply present in green tea [107]. The anticancerous activity of tea polyphenols is widely investigated [154]. Another study showed that green tea intake led to a decrease in ovarian, breast, colorectal, skin, pancreatic, and gastric cancers [155]. EGCG prevents the activity of DNMT enzyme and aids in the reactivation of numerous tumor suppressor genes. EGCG indicates substantial effects in several cancer cell lines. For instance, EGCG leads to hypomethylation and reexpression of various tumor suppressor genes such as retinoic acid receptor β (RARβ), DNA mismatch repair gene (hMLH1), $p16^{INK4a}$, and O6-methylguanine methyltransferase (MGMT), in human breast (MCF-7 and MDA-MB-231), colon (HT29), prostate (PC3), and esophageal (KYSE 150) cancer cell lines through impeding DNMT1 function [156]. Upon treatment of EGCG also produces anti-proliferative activity in invasive cancer cells. Here, EGCG reactivates cysteine-rich protein with Kazal motifs (RECK) gene through hypomethylation and prevents the invasive growth of salivary adenoid cystic carcinoma cells [157]. Numerous synthetic analogs of EGCG have been revealed to have an anticancer property [158, 159]. Few instances of EGCG-associated DNA methylation modulation are shortened in Table 6.2.

6.9.2 Quercetin

This flavonoid is rich in various types of dietary products, for example, apples, onions, or wine, and can exert a cancer-preventive effect that mediates cell cycle arrest and apoptosis in cancer cells [141]. Upon treatment with quercetin stimulates the expression of numerous tumor suppressor genes and therefore prevents cancerous growth. For instance, demethylation of the promoter of $p16^{INK4a}$ (tumor suppressor gene) triggers its function and downregulates cancer cell growth in colon cancer [179]. Similarly, quercetin decreased cancer occurrence in the DMBA-treated hamster model, considerably delaying the tumor growth via cell cycle arrest, apoptosis, repressed invasion, and angiogenesis associated with the prevention of DNMT1 and HDAC-1 [181]. The combinatorial effect of quercetin with other polyphenols, including curcumin, shows the potent inhibitory activity of DNMT and upregulated tumor suppressor gene androgen receptor (AR) demethylating AR gene promoter in AR-negative prostate cancer cell lines. Therefore, these may be a promising strategy for treating cancers [182].

Table 6.2 Polyphenols roles in DNA methylation

Sources	Dietary agent	Target genes	DNMT (-)	Type of cancer	References
Coffea	Caffeic acid	RARβ, CDKN2A	(-)	Breast	[160]
	Chlorogenic acid		(-)		
Soy	Biochanin A	Unknown	(-)	Esophageal, Prostate, breast	[161]
	Daidzein	Unknown	(-)		[162]
	Genistein	RARβ, MGMT, CDKN2A, GSTP1, HMGN5, BTG3,TERT	Decrease DNMTs, MBD1, MBD4, MeCP2 expression		[163], [164], [165]
Turmeric	Curcumin	Unknown	(-)	Esophageal, Leukemia	[166]
Acai berry, bilberry, blackberry, cranberry, and raspberry	Cyanidin	BCL-2, STAT3/ VEGF	(-)	Breast, Leukemia	[167], [168], [169]
Berries	Ellagic Acids	Unknown	(-)	Breast	[168]
	Myricetin	Unknown	(-)	Esophageal, Breast	[156], [168]
Grapes, wines, eucalyptus	Resveratrol	Unknown	(-)	Breast, Lung	[170]
Grapes, blueberries	Piceatannol (Resveratrol metabolite)	Unknown	(-)	Breast	[168]
Green tea	Epigalocatechin-3-gallate	RARβ, MGMT, MLH1, CDKN2A, RECK, TERT, RXRα, CDX2, GSTP1, WIF1	(-)	Esophageal, Oral, Prostate, Urinary, Lung, Colon, Leukemia, Lymphoma	[147], [171], [172]
	Epicatechin	Unknown	(-)	Esophageal, Breast	[173], [174]
	Epicatechin-gallate	Unknown	(-)	Esophageal	[173]
	Epigallocatechin	Unknown	(-)	Esophageal	[173]
	Catechin	RARβ	(-)	Breast	[174]
Green tea, apples, blackberries,	Catechin	Unknown	(-)		[175]

(continued)

Table 6.2 (continued)

Sources	Dietary agent	Target genes	DNMT (-)	Type of cancer	References
dark chocolate, and red wine					
Olives	Protocatechuic acid	Unknown	(-)	Breast	[168]
Broccoli	Sulforaphane	CyclinD2	Decrease DNMTs expression	Esophageal, Colon, Prostate	[176], [177]
	Isothiocyanates	GSTP1	Unknown	Esophageal, Prostate	[156], [178]
Citrus	Hesperidin	Unknown	(-)	Esophageal	[156]
	Naringenin		(-)	Esophageal	[156]
	Quercetin	CDKN2A	(-)	Esophageal, Breast, Colon	[141], [179]
Tomatoes	Lycopene	GSTP1, RARβ, HIN-1	(-)	Breast	[180]
Red grapes	Syringic Acid	Unknown	(-)	Breast	[168]
Apples	Phloretin	Unknown	(-)	Breast	[168]
Sinapis (mustard)	Sinapic acid	Unknown	(-)	Breast	[168]
Rosemary	Rosmarinic acid/ Rosmarinic	Unknown	(-)	Breast	[168]
Garcinia	Garcinol	Unknown	(-)	Esophageal	[156]
Poison ivy	Fisetin	Unknown	(-)	Esophageal, Breast	[156]
Parsley, Onion, Orange	Apigenin	Unknown	Decrease DNMTs expression		[156]

Sign abbreviations: (-): Inhibitor

6.9.3 Curcumin

Curcumin, the diferuloylmethane polyphenol from the most common Indian spice turmeric (Curcuma longa), due to which yellow coloration of curry developed, has been accompanied with several health benefits, such as prevention of tumor growth by its capability to regulate intracellular signaling pathways involved in invasion, survival, inflammation, and apoptosis as well as proliferation [183, 184]. Its anticancerous and apoptotic factors are currently stated in numerous cancers [185]. Curcumin could exert an inhibitory effect on DNMT1 by hindering its catalytic activity. Furthermore, it could induce global DNA hypomethylation in a leukemia cell line [186]. Curcumin prevents the expression of Sp1, decreasing the expression of DNMT1 and followed by induction of demethylation of DLC1 to increase DLC1. Upregulation of DLC1 expression inhibits the levels of RhoA-GTP and Cdc-GTP and subsequently impedes cancer cell proliferation. Therefore, studies have shown that curcumin may be a promising strategy for treating breast cancers [187]. FN1 [(3E,5E)-3,5-Bis(pyridin-2-methylene)-tetrahydrothiopyran-4-one], which is similar to curcumin, indicated antitumor activity by enhancing nuclear factor erythroid-2 related factor 2 (Nrf2) gene expression. FN1 induces hypomethylation of Nrf2 gene through decreasing DNMT expression and therefore increases the anti-oxidative defense mechanism of cancer cells. Thus, it may be a promising tool for cancer therapy in prostate cancers [188]. Other demethylating activities of curcumin are summarized in Table 6.2.

6.9.4 Genistein (Isoflavones)

Estrogens are a critical class of hormones, which directly interact with various growth and inflammation-modulating hormones as well as signaling pathways at different pathological stages, in differential manners [189, 190]. Among phytoestrogens, genistein is the most investigated bioactive compound, usually derived from soybeans. Briefly, owing to analogs to structure of estrogens, these phytoestrogens are mimicking as estrogens at target receptors so are popularly known as plant-based estrogens. Being structurally analogs to estrogens, phytoestrogens type of species may interfere in intrinsic activities of estrogens and may modulate various physiological functioning as well [191, 192] and so prevents the DNMT activity; therefore, it emerges as a novel promising natural product for cancer therapy [193]. Genistein works via various mechanisms in several cancer cells. It partially demethylates the promoter of the Glutathione S-Transferase P1 (GSTP1) tumor suppressor gene in MDA-MB-468 MCF-7 breast cancer cells [180]. Genistein prevents cell viability in breast cancer cells and inhibits global DNA methylation factor [165]. The current studies showed that a reduced susceptibility accompanies flavonoids to breast cancer and that microRNAs have a crucial role in breast carcinogenesis [194]. Genistein-induced apoptosis in several cancerous cells is well-known. Genistein induced apoptosis through upregulated estrogen receptor alpha and mediated along with inhibition of DNMT1 expression, followed by prevention of proliferation in human hepatocellular carcinoma (HCC) cell lines. Such a therapeutically substantial alteration of epigenetic mechanism can be a promising tool to develop HCC therapeutics [163]. Genistein also favors estrogen receptor alpha-mediated apoptosis and repressed cell viability [163]. Additional reports on genistein are shown in Table 6.2.

6.9.5 Resveratrol

Resveratrol (trans-3,4,5-trihydroxystilbene) is a polyphenol obtained from peanuts, berries, grapes, and diverse plant sources. Resveratrol has been revealed to show various health-promoting benefits for the hepatic, cardiovascular, coronary, and neurological systems [195, 196]. It has been demonstrated to prevent viral infection, platelet aggregation, inflammation, oxidative stress and hinder the growth of several types of cancer cells [195, 197]. It exerts potent anti-inflammatory activities so may be effective against various types of cancers and neuronal disorders [195, 198]. Resveratrol demonstrates anti-proliferative activity by blocking cell cycle progression in several cancers [199]. Limited studies stated resveratrol-associated hypomethylation and upregulation of tumor suppressor genes such as treatments with resveratrol decrease the expression of DNMT1/3b and upregulate tumor suppressor gene RASSF-1α in breast cancer cells. Therefore, it acts as promising molecule in the antimetastatic growth of tumors [170].

6.9.6 Apigenin

Flavones and isoflavones play a critical role in preventing growth and progression of cancer cells. Meanwhile, these natural products are found in several plants accompanied by decreased cancer growths [200]. Apigenin (4,5,7,-trihydroxyflavone) is characterized as a plant flavonoid (Matricariarecutita L.) and found in chamomile, parsley, wheat sprouts, onions, oranges, and tea [200]. Apigenin a potent cancer chemopreventive agent, defense against skin carcinogenesis [201] and stimulates numerous molecular signaling pathways, including arresting of G-1 phase in the cell cycle with the induction of $p21^{WAF1}$ [202] and arresting of G2/M phase in the cell cycle prevent p34 (cdk2) kinase [203] and Src kinase [204, 205]. Upon treatment with apigenin inhibits DNMT activity in vitro [156]. Nrf2 is an essential transcription factor which modulates a crucial antioxidative stress defense system as well as regulates skin homeostasis [205]. Anti-proliferative activity of Apigenin treatment reported in skin cancer cells, owing to increased hypomethylation as well as reactivation of nuclear factor erythroid 2 [NF-E2]-related factor 2 (Nrf2) gene promoter. Thus, it may be a new promising tool for cancer therapy in skin cancers [205].

6.9.7 Lycopene

Lycopene, a tetra-terpenoid, is a common phytoconstituent of many red-colored fruits and vegetables, such as tomatoes, which plays a crucial role in cell cycle regulation, cell growth, apoptosis, and DNA repairing process, in many cancerous cells, more specifically in breast cancer [206]. In breast cancer cells, promoter of glutathione S-transferase (GSTP1) tumor suppressor gene is reported to be demethylated with increased activity [180]. Other instances of lycopene-associated DNA methylation regulation are presented in Table 6.2.

6.9.8 Sulforaphane

Sulforaphane, an isothiocyanate extracted from kale, broccoli, cabbage, and cauliflower, involves the inhibition of HDAC activities [88, 107]. The limited studies reported regarding the role of sulforaphane on demethylation. Sulforaphane, a natural polyphenol, exhibits anticancer activities in numerous cancers, such as breast cancer, prostate, lymphocyte, as well as colon cancer through induction cell cycle arrest as well as favoring apoptosis [207, 208]. A significant reduction in aggressiveness of CaCo-2 colon cancer cells was reported with sulforaphane treatment, owing to decreased DNMT1 expression and activities [177]. Sulforaphane induces tumor suppressor genes through repression of DNMT3b to mediate promoter hypomethylation in cervical cancer [209].

6.9.9 Rosmarinic Acid

Rosmarinic acid (RA) was derived from Rosmarinus officinalis L. (Lamiaceae). Natural polyphenol exhibits anticancer activities in numerous cancers such as in breast, skin, prostate, ovarian, gastric, and colon cancer through induction apoptosis [210, 211]. Rosmarinic acid, carboxylic acid, and an antioxidant are present in several Lamiaceae herbs, such as peppermint, rosemary, and thyme, which have therapeutic effects against cancer [211]. Rosmarinic acid downregulates the expression of the DNMT1 activity with chemopreventive effects in the MCF7 breast cancer cells [168].

6.10 Polyphenols Induced Histone Modifications

The histone status is controlled by the polyphenols mainly by monitoring HAT/and/HDAC activity. These modifications are briefly discussed here.

6.10.1 EGCG

Histone modifications mediated by EGCG are extensively studied and reported in the literature [13]. The acetylation/deacetylation status of histone is modulated by EGCG by activities (enzymatic) of HAT/and/HDAC. Possibly enzyme inhibition of HAT by treating with EGCG leads to suppressing tumor growth and survival [212]. The inhibition of tumor cell growth mediated by HDAC inhibitor (HDACi) is broadly studied. The work of Pandey et al. effectively demonstrates polyphenol-mediated (obtained from green tea) increase of acetylation (H3 and H4) mainly by inhibition of HDAC activity concurrently follows with drop of HDAC (1, 2, and 3) level of expressions [213]. EGCG, when combined with other chemicals, has demonstrated higher antitumor-inducing activity. For instance, in breast and colorectal tumor cells, the mixture of EGCG and sodium butyrate (fermentation product obtain from dietary fibers) shows enhanced anticancer activity mainly through reducing HDAC and surviving activity [214]. The regulation of histone phosphorylation status by EGCG is effectively demonstrated in vitro and in vivo. The work of Li GX et al. showed that DNA damage and (tumor) programmed cell death is controlled by gamma-H2X (phosphorylated H2A variant X) [215]. The other modifications of histone mediated by EGCG are given in Table 6.3.

6.10.2 Quercetin

The quercetin represents a pigment (extract) obtained from the plants of onions, wine, or apples and possesses an antitumorigenic effect along with an inhibitory effect against HAT. The quercetin downregulates COX-2 (cyclooxygenase-2) mRNA along with an expression of protein mainly by suppressing p300 HAT (histone acetyltransferase) action in endothelial cells of humans [238]. The quercetin contains both HDAC as well as activity (inhibitory) against HAT. For instance, in HL-60 (leukemia cells in humans), upregulates apoptosis mediated by Fas ligand (FasL) mainly by inducing acetylation (of H3 histone) and by reducing the HDAC activity [246].

6.10.3 Curcumin

Curcumin performs several modifying activities ranging from DNA methylation and histone-regulation activity. From the clinical significance point of view, curcumin exhibits an inhibitory role to p300/CBP HAT activity mainly through covalent binding to HAT enzyme [247]. The inhibition of p300 HAT/CB mediated by curcumin suppresses histone acetylation and acetylation of several nonhistone proteins, mainly apoptosis inducers such as p53. Curcumin treatment does not affect PCAF and GCN5 proteasomal degradation while causing significant proteasomal degradation of proteins such as CBP and p300. This indicates the selective and more specific nature of curcumin activity [234]. Apart from the inhibitory activity against CBP and p300, it also shows inhibitory activity against HDAC. The inhibition of HDAC activity by curcumin is established in medulloblastoma cell lines, mainly connected with suppression of HDAC4 protein expression [248]. The curcumin response dramatically varies with the change of its structure and anticancer activity. For instance, selectivity towards E2 synthase-1 (mPGES-1) (which is a microsomal prostaglandin) and HDAC of different curcumin scaffold varies with substitution at various positions, such as 1) C-1, 2) C-8, and/or C-8′ [C5 (isopentenyl, 5–8), 3) C10 (geranyl, 9–12), and 4) C15 (farnesyl, 13, 14)], in contrast to parent molecule [249]. The other histone modifications by Curcumin are being discussed in Table 6.3.

Table 6.3 Polyphenols and histone modifications

Polyphenols	Dietary agent	Target	HDAC (-)	Type of cancer	References
Broccoli	3,3-diindolylmethane	COX-2	↓ HDAC expression	Colon, Breast	[216]
	Sulforaphane	H3/H4 acetylation, RARβ, HBD-2, $p21^{CIP1}$, BAX	(-)	Esophageal, Prostate, Colon, Kidney, Breast	[217], [218]
Broccoli, wasabi	Isothiocyanates	H3/H4 acetylation, $p21^{CIP1}$, GSTP1	(-)		[219], [178]
Ginger	6-methoxy-2E,9E-humuladien-8-one	H3/H4 acetylation, $p21^{CIP1}$, GSTP1	(-)	Prostate, Erythroleukemia, Leukemia, Prostate	[220]
Garlic	Allicin	H4 acetylation	Unknown	Erythroleukemia	[221]
	Allyl mercaptan	H3/H4 acetylation, $p21^{WAF1}$	(-)	Erythroleukemia, Liver, Colon	[222]
	Diallyl disulfide	H3/H4 acetylation, $p21^{WAF1}$	(-)	Erythroleukemia, Leukemia, Liver, Colon, Prostate, Fibroblasts	[223], [224]
	S-allyl mercapto cysteine	H3/H4 acetylation	(-)	Erythroleukemia, Colon	[225]
Anacardic acid	Cashew nuts	H3K9 and H3K14, deacetylation, NF-kB activation	(-)	Leukemia, Plasmodium, Cervix, Embryonic kidney, Breast, Lymphoma, Prostate, Lung, Esophageal, Skin	[226], [227], [228]
Soy	Biochanin A	RARβ	(-)	Esophageal, Prostate	[156], [161]
	Daidzein	Histones acetylation, ARβ	(-)	Esophageal, Prostate	[229]
	Equol	H2A/H2B/H3/H4 acetylation	(-)	Drosophila	[230]
	Genistein	H2A/H2B/H3/H4 acetylation $p21^{CIP1}$, $p16^{INK4a}$, PTEN, CCLD, p53, FOXA3, SIRT1, BTG3, hTERT, RARβ	(-), HAT activator	Esophageal, Prostate, Breast, Renal	[116], [231], [232]
Coffea	Caffeic acid	Unknown	(-)	Cervix, Colon	[160]

	Chlorogenic acid	Unknown	(-)	Cervix	[160]
Curcumin	Turmeric	H3/H4 deacetylation, GATA4, EOMES, GZMB, PRF1	(-), HAT inhibitor	Cervix, HIV, Hepatoma, Leukemia, Prostate, Brain, Lymphoma, Lymphocytes	[233], [234], [166]
Yellow Sweet Clover	Dihydrocoumarin	p53 acetylation	SIRT1 and SIRT2 inhibitor	Lymphoblastoid cell line	[235]
Poison ivy	Fisetin	Unknown	SIRT1 activator	Cervix, Drosophila	[236]
Liquorice	Isoliquiritigenin	Unknown	SIRT1 activator	Cervix, Drosophila	[236]
Grapes, blueberries	Piceatannol	Unknown	SIRT1 activator	Cervix, Drosophila	[236]
Citrus, apple, berries	Quercetin	IP-10, MIP-2, NF-κB/COX-2	SIRT1 activator, HAT inhibitor	Cervix, Drosophila, Small intestine, Breast	[237], [238]
Grapes, wine, eucalyptus	Resveratrol	TNFα, IL-8, RBP	SIRT1 activator	Cervix, Endothelial, Embryonic kidney, Macrophages, Lung, Liver, Cardiomyocytes, Hepatoblastoma	[239], [240], [241]
Green tea	Epicatechin	Unknown	HAT inhibitor	Lymphocytes	[212]
	Epicatechin-gallate	Unknown	HAT inhibitor	Lymphocytes	[212]
	Epigallocatechin	Unknown	HAT inhibitor	Lymphocytes, Colon	[217]
	Epigallocatechin-3-gallate	H3/H4 acetylation, H3K27 trimethylation, NF-κβ, IL-6, BMI-1, EZH2, SUZ12	HAT and HMT inhibitor	Lymphocytes, Colon, Keratinocytes, Prostate	[212], [217]
Black and green tea	Theophylline	Unknown	(-)	Alveolar macrophages, Epithelial cells, Blood, monocytes	[242]
	Polyphenon B	Unknown	↑ HDAC1 expression		[243]

(continued)

Table 6.3 (continued)

Polyphenols	Dietary agent	Target	HDAC (-)	Type of cancer	References
Garcinia	Garcinol	Global gene expression, downregulation	HAT inhibitor	Leukemia, Cervix, Lymphocytes, HIV	[244]
Opium poppy	Sanguinarine	H3K9/H3K4 demethylation, H3/H4 deacetylation	Histone Methylation inhibitor, HAT inhibitor	Liver, Cervix	[225]
Basil	Ursolic Acid	Histone acetylation	(-)	Leukemia	[245]

Sign abbreviations: (-): Inhibitor, (↑): upregulation, (↓): downregulation

6.10.4 Genistein

The genistein represents isoflavone obtained from soy possessing extreme modifying activity against histone when compare with other isoflavones namely daidzein and biochin A. it modulates activity of chromatin by controlling the condition of histone proteins. For instance, a substantial increase of trimethyl-H3K4 and acetyl-H3 (chromatin activators), downregulation of chromatin repressor symbols trimethyl-H3K27 and trimethyl-H3K9 present in agents of $p16^{INK4a}$ and p21WAF1 (examples of cancer-suppressor genes which are present in the cells of breast cancer) are controlled/regulated by the treatment of genistein [116]. Another reported role of genistein in prostate cancer cells is to suppress cancer gene expression mainly by upregulating HAT activity [250]. Genistein treatment also results in SIRT1 inhibition, a histone deacetylase (class III) [251]. Genistein when administered in combinations with other compounds is found to be more effective. For instance, the work of Pong et al. reports combinatory treatment effect of genistein with inhibitor FK228 (of histone deacetylase). The obtained results also report enhanced expression of CAR (coxsackie and adenovirus) receptor thus leading to suppress the growth of tumor in cancer cells of the bladder [252]. Some additional examples of histone modifications mediated by genistein are given in Table 6.3.

6.10.5 Resveratrol

Resveratrol demonstrates antitumor activity by controlling expression pattern of enzymes responsible for histone modifications. Resveratrol upregulates SIRT1 expression (silent information regulator 2 present in yeast, a mammalian ortholog), a type of HDAC molecules (class III) in many cancers [116, 135, 253, 254]. The resveratrol acts by inducing p53 (tumor-suppressing gene) mainly through acetylation thus suppressing MTA1 (represents protein 1 which is metastasis-associated) or NuRD (nucleosome remodeling deacetylation) which is a corepressor (as complex) found in prostate tumor cells [255]. Resveratrol, when administered in the mixture with pterostilbene leads to induction of ERα expression (estrogen receptor-α) through changes in DNA methylation and acetylation status of H3 and H4 (ER-α-negative) thus aggressively multiplying cancer cells of the breast [256].

6.10.6 Apigenin

Apigenin downregulates the activity of HDAC in addition to suppressing DNMT activity. The inhibition of HDAC1/3 followed by stimulation of histone (H3/H4) further leads to $p21^{waf1}$ protein apoptosis and favors BAX in cancer cells of the prostate [257]. Recurrence of Nrf2 (erythroid 2p45 (NF-E2)-related factor 2) gene through hypomethylation (transcription factor which regulates skin homeostasis and antioxidative defense mechanism) following administration with apigenin mainly in epidermal cells of mouse skin [205].

6.10.7 Sulforaphane

Sulforaphane possesses inhibitory activity against HDAC and belongs to Isothiocyanate group [258]. Multiple reports stated HDAC inhibition is mediated by sulforaphane along with an increase in acetylation of histone. In prostate cancer, sulforaphane also induces caspase-dependent apoptosis [258]. While, sulforaphane treatment downregulates HMT (histone methyltransferase) expression, which is leading to induce apoptosis. For instance, treating prostate cancer with sulforaphane leads to SUV39H1 (histone methyltransferase) expression through acetylation and ubiquitination reduces global H3K9me3 (trimethyl-histone H3 lysine 9). By doing this, sulforaphane-treated cells regulate positive signals responsible for apoptosis [259].

6.11 Polyphenols and miRNA Expression

miRNAs represent a group of RNAs (noncoding) that are associated with regulation (epigenetic) of tumor cells and thus are identified as epi-miRNAs [260]. These RNAs are being controlled epigenetically by various dietary nutrients so they may control carcinogenesis progression. The recent study shows an important role played by dietary polyphenols in cancer progression mediated by miRNA. The polyphenols (dietary) are believed to influence several tumor-suppressive or oncogenic miRNAs thus controlling the carcinogenic progression.

6.11.1 EGCG

EGCG plays a critical alter cancer progression through modulation in miRNA expression level, for example, by upregulating miRNA in hepatocellular carcinoma [261]. It also induces miR-16-mediated apoptosis by decreasing BCL2 oncogene expression [261]. In malignant neuroblastoma; EGCG treatment (50μM) mediates apoptosis by inducing upregulated states of various tumor-suppressing miRNAs such as miR-7-1, miR-34a, and miR-99a along with decreased oncogenic miRNAs expression namely, miR-92, miR-93, as well as miR-106b, [262]. In the CL13 cell line and preclinical lung adenocarcinoma, EGCG treatment reduced cell growth via upregulation of miR-210 [263].

6.11.2 Quercetin

Quercetin shows most likely cancer effects against various cancerous cells via inhibition of cell cycle growth in G1/G2, apoptosis as well as repression of angiogenesis through modulation in miRNAs level [238, 264, 265]. It exerts potent antitumor effects by regulating miR-34a in hepatocellular carcinoma cells (HepG2 cell line), primarily via the p53 associated pathway [266]. In lung tissue, relationship of dietary quercetin and lung carcinogenesis was also observed. Quercetin-rich diets favor elevated levels of cancer-suppressor miRNAs (let-7 group) and decreased miRNAs with cancerous growth and proliferation attributes [267]. Quercetin treatment-induced miR-143 upregulation followed by subsequent inhibition of autophagy in AGS and MKN28 cells (variants of human gastric cancer cell lines) through targeting GABARAPL-1 or autophagy-associated protein 8 (ATG-8), supporting autophagosome membrane formation [268]. The combinatorial effect of quercetin with various polyphenols exhibited an increased anticancerous activity. viability, as well as migration of breast cancer cell lines, is reduced with sulforaphane treatment, in combination with both quercetins as well as catechins; owing to trigger of miR-let-7 induction as well as kras inhibition [124]. Similarly, quercetin in combination with resveratrol potently inhibits miR-27a oncogene in colon cancer cells for anticancer activities [269].

6.11.3 Curcumin

Curcumin exerts a potential anticancer effect through modulating miRNA activity. In cancer cells, several findings showed a direct correlation between curcumin and miRNAs levels. Curcumin-treated pancreatic cancer cells downregulated at least 18 miRNAs while upregulation of around 11 miRNAs also reported. Curcumin-induced decreases the expression of tumor suppressor miR-22 through targeting genes SP1 transcription factor (SP1) as well as estrogen receptor 1 (ESR1) [270]. In melanoma cell lines, numerous curcumin analogs play a significant role in activating/inhibiting miRNA expression, followed by arresting cell cycles as well as in apoptosis. In melanoma cells, Diphenyl difluoroketone (EF24), a curcumin analog, decreases EMT, i.e., epithelial-to-mesenchymal-transition; through upregulation of miR-33b. It also concurrently decreases the expression of high mobility group AT-hook 2 (HMGA2) [271].

6.11.4 Genistein

Genistein as well as some other types of soy isoflavones have been revealed to regulate miRNAs activities. Furthermore, genistein by modulating miRNAs also regulates invasiveness, proliferation, as well as metastasis properties of various cancerous cells [272]. Genistein modulates carcinogenesis via several mechanisms in different cells. For instance, invasiveness property of colorectal cancers was reduced owing to genistein-mediated decrease in miR-95 level, accompanied by the reduced expression of Akt as well as SGK1 [273]. Nonetheless, reduction in proliferation of breast cancer cells was observed in genistein treatment, possibly due to augmented miR-23b level [274]. Growth of human uveal melanoma cells, also inhibited by the action of Genistein on oncogenic miR-27a as well as its target gene zinc finger and BTB domain containing 10 (ZBTB10) [275].

6.11.5 Resveratrol

In colon cancer, Resveratrol regulates the functionalities of around 50 different miRNAs [276]. While, in leukemia, Resveratrol treatment favor apoptosis by dose and time-dependent rise in miR-16-1 and miR-15alevel [277]. Combinatorial effect of resveratrol and pterostilbene (stilbenes) in prostate cancer reported higher apoptosis through targeted action on oncomirs, reducing expression of miR-17 and upregulation of TSG PTEN expression [278].

6.11.6 Apigenin

Apigenin-induced miRNA regulation in cancer cells is currently studied. The role of apigenin and overexpression of TSG miR-138 exert a synergistic therapeutic effect against malignant neuroblastoma. Thus, it is emerging in development of nutraceuticals based synergistic anticancer therapeutics [279].

6.11.7 Sulforaphane

The effect of sulforaphane-induced epigenetic regulation is rarely found. Sulforaphane induces EMT inhibition and miR-200c, to decrease the expression of metastatic factor ZEB1 in tumors. Therefore, it works as a therapeutic agent in bladder cancer owing to decreased metastatic growth, and synergistic anticancer properties [280]. For instance, temozolomide in combination with sulforaphane exerts a superior anticancer property in glioblastoma. Here, combinational is believed to exert therapeutic response via Wnt/β-catenin pathway-mediated miR-21 downstream [281]. Table 6.4 discussed polyphenol's roles with miRNA expression.

6.12 Polyphenols and lncRNA

The recent study shows an important role played by dietary polyphenols in cancer progression mediated by miRNA. The polyphenols (dietary) are believed to influence several tumor-suppressive or oncogenic miRNAs thus controlling the carcinogenic progression. The lncRNA regulation and expression by dietary phytochemicals are yet to be explored fully. However, still, some reports support this notion and are explained in this section.

6.12.1 Curcumin

The functional variation of lncRNAs mediated through curcumin is studied recently. Yoshida et al. showed an underlying mechanism of enhanced sensitivity of PDAC cells (pancreatic ductal adenocarcinoma) mediated by curcumin in chemotherapy. In chemoresistant PDAC cells, Zeste Homolog-2 Enhancer (EZH2) subunit of PRC2 (Polycomb Repressive Complex 2) is believed to serve backbone functions. However, Curcumin is believed to act on this histone methyltransferase followed by exerting a controlling effect on lncRNA PVT1, a critical oncogene that modulates EZH2 jobs. This fact establishes a correlation among the PDAC cells (for increased sensitivity) against chemoresistance and concurrently downregulates the PRC2-PVT1-c-Myc axis [289]. The curcumin also suppresses malignancy by HOTAIR (HOX transcript antisense RNA) downregulation, a main oncogenic aspect in metastasis of breast cancer [290].

6.12.2 Genistein

The treatment with genistein modulates the carcinogenesis process mediated by lncRNA. Chiyomaru et al. verified the downregulation of oncogene HOTAIR (HOX transcript antisense RNA) in tumor cells of the prostate when treated with genistein. The same study also supports miR-34a (tumor suppressor) activation on genistein treatment, wherein it also downregulates HOTAIR [122]. The downregulation of HOTAIR and tumor suppression is studied mainly in different tumors, including breast cancer [291].

6.12.3 Resveratrol

The inhibition of cell growth targeting different lncRNAs is reported by resveratrol. For instance, the expression of AK001796 (lncRNA) is downregulated with resveratrol treatment, a crucial factor in lung cancer proliferation [292]. Resveratrol treatment suppressed prolonging metastasis (noncoding) related to RNAMALAT1 (lung adenocarcinoma transcript 1). The targeted lncRNA is associated with the oncogenic pathway (Wnt/β-catenin), serving an essential part in colorectal cancer metastasis [293].

Table 6.4 Polyphenols and miRNA Expression

Source	Target genes	miRNA	Biological Function	Type of cancer	References
EGCG	BCL2; c-MET	Upregulates miR16 and miR-1	Apoptosis	Hepatocellular, Osteosarcoma	[261], [282]
Quercetin	EGFR, Cleaved caspase 3	Upregulates miR-146a and miR-145	Proliferation, Apoptosis	Breast, Ovarian	[266], [283]
Curcumin	PI3/AKT, CDKN1A, SET8	Upregulates miR-192-5p and miR-7, while decreases the expression of miR208	Proliferation, Apoptosis, Invasion	Lungs, Pancreas	[284], [130]
Genistein	P27, PTEN, NF-κB, Wnt	Upregulates miR-29b while decreases the expression of miR-155 miR-1260b	Proliferation, Invasion, Metastasis Proliferation	Breast, Myeloma, Renal	[126], [285], [286]
Resveratrol	IL-6/STAT3, pAKT/BCL2	Upregulates miR-34c while downregulates miR-21	Apoptosis	Colorectal, Bladder	[287], [288]
Apigenin	Unknown	Upregulates miR-138	Apoptosis	Neuroblastoma	[279]
Sulforaphane	Kras	Upregulates miR-let-7	Malignancy	Pancreas	[124]

6.12.4 Sulforaphane

The data availability related to lncRNA regulation mediated by sulforaphane is scarce. At transcriptional level, sulforaphane mediated downregulation of LINC01116. Thus, lncRNA performs the role of a promoting factor and favors proliferating. The targeted lncRNA is associated with the oncogenic pathway cells [294]. Hence, some more comprehensive analysis to understand sulforaphane effects on different cancer-related lncRNA activity is a requirement of current time [107].

6.13 Summary and Conclusion

The use of dietary polyphenols is known to be traditional and widespread across the world. Several pieces of evidence support the benefits of dietary polyphenols on multiple health conditions, including cancer. This chapter discusses the perspective of chemoprevention-regulated by dietary agents, with special consideration of epigenetic properties, histone modification, alteration in DNA methylation, and changes in miRNAs expressions, etc. The epigenetic network regulation mediated by polyphenols is reported in several in vitro models. However, there is an evident lack of in vivo data supporting such findings. Due to insufficient clinical and preclinical data on epigenetic changes by dietary polyphenols, the in vitro evidence should be carefully extrapolated and interpreted. The next step should be to estimate the optimum doses of these nutraceuticals (obtained from the diet) to manage cancer related events.

Additionally, clinical testing is needed to further study the safety/toxicity and molecular mechanism of different combinations of polyphenols, to find out chemopreventive effect. The good news is that scientists have started to discover the mechanisms (at a molecular level) supporting the "goodness" of diet-related factors that existed for centuries. Presently, several polyphenols (of dietary sources) are categorized from an "epigenomics" viewpoint. This echoes our trust and interest in the notion of natural and safe mediators for tumor chemoprevention. We believe that potential of polyphenolic compounds will become an integral part of cancer chemoprevention soon.

The experimental evidence describes the importance of nutrients in treating tumors and/or chemoprevention. These phytochemicals have also shown better potential in fighting cancer progression (multistep) either alone or in combination. A more comprehensive study is anticipated to assess the genome-wide consequence of several such phytoconstituents. A safer dose for human use will undoubtedly require further clinical studies.

Acknowledgment Authors express their sincere thanks to Dr. Salman Hosawi, Head-Department of Biochemistry and Prof. Abdulrahman L. Al Maliki, (Dean) Faculty of Science and Dr. Anas

Hamed Al Muhammadi, Vice dean of Graduate Studies for International Students, King Abdulaziz University, Jeddah 21589, Saudi Arabia.

Competing Interests The authors declare that they have no competing interests.

References

1. Alhosin M, Sharif T, Mousli M, Etienne-Selloum N, Fuhrmann G, Schini-Kerth VB, et al. Down-regulation of UHRF1, associated with re-expression of tumor suppressor genes, is a common feature of natural compounds exhibiting anti-cancer properties [Internet]. J Exp Clin Cancer Res. 2011;30:41. Available from: https://pubmed.ncbi.nlm.nih.gov/21496237/
2. Seyfried TN, Huysentruyt LC. On the origin of cancer metastasis [Internet]. Crit Rev Oncog. 2021;18((1–2)):43–73. Available from: https://pubmed.ncbi.nlm.nih.gov/23237552/
3. Pottoo FH, Barkat MA, Ansari MA, Javed MN, Jamal QM, Kamal MA. Nanotechnological based miRNA intervention in the therapeutic management of neuroblastoma. In: Seminars in cancer biology, vol. 69. Cambridge, MA: Academic Press; 2021. p. 100–8.
4. Henning SM, Wang P, Carpenter CL, Heber D. Epigenetic effects of green tea polyphenols in cancer. Epigenomics. 2013;5(6):729–41.
5. Wu JC, Lai CS, Lee PS, Ho CT, Liou WS, Wang YJ, et al. Anti-cancer efficacy of dietary polyphenols is mediated through epigenetic modifications. Curr Opin Food Sci. 2016;8:1–7.
6. Bray F, Ferlay J, Soerjomataram I, Siegel RL, Torre LA, Jemal A. Global cancer statistics 2018: GLOBOCAN estimates of incidence and mortality worldwide for 36 cancers in 185 countries [Internet]. CA Cancer J Clin. 2018;68(6):394–424. Available from: https://pubmed.ncbi.nlm.nih.gov/30207593/
7. Lin HJL, Zuo T, Chao JR, Peng Z, Asamoto LK, Yamashita SS, et al. Seed in soil, with an epigenetic view. Biochim Biophys Acta. 2009;1790:920–4.
8. Aggarwal R, Jha M, Shrivastava A, Jha AK. Natural compounds: role in reversal of epigenetic changes [Internet]. Biochem. 2015;80(8):972–89. Available from: https://pubmed.ncbi.nlm.nih.gov/26547065/
9. Audia JE, Campbell RM. Histone modifications and cancer [Internet]. Cold Spring Harb Perspect Biol. 2016;8(4):a019521. Available from: https://pubmed.ncbi.nlm.nih.gov/27037415/
10. Lin S, Gregory RI. MicroRNA biogenesis pathways in cancer [Internet]. Nat Rev Cancer. 2015;15(6):321–33. Available from: https://pubmed.ncbi.nlm.nih.gov/25998712/
11. Sager R. Expression genetics in cancer: shifting the focus from DNA to RNA [Internet]. Proc Natl Acad Sci U S A. 1997;94(3):952–5. Available from: https://pubmed.ncbi.nlm.nih.gov/9023363/
12. Ducasse M, Brown MA. Epigenetic aberrations and cancer [Internet]. Mol Cancer. 2006;5:60. Available from: https://pubmed.ncbi.nlm.nih.gov/17092350/
13. Link A, Balaguer F, Goel A. Cancer chemoprevention by dietary polyphenols: Promising role for epigenetics [Internet]. Biochem Pharmacol. 2010;80(12):1771–92. Available from: /pmc/articles/PMC2974019/?report=abstract
14. Pottoo FH, Javed MN, Rahman JU, Abu-Izneid T, Khan FA. Targeted delivery of miRNA based therapeuticals in the clinical management of Glioblastoma Multiforme. In: Seminars in cancer biology, vol. 69. Cambridge, MA: Academic Press; 2021. p. 391–8.
15. Abu-Izneid T, AlHajri N, Ibrahim AM, Javed MN, Salem KM, Pottoo FH, Kamal MA. Micro-RNAs in the regulation of immune response against SARS COV-2 and other viral infections. J Adv Res. 2020; https://doi.org/10.1016/j.jare.2020.11.013.
16. Bravo L. Polyphenols: chemistry, dietary sources, metabolism, and nutritional significance. Nutr Rev [Internet]. 2009;56(11):317–33. Available from: https://academic.oup.com/nutritionreviews/article-lookup/doi/10.1111/j.1753-4887.1998.tb01670.x

17. Yi J, Li S, Wang C, Cao N, Qu H, Cheng C, et al. Potential applications of polyphenols on main ncRNAs regulations as novel therapeutic strategy for cancer. Biomed Pharmacother. 2019;113:108703.
18. Arora I, Sharma M, Tollefsbol TO. Combinatorial epigenetics impact of polyphenols and phytochemicals in cancer prevention and therapy [Internet]. Int J Mol Sci. 2019;20(18):4567. Available from: /pmc/articles/PMC6769666/?report=abstract
19. Javed MN, Ashraf GM, Barreto GE, Naim M. Current trends for rationalizing brain targeting nanoparticles in neurological disorders (Part-I). Curr Drug Metab. 2020;21(9):648.
20. Scalbert A, Manach C, Morand C, Rémésy C, Jiménez L. Dietary polyphenols and the prevention of diseases [Internet]. Crit Rev Food Sci Nutr. 2005;45(4):287–306. Available from: https://pubmed.ncbi.nlm.nih.gov/16047496/
21. Fantini M, Benvenuto M, Masuelli L, Frajese GV, Tresoldi I, Modesti A, et al. In vitro and in vivo antitumoral effects of combinations of polyphenols, or polyphenols and anticancer drugs: Perspectives on cancer treatment [Internet]. Int J Mol Sci. 2015;16(5):9236–82. Available from: https://pubmed.ncbi.nlm.nih.gov/25918934/
22. Tsao R. Chemistry and biochemistry of dietary polyphenols [Internet]. Nutrients. 2010;2(12):1231–46. Available from: https://pubmed.ncbi.nlm.nih.gov/22254006/
23. Ramos S. Cancer chemoprevention and chemotherapy: dietary polyphenols and signalling pathways [Internet]. Mol Nutr Food Res. 2008;7(32):507–26. Available from: https://pubmed.ncbi.nlm.nih.gov/18435439/
24. Pottoo FH, Abu-Izneid T, Sudqi AM, Javed MN, AlHajri N, Hamrouni AM. Immune system response during viral infections: immunomodulators, cytokine storm (CS) and immunotherapeutics in COVID-19. Saudi Pharm J. 2021; https://doi.org/10.1016/j.jsps.2020.12.018.
25. Mohanta BC, Javed MN, Hasnain MS, Nayak AK. Polyelectrolyte complexes of alginate for controlling drug release. In: Alginates in drug delivery. Cambridge, MA: Academic Press; 2020. p. 297–321.
26. Raman S, Mahmood S, Hilles AR, Javed MN, Azmana M, Saeed Al-Japairai KA. Polymeric nanoparticles for brain drug delivery a review. Curr Drug Metab. 2020;3(2):133–49.
27. Alam MS, Javed MN, Pottoo FH, Waziri A, Almalki FA, Hasnain MS, Garg A, Saifullah MK. QbD approached comparison of reaction mechanism in microwave synthesized gold nanoparticles and their superior catalytic role against hazardous nirto-dye. Appl Organomet Chem. 2019;33(9):e5071.
28. Hasnain MS, Javed MN, Alam MS, Rishishwar P, Rishishwar S, Ali S, Nayak AK, Beg S. Purple heart plant leaves extract-mediated silver nanoparticle synthesis: optimization by Box-Behnken design. Mater Sci Eng C. 2019;99:1105–14.
29. Pottoo FH, Sharma S, Javed MN, Barkat MA, Harshita, Alam MS, Naim MJ, Alam O, Ansari MA, Barreto GE, Ashraf GM. Lipid-based nanoformulations in the treatment of neurological disorders. Drug Metab Rev. 2020;52(1):185–204.
30. Javed MN, Kohli K, Amin S. Risk assessment integrated QbD approach for development of optimized bicontinuous mucoadhesive limicubes for oral delivery of rosuvastatin. AAPS Pharm Sci Tech. 2018;3:1377–91.
31. Javed MN, Pottoo FH, Shamim A, Hasnain MS, Alam MS. Design of experiments for the development of nanoparticles, nanomaterials, and nanocomposites. In: Design of experiments for pharmaceutical product development. Singapore: Springer; 2021. p. 151–69.
32. Alam MS, Garg A, Pottoo FH, Saifullah MK, Tareq AI, Manzoor O, Mohsin M, Javed MN. Gum ghatti mediated, one pot green synthesis of optimized gold nanoparticles: investigation of process-variables impact using Box-Behnken based statistical design. Int J Biol Macromol. 2017;104:758–67.
33. Javed MN, Alam MS, Waziri A, Pottoo FH, Yadav AK, Hasnain MS, Almalki FA. QbD applications for the development of nanopharmaceutical products. In: Pharmaceutical quality by design. Cambridge, MA: Academic Press; 2019. p. 229–53.

34. Van den Berghe W. Epigenetic impact of dietary polyphenols in cancer chemoprevention: lifelong remodeling of our epigenomes. Pharmacol Res [Internet]. 2012;65(6):565–76. Available from: https://pubmed.ncbi.nlm.nih.gov/22465217/
35. Kumar A, Walia H, Pottoo FH, Javed MN. Insights of nanophytomedicines as a combinatorial therapy in disease diagnosis and treatment. In: Nanophytomedicine. Singapore: Springer; 2020. p. 113–32.
36. Li X, Oprea-Ilies GM, Krishnamurti U. New developments in breast cancer and their impact on daily practice in pathology. Arch Pathol Lab Med. 2017;141(4):490–8.
37. Kawada M, Atsumi S, Wada SI, Sakamoto S. Novel approaches for identification of anti-tumor drugs and new bioactive compounds [Internet]. J Antibiot. 2018:39–44. https://doi.org/10.1038/ja.2017.97. Available from: www.nature.com/ja
38. Ruiz-Torres V, Encinar J, Herranz-López M, Pérez-Sánchez A, Galiano V, Barrajón-Catalán E, et al. An updated review on marine anticancer compounds: the use of virtual screening for the discovery of small-molecule cancer drugs [Internet]. Molecules. 2017;22 (7):1037. Available from: http://www.mdpi.com/1420-3049/22/7/1037
39. Mishra S, Sharma S, Javed MN, Pottoo FH, Barkat MA, Alam MS, Amir M, Sarafroz M. Bioinspired nanocomposites: applications in disease diagnosis and treatment. Pharm Nanotechnol. 2019;7(3):206–19.
40. Sharma S, Javed MN, Pottoo FH, Rabbani SA, Barkat M, Sarafroz M, Amir M. Bioresponse inspired nanomaterials for targeted drug and gene delivery. Pharm Nanotechnol. 2019;7 (3):220–33.
41. Chun SW, Cha BY, Ko KS, Ryu AJ, Kim YJ, Kim SJ. PO227 gender differences of diabetic peripheral neuropathy in Korea [Internet]. Diabetes Res Clin Pract. 2014;106:S164–5.
42. Jagtap S, Meganathan K, Wagh V, Winkler J, Hescheler J, Sachinidis A. Chemoprotective mechanism of the natural compounds, epigallocatechin-3-O-gallate, quercetin and curcumin against cancer and cardiovascular diseases [Internet]. Curr Med Chem. 2009;16(12):1451–62. Available from: http://www.eurekaselect.com/openurl/content.php?genre=article&issn=0929-8673&volume=16&issue=12&spage=1451
43. Pan MH, Lai CS, Tsai ML, Ho CT. Chemoprevention of nonalcoholic fatty liver disease by dietary natural compounds [Internet]. Mol Nutr Food Res. 2014;58(1):147–71. Available from: https://pubmed.ncbi.nlm.nih.gov/24302567/
44. Chen S. Natural products triggering biological targets- a review of the anti-inflammatory phytochemicals targeting the arachidonic acid pathway in allergy asthma and rheumatoid arthritis [Internet]. Curr Drug Targets. 2012;12(3):288–301. Available from: https://pubmed.ncbi.nlm.nih.gov/20955151/
45. Albarracin SL, Stab B, Casas Z, Sutachan JJ, Samudio I, Gonzalez J, et al. Effects of natural antioxidants in neurodegenerative disease [Internet]. Nutr Neurosci. 2012;15(1):1–9. Available from: https://www.tandfonline.com/doi/abs/10.1179/1476830511Y.0000000028
46. Javed MN, Dahiya ES, Ibrahim AM, Alam MS, Khan FA, Pottoo FH. Recent advancement in clinical application of nanotechnological approached targeted delivery of herbal drugs. In: Nanophytomedicine. Singapore: Springer; 2020. p. 151–72.
47. An J, Yang H, Zhang Q, Liu C, Zhao J, Zhang L, et al. Natural products for treatment of osteoporosis: the effects and mechanisms on promoting osteoblast-mediated bone formation [Internet]. Life Sci. 2016;147:46–58. Available from: https://pubmed.ncbi.nlm.nih.gov/26796578/
48. Huang WY, Cai YZ, Zhang Y. Natural phenolic compounds from medicinal herbs and dietary plants: potential use for cancer prevention [Internet]. Nutr Cancer. 2010;62(1):1–20. Available from: https://pubmed.ncbi.nlm.nih.gov/20043255/
49. Grienke U, Schmidtke M, Von Grafenstein S, Kirchmair J, Liedl KR, Rollinger JM. Influenza neuraminidase: a druggable target for natural products [Internet]. Nat Prod Rep. 2012;29 (1):11–36.
50. Carocho M, Ferreira ICFR. A review on antioxidants, prooxidants and related controversy: natural and synthetic compounds, screening and analysis methodologies and future

perspectives [Internet]. Food Chem Toxicol. 2013;51:15–25. Available from: https://pubmed.ncbi.nlm.nih.gov/23017782/
51. Maqbool F, Mostafalou S, Bahadar H, Abdollahi M. Review of endocrine disorders associated with environmental toxicants and possible involved mechanisms [Internet]. Life Sci; 2016;145:265–273. Available from: https://pubmed.ncbi.nlm.nih.gov/26497928/
52. Tozsér J, Benko S. Natural compounds as regulators of NLRP3 inflammasome-mediated IL-1 β production. Mediators Inflamm. 2016;38(3):912–8.
53. Souza AB, De Souza MGM, Moreira MA, Moreira MR, Furtado NAJC, Martins CHG, et al. Antimicrobial evaluation of diterpenes from copaifera langsdorffii oleoresin against periodontal anaerobic bacteria [Internet]. Molecules. 2011;16(11):9611–9. Available from: https://pubmed.ncbi.nlm.nih.gov/22101836/
54. Nileeka Balasuriya BW, Vasantha Rupasinghe HP. Plant flavonoids as angiotensin converting enzyme inhibitors in regulation of hypertension [Internet]. Funct Foods Heal Dis. 2011;1(5):172–88. Available from: https://ffhdj.com/index.php/ffhd/article/view/132/270
55. Działo M, Mierziak J, Korzun U, Preisner M, Szopa J, Kulma A. The potential of plant phenolics in prevention and therapy of skin disorders [Internet]. Int J Mol Sci. 2016;17:60. Available from: https://pubmed.ncbi.nlm.nih.gov/26901191/
56. Jakobek L. Interactions of polyphenols with carbohydrates, lipids and proteins [Internet]. Food Chem. 2015;175:556–67. Available from: https://pubmed.ncbi.nlm.nih.gov/25577120/
57. Deaton AM, Bird A. CpG islands and the regulation of transcription. Genes Dev. 2011;25(10):1010–22.
58. Takai D, Jones PA. Comprehensive analysis of CpG islands in human chromosomes 21 and 22. Proc Natl Acad Sci U S A. 2002;99(6):3740–5.
59. Wang Y, Feung FCC. An evaluation of new criteria for CpG islands in the human genome as gene markers [Internet]. Bioinformatics. 2021;20(7):1170–7. Available from: http://www.ncbi.nlm.nih.gov
60. Jang HS, Shin WJ, Lee JE, Do JT. CpG and non-CpG methylation in epigenetic gene regulation and brain function. Genes (Basel). 2017;8(6):148.
61. Feinberg AP, Ohlsson R, Henikoff S. The epigenetic progenitor origin of human cancer [Internet]. Nat Rev Genet. 2006;7(1):21–33. Available from: www.nature.com/reviews/genetics
62. Szarc vel Szic K, Ndlovu MN, Haegeman G, Vanden Berghe W. Nature or nurture: let food be your epigenetic medicine in chronic inflammatory disorders. Biochem Pharmacol. 2010;80(12):1816–32.
63. Law JA, Jacobsen SE. Establishing, maintaining and modifying DNA methylation patterns in plants and animals [Internet]. Nat Rev Genet. 2010;11(3):204–20. Available from: www.nature.com/reviews/genetics
64. Kulis M, Esteller M. DNA methylation and cancer [Internet]. Adv Genet. 2021;70:27–56. Available from: https://pubmed.ncbi.nlm.nih.gov/20920744/
65. Drexler HG. Review of alterations of the cyclin-dependent kinase inhibitor INK4 family genes p15, p16, p18 and p19 in human leukemia-lymphoma cells. Leukemia. 1998;12:845–59.
66. Jacinto FV, Esteller M. MGMT hypermethylation: a prognostic foe, a predictive friend. DNA Repair (Amst). 2007;6(8):1155–60.
67. Ehrlich M. DNA hypomethylation in cancer cells. Epigenomics. 2009;1:59–177.
68. Gama-sosa MA, Slagel VA, Trewyn RW, Oxenhandler R, Kuo KC, Gehrke CW, et al. The 5-methylcytosine content of DNA from human tumors [Internet]. Nucleic Acids Res. 1983;11:6883–94. Available from: https://academic.oup.com/nar/article/11/19/6883/1067105
69. De Capoa A, Musolino A, Della Rosa S, Caiafa P, Mariani L, Del Nonno F, et al. DNA demethylation is directly related to tumour progression: evidence in normal, pre-malignant and malignant cells from uterine cervix samples. Oncol Rep. 2003;10(3):545–9. Available from: http://www.spandidos-publications.com/10.3892/or.10.3.545/abstract
70. Klutstein M, Nejman D, Greenfield R, Cedar H. DNA methylation in cancer and aging. Cancer Res. 2016;76(12):3446–50.

71. Costa FF, Paixão VA, Cavalher FP, Ribeiro KB, Cunha IW, Rinck JAD, et al. SATR-1 hypomethylation is a common and early event in breast cancer. Cancer Genet Cytogenet. 2006;165(2):135–43.
72. Widschwendter M, Jiang G, Woods C, Mü Ller HM, Fiegl H, Goebel G, et al. DNA hypomethylation and ovarian cancer biology [Internet]. Cancer Res. 2004;64(13):4472–80. Available from: http://cancerres.aacrjournals.org
73. Ribeiro AS, Albergaria A, Sousa B, Correia AL, Bracke M, Seruca R, et al. Extracellular cleavage and shedding of P-cadherin: a mechanism underlying the invasive behaviour of breast cancer cells [Internet]. Oncogene. 2010;29(3):392–402. Available from: www.nature.com/onc
74. Esteller M. Epigenetics in cancer. N Engl J Med. 2008;358(11):1148–59.
75. Serman L, Martic TN, Serman A, Vranic S. Epigenetic alterations of the Wnt signaling pathway in cancer: a mini review. Basic Med Sci. 2014;14(4):191–4.
76. Jones PA, Issa JPJ, Baylin S. Targeting the cancer epigenome for therapy [Internet]. Nat Rev Genet. 2016;17(10):630–41. Available from: www.nature.com/nrg
77. Luger K, Mäder AW, Richmond RK, Sargent DF, Richmond TJ. Crystal structure of the nucleosome core particle at 2.8 Å resolution [Internet]. Nature. 1997;389(6648):251–60. Available from: https://pubmed.ncbi.nlm.nih.gov/9305837/
78. Cutter AR, Hayes JJ. A brief review of nucleosome structure [Internet]. FEBS Lett. 2015;589:2914–22. Available from: https://pubmed.ncbi.nlm.nih.gov/25980611/
79. Hergeth SP, Schneider R. The H1 linker histones: multifunctional proteins beyond the nucleosomal core particle. EMBO Rep. 2015;16(11):1439–53. Available from: https://pubmed.ncbi.nlm.nih.gov/26474902/
80. Füllgrabe J, Kavanagh E, Joseph B. Histone onco-modifications [Internet]. Oncogene. 2011;30(31):3391–403. Available from: https://pubmed.ncbi.nlm.nih.gov/21516126/
81. Kouzarides T. Chromatin modifications and their function [Internet]. Cell. 2007;128 (4):693–705. Available from: https://pubmed.ncbi.nlm.nih.gov/17320507/
82. Taby R, Issa J-PJ. Cancer epigenetics [Internet]. CA Cancer J Clin. 2010;60(6):376–92. Available from: http://doi.wiley.com/10.3322/caac.20085
83. Yang XJ. The diverse superfamily of lysine acetyltransferases and their roles in leukemia and other diseases [Internet]. Nucleic Acids Res. 2004;32(3):959–76. Available from: https://pubmed.ncbi.nlm.nih.gov/14960713/
84. Yang XJ, Seto E. HATs and HDACs: From structure, function and regulation to novel strategies for therapy and prevention [Internet]. Oncogene. 2007;26(37):5310–8. Available from: https://pubmed.ncbi.nlm.nih.gov/17694074/
85. Albert M, Helin K. Histone methyltransferases in cancer [Internet]. Semin Cell Dev Biol. 2010;21:209–20. Available from: https://pubmed.ncbi.nlm.nih.gov/19892027/
86. Liu L, Kimball S, Liu H, Holowatyj A, Yang ZQ. Genetic alterations of histone lysine methyltransferases and their significance in breast cancer [Internet]. Oncotarget. 2015;6 (4):2466–82. Available from: https://pubmed.ncbi.nlm.nih.gov/25537518/
87. Sasidharan Nair V, El Salhat H, Taha RZ, John A, Ali BR, Elkord E. DNA methylation and repressive H3K9 and H3K27 trimethylation in the promoter regions of PD-1, CTLA-4, TIM-3, LAG-3, TIGIT, and PD-L1 genes in human primary breast cancer [Internet]. Clin Epigenetics 2018;10(1):40–53. Available from: https://pubmed.ncbi.nlm.nih.gov/29983831/
88. Okonkwo A, Mitra J, Johnson GS, Li L, Dashwood WM, Hegde ML, et al. Heterocyclic analogs of sulforaphane trigger DNA damage and impede DNA repair in colon cancer cells: interplay of HATs and HDACs. Mol Nutr Food Res. 2018;62(18):e1800228. Available from: https://pubmed.ncbi.nlm.nih.gov/29924908/
89. Lu J, Getz G, Miska EA, Alvarez-Saavedra E, Lamb J, Peck D, et al. MicroRNA expression profiles classify human cancers. Nature. 2015;435(7043):834–8. Available from: https://pubmed.ncbi.nlm.nih.gov/15944708/

90. Iorio MV, Piovan C, Croce CM. Interplay between microRNAs and the epigenetic machinery: an intricate network [Internet]. Biochim Biophys Acta Gene Regul Mech. 2010;1799 (10–12):694–701. Available from: https://pubmed.ncbi.nlm.nih.gov/20493980/
91. Lopez-Serra P, Esteller M. DNA methylation-associated silencing of tumor-suppressor microRNAs in cancer [Internet]. Oncogene. 2012;31(13):1609–22. Available from: https://pubmed.ncbi.nlm.nih.gov/21860412/
92. Calin GA, Ferracin M, Cimmino A, Di Leva G, Shimizu M, Wojcik SE, et al. A MicroRNA signature associated with prognosis and progression in chronic lymphocytic leukemia [Internet]. N Engl J Med. 2005;353(17):1793–801. Available from: https://pubmed.ncbi.nlm.nih.gov/16251535/
93. Chang TC, Wentzel EA, Kent OA, Ramachandran K, Mullendore M, Lee KH, et al. Transactivation of miR-34a by p53 broadly influences gene expression and promotes apoptosis [Internet]. Mol Cell. 2007;26(5):745–52. Available from: https://pubmed.ncbi.nlm.nih.gov/17540599/
94. Raver-Shapira N, Marciano E, Meiri E, Spector Y, Rosenfeld N, Moskovits N, et al. Transcriptional activation of miR-34a contributes to p53-mediated apoptosis [Internet]. Mol Cell. 2007;26(5):731–43. Available from: https://pubmed.ncbi.nlm.nih.gov/17540598/
95. Lehmann U, Hasemeier B, Christgen M, Müller M, Römermann D, Länger F, et al. Epigenetic inactivation of microRNA gene hsa-mir-9-1 in human breast cancer [Internet]. J Pathol. 2008;214(1):17–24. Available from: https://pubmed.ncbi.nlm.nih.gov/17948228/
96. Lujambio A, Calin GA, Villanueva A, Ropero S, Sánchez-Céspedes M, Blanco D, et al. A microRNA DNA methylation signature for human cancer metastasis [Internet]. Proc Natl Acad Sci U S A. 2008;105(36):13556–61. Available from: https://pubmed.ncbi.nlm.nih.gov/18768788/
97. Weber B, Stresemann C, Brueckner B, Lyko F. Methylation of human MicroRNA genes in normal and neoplastic cells [Internet]. Cell Cycle. 2007;6(9):1001–5. Available from: https://pubmed.ncbi.nlm.nih.gov/17457051/
98. Cao J. The functional role of long non-coding RNAs and epigenetics [Internet]. Biol Proced Online. 2014;1–13. Available from: http://www.biologicalproceduresonline.com/content/16/1/11
99. Grote P, Wittler L, Hendrix D, Koch F, Währisch S, Beisaw A, et al. The tissue-specific lncRNA fendrr is an essential regulator of heart and body wall development in the mouse. Dev Cell. 2013;24(2):206–14.
100. Arab K, Park YJ, Lindroth AM, Schäfer A, Oakes C, Weichenhan D, et al. Long noncoding RNA TARID directs demethylation and activation of the tumor suppressor TCF21 via GADD45A. Mol Cell. 2014;55(4):604–14.
101. Fang Y, Fullwood MJ. Roles, functions, and mechanisms of long non-coding RNAs in cancer. Genomics Proteomics Bioinformatics. 2016;14(1):42–54.
102. Huarte M. The emerging role of lncRNAs in cancer [Internet]. Nat Med. 2015;21 (11):1253–61. Available from: https://www.nature.com/articles/nm.3981
103. Qi P, Du X. The long non-coding RNAs, a new cancer diagnostic and therapeutic gold mine [Internet]. Mod Pathol. 2013;26(2):155–65. Available from: www.modernpathology.org
104. Kondo Y, Shinjo K, Katsushima K. Long non-coding <scp>RNA</scp> s as an epigenetic regulator in human cancers [Internet]. Cancer Sci. 2017;108(10):1927–33. https://doi.org/10.1111/cas.13342.
105. Peng WX, Koirala P, Mo YY. LncRNA-mediated regulation of cell signaling in cancer [Internet]. Oncogene. 2017;36(41):5661–7. Available from: http://www.noncode.org
106. Zhang R, Guo Y, Ma Z, Ma G, Xue Q, Li F, et al. Long non-coding RNA PTENP1 functions as a ceRNA to modulate PTEN level by decoying miR-106b and miR-93 in gastric cancer [Internet]. Oncotarget. 2017;8(16):26079–89. Available from: /pmc/articles/PMC5432239/?report=abstract
107. Khan MI, Rath S, Adhami VM, Mukhtar H. Targeting epigenome with dietary nutrients in cancer: current advances and future challenges. Pharmacol Res. 2018;129:375–87.

108. Arablou T, Kolahdouz-Mohammadi R. Curcumin and endometriosis: review on potential roles and molecular mechanisms [Internet]. Biomed Pharmacother. 2018;97:91–7. Available from: https://pubmed.ncbi.nlm.nih.gov/29080464/
109. Danciu C, Vlaia L, Fetea F, Hancianu M, Coricovac DE, Ciurlea SA, et al. Evaluation of phenolic profile, antioxidant and anticancer potential of two main representants of Zingiberaceae family against B164A5 murine melanoma cells [Internet]. Biol Res. 2015;48 (1):1. Available from: http://www.biolres.com/content/48/1/1
110. Park W, Ruhul Amin ARM, Chen ZG, Shin DM. New perspectives of curcumin in cancer prevention [Internet]. Cancer Prev Res. 2013;6(5):387–400. Available from: https://pubmed.ncbi.nlm.nih.gov/23466484/
111. Guo H, Xu Y, Fu Q. RETRACTED ARTICLE: curcumin inhibits growth of prostate carcinoma via miR-208-mediated CDKN1A activation. Tumor Biol. 2015;36(11):8511–7.
112. Sharma V, Jha AK, Kumar A, Bhatnagar A, Narayan G, Kaur J. Curcumin-mediated reversal of p15 gene promoter methylation: implication in anti-neoplastic action against acute lymphoid leukaemia cell line. Folia Biol (Czech Republic). 2015;61(2):81–9.
113. Toden S, Okugawa Y, Buhrmann C, Nattamai D, Anguiano E, Baldwin N, et al. Novel evidence for curcumin and boswellic acid-induced chemoprevention through regulation of miR-34a and miR-27a in colorectal cancer. Cancer Prev Res. 2015;8(5):431–43.
114. Prasad R, Katiyar SK. Polyphenols from green tea inhibit the growth of melanoma cells through inhibition of class I histone deacetylases and induction of DNA damage. Genes and Cancer. 2015;6(1–2):49–61.
115. Sinha S, Shukla S, Khan S, Tollefsbol TO, Meeran SM. Epigenetic reactivation of p21CIP1/WAF1 and KLOTHO by a combination of bioactive dietary supplements is partially ER-α-dependent in ERα-negative human breast cancer cells. Mol Cell Endocrinol. 2015;406:102–14.
116. Li Y, Chen H, Hardy TM, Tollefsbol TO. Epigenetic regulation of multiple tumor-related genes leads to suppression of breast tumorigenesis by dietary genistein. PLoS One. 2013;8(1): e54369.
117. Khan MA, Hussain A, Sundaram MK, Alalami U, Gunasekera D, Ramesh L, et al. (-)-Epigallocatechin-3-gallate reverses the expression of various tumor-suppressor genes by inhibiting DNA methyltransferases and histone deacetylases in human cervical cancer cells. Oncol Rep. 2015;33(4):1976–84.
118. Wu DS, Shen JZ, Yu AF, Fu HY, Zhou HR, Shen SF. Epigallocatechin-3-gallate and trichostatin A synergistically inhibit human lymphoma cell proliferation through epigenetic modification of p16 INK4a. Oncol Rep. 2013;30(6):2969–75.
119. Thakur VS, Gupta K, Gupta S. Green tea polyphenols causes cell cycle arrest and apoptosis in prostate cancer cells by suppressing class I histone deacetylases. Carcinogenesis. 2012;33 (2):377–84.
120. Sopjani M, Rinnerthaler M, Kruja J, Dermaku-Sopjani M. Intracellular signaling of the aging suppressor protein klotho. Curr Mol Med. 2015;15(1):27–37.
121. Yang Y, Liu J, Li X, Li JC. PCDH17 gene promoter demethylation and cell cycle arrest by genistein in gastric cancer. Histol Histopathol. 2012;27(2):217–24.
122. Chiyomaru T, Yamamura S, Fukuhara S, Yoshino H, Kinoshita T, Majid S, et al. Genistein inhibits prostate cancer cell growth by targeting miR-34a and oncogenic HOTAIR. PLoS One. 2013;8(8):e70372.
123. Mallucci L, Wells V. The end of KRAS, and other, cancers? A new way forward. Drug Discov Today. 2014;19(4):383–7.
124. Appari M, Babu KR, Kaczorowski A, Gross W, Herr I. Sulforaphane, quercetin and catechins complement each other in elimination of advanced pancreatic cancer by miR-let-7 induction and K-ras inhibition. Int J Oncol. 2014;45(4):1391–400.
125. Saud SM, Li W, Morris NL, Matter MS, Colburn NH, Kim YS, et al. Resveratrol prevents tumorigenesis in mouse model of Kras activated sporadic colorectal cancer by suppressing oncogenic Kras expression. Carcinogenesis. 2014;35(12):2778–86.

126. Hirata H, Ueno K, Nakajima K, Tabatabai ZL, Hinoda Y, Ishii N, et al. Genistein downregulates onco-miR-1260b and inhibits Wnt-signalling in renal cancer cells. Br J Cancer. 2013;108(10):2070–8.
127. Wang N, Wang Z, Wang Y, Xie X, Shen J, Peng C, et al. Dietary compound isoliquiritigenin prevents mammary carcinogenesis by inhibiting breast cancer stem cells through WIF1 demethylation. Oncotarget. 2015;6(12):9854–76.
128. Shimizu S. Development of anti-cancer drugs mediated by apoptosis and autophagy. Nihon Rinsho. 2015;73:1302–7.
129. Kronski E, Fiori ME, Barbieri O, Astigiano S, Mirisola V, Killian PH, et al. MiR181b is induced by the chemopreventive polyphenol curcumin and inhibits breast cancer metastasis via down-regulation of the inflammatory cytokines CXCL1 and -2. Mol Oncol. 2014;8(3):581–95.
130. Ma J, Fang B, Zeng F, Pang H, Zhang J, Shi Y, et al. Curcumin inhibits cell growth and invasion through up-regulation of miR-7 in pancreatic cancer cells. Toxicol Lett. 2014;231(1):82–91.
131. Ye M, Zhang J, Zhang J, Miao Q, Yao L, Zhang J. Curcumin promotes apoptosis by activating the p53-miR-192-5p/215-XIAP pathway in non-small cell lung cancer. Cancer Lett. 2015;357(1):196–205.
132. Zheng J, Wu C, Lin Z, Guo Y, Shi L, Dong P, et al. Curcumin up-regulates phosphatase and tensin homologue deleted on chromosome 10 through microRNA-mediated control of DNA methylation - A novel mechanism suppressing liver fibrosis. FEBS J. 2014;281(1):88–103.
133. Wang SH, Lin PY, Chiu YC, Huang JS, Kuo YT, Wu JC, et al. Curcumin-mediated HDAC inhibition suppresses the DNA damage response and contributes to increased DNA damage sensitivity. PLoS One. 2015;10(7):e0134110.
134. Chiyomaru T, Yamamura S, Fukuhara S, Hidaka H, Majid S, Saini S, et al. Genistein up-regulates tumor suppressor MicroRNA-574-3p in prostate cancer. PLoS One. 2013;8(3):e58929.
135. Li H, Jia Z, Li A, Jenkins G, Yang X, Hu J, et al. Resveratrol repressed viability of U251 cells by miR-21 inhibiting of NF-κB pathway. Mol Cell Biochem. 2013;382(1–2):137–43.
136. Ren X, Bai X, Zhang X, Li Z, Tang L, Zhao X, et al. Quantitative nuclear proteomics identifies that miR-137-mediated EZH2 reduction regulates resveratrol-induced apoptosis of neuroblastoma cells. Mol Cell Proteomics. 2015;14(2):316–28.
137. Wu JC, Wang FZ, Tsai ML, Lo CY, Badmaev V, Ho CT, et al. Se-Allylselenocysteine induces autophagy by modulating the AMPK/mTOR signaling pathway and epigenetic regulation of PCDH17 in human colorectal adenocarcinoma cells. Mol Nutr Food Res. 2015;59(12):2511–22.
138. Yang SF, Lee WJ, Tan P, Tang CH, Hsiao M, Hsieh FK, et al. Upregulation of miR-328 and inhibition of CREB-DNA-binding activity are critical for resveratrol-mediated suppression of matrix metalloproteinase-2 and subsequent metastatic ability in human osteosarcomas. Oncotarget. 2015;6(5):2736–53.
139. Yu YH, Chen HA, Chen PS, Cheng YJ, Hsu WH, Chang YW, et al. MiR-520h-mediated FOXC2 regulation is critical for inhibition of lung cancer progression by resveratrol. Oncogene. 2013;32(4):431–43.
140. Deb G, Thakur VS, Limaye AM, Gupta S. Epigenetic induction of tissue inhibitor of matrix metalloproteinase-3 by green tea polyphenols in breast cancer cells. Mol Carcinog. 2015;54(6):485–99.
141. Cossarizza A, Gibellini L, Pinti M, Nasi M, Montagna JP, De Biasi S, et al. Quercetin and cancer chemoprevention. Evidence-based Complem Altern Med. 2011;2011:591356.
142. Li Y, Li W, Yang Y, Lu Y, He C, Hu G, et al. MicroRNA-21 targets LRRFIP1 and contributes to VM-26 resistance in glioblastoma multiforme. Brain Res. 2009;1286:13–8.
143. Miyamoto K, Ushijima T. Diagnostic and therapeutic applications of epigenetics [Internet]. Jpn J Clin Oncol. 2005;35(6):293–301. Available from: https://pubmed.ncbi.nlm.nih.gov/15930038/

144. Gilbert J, Gore SD, Herman JG, Carducci MA. The clinical application of targeting cancer through histone acetylation and hypomethylation [Internet]. Clin Cancer Res. 2004;10 (14):4589–96. Available from: https://pubmed.ncbi.nlm.nih.gov/15269129/
145. Horrobin DF. Are large clinical trials in rapidly lethal diseases usually unethical? [Internet]. Lancet. 2003;361(9358):695–7. Available from: https://pubmed.ncbi.nlm.nih.gov/12611394/
146. Komashko VM, Farnham PJ. 5-azacytidine treatment reorganizes genomic histone modification patterns [Internet]. Epigenetics. 2010;5(3):229–40. Available from: https://pubmed.ncbi.nlm.nih.gov/20305384/
147. Gao Z, Xu Z, Hung MS, Lin YC, Wang T, Gong M, et al. Promoter demethylation of WIF-1 by epigallocatechin-3-gallate in lung cancer cells. Anticancer Res. 2009;29(6):2025–30.
148. Choo QY, Ho PC, Tanaka Y, Lin HS. Histone deacetylase inhibitors MS-275 and SAHA induced growth arrest and suppressed lipopolysaccharide-stimulated NF-KB p65 nuclear accumulation in human rheumatoid arthritis synovial fibroblastic E11 cells [Internet]. Rheumatology. 2010;49(8):1447–60. Available from: https://pubmed.ncbi.nlm.nih.gov/20421217/
149. Kim SH, Kang HJ, Na H, Lee MO. Trichostatin A enhances acetylation as well as protein stability of ERα through induction of p300 protein [Internet]. Breast Cancer Res. 2010;12(2): R22. Available from: https://pubmed.ncbi.nlm.nih.gov/20388208/
150. Zelent A, Waxman S, Carducci M, Wright J, Zweibel J, Gore SD. State of the translational science: Summary of Baltimore workshop on gene re-expression as a therapeutic target in cancer January 2003 [Internet]. Clin Cancer Res. 2004;10(14):4622–9. Available from: https://pubmed.ncbi.nlm.nih.gov/15269133/
151. Sato N, Maitra A, Fukushima N, Van Heek NT, Matsubayashi H, Iacobuzio-Donahue CA, et al. Frequent hypomethylation of multiple genes overexpressed in pancreatic ductal adenocarcinoma. Cancer Res. 2003;63(14):4158–66.
152. Costello JF, Plass C. Methylation matters [Internet]. J Med Genet. 2001;38:285–303. Available from: https://pubmed.ncbi.nlm.nih.gov/11333864/
153. Russo GL, Vastolo V, Ciccarelli M, Albano L, Macchia PE, Ungaro P. Dietary polyphenols and chromatin remodeling [Internet]. Crit Rev Food Sci. 2017;57(12):2589–99. Available from: https://pubmed.ncbi.nlm.nih.gov/26357880/
154. Khan N, Mukhtar H. Tea and health: studies in humans [Internet]. Curr Pharm Des. 2013;19 (4):6141–7. Available from: https://pubmed.ncbi.nlm.nih.gov/23448443/
155. Li Y, Tollefsbol TO. Impact on DNA methylation in cancer prevention and therapy by bioactive dietary components. Curr Med Chem. 2010;17(20):2141–51.
156. Fang M, Chen D, Yang CS. Dietary polyphenols may affect DNA methylation [Internet]. J Nutr. 2007;137(1 Suppl):223–8. Available from: https://pubmed.ncbi.nlm.nih.gov/17182830/
157. Zhou XQ, Xu XN, Li L, Ma JJ, Zhen EM, Han CB. Epigallocatechin-3-gallate inhibits the invasion of salivary adenoid cystic carcinoma cells by reversing the hypermethylation status of the RECK gene [Internet]. Mol Med Rep. 2015;12(4):6031–6. Available from: https://pubmed.ncbi.nlm.nih.gov/26299812/
158. Dou QP. Computational modeling of the potential interactions of the proteasome β5 subunit and catechol-O-methyltransferase-resistant EGCG analogs [Internet]. Int J Mol Med. 2010;26 (2):209–15. Available from: https://pubmed.ncbi.nlm.nih.gov/20596600/
159. Huo C, Yang H, Cui QC, Dou QP, Chan TH. Proteasome inhibition in human breast cancer cells with high catechol-O-methyltransferase activity by green tea polyphenol EGCG analogs. Bioorg Med Chem. 2010;18(3):1252–8.
160. Lee WJ, Zhu BT. Inhibition of DNA methylation by caffeic acid and chlorogenic acid, two common catechol-containing coffee polyphenols. Carcinogenesis. 2006;27(2):269–77.
161. Vandegehuchte MB, Lemière F, Vanhaecke L, Vanden Berghe W, Janssen CR. Direct and transgenerational impact on Daphnia magna of chemicals with a known effect on DNA methylation. Comp Biochem Physiol C Toxicol Pharmacol. 2010;151(3):278–85.
162. Guerrero-Bosagna CM, Sabat P, Valdovinos FS, Valladares LE, Clark SJ. Epigenetic and phenotypic changes result from a continuous pre and post natal dietary exposure to phytoestrogens in an experimental population of mice. BMC Physiol. 2008;8(1):17.

163. Kavoosi F, Dastjerdi M, Valiani A, Esfandiari E, Sanaei M, Hakemi M. Genistein potentiates the effect of 17-beta estradiol on human hepatocellular carcinoma cell line [Internet]. Adv Biomed Res. 2016;5(1):133. Available from: /pmc/articles/PMC5025906/?report=abstract
164. Majid S, Dar AA, Shahryari V, Hirata H, Ahmad A, Saini S, et al. Genistein reverses hypermethylation and induces active histone modifications in tumor suppressor gene B-cell translocation gene 3 in prostate cancer. Cancer. 2010;116(1):66–76.
165. Xie Q, Bai Q, Zou L-Y, Zhang Q-Y, Zhou Y, Chang H, et al. Genistein inhibits DNA methylation and increases expression of tumor suppressor genes in human breast cancer cells [Internet]. Genes Chromosom Cancer. 2014;53(5):422–31. Available from: http://doi.wiley.com/10.1002/gcc.22154
166. Kuck D, Singh N, Lyko F, Medina-Franco JL. Novel and selective DNA methyltransferase inhibitors: docking-based virtual screening and experimental evaluation. Bioorg Med Chem. 2010;18(2):822–9.
167. Khoo HE, Azlan A, Tang ST, Lim SM. Anthocyanidins and anthocyanins: colored pigments as food, pharmaceutical ingredients, and the potential health benefits [Internet]. Food Nutr Res. 2017;61(4):1361779. https://doi.org/10.1080/16546628.2017.1361779.
168. Paluszczak J, Krajka-Kuźniak V, Baer-Dubowska W. The effect of dietary polyphenols on the epigenetic regulation of gene expression in MCF7 breast cancer cells [Internet]. Toxicol Lett. 2010;192(2):119–25. Available from: https://pubmed.ncbi.nlm.nih.gov/19840838/
169. Ma X, Ning S. Cyanidin-3-glucoside attenuates the angiogenesis of breast cancer via inhibiting STAT3/VEGF pathway. Phyther Res. 2019;33(1):81–9.
170. Qin W, Zhang K, Clarke K, Weiland T, Sauter ER. Methylation and miRNA effects of resveratrol on mammary tumors vs. normal tissue. Nutr Cancer. 2014;66(2):270–7.
171. Morey Kinney SR, Zhang W, Pascual M, Greally JM, Gillard BM, Karasik E, et al. Lack of evidence for green tea polyphenols as DNA methylation inhibitors in murine prostate. Cancer Prev Res. 2009;2(12):1065–75.
172. Volate SR, Muga SJ, Issa AY, Nitcheva D, Smith T, Wargovich MJ. Epigenetic modulation of the retinoid X receptor α by green tea in the azoxymethane-ApcMin/+ mouse model of intestinal cancer. Mol Carcinog. 2009;48(10):920–33.
173. Fang MZ, Wang Y, Ai N, Hou Z, Sun Y, Lu H, et al. Tea polyphenol (-)-epigallocatechin-3-gallate inhibits DNA methyltransferase and reactivates methylation-silenced genes in cancer cell lines. Cancer Res. 2003;63(22):7563–70.
174. Won JL, Shim JY, Zhu BT. Mechanisms for the inhibition of DNA methyltransferases by tea catechins and bioflavonoids. Mol Pharmacol. 2005;68(4):1018–30.
175. Clarke KA, Dew TP, Watson REB, Farrar MD, Osman JE, Nicolaou A, et al. Green tea catechins and their metabolites in human skin before and after exposure to ultraviolet radiation [Internet]. J Nutr Biochem. 2016;27:203–10. Available from: https://pubmed.ncbi.nlm.nih.gov/26454512/
176. Hsu A, Wong CP, Yu Z, Williams DE, Dashwood RH, Ho E. Promoter de-methylation of cyclin D2 by sulforaphane in prostate cancer cells [Internet]. Clin. Epigenetics. 2011;3(1):3. Available from: http://clinicalepigeneticsjournal.biomedcentral.com/articles/10.1186/1868-7083-3-3
177. Traka M, Gasper AV, Smith JA, Hawkey CJ, Bao Y, Mithen RF. Transcriptome analysis of human colon Caco-2 cells exposed to sulforaphane [Internet]. J Nutr. 2005;135(8):1865–72. Available from: https://academic.oup.com/carcin/article/32/4/537/2463635
178. Wang LG, Beklemisheva A, Liu XM, Ferrari AC, Feng J, Chiao JW. Dual action on promoter demethylation and chromatin by an isothiocyanate restored GSTP1 silenced in prostate cancer. Mol Carcinog. 2007;46(1):24–31.
179. Tan S, Wang C, Lu C, Zhao B, Cui Y, Shi X, et al. Quercetin is able to demethylate the p16INK4a gene promoter [Internet]. Chemotherapy. 2009;55(1):6–10. Available from: https://www.karger.com/Article/FullText/166383
180. King-Batoon A, Leszczynska JM, Klein CB. Modulation of gene methylation by genistein or lycopene in breast cancer cells. Environ Mol Mutagen. 2008;49(1):36–45.

181. Priyadarsini RV, Vinothini G, Murugan RS, Manikandan P, Nagini S. The flavonoid quercetin modulates the hallmark capabilities of hamster buccal pouch tumors. Nutr Cancer. 2011;63 (2):218–26.
182. Sharma V, Kumar L, Mohanty SK, Maikhuri JP, Rajender S, Gupta G. Sensitization of androgen refractory prostate cancer cells to anti-androgens through re-expression of epigenetically repressed androgen receptor - Synergistic action of quercetin and curcumin. Mol Cell Endocrinol. 2016;431:12–23.
183. Prasad S, Gupta SC, Tyagi AK, Aggarwal BB. Curcumin, a component of golden spice: From bedside to bench and back. Biotechnol Adv. 2014;32(6):1053–64.
184. Teiten MH, Eifes S, Dicato M, Diederich M. Curcumin-the paradigm of a multi-target natural compound with applications in cancer prevention and treatment. Toxins (Basel). 2010;2 (1):128–62.
185. Fu S, Kurzrock R. Development of curcumin as an epigenetic agent. Cancer. 2010;116 (20):4670–6. https://doi.org/10.1002/cncr.25414.
186. Liu Z, Xie Z, Jones W, Pavlovicz RE, Liu S, Yu J, et al. Curcumin is a potent DNA hypomethylation agent. Bioorg Med Chem Lett. 2009 Feb 1;19(3):706–9.
187. Liu Y, Zhou J, Hu Y, Wang J, Yuan C. Curcumin inhibits growth of human breast cancer cells through demethylation of DLC1 promoter [Internet]. Mol Cell Biochem. 2017;425:47–58. Available from: https://idp.springer.com/authorize/casa?redirect_uri=https://link.springer.com/content/pdf/10.1007/s11010-016-2861-4.pdf&casa_token=CyxBwpKuPbsAAAAA:Gc8M7hD0MaRuZC_OgnYEIQk6XfteOPvlVVg-z6AG5_0QVSrcg6X41eGRKziOHtNxVVQfuZEgzocFphc
188. Li W, Pung D, Su ZY, Guo Y, Zhang C, Yang AY, et al. Epigenetics reactivation of Nrf2 in prostate TRAMP C1 cells by curcumin analogue FN1 [Internet]. Chem Res Toxicol. 2016;29 (4):694–703. Available from: https://pubmed.ncbi.nlm.nih.gov/26991801/
189. Pottoo FH, Javed M, Barkat M, Alam M, Nowshehri JA, Alshayban DM, Ansari MA. Estrogen and serotonin: complexity of interactions and implications for epileptic seizures and epileptogenesis. Curr Neuropharmacol. 2019;17(3):214–31.
190. Pottoo FH, Tabassum N, Javed MN, Nigar S, Sharma S, Barkat MA, Alam MS, Ansari MA, Barreto GE, Ashraf GM. Raloxifene potentiates the effect of fluoxetine against maximal electroshock induced seizures in mice. Eur J Pharm Sci. 2020;146:105261.
191. Pandey M, Saleem S, Nautiyal H, Pottoo FH, Javed MN. PINK1/Parkin in neurodegenerative disorders: crosstalk between mitochondrial stress and neurodegeneration. In: Quality control of cellular protein in neurodegenerative disorders. Hershey, PA: IGI Global; 2020. p. 282–301.
192. Pottoo FH, Tabassum N, Javed MN, Nigar S, Rasheed R, Khan A, Barkat MA, Alam MS, Maqbool A, Ansari MA, Barreto GE. The synergistic effect of raloxifene, fluoxetine, and bromocriptine protects against pilocarpine-induced status epilepticus and temporal lobe epilepsy. Mol Neurobiol. 2019;56(2):1233–47.
193. Fenaux P, Mufti GJ, Hellstrom-Lindberg E, Santini V, Finelli C, Giagounidis A, et al. Efficacy of azacitidine compared with that of conventional care regimens in the treatment of higher-risk myelodysplastic syndromes: a randomised, open-label, phase III study. Lancet Oncol. 2009;10 (3):223–32.
194. Hui C, Yujie F, Lijia Y, Long Y, Hongxia X, Yong Z, et al. MicroRNA-34a and microRNA-21 play roles in the chemopreventive effects of 3,6-dihydroxyflavone on 1-methyl-1-nitrosourea-induced breast carcinogenesis. Breast Cancer Res. 2012;14(3):R80.
195. Athar M, Back JH, Kopelovich L, Bickers DR, Kim AL. Multiple molecular targets of resveratrol: Anti-carcinogenic mechanisms. Arch Biochem Biophys. 2009;486:95–102.
196. Athar M, Back JH, Tang X, Kim KH, Kopelovich L, Bickers DR, et al. Resveratrol: a review of preclinical studies for human cancer prevention. Toxicol Appl Pharmacol. 2007;224:274–83.
197. Jang DS, Kang BS, Ryu SY, Chang IM, Min KR, Kim Y. Inhibitory effects of resveratrol analogs on unopsonized zymosan-induced oxygen radical production. Biochem Pharmacol. 1997;576(6):705–12.

198. Nigar S, Pottoo FH, Tabassum N, Verma SK, Javed MN. Molecular insights into the role of inflammation and oxidative stress in epilepsy. J Adv Med Pharm Sci. 2016:1–9. https://doi.org/10.9734/JAMPS/2016/24441.
199. Mao Q-Q, Bai Y, Lin Y-W, Zheng X-Y, Qin J, Yang K, et al. Resveratrol confers resistance against taxol via induction of cell cycle arrest in human cancer cell lines [Internet]. Mol Nutr Food Res. 2010;54(11):1574–84. https://doi.org/10.1002/mnfr.200900392.
200. Birt DF, Hendrich S, Wang W. Dietary agents in cancer prevention: flavonoids and isoflavonoids. Pharmacol Ther Pergamon. 2001;90(2–3):157–77.
201. Kashyap D, Sharma A, Tuli HS, Sak K, Garg VK, Buttar HS, et al. Apigenin: a natural bioactive flavone-type molecule with promising therapeutic function. J Funct Foods. 2018;48:457–71.
202. Lepley DM, Pelling JC. Induction of p21/WAF1 and G1 cell-cycle arrest by the chemopreventive agent apigenin. Mol Carcinog. 1997;19(2):74–82.
203. McVean M, Weinberg WC, Pelling JC. A p21waf1-independent pathway for inhibitory phosphorylation of cyclin-dependent kinase p34cdc2 and concomitant G2/m arrest by the chemopreventive flavonoid apigenin. Mol Carcinog. 2002;33(1):36–43.
204. Byun S, Park J, Lee E, Lim S, Yu JG, Lee SJ, et al. Src kinase is a direct target of apigenin against UVB-induced skin inflammation. Carcinogenesis. 2013;34(2):397–405.
205. Paredes-Gonzalez X, Fuentes F, Su ZY, Kong ANT. Apigenin reactivates Nrf2 anti-oxidative stress signaling in mouse skin epidermal JB6 P + cells through epigenetics modifications. AAPS J. 2014;16(4):727–35. Available from: https://link.springer.com/article/10.1208/s12248-014-9613-8
206. Chalabi N, Satih S, Delort L, Bignon YJ, Bernard-Gallon DJ. Expression profiling by whole-genome microarray hybridization reveals differential gene expression in breast cancer cell lines after lycopene exposure. Biochim Biophys Acta. 2007;1769(2):124–30.
207. Arumugam A, Razis AFA. Apoptosis as a mechanism of the cancer chemopreventive activity of glucosinolates: a review [Internet]. Asian Pac J Cancer Prev. 2018;19(6):1439–48. Available from: /pmc/articles/PMC6103590/
208. Trachootham D, Zhang H, Zhang W, Feng L, Du M, Zhou Y, et al. Effective elimination of fludarabine-resistant CLL cells by PEITC through a redox-mediated mechanism [Internet]. Blood. 2008;112(5):1912–22. Available from: https://pubmed.ncbi.nlm.nih.gov/18574029/
209. Ali Khan M, Kedhari Sundaram M, Hamza A, Quraishi U, Gunasekera D, Ramesh L, et al. Sulforaphane reverses the expression of various tumor suppressor genes by targeting DNMT3B and HDAC1 in human cervical cancer cells. Evidence-based Complem Altern Med. 2015;2015:412149.
210. Khojasteh A, Mirjalili MH, Alcalde MA, Cusido RM, Eibl R, Palazon J. Powerful plant antioxidants: a new biosustainable approach to the production of rosmarinic acid. Antioxidants. 2020;9(12):1273.
211. Moore J, Yousef M, Tsiani E. Anticancer effects of rosemary (Rosmarinus officinalis L.) extract and rosemary extract polyphenols. Nutrients. 2016;8(11):731.
212. Choi KC, Myung GJ, Lee YH, Joo CY, Seung HK, Kang HB, et al. Epigallocatechin-3-gallate, a histone acetyltransferase inhibitor, inhibits EBV-induced B lymphocyte transformation via suppression of RelA acetylation [Internet]. Cancer Res. 2009;69(2):583–92. Available from: http://cancerres.aacrjournals.org/
213. Pandey M, Shukla S, Gupta S. Promoter demethylation and chromatin remodeling by green tea polyphenols leads to re-expression of GSTP1 in human prostate cancer cells. Int J Cancer; 2010;126(11): https://doi.org/10.1002/ijc.24988
214. Saldanha SN, Kala R, Tollefsbol TO. Molecular mechanisms for inhibition of colon cancer cells by combined epigenetic-modulating epigallocatechin gallate and sodium butyrate. Exp Cell Res. 2014;324(1):40–53.
215. Li G-X, Chen Y-K, Hou Z, Xiao H, Jin H, Lu G, et al. Pro-oxidative activities and dose–response relationship of (−)-epigallocatechin-3-gallate in the inhibition of lung cancer cell growth: a comparative study in vivo and in vitro [Internet]. Carcinogenesis. 2010;31

(5):902–10. Available from: https://academic.oup.com/carcin/article-lookup/doi/10.1093/carcin/bgq039
216. Li Y, Li X, Guo B. Chemopreventive agent 3,3′-diindolylmethane selectively induces proteasomal degradation of class I histone deacetylases. Cancer Res. 2010;70(2):646–54.
217. Nair S, Hebbar V, Shen G, Gopalakrishnan A, Khor TO, Yu S, et al. Synergistic effects of a combination of dietary factors sulforaphane and (-) epigallocatechin-3-gallate in HT-29 AP-1 human colon carcinoma cells. Pharm Res. 2008;25(2):387–99.
218. Schwab M, Reynders V, Loitsch S, Steinhilber D, Schröder O, Stein J. The dietary histone deacetylase inhibitor sulforaphane induces human β-defensin-2 in intestinal epithelial cells [Internet]. Immunology. 2008;125(2):241–51. Available from: https://pubmed.ncbi.nlm.nih.gov/18373608/
219. Wang LG, Liu XM, Fang Y, Dai W, Chiao FB, Puccio GM, et al. De-repression of the p21 promoter in prostate cancer cells by an isothiocyanate via inhibition of HDACs and c-Myc. Int J Oncol. 2008;33(2):375–80.
220. Chung IM, Kim MY, Park WH, Moon HI. Histone deacetylase inhibitors from the rhizomes of Zingiber zerumbet. Pharmazie. 2008;63(10):774–6.
221. Lea MA, Rasheed M, Randolph VM, Khan F, Shareef A, DesBordes C. Induction of histone acetylation and inhibition of growth of mouse erythroleukemia cells by S-allylmercaptocysteine. Nutr Cancer. 2002;43(1):90–102.
222. Nian H, Delage B, Pinto JT, Dashwood RH. Allyl mercaptan, a garlic-derived organosulfur compound, inhibits histone deacetylase and enhances Sp3 binding on the P21WAF1 promoter. Carcinogenesis. 2008;29(9):1816–24.
223. Arunkumar A, Vijayababu MR, Gunadharini N, Krishnamoorthy G, Arunakaran J. Induction of apoptosis and histone hyperacetylation by diallyl disulfide in prostate cancer cell line PC-3. Cancer Lett. 2007;251(1):59–67.
224. Druesne-Pecollo N, Chaumontet C, Pagniez A, Vaugelade P, Bruneau A, Thomas M, et al. In vivo treatment by diallyl disulfide increases histone acetylation in rat colonocytes. Biochem Biophys Res Commun. 2007;354(1):140–7.
225. Selvi BR, Pradhan SK, Shandilya J, Das C, Sailaja BS, Shankar GN, et al. Sanguinarine interacts with chromatin, modulates epigenetic modifications, and transcription in the context of chromatin. Chem Biol. 2009;16(2):203–16.
226. Chandregowda V, Kush A, Reddy GC. Synthesis of benzamide derivatives of anacardic acid and their cytotoxic activity. Eur J Med Chem. 2009;44(6):2711–9.
227. Kim MK, Shin JM, Eun HC, Chung JH. The role of p300 histone acetyltransferase in UV-induced histone modifications and MMP-1 gene transcription. PLoS One. 2009;4(3):e4864.
228. Rangappa DB, Rangappa D, Thanuja KN, Rangappa KS, Rani MN, et al. Synthesis, characterization and cytotoxic studies of benzamide derivatives of anacardic acid using human liver cancer cells. Clin Oncol Res. 2020.
229. Fang MZ, Chen D, Sun Y, Jin Z, Christman JK, Yang CS. Reversal of hypermethylation and reactivation of p16INK4a, RARβ, and MGMT genes by genistein and other isoflavones from soy [Internet]. Clin Cancer Res. 2005;11(19 I):7033–41. Available from: https://pubmed.ncbi.nlm.nih.gov/16203797/
230. Hong T, Nakagawa T, Pan WJ, Kim MY, Kraus WL, Ikehara T, et al. Isoflavones stimulate estrogen receptor-mediated core histone acetylation. Biochem Biophys Res Commun. 2004;317(1):259–64.
231. Li Y, Liu L, Andrews LG, Tollefsbol TO. Genistein depletes telomerase activity through cross-talk between genetic and epigenetic mechanisms. Int J Cancer. 2009;125(2):286–96.
232. Majid S, Dar AA, Ahmad AE, Hirata H, Kawakami K, Shahryari V, et al. BTG3 tumor suppressor gene promoter demethylation, histone modification and cell cycle arrest by genistein in renal cancer. Carcinogenesis. 2009;30(4):662–70.

233. Araki Y, Fann M, Wersto R, Weng N. Histone acetylation facilitates rapid and robust memory CD8 T cell response through differential expression of effector molecules (eomesodermin and its targets: perforin and granzyme B). J Immunol. 2008;180(12):8102–8.
234. Balasubramanyam K, Varier RA, Altaf M, Swaminathan V, Siddappa NB, Ranga U, et al. Curcumin, a novel p300/CREB-binding protein-specific inhibitor of acetyltransferase, represses the acetylation of histone/nonhistone proteins and histone acetyltransferase-dependent chromatin transcription. J Biol Chem. 2004;279(49):51163–71.
235. Olaharski AJ, Rine J, Marshall BL, Babiarz J, Zhang L, Verdin E, et al. The flavoring agent dihydrocoumarin reverses epigenetic silencing and inhibits sirtuin deacetylases. PLoS Genet. 2005;1(6):e77.
236. Wood JG, Regina B, Lavu S, Hewitz K, Helfand SL, Tatar M, et al. Sirtuin activators mimic caloric restriction and delay ageing in metazoans. Nature. 2004;430(7000):686–9.
237. Ruiz PA, Braune A, Hölzlwimmer G, Quintanilla-Fend L, Haller D. Quercetin inhibits TNF-induced NF-κB transcription factor recruitment to proinflammatory gene promoters in murine intestinal epithelial cells [Internet]. J Nutr. 2007;137(5):1208–15. Available from: https://pubmed.ncbi.nlm.nih.gov/17449583/
238. Xiao X, Shi D, Liu L, Wang J, Xie X, Kang T, et al. Quercetin suppresses cyclooxygenase-2 expression and angiogenesis through inactivation of P300 signaling. PLoS One. 2011;6(8): e22934.
239. Gracia-Sancho J, Villarreal G, Zhang Y, García-Cardeña G. Activation of SIRT1 by resveratrol induces KLF2 expression conferring an endothelial vasoprotective phenotype. Cardiovasc Res. 2010;85(3):514–9.
240. Venturelli S, Berger A, Böcker A, Busch C, Weiland T, Noor S, et al. Resveratrol as a Pan-HDAC inhibitor alters the acetylation status of jistone proteins in human-derived hepatoblastoma cells [Internet]. PLoS One. 2013;8(8):e73097. Available from: https://pubmed.ncbi.nlm.nih.gov/24023672/
241. Yang J, Kong X, Martins-Santos MES, Aleman G, Chaco E, Liu GE, et al. Activation of SIRT1 by resveratrol represses transcription of the gene for the cytosolic form of phosphoenolpyruvate carboxykinase (GTP) by deacetylating hepatic nuclear factor 4α [Internet]. J Biol Chem. 2009;284(40):27042–53. Available from: https://pubmed.ncbi.nlm.nih.gov/19651778/
242. Cosío BG, Mann B, Ito K, Jazrawi E, Barnes PJ, Chung KF, et al. Histone acetylase and deacetylase activity in alveolar macrophages and blood mononocytes in asthma. Am J Respir Crit Care Med. 2004;170(2):141–7.
243. Murugan RS, Vinothini G, Hara Y, Nagini S. Black tea polyphenols target matrix metalloproteinases, RECK, proangiogenic molecules and histone deacetylase in a rat hepatocarcinogenesis model. Anticancer Res. 2009;29(6):2301–5.
244. Balasubramanyam K, Altaf M, Varier RA, Swaminathan V, Ravindran A, Sadhale PP, et al. Polyisoprenylated benzophenone, garcinol, a natural histone acetyltransferase inhibitor, represses chromatin transcription and alters global gene expression. J Biol Chem. 2004;279 (32):33716–26.
245. Chen IH, Lu MC, Du YC, Yen MH, Wu CC, Chen YH, et al. Cytotoxic triterpenoids from the stems of Microtropis japonica. J Nat Prod. 2009;72(7):1231–6.
246. Lee WJ, Chen YR, Tseng TH. Quercetin induces FasL-related apoptosis, in part, through promotion of histone H3 acetylation in human leukemia HL-60 cells. Oncol Rep. 2011;25 (2):583–91.
247. Singh N, Misra K. Computational screening of molecular targets in Plasmodium for novel non resistant anti-malarial drugs. Bioinformation. 2009;3(6):255–62.
248. Lee SJ, Krauthauser C, Maduskuie V, Fawcett PT, Olson JM, Rajasekaran SA. Curcumin-induced HDAC inhibition and attenuation of medulloblastoma growth in vitro and in vivo. BMC Cancer. 2011;11:44.
249. Iranshahi M, Chini MG, Masullo M, Sahebkar A, Javidnia A, Chitsazian Yazdi M, et al. Can small chemical modifications of natural pan-inhibitors modulate the biological selectivity? The

case of curcumin prenylated derivatives acting as HDAC or mPGES-1 inhibitors. J Nat Prod. 2015;78(1):2867–79.
250. Majid S, Kikuno N, Nelles J, Noonan E, Tanaka Y, Kawamoto K, et al. Genistein induces the p21WAF1/CIP1 and p16INK4a tumor suppressor genes in prostate cancer cells by epigenetic mechanisms involving active chromatin modification. Cancer Res. 2008;68(8):2736–44.
251. Kikuno N, Shiina H, Urakami S, Kawamoto K, Hirata H, Tanaka Y, et al. Genistein mediated histone acetylation and demethylation activates tumor suppressor genes in prostate cancer cells. Int J Cancer. 2008;141(7):1492.
252. Pong RC, Roark R, Ou JY, Fan J, Stanfield J, Frenkel E, et al. Mechanism of increased coxsackie and adenovirus receptor gene expression and adenovirus uptake by phytoestrogen and histone deacetylase inhibitor in human bladder cancer cells and the potential clinical application. Cancer Res. 2006;66(17):8882–8.
253. Li G, Rivas P, Bedolla R, Thapa D, Reddick RL, Ghosh R, et al. Dietary resveratrol prevents development of high-grade prostatic intraepithelial neoplastic lesions: involvement of SIRT1/S6K axis. Cancer Prev Res. 2013;6(1):27–39.
254. Scuto A, Kirschbaum M, Buettner R, Kujawski M, Cermak JM, Atadja P, et al. SIRT1 activation enhances HDAC inhibition-mediated upregulation of GADD45G by repressing the binding of NF-κB/STAT3 complex to its promoter in malignant lymphoid cells. Cell Death Dis. 2013;4(5):e635. Available from: https://pubmed.ncbi.nlm.nih.gov/23681230/
255. Kai L, Samuel SK, Levenson AS. Resveratrol enhances p53 acetylation and apoptosis in prostate cancer by inhibiting MTA1/NuRD complex [Internet]. Int J Cancer. 2010;126(7):1538–48. Available from: https://pubmed.ncbi.nlm.nih.gov/19810103/
256. Kala R, Tollefsbol TO. A novel combinatorial epigenetic therapy using resveratrol and pterostilbene for restoring estrogen receptor-α (ERα) expression in ERα-negative breast cancer cells [Internet]. PLoS One. 2016;11(6):e0155057. Available from: https://pubmed.ncbi.nlm.nih.gov/27159275/
257. Pandey M, Kaur P, Shukla S, Abbas A, Fu P, Gupta S. Plant flavone apigenin inhibits HDAC and remodels chromatin to induce growth arrest and apoptosis in human prostate cancer cells: In vitro and in vivo study. Mol Carcinog. 2012;51(12):952–62.
258. Myzak MC, Hardin K, Wang R, Dashwood RH, Ho E. Sulforaphane inhibits histone deacetylase activity in BPH-1, LnCaP and PC-3 prostate epithelial cells. Carcinogenesis. 2006;27(4):811–9.
259. Watson GW, Wickramasekara S, Palomera-Sanchez Z, Black C, Maier CS, Williams DE, et al. SUV39H1/H3K9me3 attenuates sulforaphane-induced apoptotic signaling in PC3 prostate cancer cells. Oncogenesis. 2014;3(12):e131.
260. Valeri N, Vannini I, Fanini F, Calore F, Adair B, Fabbri M. Epigenetics, miRNAs, and human cancer: a new chapter in human gene regulation. Mamm Genome. 2009;20(9–10):573–80.
261. Tsang WP, Kwok TT. Epigallocatechin gallate up-regulation of miR-16 and induction of apoptosis in human cancer cells. J Nutr Biochem. 2010;21(2):140–6.
262. Chakrabarti M, Khandkar M, Banik NL, Ray SK. Alterations in expression of specific microRNAs by combination of 4-HPR and EGCG inhibited growth of human malignant neuroblastoma cells. Brain Res. 2012;1454:1–13.
263. Wang H, Bian S, Yang CS. Green tea polyphenol EGCG suppresses lung cancer cell growth through upregulating miR-210 expression caused by stabilizing HIF-1α [Internet]. Carcinogenesis. 2011;32(12):1881–9. Available from: https://pubmed.ncbi.nlm.nih.gov/21965273/
264. Vidya Priyadarsini R, Senthil Murugan R, Maitreyi S, Ramalingam K, Karunagaran D, Nagini S. The flavonoid quercetin induces cell cycle arrest and mitochondria-mediated apoptosis in human cervical cancer (HeLa) cells through p53 induction and NF-κB inhibition. Eur J Pharmacol. 2010;649(1–3):84–91.
265. Zhang Q, Zhao XH, Wang ZJ. Cytotoxicity of flavones and flavonols to a human esophageal squamous cell carcinoma cell line (KYSE-510) by induction of G2/M arrest and apoptosis. Toxicol Vitr. 2009;23(5):797–807.

266. Lou G, Liu Y, Wu S, Xue J, Yang F, Fu H, et al. The p53/miR-34a/SIRT1 positive feedback loop in quercetin-induced apoptosis. Cell Physiol Biochem. 2015;35(6):2192–202.
267. Lam TK, Shao S, Zhao Y, Marincola F, Pesatori A, Bertazzi PA, et al. Influence of quercetin-rich food intake on microRNA expression in lung cancer tissues. Cancer Epidemiol Biomarkers Prev. 2012;21(12):2176–84.
268. Du F, Feng Y, Fang J, Yang M. MicroRNA-143 enhances chemosensitivity of Quercetin through autophagy inhibition via target GABARAPL1 in gastric cancer cells. Biomed. Pharmacother. 2015;74:169–77.
269. Del Follo-Martinez A, Banerjee N, Li X, Safe S, Mertens-Talcott S. Resveratrol and quercetin in combination have anticancer activity in colon cancer cells and repress oncogenic microRNA-27a. Nutr Cancer. 2013;65(3):494–504.
270. Sun M, Estrov Z, Ji Y, Coombes KR, Harris DH, Kurzrock R. Curcumin (diferuloylmethane) alters the expression profiles of microRNAs in human pancreatic cancer cells. Mol Cancer Ther. 2008;7(3):764–73.
271. Zhang P, Bai H, Liu G, Wang H, Chen F, Zhang B, et al. MicroRNA-33b, upregulated by EF24, a curcumin analog, suppresses the epithelial-to-mesenchymal transition (EMT) and migratory potential of melanoma cells by targeting HMGA2. Toxicol Lett. 2015;234 (3):151–61.
272. Li Y, Vandenboom TG, Kong D, Wang Z, Ali S, Philip PA, et al. Up-regulation of miR-200 and let-7 by natural agents leads to the reversal of epithelial-to-mesenchymal transition in gemcitabine-resistant pancreatic cancer cells. Cancer Res. 2009;69(16):6704–12.
273. Qin J, Chen JX, Zhu Z, Teng JA. Genistein inhibits human colorectal cancer growth and suppresses MiR-95, Akt and SGK1. Cell Physiol Biochem. 2015;35(5):2069–77.
274. Avci CB, Susluer SY, Caglar HO, Balci T, Aygunes D, Dodurga Y, et al. Genistein-induced mir-23b expression inhibits the growth of breast cancer cells. Wspolczesna Onkol. 2015;19 (1):32–5.
275. Sun Q, Cong R, Yan H, Gu H, Zeng Y, Liu N, et al. Genistein inhibits growth of human uveal melanoma cells and affects microRNA-27a and target gene expression. Oncol Rep. 2009;22 (3):563–7.
276. Tili E, Michaille JJ, Alder H, Volinia S, Delmas D, Latruffe N, et al. Resveratrol modulates the levels of microRNAs targeting genes encoding tumor-suppressors and effectors of TGFβ signaling pathway in SW480 cells [Internet]. Biochem Pharmacol. 2010;80(12):2057–65. Available from: https://pubmed.ncbi.nlm.nih.gov/20637737/
277. Azimi A, Hagh MF, Talebi M, Yousefi B, Hossein Pour Feizi AA, Baradaran B, et al. Time - and concentration - dependent effects of resveratrol on miR 15a and miR16-1 expression and apoptosis CCRF-CEM acute lymphoblastic leukemia cell line. Asian Pac J Cancer Prev. 2015;16(15):6463–8.
278. Dhar S, Kumar A, Rimando AM, Zhang X, Levenson AS. Resveratrol and pterostilbene epigenetically restore PTEN expression by targeting oncomiRs of the miR-17 family in prostate cancer. Oncotarget. 2015;6(29):27214–26.
279. Chakrabarti M, Banik NL, Ray SK. MiR-138 overexpression is more powerful than hTERT knockdown to potentiate apigenin for apoptosis in neuroblastoma in vitro and in vivo. Exp Cell Res. 2013;319(10):1575–85.
280. Shan Y, Zhang L, Bao Y, Li B, He C, Gao M, et al. Epithelial-mesenchymal transition, a novel target of sulforaphane via COX-2/MMP2, 9/Snail, ZEB1 and miR-200c/ZEB1 pathways in human bladder cancer cells. J Nutr Biochem. 2013;24(6):1062–9.
281. Lan F, Pan Q, Yu H, Yue X. Sulforaphane enhances temozolomide-induced apoptosis because of down-regulation of miR-21 via Wnt/β-catenin signaling in glioblastoma [Internet]. J Neurochem. 2015;134(5):811–8. https://doi.org/10.1111/jnc.13174.
282. Zhu K, Wang W. Green tea polyphenol EGCG suppresses osteosarcoma cell growth through upregulating miR-1. Tumor Biol. 2016;37(4):4373–82.
283. Zhou J, Gong J, Ding C, Chen G. Quercetin induces the apoptosis of human ovarian carcinoma cells by upregulating the expression of microRNA-145. Mol Med Rep. 2015;12(2):3127–31.

284. Jin H, Qiao F, Wang Y, Xu Y, Shang Y. Curcumin inhibits cell proliferation and induces apoptosis of human non-small cell lung cancer cells through the upregulation of miR-192-5p and suppression of PI3K/Akt signaling pathway. Oncol Rep. 2015;34(5):2782–9.
285. De La Parra C, Castillo-Pichardo L, Cruz-Collazo A, Cubano L, Redis R, Calin GA, et al. Soy isoflavone genistein-mediated downregulation of miR-155 contributes to the anticancer effects of genistein. Nutr Cancer. 2016;68(1):154–64.
286. Xie J, Wang J, Zhu B. Genistein inhibits the proliferation of human multiple myeloma cells through suppression of nuclear factor-κB and upregulation of microRNA-29b [Internet]. Mol Med Rep. 2016;13(2):1627–32. Available from: http://www.spandidos-publications.com/10.3892/mmr.2015.4740/abstract
287. Yang S, Li W, Sun H, Wu B, Ji F, Sun T, et al. Resveratrol elicits anti-colorectal cancer effect by activating miR-34c-KITLG in vitro and in vivo. BMC Cancer. 2015;15(1):969.
288. Zhou C, Ding J, Wu Y. Resveratrol induces apoptosis of bladder cancer cells via miR-21 regulation of the Akt/Bcl-2 signaling pathway [Internet]. Mol Med Rep. 2014;9(4):1467–73. Available from: http://www.spandidos-publications.com/10.3892/mmr.2014.1950/abstract
289. Yoshida K, Toden S, Ravindranathan P, Han H, Goel A. Curcumin sensitizes pancreatic cancer cells to gemcitabine by attenuating PRC2 subunit EZH2, and the lncRNA PVT1 expression. Carcinogenesis. 2017;38(10):1036–46.
290. Pei CS, Wu HY, Fan FT, Wu Y, Shen CS, Pan LQ. Influence of curcumin on HOTAIR-mediated migration of human renal cell carcinoma cells. Asian Pac J Cancer Prev. 2014;15 (10):4239–43.
291. Chen J, Lin C, Yong W, Ye Y, Huang Z. Calycosin and genistein induce apoptosis by inactivation of HOTAIR/p-akt signaling pathway in human breast cancer MCF-7 cells. Cell Physiol Biochem. 2015;35(2):722–8.
292. Yang Q, Xu E, Dai J, Liu B, Han Z, Wu J, et al. A novel long noncoding RNA AK001796 acts as an oncogene and is involved in cell growth inhibition by resveratrol in lung cancer. Toxicol Appl Pharmacol. 2015;285(2):79–88.
293. Ji Q, Liu X, Fu X, Zhang L, Sui H, Zhou L, et al. Resveratrol inhibits invasion and metastasis of colorectal cancer cells via MALAT1 mediated Wnt/β-catenin signal pathway. PLoS One. 2013;8(11):e78700. https://doi.org/10.1371/journal.pone.0078700.
294. Ho E, Ho E, Hendrix DA, Ho E, Ho E. Long noncoding RNAs and sulforaphane: a target for chemoprevention and suppression of prostate cancer. J Nutr Biochem. 2017;42:72–83.

Flavonoids Targeting Cancer Stem Cells: A Paradigm to Anticancer Efficacy

7

Nahida Siddiqui, Lubna Abidin, Nazima Nisar, Irfan Ahmad, and Ali Nasir Siddiqui

Abstract

Cancer stem cells (CSCs) are sub-populated cells in the tumor and responsible for tumor growth, heterogeneity, relapse, and progression of cancer. They play a dynamic role in developing resistance of chemotherapeutics and promoting epithelial mesenchymal transition (EMT) and metastasis in tumors, which are accountable for approximately 90% of mortality. Thus, agents targeting CSCs or chemosensitizing CSCs have now gained significant importance in the regulation and inhibition of various malignancies. Nowadays, numerous dietary polyphenolic compounds such as flavonoids are being explored as potential candidates to be utilized in chemoprevention and treatment of various cancers by targeting CSCs. In multiple studies, flavonoids have shown an inhibitory effect on the self-renewal potential, stemness characteristics, EMT process, and survival of CSCs in different tumors. Literature shows that few flavonoids like genistein, quercetin, silibinin, and apigenin have been explored substantially for their role in inhibition of CSCs. However, there is paucity of data for some of the flavonoids such as broussoflavonol B, icaritin, morusin, casticin, wogonin, baicalein, luteolin, ugonin J and K, naringine, and pomiferin though they have also shown inhibition

N. Siddiqui (✉)
HIMT College of Pharmacy, Greater Noida, Uttar Pradesh, India

L. Abidin
Department of Pharmacognosy and Phytochemistry, Plant Biotechnology Laboratory, School of Pharmaceutical Research & Education, Jamia Hamdard University, New Delhi, India

N. Nisar · I. Ahmad
Department of Clinical Laboratory Sciences, College of Applied Medicinal Sciences, King Khalid University, Abha, Kingdom of Saudi Arabia

A. N. Siddiqui
Independent Researcher, New Delhi, India

S. Tabrez, M. Imran Khan (eds.), *Polyphenols-based Nanotherapeutics for Cancer Management*, https://doi.org/10.1007/978-981-16-4935-6_7

of CSCs. This chapter illustrates a descriptive information about CSCs, their characteristics, biomarkers, and pathways involved in their maintenance (Notch, Hedgehog, Wnt/β-catenin, PI3K/Akt, and NF-κB). In addition, the literature around several flavonoids and their effect in reduction or eradication of CSCs via attenuation of different signaling pathways have been reviewed.

Keywords

Cancer stem cells (CSCs) · Epithelial Mesenchymal Transition (EMT) · Flavonoids · Hedgehog · Notch · Polyphenolic compounds · Wnt/β-catenin

7.1 Introduction

Cancer Stem Cells (CSCs), also known as cancer-initiating cells (CICs) or tumor-initiating cells (TICs), are sub-populated cells (0.1–10%) of the tumor and are mainly responsible for tumor heterogeneity, tumor growth, recurrence, self-renewal, and progression of various types of cancer depicted in Fig. 7.1 [1, 2]. Unlike normal stem cells, CSCs have indefinite potential of self-renewal that leads to tumorigenesis. The alteration in the metabolic and phenotypic characteristics of CSCs, mainly because of various genetic and epigenetic modifications, leads to the emergence of tumor heterogeneity which increases tumor survival and invasion into other tissues and further complicates the cancer treatment [1, 3]. CSCs were first identified in acute myeloid leukemia (AML) by Bonnet and Dick in 1994 [4]. In solid tumors, it was first derived from breast cancer cells in 2003 when a group of researchers injected the $CD44^{+}$, $CD24^{-/low}$ populated cells in immune-deficient mice [5]. Thereafter, CSCs have also been found in brain, lung, prostate, colon, multiple myeloma, pancreatic, liver, head and neck, ovarian, cervical, gastric, and other cancers [1, 6–9].

The CSCs are accountable for the resistance development against chemoradiotherapies, epithelial mesenchymal transitions (EMT), and metastasis which are the main cause of approximately 90% of mortality [4, 10]. The resistance against treatments and disease progression may occur partly due to the lower proliferative rate of CSCs compared to non-CSCs [11]. They are nowadays targeted for cancer treatment due to their capability to initiate and propagate tumor growth and develop resistance [12].

In several in vitro and in vivo studies, dietary phytocompounds have been shown to inhibit tumor formation and progression in various malignancies [8, 13, 14]. The studies showing the potential role of phytocompounds against CSCs are limited. However, in recent years, studies have been conducted and demonstrated the anti-CSCs effect of some phytocompounds [8, 13–17]. Polyphenolic compounds, especially flavonoids have shown their role in inhibiting tumorigenesis due to their anti-CSCs effect indicating that they can be an attractive chemopreventive and chemotherapeutic candidate for cancer treatment [18–20]. In this chapter, the effects of

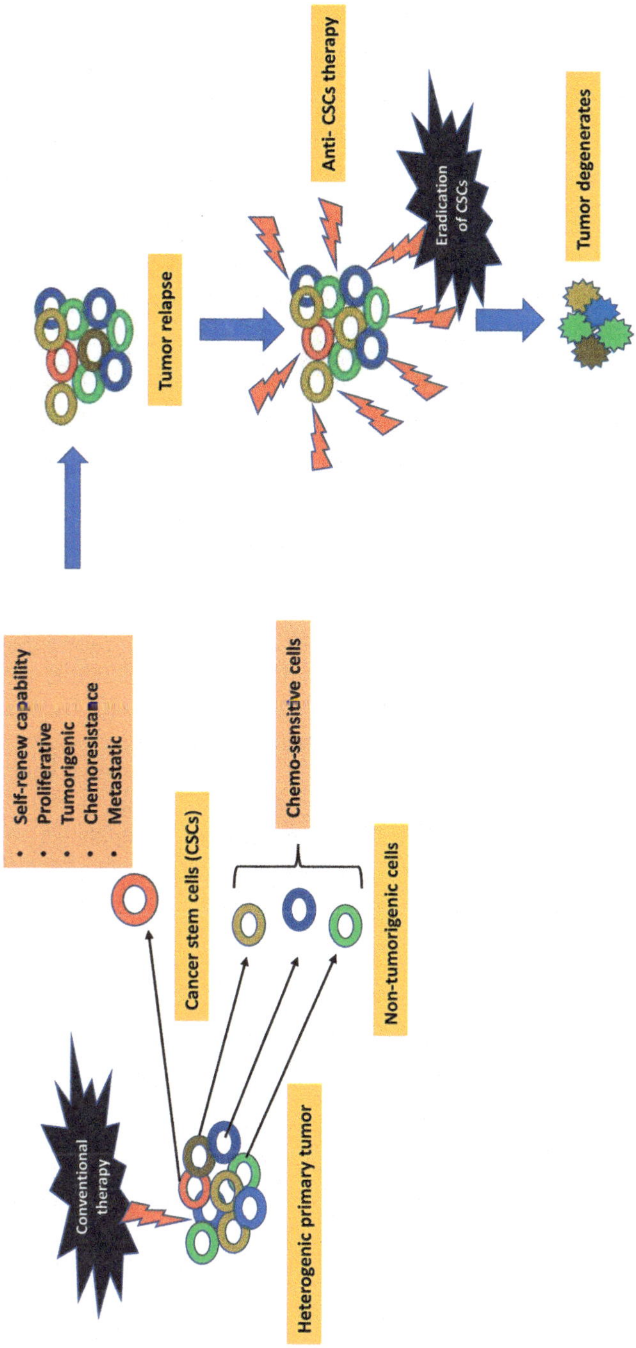

Fig. 7.1 Tumor initiation through cancer stem cells (CSCs)

different flavonoids and their derivatives on CSCs derived from various types of cancers have been illustrated.

7.2 Characteristics of Cancer Stem Cells (CSCs)

7.2.1 Salient Features

CSCs possess three unique characteristics that enable them for tumor initiation, propagation, and spread [2, 14, 18, 21–24]:

1. The self-renewal capacity helps CSCs to preserve their pool.
2. CSCs are multipotent and give rise to the heterogeneous population of cells through asymmetric division.
3. The uncontrolled proliferative potential of CSCs supports the sustained development of tumors.

7.2.2 Promotion of Epithelial Mesenchymal Transition (EMT)

Epithelial mesenchymal transition is found as one of the significant characteristics of CSCs. During EMT, the features of epithelial cells converts to mesenchymal cell-like phenotypes (spindle-shaped appearance) which also enhances the invasive potential and motility of the cells [4, 25, 26]. During EMT progression, E-cadherin which is epithelial cell marker is downregulated whereas mesenchymal markers like N-cadherin and vimentin are upregulated [26]. EMT is a reversible change as it can induce intravasation to invade healthy group of cells followed by extravasation to form new tumors (Fig. 7.2). In intravasation process, the epithelial cancer cells change their phenotype to mesenchymal cells while entering into the bloodstream. Mesenchymal-epithelial transition (MET) is the reverse form of EMT occurring along with these changes after extravasation and can boost new tumors formation [26, 27].

The molecular mechanism of EMT includes inducers, regulators, and effectors. When the tumors start to grow due to signal the transition order by the inducers like TGF- β, VEGF, IGF, Wnt, and Notch causes nutrient deficit and hypoxia in the cells of the tumor at the center [28]. The regulators are transcription factors or drivers that change the cell shape and make them more favorable to invade other healthy tissues by regulating the cytoskeleton [29]. Master regulators of the EMT are Twist and Snail1 which regulate repression of E-cadherin and enhances the tumor-initiating capacity of cells, respectively. Other regulators of EMT are SMAD, BMP, Slug, ZEB1, and ZEB2 which are found helpful in suppressing transcription by binding directly to E-cadherin at the promoter region [26, 30]. Vimentin and keratin act as a regulator to maintain overall cell shape towards mesenchymal cells which are more motile [3]. Enzymes such as collagenases and matrix metalloproteinases (MMPs) promote the escape of tumor cells from the primary tumor site and help them to enter

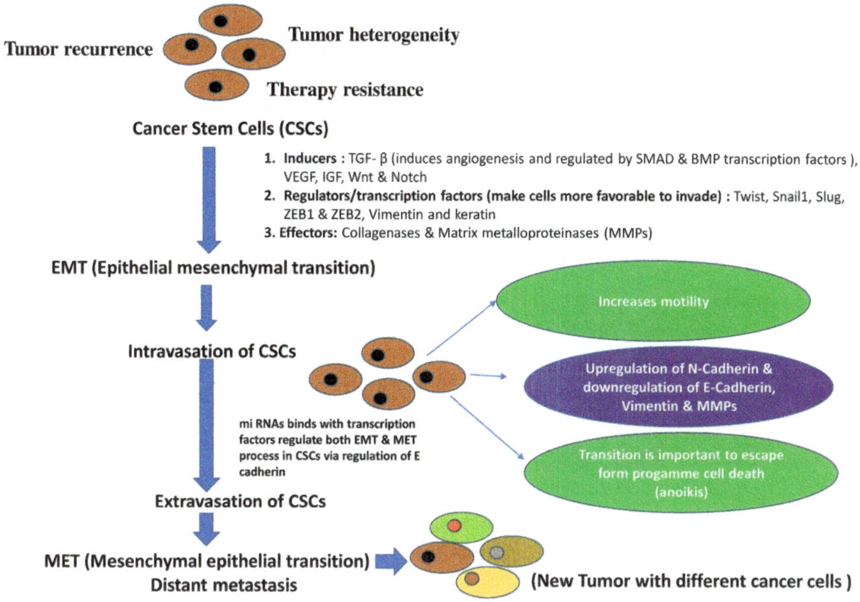

Fig. 7.2 Epithelial mesenchymal transition (EMT)

the bloodstream [31]. Moreover, the transition of EMT to MET is an essential step in tumor formation to escape the CSCs from programmed cell death, an apoptosis that kills epithelial cells in the blood circulation [32].

7.2.3 Chemoradiotherapy Resistance

One of the significant characteristics of CSCs is the development of resistance against chemoradiotherapy. Resistance attained by CSCs is generally regulated by the high capacity for DNA repair mechanism and increased protection against reactive oxygen species (ROS). CSCs stay dormant during chemoradiotherapy and can regenerate cancer after therapy. Dormancy of CSCs is associated with multiple genes (e.g., TGF-β2) [29, 33] which are responsible for therapy resistance and contribute to cancer relapse [33, 34]. It has also been shown that conventional therapies target the high proliferative stem cells instead of dormant CSCs of tumor that can cause a recurrence of cancer [26]. Additionally, chemoradiotherapy resistance also develops due to the upregulation of anti-apoptotic pathways.

Recent studies suggested that abnormal chromatin package density is correlated with the survival rate of cancer cells which are resistant to chemotherapies [35]. Moreover, studies have indicated that the growing number of EMT cell states are regulated by epigenetic mechanisms [36].

Tumor heterogeneity is defined as a state when cancer cells possess distinct genotypes and phenotypes within a single tumor (intra-tumor heterogeneity) and are also responsible for complication or resistance to chemotherapy. An epigenetic mechanism is involved to cause the phenotypic differences between the CSCs and non-CSCs. In studies, CSCs have shown to cause tumor heterogeneity and promote new tumor development as compared to normal cancer cells [33, 37, 38]. In the present scenario, intra-tumor heterogeneity is a big challenge in the development of cancer therapy.

The overexpression of the telomerase enzyme, regulated by mutated hTERT gene, may cause unstable chromosome length in CSCs. Telomere repeats are akin to the self-renewal capacity of CSCs which is controlled by telomerase activity. Moreover, it has been shown that mitochondrial telomerase activity in CSCs protects nuclear DNA by reducing the level of ROS and causing therapy resistance [39, 40].

7.3 Biomarkers of CSCs

Biomarkers, proteins or glycoproteins, define the properties of CSCs and are upregulated, downregulated, or mutated in malignancies. The enhanced activity of these biomarkers is well correlated with CSCs biology and help in developing new strategies to treat various malignancies and resistance cases [29, 33, 41]. Few of the biomarkers of CSCs are cell surface antigens while others are located in the cytoplasm such as Aldehyde dehydrogenase 1 (ALDH1). ALDH1 oxidizes aldehyde into carboxylic acid to protect CSCs and increases their chemoresistance by detoxification of chemotherapeutics. It has three main isotypes such as ALDH1A1, ALDH1A2, and ALDH1A3 which are involved in self-renewal, differentiation, and self-protection of CSCs. CD44 is a hyaluronic acid receptor and is responsible for invasiveness, metastatic potential, and development of drug resistance in CD44 expressing CSCs. It has several isoforms with different significant roles in CSCs. CD44, CD24, and EpCAM have stemness properties and causing chemoresistance. CD117 is the stem cell growth factor receptor, encoded by the c-KIT gene and CD133 is a common marker of CSCs associated with a poor prognosis and chemoresistance [42]. Table 7.1 refers to the list of some common surface biomarkers of CSCs in various types of cancer [1, 32, 41, 43–51].

Specific biomarkers can be used to differentiate CSCs from normal cells and other tumor cells [52]. It is further difficult to identify CSCs by a single biomarker and understanding the role of specific biomarkers is pivotal to treat current issues of cancer. Moreover, to date, no universal CSCs biomarker has been discovered. The current methodologies to isolate and detect functional differences of CSCs from non-CSCs population are image-based, sphere formation, cytological sorting using flow cytometry, CRISPR-Cas9 3D sphere culture systems, magnetic-activated cell sorting (MACS), and xenotransplantation. Among all, xenotransplantation is the best method to confirm the existence of CSCs [53]. Thus, identifying and isolating specific CSCs biomarkers in conjunction with new technologies is imperative for the treatment of various malignancies [4]. This further promotes findings of the novel therapeutics in eradicating highly tumorigenic and therapy-resistant CSCs.

Table 7.1 Common surface biomarkers of CSCs in various types of human cancers

Types of cancer	Biomarkers
Hematological	CD34, CD38, CD19, CD26
Breast	ABCG2, AC133, $CD44^+$/ $CD24^{-low}$, CD133, CD61, ALDH1, $CD338^+$, α6/β3 integrin, EPCAM
Colon	AC133, CD44, CD24, CD29, CD133, CD166, EpCAM
Brain	CD90, CD133, CD15, AC133
Head and Neck	ALDH1, CD44, CD271
Skin	CD20, CD271
Liver	$CD133^+$/$CD44^+$, EpCAM, $CD45^-$, $CD90^+$, ABCG2, CD44, CD90, CD13
Endometrial	CD133, ALDH1
Intestine	Lrg5
Prostate	Integrin α2/β1, BMI-1, integrin α6, $CD133^+$, $CD44^+$, ABCG2/Hoechst 33342, SCA-1, $CD166^+$, $CD151^+$, $p63^+$CD133
Ovarian	$CD133^+$, $CD44^+$, $CD117^+$, $CD24^+$, AC133
Lung	ABCG2, CD44, CD133, CD166
Bladder	$CD44^+$, $CD47^+$, $CK5^+$
Glioblastoma	$CD133^+$ and $CD15^+$
Renal	$CD133^+$
Pancreatic	CD44+, $CD24^+$
Osteosarcoma	$CD117^+$, $CD133^+$, Stro-1^+
Multiple myeloma	$CD38^-$, $CD34^+$, $CD138^+$
Colorectal cancer	$CD133^+$, $CD44^+$, $CD26^+$, ALDH

7.4 Possible Pathways Involved in Regulation of CSCs

The Wnt, Hedgehog, and Notch are the major evolutionarily conserved signaling pathways responsible for stemness and differentiation of CSCs. Other signaling pathways such as PI3K/AKT and NF-κB also play important role in the regulation of CSCs characteristics. The aberrant activation of these signaling pathways stimulates CSCs proliferation, restricts differentiation, and prevents apoptosis [54]. Therapeutic approaches targeting these aberrant signaling pathways are required to treat the various types of cancer [55]. Moreover, transcription factors such as SOX2, NANOG, OCT-4, KLF-4, and c-MYC are important for the self-renewal capacity of CSCs. These transcription factors also stands out as potential targets for cancer therapy [33, 56].

7.4.1 The Notch Pathway

The Notch signaling pathway is complex and multifaceted, reflecting its roles in diverse functional activities. The loss of Notch activity favors the EMT process [1]. For the maintenance of stemness of CSCs, upregulation of Notch pathway is responsible along with overexpression of Notch signaling genes (Notch1, Notch3, Jag1, and Jag2) and Notch target gene (Hes1) [57]. Notch signaling via transmembrane ligands and receptors is primarily involved in the communication between adjoining cells. Interaction between ligand on one cell and a transmembrane receptor on a neighboring cell triggers a two-step proteolytic cleavage of the receptor [58]. The first cleavage is mediated by a disintegrin and metalloproteinase enzymes (ADAM 10 or 17) also known as tumor necrosis factor-α converting enzyme (TACE) and the second cleavage is mediated by γ-secretase. This cleavage releases an intracellular fragment which interacts with nuclear factors to regulate target gene expression. The Notch pathway comprises of five canonical Notch ligands (Delta-like ligand 1 [DLL1], DLL3, DLL4, Jagged1, and Jagged2) and four Notch receptor paralogues (Notch1–4) [59]. Different tumors and tumor subtypes can express different Notch receptors and ligands. Furthermore, posttranslational modifications of Notch receptors can change their affinity for ligands and their intracellular half-lives. The non-canonical Notch signaling pathway also has relevance in cancer. Thus, targeting Notch signaling has the potential to simultaneously affect multiple cell types within a tumor, from CSCs to immune cells, vascular endothelial cells, and tumor cells. Additionally, the mechanistic understanding of the role of Notch signaling in specific cancers is required for the successful development of agents targeting the Notch pathway.

The Notch pathway is associated with CSCs in various cancers such as breast cancer, medulloblastoma, and other gliomas. CSCs can be eliminated by Gamma-secretase inhibitors (GSIs) which decrease the subpopulation and tumor sphere formation frequency of CSCs. However, GSIs are relatively nonselective drugs and sometimes also produce toxicity like secretory diarrhea. Highly specialized monoclonal antibodies (mAbs) that specifically antagonize Notch ligands and receptors provide single-target specificity. Knockdown of Hes1 of the CSCs decreases tumor sphere formation, suggesting that Notch signaling activity is required for stemness and promoting cell survival of CSCs.

Hence, it can be speculated that inhibition of Notch signaling pathway in CSCs can play a great role in the treatment of various types of tumors via reducing the population of CSCs. With anti-Delta-like 4 ligand antibodies, either alone or in combination with the chemotherapeutic agents, we can reduce the frequency of CSCs ($EpCAM^+/CD44^+/CD166^+$). Si-RNA targeted to Notch4 is also found active in suppressing breast cancer recurrence [60].

Flavonoids also target the Notch signaling pathway for eradication and reduction of CSCs. This activity of flavonoids might be due to the regulation of Υ-secretase, Notch ligands and receptors, knockdown of Hes1, si-RNA targeted to Notch4, or inhibition of DLL-4 ligand.

7.4.2 The Hedgehog Pathway

The Hedgehog pathway is considered to modulate tumorigenesis through tissue patterning, propagation, differentiation, and EMT [61, 62]. Atypical activation of this pathway is responsible for maintenance and tumorigenesis of CSCs as seen in various cancers like myeloid leukemia, myeloma, glioma, colorectal, and gastric cancer [63, 64].

The major troupes in the Hedgehog pathway are the three secreted ligands including Sonic, Desert, and Indian. Smoothened (transmembrane protein) and 3 Gli transcription factors (Gli1-3) along with ligands regulate the suppression or activation of Hedgehog pathway. Islam and team have demonstrated the indispensable role of Sonic hedgehog pathway in the promotion of the EMT, tumorigenicity, and stemness in both in vitro and in vivo studies [65].

When Patched receptor is unoccupied, it acts as a constitutive inhibitor of Smoothened. At this state, Gli3 and Gli2-R repress the target gene transcription. However, when the ligand binds to Patched receptor, the suppression on Smoothened is released allowing transcription of target genes [66]. Overexpression of Smoothened, Gli1, Sonic hedgehog, and Patched1 gene with decreased expression of the stemness genes (SOX-2, NANOG, and OCT-4) are found to be responsible for survival, stemness, proliferation, self-renewal, and clonogenicity of CSCs both in vivo and in vitro [67].

Cyclopamine and IPI269609, which are antagonist of Smoothened, have been shown to reduce the populations or eradicate CSCs and induce tumor suppression in pancreatic and brain cancer [68–70]. The combined chemotherapeutics targeting Hedgehog pathway to eradicate CSCs have attracted general attention [71, 72]. In studies, flavonoids alone or in combination with chemotherapeutic agents have shown to target CSCs or sensitize CSCs possibly via hedgehog signaling pathway by regulating their receptors, ligands, smoothened, or transcriptional factors. This has been further described in section 5.

7.4.3 The Wnt/β-catenin Pathway

It is an enormously evolutionarily conserved signaling pathway which plays a dynamic role in modulating cell propagation and differentiation. In carcinogenesis, the aberrant signaling of this pathway facilitates the clonal expansion or tumor heterogeneity which ultimately causes self-renewal, metastasis, multidrug resistance, and invasiveness of CSCs [54, 73, 74].

This is a highly complex pathway comprising of 19 different Wnt ligands and more than 15 receptors. Conventionally, this pathway comprises of 2 signaling pathways: canonical (mediated through β-catenin, a transcriptional regulator) and non-canonical (independent to β-catenin) [74]. The canonical pathway gets triggered when one cell secreted Wnt ligands binds to Frizzled receptors or LRP 5 (low-density lipoprotein-related protein) and LRP 6 co-receptors of the adjacent cell [75]. Signaling through these two Wnt pathways is necessary for embryonic development and homeostasis of various tissues [74, 76]. In general, the canonical Wnt pathway is involved in regulation of proliferation, survival, and cell fate decisions while the non-canonical pathway is involved in regulation of asymmetrical divisions in cells, cell polarity, and migration. It is observed that stem cells of various postnatal tissues are controlled through the canonical signaling pathway [75].

Along with tumorigenesis, Wnt signaling has been associated with CSCs-mediated metastasis and maintenance of its stemness. A significantly higher level of Wnt signaling proteins such as LEF-1, cyclin D1, β-catenin, and TCF-4 along with Wnt-responsive gene transcription are found in breast CSCs compared with normal cancer cells. Moreover, the knockdown of canonical Wnt pathway in CSCs diminishes the expression of genes involved in stemness (CD44, ALDH1, and Sca-1), CSCs subpopulation, and inhibits tumor sphere formation. This indicates that Wnt signaling is essential for CSCs stemness maintenance [77]. Furthermore, a higher expression of Wnt genes (TCF-4 and Disheveled) is present in metastatic CSCs [78].

Non-canonical pathway may also be responsible for tumor instigation through Wnt5a actions, a non-canonical Wnt ligand. An in vivo study (ErbB2-driven mammary tumorigenesis on mouse model) showed that Wnt5a ligand limited the expansion of basally located CSCs in tumor [79].

The canonical Wnt signaling cascade is involved in self-renewal of stem cells and production or differentiation of ancestor cells [80–82] whereas non-canonical Wnt signaling pathway is involved in the conservation of stem cells, guidance of cell movement, or inhibition of the canonical signaling cascade [9, 83–85]. Both Wnt signaling cascades play crucial roles in the growth and progression of CSCs [86].

Deviant activation of this pathway in CSCs was severely linked with tumorigenesis in various tissues. Chemotherapeutic agents that can be specific to a Wnt receptor frizzled7, essential co-receptor binder for LRP6, and Wnt signaling antagonist are responsible for depletion of clonal expansion and tumorigenicity of CSCs in various kinds of tumors [87]. Knocking down miR-142, which is a potent effector for activating this signaling is also helpful in diminishing tumor-initiating ability and sphere formation of CSCs [88]. Moreover, suppressors of Wnt/β-catenin pathway significantly lessen the population, stemness, and self-renewal capacity of CSCs [89]. Additionally, inhibiting Wnt/β-catenin makes CSCs more chemosensitive to conventional drugs along with reduction of self-renewal and tumorigenic ability [90]. Thus, targeting Wnt/β-catenin signaling would be a promising approach to conquer CSCs.

7.4.4 Role of PI3K/Akt and NF-kB Pathways in CSCs

The aberrant PI3K/Akt signaling pathway boosts up the cellular proliferation and survival of the CSCs [91, 92]. PI3K is a heterodimer consisting of a regulatory subunit—p85 and a catalytic subunit—p110 and Akt, a protein kinase. Both can regulate the EMT process by modulating a series of relevant transcription factors such as Twist, Snail, and Slug; inducing integrin-linked kinase activities and stimulating MMPs. Moreover, PI3K/Akt might induce the EMT in CSCs in cooperation with TGF-β, NF-κB, RAS, and Wnt/β-catenin [93].

Studies reported that microRNAs (miR-126, miR-10b) are helpful in the maintenance of CSCs state via PI3K signaling through inhibition of PTEN. They promote maintenance of CSCs by increasing tumor sphere formation along with overexpression of stemness genes OCT-4 and Snail1 [94, 95]. These findings show that PTEN signaling plays a suppressive role in the maintenance of CSCs stemness [95].

Aberrant activation and overexpression of the proinflammatory transcription factor (NF-κB) protect CSCs from the programmed cell death (apoptosis) by direct upregulation of anti-apoptotic genes or antagonistic effect on p53 pathway and promote self-renewal characteristics of CSCs [58]. Transcription factors consist of five different proteins that function as dimers which are normally inactivated in the cytoplasm through binding to IκB proteins. Activation of this pathway occurs due to binding of tumor necrosis factor alpha (TNF-α), IL-1β, and bacterial cell wall components to their respective receptors (TNF receptor, IL-1 receptor, and toll-like receptors also known as TLRs), respectively [96]. In case of canonical NF-κB pathway, adapter proteins are recruited, facilitating the phosphorylation and activation of IκB kinase (IKKβ) proteins which subsequently initiate the phosphorylation of IκB proteins, marking them for ubiquitination and degradation [96]. Degradation of IκB releases NF-κB which translocates to the nucleus and activates transcription of target genes [58]. In case of non-canonical NF-κB pathway, activation occurs through different receptors, such as receptor activator of NF-κB (RANK) and CD40, signaling through NF-κB inducing kinase and IKKα. Then p100/RelB dimers are processed into p52/RelB dimers which translocate to the nucleus and activates transcription. The NF-kB pathway is a highly complex and critical signaling pathway and has role in cellular proliferation, survival, and differentiation of CSCs [96]. Hence, we can conclude that NF-κB signaling constitutes an important pathway controlling the self-renewal and tumorigenesis of CSCs [97, 98]. NF-κB signaling has also been implicated in enabling CSCs to facilitate metastasis by downregulation of IKKβ. Genetic silencing or chemical inhibition of IKKβ reduced the expression of the stemness proteins LIN-28, OCT-4, SOX-2, and NANOG. The NF-κB signaling pathway may support CSCs stemness and promote tumor metastasis in cancers [99].

7.5 Flavonoids Targeting CSCs

In recent years, several dietary compounds derived from natural sources have been found effective in chemoprevention and treatment of various types of cancers. Flavonoids are a class of polyphenolic secondary metabolites consisting of a C6-C3-C6 skeleton (15-carbon structure that consists of two phenyl rings and a heterocyclic ring) that are found abundantly in dietary plants and some medicinal herbs. On the basis of their chemical structures, they are categorized as flavones, flavanones, flavonols, and isoflavones which are commonly present in the human

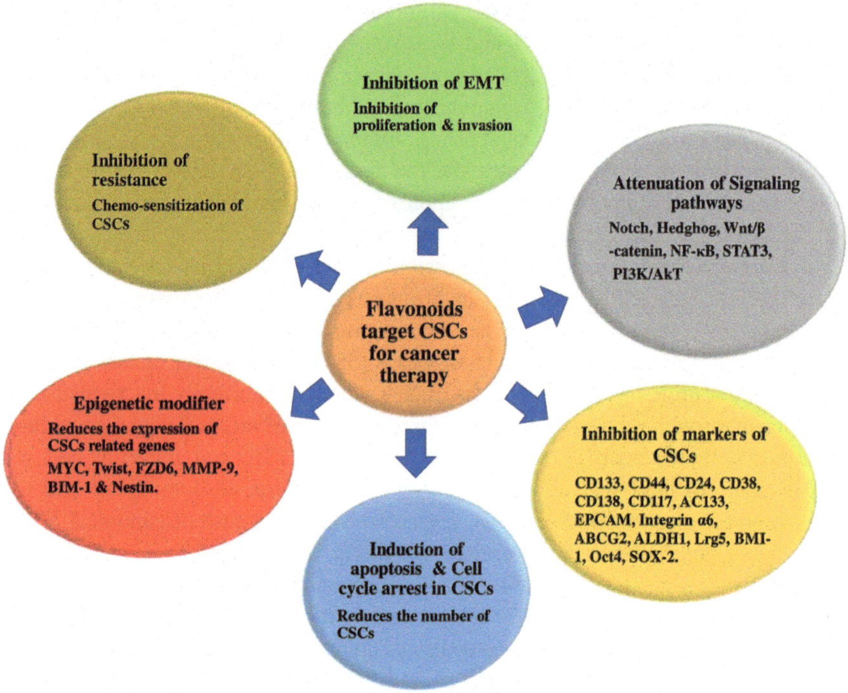

Fig. 7.3 Flavonoids targeting CSCs

diet [1, 100–102]. They possess anticancer activity both in preclinical and cellular model systems (Fig. 7.3). They have also shown an inhibitory effect on the self-renewal potential and survival of CSCs in various tumors [1, 54]. Moreover, several recent studies have suggested that flavonoids can also play important role in targeting the CSCs and may sensitize them towards conventional anticancer therapies [58, 103–105]. We have reviewed the available literature of flavonoids targeting CSCs responsible for progression of disease along with their attenuating signaling pathways.

Mostly flavonoids regulate or eradicate CSCs of tumors by targeting various pathways which might be associated with maintenance of CSCs such as Wnt/β-catenin, Hedgehog, Notch, PI3K/Akt, and NF-κB signaling pathways. Few of the flavonoids such as genistein, quercetin, silibinin, and apigenin have been explored substantially in the literature for their role in inhibition of CSCs. However, there is paucity of data for some of the flavonoids such as broussoflavonol B, icaritin, morusin, casticin, wogonin, baicalein, luteolin, ugonin J and K, naringine, and pomiferin though they have also shown inhibition of CSCs. These flavonoids have been shown to directly or indirectly modulate these signaling pathways and contribute to the reduction of CSCs growth and maintenance.

7.5.1 Genistein

Genistein or Prunetol (4',5,7-Trihydroxyisoflavone) is an isoflavone type of flavonoid. Perkin and Newbury were the first to isolate genistein in 1899 from *Genista tinctoria* (Leguminosae) [106–109]. Genistein is a highly active anticancer phytocompound used in the treatment of various types of malignancies [110–112].

Genistein is known to act via attenuating some signaling pathways like Notch, Hedgehog, and Wnt/β-catenin of CSCs. Moreover, there are other cellular targets of genistein through which it can inhibit stemness of CSCs. In recent years, the inhibitory action of genistein against CSCs was established in colon, breast, prostate, and pancreatic cancer [16, 113–115]. Downregulation of expression of cyclin B1, Bcl-2, and Bcl-xL via Notch pathway in breast cancer was also exemplified [114]. In one in vitro study, Chen and colleagues demonstrated that genistein can cause overexpression of ARHI tumor suppressor gene thereby inhibiting cell proliferation and inducing apoptosis in CSCs in prostate cancer [15]. It has also exhibited an antagonistic role against prostate CSCs through inhibition of Hedgehog-Gli1 pathway [16]. Sekar and coworkers conducted in vivo experiment in 1, 2-dimethyl hydrazine (DMH) induced colon cancer model in mice. They observed that genistein had reduced Argyrophilic nuclear organizer region (AgNOR) and proliferating cell nucleolar antigen (PCNA) along with suppression of colonic stem cell markers [113]. Xia and colleagues showed that genistein was capable to upregulate miR-34a along with downregulation of Notch-1 in pancreatic cancer [115].

The inhibitory role of genistein on Wnt/β-catenin signaling pathway in CSCs has also been well-established in various studies. In an ex vivo study, genistein was found to have an inhibitory effect on Wnt/β-catenin pathway by regulating miR-1260b expression in renal cancer cells [116]. In a study, genistein prevented self-renewal of breast CSCs via attenuation of Wnt/β-catenin pathway [117].

Furthermore, genistein has the potential to inhibit ovarian CSCs via suppression of FOXO3a and FOXM1 along with downregulation of expression of stem cell markers (CD133, CD44, and ALDH1) responsible for self-renewal [14]. This finding was further supported by another study in which ovarian tumor suppression was due to decreased expression of CD163 and p-STAT3 [118]. Genistein also inhibited the self-renewal capacity and reduced the resistance of therapy in gastric cancer by suppression of CSCs markers [119]. It has the ability to reverse EMT process in colon cancer by inhibiting cell migration via downregulation of EMT markers (ZEB1, ZEB2, FOXC1, FOXC2, Snail2/slug, and TWIST1) along with suppression of Notch-1, p-NF-κB, and NF-κB signaling in in vitro study [120]. The inhibitory role of genistein in CSCs was tested in renal and nasopharyngeal cancer and was found to suppress of Hedgehog signaling pathway [121, 122].

Recently, genistein has also shown an inhibitory effect in lung cancer by decreasing cell viability, migration, and invasion of lung CSCs through suppression of protein expression levels of CD133, CD44, Bmi1, and Nanog [123]. The role of genistein in head and neck cancer was too studied and was found to downregulate EMT. It also synergized the effect of doxorubicin, cisplatin, and 5-flourouracil to cause cell death in CSCs [124] (Table 7.2). Genistein has also produced a synergistic

Table 7.2 Anticancer potential of Genistein targeting CSCs

Treatment	Cancer target	Cell line/Model used	Assay used	Conclusion	Refs.
Genistein	Renal cancer	Ex vivo study in A-498, 786-O, and Caki-2 cell line	MicroRNA transfection, Viability assay, Invasion assay, Apoptosis analysis, Plasmid construction, Luciferase assay, RT-qPCR, and Western blotting	Blocking of Wnt/β-catenin pathway and miR-1260b was downregulated, induction of apoptosis, inhibition of cell proliferation and invasion	[116]
Genistein	Renal cancer	In vitro study in 768-O and ACHN cell line	Sphere formation assay, Cell cycle analysis, Flow cytometry analysis, Western blotting, and RT- qPCR	Activation of Sonic hedgehog pathway, inhibiting proliferation and induction of apoptosis	[122]
Genistein	Colon cancer	In vitro study in HT-29 cell line	Cell proliferation assay, Flow cytometry analysis, Invasion assays, DAPI staining, Cell apoptosis analysis, Immunofluorescence staining, and RT-PCR	Suppression of Notch pathway leading to reversal of EMT, induction of apoptosis and inhibition of cell invasion	[120]
Genistein	Colon cancer	In vivo study in 1,2-dimethyl hydrazine-induced colon cancer model	Alcian blue staining, AgNOR, and PCNA analysis	Wnt/β-catenin pathway was downregulated along with restoration of colonic niche and suppression of stem cell markers (CD133, CD44, and β-catenin)	[113]
Genistein	Colon cancer	In vitro study in MGC-803 and SGC-7901 cell line followed by in vivo study in Nude mice xenograft model	Soft agar colony formation assay, Tumor sphere formation assay, MTT assay, RNA extraction, RT-PCR, RT-qPCR, and Tumor growth in xenografts	Inhibition of self-renewal capacity in cancer cells along with reduced chemoresistance via downregulation of ABCC1, ABCC5, ABCG2, and ERK 1/2 activity (Notch pathway) and inhibition of ABCG2 mRNA expression	[119]
Genistein	Breast cancer	In vitro study in transfected MSF cell line	Red oil O staining, RT-qPCR, Triglyceride quantification assay,	Cell growth prevented by repression of Wnt/β-catenin	[117]

			Western blotting, Cell viability assay, Tumor sphere formation assay		
Genistein	Breast cancer	In vitro study in transfected MDA-MB-231 cell	Quantitative apoptotic cell death assay, MTT assay, Cell cycle analysis, and Western blotting	Inhibition of Notch-1 pathway causing inhibition of NF-Kb Leading to downregulation of cyclinB1, inhibition of proliferation, and induction of apoptosis	[114]
Genistein + Doxorubicin	Breast cancer	In vitro study in doxorubicin-resistant CSCs derived from parental MCF-7 cells	MTT assay, Fluoro-spectrophotometry, Cell cycle analysis, Apoptosis analysis, Flow cytometry, RT-PCR, and Western blotting	Suppression of mRNA and protein expression of c-erbB2, chemosensitized the CSCs to doxorubicin via P-gp-independent mechanism, induction of cell cycle arrest and apoptosis	[128]
Genistein	Prostate cancer	In vitro study in PC-3 cell line	Tumorsphere formation assay and Colony formation assay	Inhibition of Gli1 gene suppressing CD44 marker causing decreased tumorigenicity through modulation in Hedgehog pathway	[16]
Genistein	Prostate cancer	In vitro study in CSCs isolated from PC-3, LNCap, and Du145	RT-PCR, Cell proliferation assay, Invasion assay, Luciferase activity assay, Flow cytometry, Western blotting, and Immunohistochemistry	Activation of Hedgehog pathway caused overexpression of ARHI tumor suppressor gene, inhibited cell proliferation, and induced apoptosis	[15]
Genistein	Prostate cancer	In vitro study in AsPC-1 cell line	MTT assay, Clonogenic assay, Histone/DNA ELISA, RT-PCR, Sphere formation assay, Western blot analysis, and miRNA-34a Transfection	Reexpression of miR-34a through downregulation of Notch-1 causing induction of apoptosis in CSCs	[115]
Genistein	Nasopharyngeal cancer	In vitro study in human nasopharyngeal cancer cell lines	Tumor sphere forming assay	Sonic hedgehog was suppressed leading to inhibition of	[121]

(continued)

Table 7.2 (continued)

Treatment	Cancer target	Cell line/Model used	Assay used	Conclusion	Refs.
		CNE2 and HONE1 enriched CSCs		tumorsphere formation capacity, cell proliferation, and induction of apoptosis. Decreased the number of EpCAM+ cells, suppressed expression of stem cell markers	
Genistein	Lung cancer	In vitro study in IMR-90, H460, and A549 cell lines	Sphere formation assay, Cell viability assay, Wound-healing assay, Transwell invasion assay, Western blotting, and Cell transduction analysis	Downregulation of FoxM1 causing inhibition of CSCs migration and invasion via suppression of Wnt/β-catenin	[123]
Gensitein + Oxaliplatin	Oral cancer	In vivo study in Dimethylbenz[a] anthracene (DMBA)-induced oral carcinoma model	Histopathological analysis	Downregulation of Wnt/β-catenin caused decreased CD44 expression and thus decreased cell proliferation	[126]
Genistein	Head and neck cancer	Ex vivo in head and neck cancer tissues resected from head and neck cancer patients	Cell proliferation assay, Sphere formation assay, Migration and invasion assay, Luciferase assay, Flow cytometry, Colony formation analysis, RT-PCR, and Western blotting	Activation of Notch caused inhibition of stemness characteristics including migration, invasion, and colony-forming abilities	[124]
Genistein	Ovarian cancer	In vitro study in SKOV3 and OVCAR-3 cell lines along with in vivo in nude mice xenograft model	In vivo tumorigenicity assay, MTT assay, and Western blotting.	Activation of FOXO3a and downregulation of FOXM1 and stem cell markers (CD133, CD44, and ALDH1) by which significantly inhibiting proliferation and self-renewal capacity of CSCs.	[14]
Genistein	Ovarian cancer	In vitro study in SKOV3, A2780, and OVCAR-3 cell lines followed	Sphere formation assay, Colony formation test, Enzyme-linked	Activation of hedgehog pathway caused blocking IL-8/STAT3	[118]

		by in vivo study in nude mice xenograft model	immunosorbent assay, western blotting, and in vivo tumorigenicity experiment	signaling which leads to inhibition of self-renewal capacity of CSCs	
Gensitein + Tamoxifen	Hepatic cancer	In vitro study in HepG2 cell line	Cell growth assay, Cell viability assay, Cell cycle analysis, and Flow cytometry	Synergistically inhibited proliferation and induced apoptosis	[125]
Gensitein + 5-fluorouracil	Colorectal cancer	In vitro study in HT 29 cell line	Colonosphere formation, Cell viability, Cell cycle analysis, Flow cytometry, and Western blotting	Reductions in $CD133^{+}CD44^{+}$ subpopulation along with reduced colonosphere formation through upregulation of Notch pathway	[127]

effect with other chemotherapeutic drugs and is helpful in chemosensitizing the CSCs to treat resistance cases. Sanaei *et al.* studied the combined effect of genistein and Tamoxifen in hepatocellular cancer cell line (HepG2). It showed that the combination synergistically inhibited proliferation and induced apoptosis [125]. Genistein has a synergistic effect when used in combination with oxaliplatin since the combination exhibited suppression of the expression of CSCs marker (CD44) and inhibited cell proliferation in oral squamous cell carcinoma [126]. Genistein has also shown a synergistic effect when given in combination with doxorubicin and 5-FU. They targeted CSCs and chemosensitize them [127, 128]. The role of genistein to retard CSCs has been explored in various studies which are presented in Table 7.2 with their cellular pathways.

7.5.2 Quercetin

Quercetin ($C_{15}H_{10}O_7$), a flavonol from the class of flavonoids, is dietary polyphenolic compound found in many dietary plants and also found in medicinal botanicals [*Ginkgo biloba* (Ginkgoaceae) and *Hypericum perforatum* (Hypericaceae)] displays excellent antitumor activity [129]. It induces apoptosis and downregulates protein expression of EMT, angiogenesis, and stemness of CSCs population in many cancer [130, 131]. In studies, quercetin has been shown to inhibit breast cancer via targeting CSCs. Recently, upregulation of small heat shock proteins 27 (Hsp27) was found to be beneficial in maintaining CSCs along with their stemness [131–133]. Quercetin could act as an inhibitor of Hsp27 which causes a decrease in self-renewal capacity of CSCs which eventually reduces the population of $ALDH^+$ breast CSCs. Quercetin further displayed the synergistic effect with geldanamycin (Hsp90 inhibitor) and reduced the migration, tumorigenesis, and population of $ALDH^+$ breast CSCs via the suppression of Hsp90 and Hsp27 [134]. In another study, quercetin suppressed vascularization of tumors by targeting epidermal growth factor (EGF)/Hsp27 signaling [135]. In addition to target Hsp27, quercetin has shown an inhibitory effect on PI3K/Akt/mTOR signaling pathway which is responsible for self-renewal and stemness of CSCs in breast cancer [136]. Quercetin has also demonstrated an improvement in chemosensitivity of resistance cases and inhibited population of breast CSCs by blocking nuclear translocation of Y-box binding protein 1 and hence downregulating P-glycoprotein. This is one of the reasons for its effect in reducing the multidrug resistance and stemness of CSCs [136, 137]. The use of anticancer agents in combination with quercetin has resulted in reduced target toxicity, induction of apoptosis, lowering the cancer recurrence, and inhibition of EMT in CSCs.

Quercetin has also shown promising result in head and neck cancer by showing inhibitory effect on stemness signature, self-renewal capacity, migration ability, and EMT along with reduction in CSCs number which were derived from SAS and OECM1 cell lines (Table 7.3) [138]. It has also shown anticancer effect against teratocarcinoma via antagonizing the Wnt/β-catenin signaling pathway in CSCs of NT2/D1 human cell line [139]. When quercetin was used with other flavonoid, such as luteolin, the combination reversed the EMT process by downregulating the EMT

Table 7.3 Anticancer potential of Quercetin targeting CSCs

Treatment	Target cancer	Cell lines/Model used	Assay used	Conclusion	Refs.
Quercetin + Sulforaphane	Pancreatic Cancer	In vitro study in Human pancreatic cancer cell line—$CSCs^{high}$ MIA-PaCa2 and BxPc-3 cells In vivo xenograft model using NMRI (nu/nu) male mice—xenografted subcutaneously $CSCs^{high}$ MIA-PaCa cells	Measurement of apoptosis, MTT assay, Spheroid assay, Colony formation assays, Detection of ALDH1 activity, Caspase activity assay, Western Blot analysis. Immunohistochemistry and immunofluorescence analysis of xenograft tissue and Electrophoretic mobility shift assay	Prevented NF-κB signaling pathway responsible for EMT and tumor progression Inhibited Twist-2 and vimentin proteins involved in EMT. In vivo outcome: Inhibited growth of CSCs enriched xenografts and induction of apoptosis	[130]
Quercetin + Cisplatin	Oral cancer	In vitro study in Drug resistant sphere (DRSP) model. Human tongue cancer cell line resistant to Cisplatin—SCC25 used. In vivo study - SCC25 and spheres xenografted subcutaneously into BALB/c nude mice	MTT assay, in vivo Tumorigenic Assay, and Immunohistochemistry	Chemosensitized to CSCs and treat MDR-1 via inhibition of p38 MAPK–Hsp27 signaling and suppression of ABCG2 gene of the drug resistance. Reversed the EMT via upregulation of E-cadherin and downregulation of vimentin, Twist-1, and fascin-1	[143]
Quercetin	Head and neck cancer	Head and neck CSCs (HNC-CSCs)—$ALDH^{+}$ SAS and OECM1 cell line	Aldefluor assay, Cell migration assay, and Western blot analysis	It inhibited stemness signature, migration ability, and EMT Suppressed stemness markers expression genes (Oct-4, Nanog, and Nestin) and mesenchymal-related protein (Twist, vimentin, and N-cadherin)	[138]
Quercetin and Luteolin	Prostate cancer	In vitro study—Du145 III model using highly invasive Du145-III	Invasion assay, Wound-healing assay, Capillary formation assay, Spheroidal assay,	Significantly delayed migration, invasion, and inhibited number with volume of spheroids	[141]

(continued)

Table 7.3 (continued)

Treatment	Target cancer	Cell lines/Model used	Assay used	Conclusion	Refs.
		subline from Du145-P parental tumor cell line	Western blotting, PCR amplification, and Transfection of Si-RNA analysis	formation Also, markedly reduced expression of CD44, ABCG2, Sox2, and Nanog markers via modulation of JNK signaling pathway.	
Quercetin and Luteolin	Epidermal carcinoma	In vitro study in A431-III CSCs derived from parental A431-P	Immunofluorescence microscopy, RT-PCR, Gelatin zymography, Wound-healing assay, Invasion assay, and Transfection analysis	Suppressed EMT in CSCs via attenuating EMT markers and reduced the overexpression of MMP-9	[140]
Quercetin	Teratocarcinoma	In vitro model in NT2/D1 cells	Immunocytochemistry, Western blot analysis, Cell adhesion assay, Wound-healing migration assay, RT-PCR analysis, and Transfections and luciferase assay	Antagonized the Wnt/β-catenin signaling pathway by inhibiting β-catenin nuclear translocation and the downregulation of β-catenin-dependent transcription	[139]
Quercetin + EGCG	Prostate cancer	In vitro study —$CD44^+$ and $CD133^+$ CSCs from PC-3 and LNCaP cells	Transwell Migration and invasion assay, Soft agar colony assay, Tumor Spheroid Assay, Caspase-3/7 Assay, and Western blot analysis	Synergistically enhanced the capacity of EGCG mediated inhibition of self-renewal and metastasis in CSCs	[18]
Quercetin	Pancreatic cancer	In vitro study—CSCs enriched AsPC1 and AsPC1. Patient-derived pancreatic tissue (ex vivo study)	Immunofluorescence and time-lapse microscopy, microRNA microarray analysis, bioinformatics and computational analysis, qRT-PCR, Western blot	Inhibition of self-renewal and proliferation by converting symmetric division of CSCs in asymmetric via induction of miR-200-3p which is responsible to modulate Notch signaling	[204]

			analysis, Self-renewal and differentiation assays		
Quercetin-3 methyl ether	Breast cancer (triple-negative and hormone-sensitive breast cancer)	CSCs derived from MCF-7 and T47D cell lines	CCK-8 and colony formation assay, Flow cytometry, Wound-healing assay, Transwell assay, Mammosphere formation assay, and Western blotting analysis	Inhibited self-renewal, proliferation, and EMT process (via upregulation of E-cadherin and downregulation of vimentin and MMP-2) Also, cell cycle arrest at the G2-M phase and inhibit sphere formation and reduce stemness markers of CSCs Induces phosphorylation of PI3K/AKT signaling pathway and decreases expression of Notch 1	[205]
Quercetin	Gastric cancer	Gastric CSCs from MGC803 parental cells.	Colony formation assay, RT-qPCR, MTT assay, Flow cytometry, Caspase activity assay, and Western blotting	Triggered mitochondrial apoptotic-dependent growth inhibition by the blockade of PI3K/Akt signaling pathway	[206]
Quercetin	Pancreatic cancer	$CD133^{+}$PANC-1 cell line.	MTT assay and immunocytochemistry study	Inhibited EMT *via inhibition of* ACTA-2, IL-1β, and N-cadherin and increased level of vimentin and TNF-α markers	[207]
Quercetin	Breast cancer	CSCs in the MDA-MB-231 cell line	Cell proliferation assay, Apoptosis analysis, Cell cycle assay, Fluorescence-activated cell sorting (FACS), Soft agar colony formation assay, Mammosphere culture, and Western blotting	Suppressed breast CSCs proliferation, self-renewal, and invasiveness Also, downregulated the expression levels of proteins related to tumorigenesis and cancer progression (ALDH-1A1, C-X-C chemokine	[208]

(continued)

Table 7.3 (continued)

Treatment	Target cancer	Cell lines/Model used	Assay used	Conclusion	Refs.
				receptor type 4, mucin 1 and epithelial cell adhesion molecules)	
Quercetin + Midkine (growth factor)	Prostate cancer	$CD44^+/CD133^+$ and $CD44^+$ CSCs from PC3 and LNCaP cells	Image-based cytometer, RT-qPCR, Western blotting, and Transwell migration assay	Synergistically reduced the cell survival, induced apoptosis, and caused cell cycle arrest at G1 phase more effectively than the individual via inhibition of phosphorylation of PI3K, AKT, and ERK1/2 along with reduction of the protein expression of p38, ABCG2, and NF-κB	[209]
Quercetin + Doxorubicin	Colorectal cancer	$CD133^+$ CSCs derived from HT29 cell line	MTT cytotoxicity assay and flow cytometry analysis	Chemosensitize the CSCs and bulk tumor cells to doxorubicin in colorectal cancer	[142]
Quercetin + Sulforaphane + EGCG	Advanced pancreatic cancer	CSCs from human established PDA cell lines BxPc-3 and MIA-PaCa2 and human hTERT-HPNE immortalized pancreatic duct cells CRL-1097	Colony-forming assay, Spheroid assay, Western blot analysis, and Transwell migration assay	Induced miR-let-7 in CSCs but not in normal cells Caused inhibition of K-ras which are specifically responsible for inhibition of growth and progression in advanced pancreatic cancer	[210]
Quercetin + Ionizing radiation	Colon cancer	In vitro study in human colon CSCs—$CD133^+$ derived from DLD-1, HT-29; Normal colonic epithelial cell CCD-18co In vivo Tumor xenograft studies using Balb/c nude mice	Cell proliferation assay, DAPI staining and TUNEL assay, Fluorogenic DEVDase assay, Flow cytometry assay, Colonosphere assay, Cell proliferation assay, colony	Reduced the expressions of all five proteins of Υ-secretase complex in CSCs of HT29 and DLD-1 cells Also, reduced the expression of Hes 1 and Notch 1 signaling	[211]

			formation assay and Immunoblotting		
Quercetin + Sulforaphane	Pancreatic cancer	In vitro study using Human pancreatic CSCs ($CD44^+$/$CD24^+$/ESA^+)	Tumor spheroid assay, Soft agar colony assay, Western blot analysis, and Lentiviral vector-mediated transduction analysis	Quercetin synergized sulforaphane to inhibit self-renewal capacity and metastasis of pancreatic CSCs	[212]

markers in epidermal carcinoma [140]. These combinations are also shown to inhibit the JNK signaling pathway, which further explain their effects on stemness, vasculogenic mimicry properties, and metastatic potential in Du145-III cells (CSCs) derived from Du144-Parental cell line of prostate cancer [141].

Quercetin and EGCG (Epigallocatechin gallate) found in tea, act synergistically and inhibited self-renewal potential along with migration and invasion properties of CSCs of prostate carcinoma by inhibiting TCF/LEF and Gli activities. Quercetin with EGCG lowers the viability of prostate tumor spheroids and lessens the migratory, invasiveness, and colony-forming potential of $CD44^+/CD133^+$ prostate CSCs [18]. The anti-CSCs activity of sulforaphane in combination with quercetin has been found more effective in treatment of pancreatic cancer in the MIA-aCa2 CSCs via inhibiting tumor growth [130]. Quercetin has further drawn attention as a potential CSCs targeting therapeutic agent in colon cancer by inhibiting the proliferation of $CD133^+$ colon CSCs and also increasing the chemosensitivity to doxorubicin in in vitro study [142].

Furthermore, the combined effect of cisplatin and quercetin in head and neck cancer was found promising in drug-resistant cases of cisplatin therapy. SCC25 oral squamous cisplatin-resistant CSCs were implanted into nude mice. They significantly inhibited the tumor growth compared with cisplatin or control alone and chemosensitized the CSCs [143] (Table 7.3).

7.5.3 Silibinin

Silibinin is a flavonolignan obtained from the seeds and fruits of milk thistle plant *Silybum marianum* (Asteraceae) and has been used for the treatment of various types of liver ailment [144]. Previous investigations have shown its strong chemopreventive abilities in various types of cancers [6, 145–149] (Table 7.4). Silibinin has exemplified its action to inhibit colon CSCs in in vitro and ex vivo models and prevent the self-renewal and sphere formation of CSCs by suppressing the PP2Ac/AKT Ser473/mTOR pathway [150]. This is further supported by another study in which silibinin decreased the number and colon sphere formation of CSCs in colorectal cancer by interfering with kinetics and shifted the cell division process towards asymmetric type (generating one CSCs and one first-generation progenitor cell) [151]. Silibinin was found to be effective in colon cancer cell line via blockage of β-catenin Wnt signaling pathway. It downregulates β-catenin gene and protein expression in CSCs. Silibinin also significantly suppressed the proliferation of CSCs by inducing apoptosis by increasing the Bax/Bcl-2 ratio. It has further shown downregulation of stemness markers of CSCs like CD133, CD44, BMI1, ALDH1, and doublecortin-like kinase 1. Additionally, it has the ability to inhibit migration by attenuation of EMT through decreased expression of N-cadherin and vimentin along with increased expression of E-cadherin [152].

The nanoformulation of silibinin has inhibited proliferation and migration of CSCs by induction of apoptosis using MIA-PaCa pancreatic cell line through suppression of some onco-miRs (miR-155, miR-222, and miR-21) and upregulation

Table 7.4 Anticancer potential of silibinin targeting CSCs

Treatment	Cancer target	Cell line/Model used	Assay used	Conclusion	Refs.
Silibinin	Colorectal Cancer	In vitro study in HCT-116 cell lines	MTT assay, Colony formation assay, RT-qPCR, Western blot, Migration, and Sphere formation assay	Induction of apoptosis, suppression of migration and elimination of CSCs, attenuation of EMT-related markers via blocking of Wnt signaling pathway	[152]
Silibinin	Pancreatic cancer	In vitro study in MIA-PaCa-2 cell line	Hanging drop technique and staining of CD133, CD24, and CD44 biomarkers	Induced apoptosis by upregulation of apoptotic genes Inhibited migration and proliferation via downregulation of AKT3, MASPINE, and SERPINEA12. Suppression of some miRs such as miR-155, miR-222, and miR-21 and upregulation of miR-34a, miR-126, and miR-let7b in MIA-PaCa-2 cells	[153]
Silibinin + 5FU	Colon cancer	In vitro study in HCT116-derived $CD44^+$ CSCs	Western blotting, Sphere forming assay, Wound-healing assay, Flow cytometry analysis, Propidium Iodide staining for nuclear morphology	Inhibit cell proliferation via decreasing CD44v6, Nanog, CTNNB1, and CDKN2A expression along with increased E-cadherin. Inhibit sphere formation, cell migration, activate apoptotic and autophagy cell death May inhibit PI3K/MAPK dual activation and arrest the cell cycle at G0/G1 phase for reducing stemness of CSCs	[154]
Silibinin	Colorectal cancer	In vitro study in $CD44^+EpCAM^{high}$, $CD44^+EpCAM^{low}$, $CD44^-EpCAM^{high}$, and $CD44^-EpCAM^{low}$ from human	Sphere cluster formation assays and RT-qPCR array	Decrease the number of CSCs Inhibitory effect on both number and size of colon spheres by decreasing self-renewal properties, blockage of	[151]

(continued)

Table 7.4 (continued)

Treatment	Cancer target	Cell line/Model used	Assay used	Conclusion	Refs.
		Colorectal cancer cell lines SW480, HT29, and LoVo		IL-4/-6 signaling, and transformation of $CD44^+$ population into a CD44- phenotype	
Silibinin	Colorectal cancer	Ex vivo study in colorectal $CD133^+$ CSCs isolated from a primary tumor of a female patient with Duke C3 colorectal Adenocarcinoma and HT-29 cell line	Counting sphere numbers, Flow cytometry, and Immunofluorescence	Inhibited colon CSCs self-renewal and sphere formation by suppressing the PP2Ac/AKT Ser473/mTOR pathway	[150]
Silibinin + Sorafenib	Hepatic cancer	In vitro study in Human hepatocellular carcinoma cells SMMC-7721, Bel-7402, Bel-7404, HepG2, MHCC97H, MHCC97L, and LM-3 cells. Mouse hepatocellular carcinoma Hepa1-6 and H22 cells. In vivo subcutaneous transplantation tumor model	MTT assay, Western blot analysis, Apoptosis analysis, Clone formation assay, TUNEL assay, and Flow cytometric analysis	Inhibited the formation and self-renewal of hepatocellular CSCs by downregulating the expression of NANOG and Krueppel-like factor 4. Also, activated apoptosis by decreasing anti-apoptotic proteins Bcl-2 and Mcl-1 and inhibit proliferation. Improve resistance of sorafenib via deactivation of STAT3/AKT/ERK signaling pathway	[144]

of some tumor suppressive miRs (miR-34a, miR-126, and miR-let7b) [153]. Moreover, silibinin also has a synergistic effect with other therapeutics. Silibinin in combination with sorafenib has shown a synergistic effect through inhibition of phosphorylation of STAT3/ERK/AKT pathway. This leads to inhibited sphere formation and self-renewal of CSCs in hepatic carcinoma [144] (Table 7.4). The combination of silibinin and 5-FU has demonstrated inhibition of CD44v6 (isoform of CD44) which resulted in weakened stemness characteristic of colon CSCs. CD44v6 is a functional biomarker responsible for cancer progression, initiation of metastatic process, resistance to conventional therapeutics, relapse, and associated with poor survival in patients with colon cancer [154].

7.5.4 Apigenin

Apigenin, a common polyphenolic dietary flavone, is abundantly present in many fruits, vegetables, and Chinese medicinal herbs. Evidence from in vitro and in vivo studies has shown its anticancer potential in multiple types of malignancies such as brain tumor, ovarian cancer, lung carcinoma, prostate cancer, breast cancer, and other tumors [104, 105, 155–157]. Recently, the anticancer effect of apigenin has been widely investigated via targeting sub-populated CSCs. Also, it reduced the toxicity of chemotherapeutic agents. Apigenin has been reported to suppress various human cancers in in vitro and in vivo models by targeting multiple biological processes such as triggering cell apoptosis and autophagy, inducing cell cycle arrest, and suppressing cell migration and invasion. This chapter also includes the most recent advancement of apigenin and its synergistic effect with other chemotherapeutic agents by targeting CSCs along with attenuation of involved signaling pathways (Table 7.5). The use of apigenin with chemotherapeutics has overcome the cancer drug resistance or may reduce the toxicities [158]. The glycosidal form of apigenin, Isovitexin (apigenin-6-C-glucoside), has also exhibited its anticancer potential against CSCs in hepatic carcinoma. It decreases the progression of carcinogenicity and stemness by downregulating FoxM1 via inhibition of manganese superoxide dismutase [159]. Isovitexin also suppressed sphere, colony formation, and decreased CD44+ cell population along with suppressed the level of ABCG2, ALDH1, and NANOG mRNA in SK-Hep-1 spheroids of hepatocellular carcinoma by upregulating miR-34a expression [160]. It has the ability to inhibit osteosarcoma by decreasing CSCs population in in vivo model. It has shown to repressed sphere formation, induced apoptotic cell death, and reduced mRNA levels in CSCs derived from U2OS-SC and MG63-SC cells [161]. Studies of apigenin in CSCs are presented in Table 7.5.

7.5.5 Miscellaneous Flavonoids Targeting CSCs

There is limited evidence exists on other flavonoids which have shown their preventive effect against CSCs via modulating signaling pathways involved in the

Table 7.5 Anticancer potential of apigenin targeting CSCs

Treatment	Cancer target	Cell lines/Model used	Assay used	Conclusion	Refs.
Apigenin	Brain tumor	In vitro study in Human GBM CSCs-$CD133^+$ U87MG and U373MG cells	Cell growth assay, Invasion assay, Western blot analysis, Wound-healing assay, and migration assay	Suppressed the self-renewal capacity, cell growth, clonogenicity, and invasiveness of CSCs via suppression of c-Met Signaling pathway	[213]
Apigenin	Ovarian cancer	In vitro study in SKOV-3 cell line-derived CSCs	Tumor sphere formation assay, si-RNA and plasmid DNA transfection, and Western blot analysis	Inhibited self-renewal capacity and downregulated the expression of Gli1 via inhibition of CK2α proteins	[157]
Apigenin + Cisplatin	Lung cancer	In vitro study in Non-small cell lung CSCs—$CD133^+$ A549R cells	MTT assay, FACS analysis, Western blot analysis, and si-RNA transfection	Synergistically enhanced antitumor effect of Cisplatin in resistant cases of lung Cancer by decreasing population of CSCs via induction of p53expression	[104]
Apigenin	Breast cancer	In vitro study in MDA-MB-231 and MDA-MB-436 cells. In vivo analysis for tumorigenesis	Cell proliferation and Colony formation assay, Mammosphere formation assay, Flow cytometry analysis, Wound-healing and Transwell migration assays, Luciferase reporter assay, RT-PCR analysis. In vivo study of tumorigenic evaluation using female BALB/c nude mice injected with Apigenin-treated of MDA-MB-231	Suppressed the CSCs properties such as decrease in the $CD44^+/CD24^-$ CSCs subpopulation and inhibits mammosphere formation of triple-negative breast cancer cells by inhibiting YAP/TAZ activity	[214]
Apigenin	Head and neck cancer	In vitro study in CSCs derived from HN-30 Ex vivo and in vivo tumorigenesis study using CSCs implanted mice	Semiquantitative RT-PCR and RT-PCR, MTT assay, and flow cytometry	Effectively reduced tumor mass and prevent recurrence by CSCs	[156]

Apigenin + Cisplatin	Prostate cancer	Ex vivo study using $CD44^+$ PCa CSCs isolated from human androgen-independent PC3 PCa cells by using human $CD44^-$PE antibody	MTT assay, RT-qPCR, Western blot analysis, Wound-healing assay, and Image-based Cytometer	Suppressed the phosphorylation of p-PI3K and p-Akt Inhibited the protein expression of NF-kB, and downregulated the cell cycle by upregulating p21, as well as cyclin-dependent kinases CDK-2, -4, and -6 Sensitizes human $CD44^+$ prostate CSCs to cisplatin therapy	[105]
Apigenin	Prostate cancer	Prostate CSCs ($CD44^+$) from human prostate cancer PC3 cells	MTT assay, Annexin V/propidium iodide (PI) binding assay, RT-qPCR, Protein extraction, and Western blot analysis	Inhibited CSCs survival due to significant increase of p21 and p27 Induced apoptosis via activation of extrinsic pathway Also, suppressed migration and invasion of CSCs via inhibition of MMP-2, MMP-9, snail and slug Reduced pluripotency marker Oct3/4 protein expression via downregulation of PI3K/Akt/NF-κB signaling	[155]

maintenance of CSCs. These flavanoids are broussoflavonol B, icaritin, casticin, pomiferin, morusin, baicalein, ugonin, wogonin, luteolin, and kaempferol.

Broussoflavonol B (5,7,3′,4′- Tetrahydroxy-3-methoxy-6,8-diprenylflavone) is chemically prenylflavone isolated from *Broussonetia papyrifera* (Moraceae) commonly known as Paper mulberry. It inhibits the growth of ER-positive (estrogen positive) breast cancer in MCF7 cells probably through downregulation of ER-α36 expression. [64, 103, 162]. The knockdown of expression of ER-α36 by broussoflavonol B inhibits tumor sphere formation and reduced the count of HER2-CSCs which help in treating the therapy-resistant cases [103]. Jeong and Ryu reported its anticancer potential in pancreatic cancer via suppression of the FoxM1 and its target genes to induce G_0/G_1 phase arrest in p53 mutant PANC-1 cells. It also inhibited cell migration and invasion by reducing ERK activity and MMP-2 expression [163] Table 7.6.

Icaritin is a mono-prenylflavonoid derivative (flavonoid skeleton with a lipophilic prenyl side chain) obtained from Chinese herb *Epimedium* Genus having estrogen receptor modulator effect and hence called phytoestrogen. Icaritin and its analogs regulate cell growth of various types of cancers such as breast cancer, esophageal cancer, chronic myeloid leukemia (CML), and lung carcinoma [103, 164–167] Table 7.6.

Morusin, a prenylated flavonoids obtained from root bark of *Morus australis* (Moraceae) possess anticancer effect on various type of malignancies [168–170]. It showed inhibition of the growth and migration of human cervical CSCs from HeLa cell line through attenuation of NF-kBp65 activity mediated apoptotic induction [168]. Further, it showed promising anticancer potential in aggressive type of brain cancer, i.e., glioblastoma. Morusin inhibits glioblastoma CSCs by induction of apoptosis by upregulating the protein expressions of PPARϒ, Bax, and caspase-3. Additionally, it downregulates the expressions of Bcl-2 and stemness markers such as CD133, nestin, Oct4, and Sox2 and attenuates adipocyte trans-differentiation [171]. Recently, morusin was found to be a potential anticancer agent in laryngeal cancer by inhibiting the stemness and proliferation of CSCs [172] (Table 7.6).

Casticin (3′,5-dihydroxy-3,4′,6,7-tetramethoxyflavone) is a natural polymethoxy-flavone also called as vitexicarpin, isolated from the fruits of *Vitex trifolia* (Lamiaceae) [173]. Casticin has exemplified its anticancer potential via targeting CSCs and modulating their stemness related proteins, AMPK/FoxO3 signaling pathway activation, blocking Wnt/catenin signaling pathways and inhibiting EMT process by regulating expressions of E-cadherin, MMPs and N-cadherin in various types of cancers like liver cancer, lung cancer, and nasopharyngeal cancer [173–175] Table 7.6.

Other flavonoids having anti-CSCs effect are pomiferin which is isolated from the fruit of the *Maclura pomifera* (Moraceae) effective in glioblastoma [176]. Ugonin J and K (two cyclohexylmethyl flavonoids) isolated from the rhizomes of *Helminthostachys zeylanica* (Ophioglossaceae) are effective in breast cancer [177]. Naringenin which is obtained from tomato and citrus fruits acts as a phytoestrogen and is effective in inhibition of ER^+ breast cancer CSCs [178]. Its seminatural derivative, named 6-C-(E-phenylethenyl) naringenin was found effective in the

Table 7.6 Anticancer potential of the miscellaneous flavonoids targeting CSCs

Treatment	Cancer target	Cell lines/Model used	Assay used	Conclusion	Refs.
Broussoflavonol B	Tripple negative breast cancer	In vitro study in CSCs derived from MDA-MB-231 cell line	Western blot assay, Cell cycle, and Cell death analysis	Exhibited growth inhibitory activity via induction of differentiation of CSCs mainly into the luminal epithelial lineage	[162]
Broussoflavonol B	Breast cancer	In vitro study in transfected HER2-CSCs	Tumor sphere formation assay, Flow cytometry analysis, and Western blot analysis	ER-α36 knockdown significantly reduced the numbers of the $CD44^{+}/CD24^{-}$ CSCs and tumor sphere formation ability Treat Tamoxifen-resistant cases of ER^{+} breast cancer	[103]
Icaritin	Breast cancer	In vitro study in $ALDH^{-high}$ positive CSCs from the MDA-MB-453 and MCF7 cells	Cell growth assay, Western blot assay, Cell cycle, and cell death analysis	Reduce the number of CSCs. Chemosensitized CSCs to tamoxifen via activation of MAPK/ERK pathway	[164]
Icaritin	Esophageal cancer	In vitro study in $CD133^{+}$ ECA109 cell line	CCK-8 method and Transwell assay	Inhibit esophageal CSCs by promoting cell apoptosis Downregulated the level of Hedgehog, Smoothen and Gli in Hedgehog pathway, and upregulated GSK3β. Downregulated Wnt and β-catenin in Wnt pathway	[167]
Icaritin analog SNG1153	Lung cancer	In vitro study in H460 CSCs and in vivo study using mice injected with CSCs of H460	CCK-8 assay, Colony formation assay, Cell apoptosis assay, Tumorsphere culture, Western blot analysis, and FACS assay	Exhibited anti-growth activity and inhibited tumor shpere formation in CSCs via downregulating Wnt/β-catenin signaling pathway	[166]

(continued)

Table 7.6 (continued)

Treatment	Cancer target	Cell lines/Model used	Assay used	Conclusion	Refs.
Icaritin analog SNGI 153 +TKIs tyrosine kinase inhibitor (imatinib mesylate/dasatinib)	Chronic myeloid leukemia (CML)	In vitro study in $BCR\text{-}ABL^-$ LSCs and $BCR\text{-}ABL^-T315I$ mutant cells. In vivo study on SNG mice	Viability and apoptosis assays	Eliminate TKI-insensitive LSCs In vivo study Elimination of infiltrated $BCR\text{-}ABL^+$ blast cells and enhances survival of mice via inhibition of the downstream RAS/MAPK pathway	[165]
Morusin	Glioblastoma	In vitro study in CSCs of Human GBM cell line In vivo study in male BALB/C-nu/nu mice	Cell cytotoxicity assay, Neurosphere formation inhibition, Adipogenic differentiation, Apoptosis induction, and Tumor growth inhibition in vivo assays	Potential to inhibit human Glioblastoma CSCs growth through stemness attenuation, adipocyte trans-differentiation and apoptosis induction	[171]
Morusin	Cervical cancer	In vitro study in cervical CSCs-SFCs derived from Human cervical cancer cell line HeLa	Cell proliferation, Tumor sphere formation and transwell assay, Apoptotic death with DAPI staining, and Western blotting	Potential to kill CSCs and inhibits growth and migration through attenuation of NF-κB activity-mediated apoptosis induction	[168]
Morusin	Laryngeal cancer	In vitro study in $CD133^+$ laryngeal CSCs	Tumor sphere formation assay, Transwell assay, MTT assay and Immunofluorescence staining, RT-qPCR, and Western blot	Weakened stemness phenotype of CSCs may be due to downregulation effect on stemness-associated markers	[172]
Casticin	Liver cancer	In vitro study in liver CSCs $CD133^+$ SFCs of MHCC97 cell line In vivo study—	Sphere formation assay, MTT assay, and Western blot analysis Tumorigenic assay in vivo	Inhibited proliferation and self-renewal of liver CSCs via blocking the Wnt/β-catenin signaling pathway	[175]

		Tumorigenicity assay in Balb/c-nu mice			
Casticin	Lung cancer	In vitro study in lung CSCs-SFCs rich in CD133, CD44, and ALDH1 of A549 cell line In vivo study—Tumorigenicity assay in Balb/c-nu immunodeficient mice	Matrigel invasion assay, Sphere forming and self-renewal assay, MMP-9 activity assay, Western blot analysis, MTT assay	Suppresses self-renewal and invasion of CSCs via decreased CD133, CD44 and ALDH1 protein expression and reduced MMP-9 activity Also, downregulate AKT phosphorylation	[215]
Pomiferin	Gliobastoma	In vitro study in CSCs from human glioma tumor cell lines—$CD133^+$ U373 and U87 cells	Neurosphere Formation Assay, Flow Cytometry Analysis, quantitative RT-PCR, Matrigel Invasion Assay, MTS assay	Inhibited cell viability and reduce $CD133^+$ cell population, sphere formation, and invasion ability of glioma neurosphere cells via downregulation of stemness-associated genes (BIM1, Nestin and Nanog)	[176]
Wogonin	Multiple myeloma	In vitro study in human multiple myeloma CSCs—RPMI8226	CCK assay, Western blotting assay, Apoptosis, and cell *cycle analysis with Flow* cytometry	Modulated the expression of ABCG2 protein and decreases *the number of human multiple* myeloma CSCs	[183]
Wogonin	Osteosarcoma	In vitro study in $CD133^+$CAL72 human osteosarcoma CSCs	Cell migration and invasion assays, Colony assay, Wound-healing assay, Hoechst 33342 staining, Sphere formation assay, Western blotting, and Gelatin zymography	Inhibiting migration and invasion by suppressing metastasis and induced apoptosis in $CD133^+$CSCs via inhibiting MMP-9 expression	[192]
Wogonin	Osteosarcoma (Bone cancer)	In vitro study in $CD133^+$Cal72 osteosarcoma CSCs	MTT assay, Transwell assay, Sphere formation assay, Flow cytometry,	Increased ROS level and inhibited stemness by regulating ROS-related signaling	[194]

(continued)

Table 7.6 (continued)

Treatment	Cancer target	Cell lines/Model used	Assay used	Conclusion	Refs.
			Immunocytochemistry and Western blotting	Also, downregulated the expression of PRX5 and induced ROS Reduced the expression of CSCs-related genes MYC and OCT3/4	
Wogonoside (main in vivo metabolite of wogonin)	Cutaneous squamous cell carcinoma	In vitro study in SCL-1 and SCC12 cell lines In vivo model using male BALB/c nude mice	Colony Formation Assay, Transwell Assay, Immunofluorescence Assay, Microtube Formation Assay, Flow Cytometry, Tumor sphere formation Assay, and Western Blot Analysis	Efficiently abolished the $CD133^+$CSCs and suppress the expression of CSCs markers (ALDH1, SOX-2, Oct4 and CD44) via suppression of PI3K/AKT and Wnt/β-catenin pathways	[195]
Ugonin J and K	Breast cancer	In vivo xenograft model injecting NANOG overexpressed MCF-7 cells (CSCs) into mammary fat pads of female SCID mice	Tumor xenograft analysis	Suppressed self-renewal of CSCs via downregulation of NANOG through p53 activation	[177]
Baicalein	Pancreatic cancer	In vitro study in pancreatic CSCs—$CD44^+CD24^+$ PANC-1 cells In vivo study in female BALB/c nude mice	Cell viability and apoptosis assays, Wound-healing assay, Sphere forming assay, Colony formation assay, and Western blot analysis In vivo analysis—Xenograft tumor and Immunohistochemistry analysis	Induced apoptosis and inhibited self-renewal of CSCs via modulation of Sonic Hedgehog pathway	[180]
Baicalein	Breast cancer	In vitro study in treatment-resistant Tripple Negative	MTT assay, Clonogenic assay, Mammosphere Assay,	Inhibited CSCs and metastasis in TNBC via induction of	[182]

		breast cancer (TNBC) CSCs-MDA-MB-231/IR from parental MDA-MB-231 cells.	Wound-Healing Assay, Invasion Assay, Flow cytometry, Western blotting, Transcriptomic Analysis, and Pathway and gene expression analysis	IFIT2 which has role in apoptosis signaling Also, inhibited developing resistance and chemosensitized CSCs	
Baicalein	Liver cancer	In vitro study in Huh7 cell line Ex vivo study in CD133$^+$CSCs isolated from HCV Core Tg mice fed alcohol and Spnb$^{+/-}$ mice, NS5A Tg mice fed Western diet Ex vivo study in HCC tissues excised from alcoholic HCV infected patients	Spheroid formation and Clonogenic assays, Patient-derived xenograft analysis	Selectively inhibited self-renewal, stemness, and EMT ability of CSCs via suppression of NANOG, Sox2, and Twist gene expression Also, competitively inhibited GTP binding of SAR1B GTPase essential for autophagy and synergizes cell death caused by mTORC1 inhibition in CSCs. Selectively induced apoptosis in CSCs but not in normal hepatocytes of mice	[181]
Luteolin + Radiation therapy	Oral cancer	In vitro study in oral CSCs-SAS, and GNM cell line	MTT assay, Flow cytometric analysis, Invasion and Colony-forming assay, Enzyme-linked immunosorbent assay and Western blot analysis	Attenuated tumorigenicity of oral CSCs through IL-6/ STAT3 signaling pathway inactivation	[191]
Luteolin	Prostate cancer	In vitro study in human prostate cancer cell lines (PC-3, DU145).	Cell proliferation assay, Drug sensitivity assay, Cell migration assay, Colony formation assay, Sphere	Upregulated FZD6 (Frizzled class receptor) which is the main cause of inhibition of	[167]

(continued)

Table 7.6 (continued)

Treatment	Cancer target	Cell lines/Model used	Assay used	Conclusion	Refs.
		Ex vivo study on human sample	formation assay. q-RTPCR, Immunoblotting, Lentiviral generation and infection, Luciferase reporter assay	Wnt signaling and the stemness in PCa CSCs	
Kaempferol	Breast cancer	In vitro study in MCF-7 breast CSCs	Cell viability assay, quantitative PCR amplification	It was effective in eradication of CSCs in dose-dependent manner and found more effective than docetaxel in downregulation of Oct-4, Nanog, ABCB1, and ALDH1A1 markers of CSCs	[196]

treatment of hepatocellular carcinoma by suppressing Wnt/β-catenin signaling [179]. Baicalein is 5,6,7-trihydroxyflavone, originally isolated from the roots of *Scutellaria baicalensis* (Lamiaceae) possessing anticancer effect by targeting CSCs of pancreatic, liver, multiple myeloma, and breast cancer [180–183] Table 7.6. Luteolin is 3,4,5,7-tetrahydroxyflavone obtained from many dietary plants such as chamomile tea, celery, perilla leaf, and green peppers. The in vitro and in vivo studies showed that it inhibits cancer initiation and progression by interfering with transcription factors and kinases, regulating cell cycle, apoptosis, and inhibiting cell transformation, migration, invasion, and angiogenesis [184–189]. It also has the potential to target CSCs via attenuation of different pathways [167] and also produce a synergistic effect to enhance the anticancer potential of the other chemotherapeutic drugs [190]. Moreover, it is sensitizing the CSCs and treating therapy resistance cases of cancer [141, 191] (Tables 7.3 and 7.6).

Wogonin is an O-methylated flavone found in the roots of *Scutellaria baicalensis* (Lamiaceae). Wogonin has been also used to target CSCs in various malignancies such as osteosarcoma, multiple myeloma, and breast cancer [183, 192–194] by attenuation of EMT markers (MMP-9), regulation of ROS signaling. Wogonoside which is a glycoside of wogonin has shown anticancer potential against cutaneous squamous carcinoma via suppression of PI3K/AKT and Wnt/β-catenin pathway of CSCs [195].

Kaempferol (3,5,7-trihydroxy-2-(4-hydroxyphenyl)-4H-1-benzopyran-4-one) is a phytoestrogen, obtained abundantly from tea, broccoli, apples, strawberries, and beans. It showed an anti-CSCs effect by decreasing breast CSCs derived from MCF-7 cell line and downregulated the markers such as Oct4, Nanog, ABCB1, and ALDH1A1 [196].

The details of studies regarding the inhibitory action of miscellaneous flavonoids in CSCs have been described in Table 7.6.

7.6 Future Prospects of Flavonoids Targeting CSCs in Malignancies

In recent years, there has been much attention towards the inhibition of CSCs to reduce the severeness and resistant cases of cancer. Hence, polyphenolic flavonoids are used to prevent cancer progression via targeting CSCs. Flavonoids are regarded as multifacet phytocompounds possessing plethora of therapeutic effects [181, 197, 198]. There is substantial data available which have shown their potential to eradicate CSCs. However, no evaluation has been conducted in the clinical setting targeted CSCs. Furthermore, the major issue to target the CSCs is the identification of specific markers for a particular type of tumor. The specific markers would provide novel strategies to target the CSCs and inhibit the progression of cancer. Flavonoids also act as epigenetic modifiers by inhibiting early epigenetic alterations and inhibit cancer cell proliferation in in vitro models using cell lines. In various in vitro studies, flavonoids activate the expression of different tumor suppressor genes by epigenetic modifications [199, 200]. However, there is a lack of studies of flavonoids as epigenetic modifiers targeting CSCs maintenance. Hence, there is a need for studies on flavonoids as natural epigenetic modulators for the treatment of cancers targeting CSCs which could represent a promising and valid strategy to inhibit chemoresistance and carcinogenesis. Flavonoids are able to eradicate and chemosensitize the CSCs of various tumors via attenuating many pathways but they suffer from certain limitations such as poor solubility, poor permeability, bitter taste, extensive intestinal metabolism, and instability which diminish their bioavailability. Due to these issues, relatively high dose of flavonoids is required to produce a significant biological response. Strategies are needed to overcome these issues of solubility and thereby improving its oral bioavailability. Chemical modification in the structure of flavonoids may enhance the stability of flavonoids [109, 111, 201–203]. This will help to conduct their clinical trials and enhance their clinical usage. This chapter also described that the combination of flavonoids with conventional therapies could enhance the therapeutic effects and chemoradiosensitize the CSCs in various malignancies [182]. Hence, they may enhance the anticancer potential along with a reduction in resistance.

References

1. Sak K. Cytotoxicity of dietary flavonoids on different human cancer types. Pharmacogn Rev. 2014;8(16):122–46.
2. Chen D, Pamu S, Cui Q, Chan TH, Dou QP. Novel epigallocatechin gallate (EGCG) analogs activate AMP-activated protein kinase pathway and target cancer stem cells. Bioorg Med Chem. 2012;20(9):3031–7.
3. O'Brien-Ball C, Biddle A. Reprogramming to developmental plasticity in cancer stem cells. Dev Biol. 2017;430(2):266–74.
4. Kuşoğlu A, Biray AÇ. Cancer stem cells: a brief review of the current status. Gene. 2019;681:80–5.
5. Al-Hajj M, Wicha MS, Benito-Hernandez A, Morrison SJ, Clarke MF. Prospective identification of tumorigenic breast cancer cells. Proc Natl Acad Sci U S A. 2003;100(7):3983–8.
6. Ting H, Deep G, Agarwal R. Molecular mechanisms of silibinin-mediated cancer chemoprevention with major emphasis on prostate cancer. AAPS J. 2013;15(3):707–16.
7. Hu Y, Fu L. Targeting cancer stem cells: a new therapy to cure cancer patients. Am J Cancer Res. 2012;2(3):340–56.
8. Li Y, Wicha MS, Schwartz SJ, Sun D. Implications of cancer stem cell theory for cancer chemoprevention by natural dietary compounds. J Nutr Biochem. 2011;22(9):799–806.
9. Wang MT, Holderfield M, Galeas J, Delrosario R, To MD, Balmain A, et al. K-ras promotes tumorigenicity through suppression of non-canonical Wnt signaling. Cell. 2015;163 (5):1237–51.
10. Gooding AJ, Schiemann WP. Epithelial-mesenchymal transition programs and cancer stem cell phenotypes: mediators of breast cancer therapy resistance. Mol Cancer Res. 2020;18 (9):1257–70.
11. Visvader JE, Lindeman GJ. Cancer stem cells in solid tumours: accumulating evidence and unresolved questions. Nat Rev Cancer. 2008;8(10):755–68.
12. Wicha MS, Liu S, Dontu G. Cancer stem cells: an old idea – a paradigm shift. Cancer Res. 2006;66(4):1883–90. discussion 95-6
13. Dai Z, Nair V, Khan M, Ciolino HP. Pomegranate extract inhibits the proliferation and viability of MMTV-Wnt-1 mouse mammary cancer stem cells in vitro. Oncol Rep. 2010;24 (4):1087–91.

14. Ning Y, Luo C, Ren K, Quan M, Cao J. FOXO3a-mediated suppression of the self-renewal capacity of sphere-forming cells derived from the ovarian cancer SKOV3 cell line by 7-difluoromethoxyl-5,4'-di-n-octyl genistein. Mol Med Rep. 2014;9(5):1982–8.
15. Chen Y, Zaman MS, Deng G, Majid S, Saini S, Liu J, et al. MicroRNAs 221/222 and genistein-mediated regulation of ARHI tumor suppressor gene in prostate cancer. Cancer Prev Res (Philadelphia, PA). 2011;4(1):76–86.
16. Zhang L, Li L, Jiao M, Wu D, Wu K, Li X, et al. Genistein inhibits the stemness properties of prostate cancer cells through targeting Hedgehog-Gli1 pathway. Cancer Lett. 2012;323 (1):48–57.
17. Nishimura N, Hartomo TB, Pham TV, Lee MJ, Yamamoto T, Morikawa S, et al. Epigallocatechin gallate inhibits sphere formation of neuroblastoma BE(2)-C cells. Environ Health Prev Med. 2012;17(3):246–51.
18. Tang SN, Singh C, Nall D, Meeker D, Shankar S, Srivastava RK. The dietary bioflavonoid quercetin synergizes with epigallocatechin gallate (EGCG) to inhibit prostate cancer stem cell characteristics, invasion, migration and epithelial-mesenchymal transition. J Mol Signal. 2010;5:14.
19. Tang SN, Fu J, Nall D, Rodova M, Shankar S, Srivastava RK. Inhibition of sonic hedgehog pathway and pluripotency maintaining factors regulate human pancreatic cancer stem cell characteristics. Int J Cancer. 2012;131(1):30–40.
20. Sharif T, Auger C, Bronner C, Alhosin M, Klein T, Etienne-Selloum N, et al. Selective proapoptotic activity of polyphenols from red wine on teratocarcinoma cell, a model of cancer stem-like cell. Invest New Drugs. 2011;29(2):239–47.
21. Lin CH, Shen YA, Hung PH, Yu YB, Chen YJ. Epigallocatechin gallate, polyphenol present in green tea, inhibits stem-like characteristics and epithelial-mesenchymal transition in nasopharyngeal cancer cell lines. BMC Complement Altern Med. 2012;12:201.
22. Quan MF, Xiao LH, Liu ZH, Guo H, Ren KQ, Liu F, et al. 8-bromo-7-methoxychrysin inhibits properties of liver cancer stem cells via downregulation of β-catenin. World J Gastroenterol. 2013;19(43):7680–95.
23. Alvero AB, Montagna MK, Holmberg JC, Craveiro V, Brown D, Mor G. Targeting the mitochondria activates two independent cell death pathways in ovarian cancer stem cells. Mol Cancer Ther. 2011;10(8):1385–93.
24. Hsu HS, Lin JH, Huang WC, Hsu TW, Su K, Chiou SH, et al. Chemoresistance of lung cancer stemlike cells depends on activation of Hsp27. Cancer. 2011;117(7):1516–28.
25. Nieto MA, Huang RY, Jackson RA, Thiery JP. EMT: 2016. Cell. 2016;166(1):21–45.
26. Shibue T, Weinberg RA. EMT, CSCs, and drug resistance: the mechanistic link and clinical implications. Nat Rev Clin Oncol. 2017;14(10):611–29.
27. Chiang SP, Cabrera RM, Segall JE. Tumor cell intravasation. Am J Physiol Cell Physiol. 2016;311(1):C1–c14.
28. Jiang J, Tang YL, Liang XH. EMT: a new vision of hypoxia promoting cancer progression. Cancer Biol Ther. 2011;11(8):714–23.
29. Mitra A, Mishra L, Li S. EMT, CTCs and CSCs in tumor relapse and drug-resistance. Oncotarget. 2015;6(13):10697–711.
30. De Craene B, Berx G. Regulatory networks defining EMT during cancer initiation and progression. Nat Rev Cancer. 2013;13(2):97–110.
31. Leopold PL, Vincent J, Wang H. A comparison of epithelial-to-mesenchymal transition and re-epithelialization. Semin Cancer Biol. 2012;22(5-6):471–83.
32. Reid PA, Wilson P, Li Y, Marcu LG, Bezak E. Current understanding of cancer stem cells: Review of their radiobiology and role in head and neck cancers. Head Neck. 2017;39 (9):1920–32.
33. Batlle E, Clevers H. Cancer stem cells revisited. Nat Med. 2017;23(10):1124–34.
34. Bragado P, Estrada Y, Parikh F, Krause S, Capobianco C, Farina HG, et al. TGF-β2 dictates disseminated tumour cell fate in target organs through TGF-β-RIII and p38α/β signalling. Nat Cell Biol. 2013;15(11):1351–61.

35. You JS, Jones PA. Cancer genetics and epigenetics: two sides of the same coin? Cancer Cell. 2012;22(1):9–20.
36. Avgustinova A, Benitah SA. The epigenetics of tumour initiation: cancer stem cells and their chromatin. Curr Opin Genet Dev. 2016;36:8–15.
37. Sun XX, Yu Q. Intra-tumor heterogeneity of cancer cells and its implications for cancer treatment. Acta Pharmacol Sin. 2015;36(10):1219–27.
38. Meacham CE, Morrison SJ. Tumour heterogeneity and cancer cell plasticity. Nature. 2013;501 (7467):328–37.
39. Lipinska N, Romaniuk A, Paszel-Jaworska A, Toton E, Kopczynski P, Rubis B. Telomerase and drug resistance in cancer. Cell Mol Life Sci. 2017;74(22):4121–32.
40. Yan J, Zhou Y, Chen D, Li L, Yang X, You Y, et al. Effects of mitochondrial translocation of telomerase on drug resistance in hepatocellular carcinoma cells. J Cancer. 2015;6(2):151–9.
41. Gopalan V, Islam F, Lam AK. Surface markers for the identification of cancer stem cells. Methods Mol Biol (Clifton, NJ). 2018;1692:17–29.
42. Nunes T, Hamdan D, Leboeuf C, El Bouchtaoui M, Gapihan G, Nguyen TT, et al. Targeting cancer stem cells to overcome chemoresistance. Int J Mol Sci. 2018;19(2):4036.
43. Ailles LE, Weissman IL. Cancer stem cells in solid tumors. Curr Opin Biotechnol. 2007;18 (5):460–6.
44. Carvalho MJ, Laranjo M, Abrantes AM, Torgal I, Botelho MF, Oliveira CF. Clinical translation for endometrial cancer stem cells hypothesis. Cancer Metastasis Rev. 2015;34(3):401–16.
45. Leccia F, Del Vecchio L, Mariotti E, Di Noto R, Morel AP, Puisieux A, et al. ABCG2, a novel antigen to sort luminal progenitors of BRCA1- breast cancer cells. Mol Cancer. 2014;13:213.
46. Soltanian S, Matin MM. Cancer stem cells and cancer therapy. Tumour Biol. 2011;32 (3):425–40.
47. Vilchez V, Turcios L, Zaytseva Y, Stewart R, Lee EY, Maynard E, et al. Cancer stem cell marker expression alone and in combination with microvascular invasion predicts poor prognosis in patients undergoing transplantation for hepatocellular carcinoma. Am J Surg. 2016;212(2):238–45.
48. Kure S, Matsuda Y, Hagio M, Ueda J, Naito Z, Ishiwata T. Expression of cancer stem cell markers in pancreatic intraepithelial neoplasias and pancreatic ductal adenocarcinomas. Int J Oncol. 2012;41(4):1314–24.
49. Salnikov AV, Gladkich J, Moldenhauer G, Volm M, Mattern J, Herr I. CD133 is indicative for a resistance phenotype but does not represent a prognostic marker for survival of non-small cell lung cancer patients. Int J Cancer. 2010;126(4):950–8.
50. Svachova H, Pour L, Sana J, Kovarova L, Raja KR, Hajek R. Stem cell marker nestin is expressed in plasma cells of multiple myeloma patients. Leuk Res. 2011;35(8):1008–13.
51. Isfoss BL, Busch C, Hermelin H, Vermedal AT, Kile M, Braathen GJ, et al. Stem cell marker-positive stellate cells and mast cells are reduced in benign-appearing bladder tissue in patients with urothelial carcinoma. Virchows Arch. 2014;464(4):473–88.
52. Fisher R, Pusztai L, Swanton C. Cancer heterogeneity: implications for targeted therapeutics. Br J Cancer. 2013;108(3):479–85.
53. Fulawka L, Donizy P, Halon A. Cancer stem cells – the current status of an old concept: literature review and clinical approaches. Biol Res. 2014;47(1):66.
54. Kandhari K, Agraval H, Sharma A, Yadav UC, Singh RP. Flavonoids and cancer stem cells maintenance and growth. Functional food and human health. New York: Springer; 2018. p. 587–622.
55. Koury J, Zhong L, Hao J. Targeting signaling pathways in cancer stem cells for cancer treatment. Stem Cells Int. 2017;2017:2925869.
56. Chi HC, Tsai CY, Tsai MM, Yeh CT, Lin KH. Roles of long noncoding RNAs in recurrence and metastasis of radiotherapy-resistant cancer stem cells. Int J Mol Sci. 2017;18(9) https://doi.org/10.3390/ijms18091903.

57. Paryan M, Mohammadi-Yeganeh S, Samiee SM, Soleimani M, Arefian E, Azadmanesh K, et al. Investigation of deregulated genes of Notch signaling pathway in human T cell acute lymphoblastic leukemia cell lines and clinical samples. Mol Biol Rep. 2013;40(10):5531–40.
58. Matsui WH. Cancer stem cell signaling pathways. Medicine. 2016;95(1 Suppl 1):S8–s19.
59. Venkatesh V, Nataraj R, Thangaraj GS, Karthikeyan M, Gnanasekaran A, Kaginelli SB, et al. Targeting Notch signalling pathway of cancer stem cells. Stem Cell Investig. 2018;5:5.
60. Pan Y, Ma S, Cao K, Zhou S, Zhao A, Li M, et al. Therapeutic approaches targeting cancer stem cells. J Cancer Res Ther. 2018;14(7):1469–75.
61. Katoh Y, Katoh M. Hedgehog signaling, epithelial-to-mesenchymal transition and miRNA (review). Int J Mol Med. 2008;22(3):271–5.
62. He HC, Chen JH, Chen XB, Qin GQ, Cai C, Liang YX, et al. Expression of hedgehog pathway components is associated with bladder cancer progression and clinical outcome. Pathol Oncol Res. 2012;18(2):349–55.
63. Takezaki T, Hide T, Takanaga H, Nakamura H, Kuratsu J, Kondo T. Essential role of the Hedgehog signaling pathway in human glioma-initiating cells. Cancer Sci. 2011;102 (7):1306–12.
64. Zhang C, Li C, He F, Cai Y, Yang H. Identification of CD44+CD24+ gastric cancer stem cells. J Cancer Res Clin Oncol. 2011;137(11):1679–86.
65. Islam SS, Mokhtari RB, Noman AS, Uddin M, Rahman MZ, Azadi MA, et al. Sonic hedgehog (Shh) signaling promotes tumorigenicity and stemness via activation of epithelial-to-mesenchymal transition (EMT) in bladder cancer. Mol Carcinog. 2016;55(5):537–51.
66. Merchant AA, Matsui W. Targeting Hedgehog – a cancer stem cell pathway. Clin Cancer Res. 2010;16(12):3130–40.
67. Clement V, Sanchez P, de Tribolet N, Radovanovic I, Ruiz i Altaba A. HEDGEHOG-GLI1 signaling regulates human glioma growth, cancer stem cell self-renewal, and tumorigenicity. Curr Biol. 2007;17(2):165–72.
68. Zhang B, Jiang T, Shen S, She X, Tuo Y, Hu Y, et al. Cyclopamine disrupts tumor extracellular matrix and improves the distribution and efficacy of nanotherapeutics in pancreatic cancer. Biomaterials. 2016;103:12–21.
69. Iovine V, Mori M, Calcaterra A, Berardozzi S, Botta B. One hundred faces of cyclopamine. Curr Pharm Des. 2016;22(12):1658–81.
70. Fu Q, Liu P, Sun X, Huang S, Han F, Zhang L, et al. Ribonucleic acid interference knockdown of IL-6 enhances the efficacy of cisplatin in laryngeal cancer stem cells by down-regulating the IL-6/STAT3/HIF1 pathway. Cancer Cell Int. 2017;17:79.
71. Ulasov IV, Nandi S, Dey M, Sonabend AM, Lesniak MS. Inhibition of Sonic hedgehog and Notch pathways enhances sensitivity of CD133(+) glioma stem cells to temozolomide therapy. Mol Med (Cambridge, MA). 2011;17(1-2):103–12.
72. Bahra M, Kamphues C, Boas-Knoop S, Lippert S, Esendik U, Schüller U, et al. Combination of hedgehog signaling blockage and chemotherapy leads to tumor reduction in pancreatic adenocarcinomas. Pancreas. 2012;41(2):222–9.
73. Anastas JN, Moon RT. WNT signalling pathways as therapeutic targets in cancer. Nat Rev Cancer. 2013;13(1):11–26.
74. Kahn M. Can we safely target the WNT pathway? Nat Rev Drug Discov. 2014;13(7):513–32.
75. Clevers H, Loh KM, Nusse R. Stem cell signaling. An integral program for tissue renewal and regeneration: Wnt signaling and stem cell control. Science (New York, NY). 2014;346 (6205):1248012.
76. Holland JD, Klaus A, Garratt AN. Birchmeier WJCoicb. Wnt signal stem cancer stem cells. 2013;25(2):254–64.
77. Jang GB, Kim JY, Cho SD, Park KS, Jung JY, Lee HY, et al. Blockade of Wnt/β-catenin signaling suppresses breast cancer metastasis by inhibiting CSC-like phenotype. Sci Rep. 2015;5:12465.
78. Pandit TS, Kennette W, Mackenzie L, Zhang G, Al-Katib W, Andrews J, et al. Lymphatic metastasis of breast cancer cells is associated with differential gene expression profiles that

predict cancer stem cell-like properties and the ability to survive, establish and grow in a foreign environment. Int J Oncol. 2009;35(2):297–308.
79. Borcherding N, Kusner D, Kolb R, Xie Q, Li W, Yuan F, et al. Paracrine WNT5A signaling inhibits expansion of tumor-initiating cells. Cancer Res. 2015;75(10):1972–82.
80. Barker N. Adult intestinal stem cells: critical drivers of epithelial homeostasis and regeneration. Nat Rev Mol Cell Biol. 2014;15(1):19–33.
81. Van Camp JK, Beckers S, Zegers D, Van Hul W. Wnt signaling and the control of human stem cell fate. Stem Cell Rev Rep. 2014;10(2):207–29.
82. Yang K, Wang X, Zhang H, Wang Z, Nan G, Li Y, et al. The evolving roles of canonical WNT signaling in stem cells and tumorigenesis: implications in targeted cancer therapies. Lab Invest. 2016;96(2):116–36.
83. Qin L, Yin YT, Zheng FJ, Peng LX, Yang CF, Bao YN, et al. WNT5A promotes stemness characteristics in nasopharyngeal carcinoma cells leading to metastasis and tumorigenesis. Oncotarget. 2015;6(12):10239–52.
84. Webster MR, Kugel CH 3rd, Weeraratna AT. The Wnts of change: How Wnts regulate phenotype switching in melanoma. Biochim Biophys Acta. 2015;1856(2):244–51.
85. Kumawat K, Gosens R. WNT-5A: signaling and functions in health and disease. Cell Mol Life Sci. 2016;73(3):567–87.
86. Katoh M. Canonical and non-canonical WNT signaling in cancer stem cells and their niches: Cellular heterogeneity, omics reprogramming, targeted therapy and tumor plasticity (Review). Int J Oncol. 2017;51(5):1357–69.
87. Ribeiro AS, Paredes J. P-cadherin linking breast cancer stem cells and invasion: a promising marker to identify an "Intermediate/Metastable" EMT State. Front Oncol. 2014;4:371.
88. Isobe T, Hisamori S, Hogan DJ, Zabala M, Hendrickson DG, Dalerba P, et al. miR-142 regulates the tumorigenicity of human breast cancer stem cells through the canonical WNT signaling pathway. eLife. 2014;3:e01977.
89. Xu L, Zhang L, Hu C, Liang S, Fei X, Yan N, et al. WNT pathway inhibitor pyrvinium pamoate inhibits the self-renewal and metastasis of breast cancer stem cells. Int J Oncol. 2016;48(3):1175–86.
90. Sun X, Xu C, Xiao G, Meng J, Wang J, Tang SC, et al. Breast cancer stem-like cells are sensitized to tamoxifen induction of self-renewal inhibition with enforced Let-7c dependent on Wnt blocking. Int J Mol Med. 2018;41(4):1967–75.
91. Lunardi A, Webster KA, Papa A, Padmani B, Clohessy JG, Bronson RT, et al. Role of aberrant PI3K pathway activation in gallbladder tumorigenesis. Oncotarget. 2014;5(4):894–900.
92. Ye B, Jiang LL, Xu HT, Zhou DW, Li ZS. Expression of PI3K/AKT pathway in gastric cancer and its blockade suppresses tumor growth and metastasis. Int J Immunopathol Pharmacol. 2012;25(3):627–36.
93. Xu W, Yang Z, Lu N. A new role for the PI3K/Akt signaling pathway in the epithelial-mesenchymal transition. Cell Adh Migr. 2015;9(4):317–24.
94. Lechman ER, Gentner B, Ng SWK, Schoof EM, van Galen P, Kennedy JA, et al. miR-126 regulates distinct self-renewal outcomes in normal and malignant hematopoietic stem cells. Cancer Cell. 2016;29(4):602–6.
95. Bahena-Ocampo I, Espinosa M, Ceballos-Cancino G, Lizarraga F, Campos-Arroyo D, Schwarz A, et al. miR-10b expression in breast cancer stem cells supports self-renewal through negative PTEN regulation and sustained AKT activation. EMBO Rep. 2016;17(5):648–58.
96. Hoesel B, Schmid JA. The complexity of NF-κB signaling in inflammation and cancer. Mol Cancer. 2013;12:86.
97. Pellegrini P, Cordero A, Gallego MI, Dougall WC, Muñoz P, Pujana MA, et al. Constitutive activation of RANK disrupts mammary cell fate leading to tumorigenesis. Stem cells (Dayton, Ohio). 2013;31(9):1954–65.
98. Zhang W, Tan W, Wu X, Poustovoitov M, Strasner A, Li W, et al. A NIK-IKKα module expands ErbB2-induced tumor-initiating cells by stimulating nuclear export of p27/Kip1. Cancer Cell. 2013;23(5):647–59.

99. Chen C, Cao F, Bai L, Liu Y, Xie J, Wang W, et al. IKKβ enforces a LIN28B/TCF7L2 positive feedback loop that promotes cancer cell stemness and metastasis. Cancer Res. 2015;75 (8):1725–35.
100. Tran TA, Ahn KS, Song YW, Moon JY, Cho M, Lim Y, et al. Mechanism of 2',3'-dimethoxyflavanone-induced apoptosis in breast cancer stem cells: role of ubiquitination of caspase-8 and LC3. Arch Biochem Biophys. 2014;562:92–102.
101. Xu SL, Zhu KY, Bi CW, Yan L, Men SW, Dong TT, et al. Flavonoids, derived from traditional Chinese medicines, show roles in the differentiation of neurons: possible targets in developing health food products. Birth Defects Res C Embryo Today. 2013;99(4):292–9.
102. Haar CP, Hebbar P, Wallace GC, Das A, Vandergrift WA 3rd, Smith JA, et al. Drug resistance in glioblastoma: a mini review. Neurochem Res. 2012;37(6):1192–200.
103. Yin L, Pan X, Zhang XT, Guo YM, Wang ZY, Gong Y, et al. Downregulation of ER-α36 expression sensitizes HER2 overexpressing breast cancer cells to tamoxifen. Am J Cancer Res. 2015;5(2):530–44.
104. Li Y, Chen X, He W, Xia S, Jiang X, Li X, et al. Apigenin enhanced antitumor effect of cisplatin in lung cancer via inhibition of cancer stem cells. Nutr Cancer. 2020:1–9. https://doi.org/10.1080/01635581.2020.1802494.
105. Erdogan S, Turkekul K, Serttas R, Erdogan Z. The natural flavonoid apigenin sensitizes human CD44(+) prostate cancer stem cells to cisplatin therapy. Biomed Pharmacother. 2017;88:210–7.
106. Bansal M, Singh N, Pal S, Dev I, Ansari KM. Chemopreventive role of dietary phytochemicals in colorectal cancer, Advances in molecular toxicology, vol. 12. Amsterdam: Elsevier; 2018. p. 69–11.
107. Evans WCED. Phenols and phenolic glycosides. Trease and Evans' Pharmacognosy. Philadelphia, PA: WB Saunders; 2009.
108. Walter ED. EJJotAcS. Genistin (an isoflavone glucoside) and its aglucone, genistein, from soybeans. J Am Chem Soc. 1941;63(12):3273–6.
109. Spagnuolo C, Russo GL, Orhan IE, Habtemariam S, Daglia M, Sureda A, et al. Genistein and cancer: current status, challenges, and future directions. Adv Nutr (Bethesda, MD). 2015;6 (4):408–19.
110. Lee JY, Kim HS, Song YS. Genistein as a potential anticancer agent against ovarian cancer. J Tradit Complement Med. 2012;2(2):96–104.
111. Tuli HS, Tuorkey MJ, Thakral F, Sak K, Kumar M, Sharma AK, et al. Molecular mechanisms of action of genistein in cancer: recent advances. Front Pharmacol. 2019;10:1336.
112. Aarushi G, Sahoo P, Tejpal AJ. Genistein - a potential boon for cancer therapy. Pharm Innov. 2016;5(6, Part B):81.
113. Sekar V, Anandasadagopan SK, GanapasamSJB. Genistein regulates tumor microenvironment and exhibits anticancer effect in dimethyl hydrazine-induced experimental colon carcinogenesis. Biofactors. 2016;42(6):623–37.
114. Pan H, Zhou W, He W, Liu X, Ding Q, Ling L, et al. Genistein inhibits MDA-MB-231 triple-negative breast cancer cell growth by inhibiting NF-κB activity via the Notch-1 pathway. Int J Mol Med. 2012;30(2):337–43.
115. Xia J, Duan Q, Ahmad A, Bao B, Banerjee S, Shi Y, et al. Genistein inhibits cell growth and induces apoptosis through up-regulation of miR-34a in pancreatic cancer cells. Curr Drug Targets. 2012;13(14):1750–6.
116. Hirata H, Ueno K, Nakajima K, Tabatabai ZL, Hinoda Y, Ishii N, et al. Genistein downregulates onco-miR-1260b and inhibits Wnt-signalling in renal cancer cells. Br J Cancer. 2013;108(10):2070–8.
117. Montales MT, Rahal OM, Nakatani H, Matsuda T, Simmen RC. Repression of mammary adipogenesis by genistein limits mammosphere formation of human MCF-7 cells. J Endocrinol. 2013;218(1):135–49.

118. Ning Y, Feng W, Cao X, Ren K, Quan M, Chen A, et al. Genistein inhibits stemness of SKOV3 cells induced by macrophages co-cultured with ovarian cancer stem-like cells through IL-8/STAT3 axis. J Exp Clin Cancer Res. 2019;38(1):19.
119. Huang W, Wan C, Luo Q, Huang Z, Luo Q. Genistein-inhibited cancer stem cell-like properties and reduced chemoresistance of gastric cancer. Int J Mol Sci. 2014;15(3):3432–43.
120. Zhou P, Wang C, Hu Z, Chen W, Qi W, Li A. Genistein induces apoptosis of colon cancer cells by reversal of epithelial-to-mesenchymal via a Notch1/NF-κB/slug/E-cadherin pathway. BMC Cancer. 2017;17(1):813.
121. Zhang Q, Cao WS, Wang XQ, Zhang M, Lu XM, Chen JQ, et al. Genistein inhibits nasopharyngeal cancer stem cells through sonic hedgehog signaling. Phytother Res. 2019;33(10):2783–91.
122. Li E, Zhang T, Sun X, Li Y, Geng H, Yu D, et al. Sonic hedgehog pathway mediates genistein inhibition of renal cancer stem cells. Oncol Lett. 2019;18(3):3081–91.
123. Fu Z, Cao X, Liu L, Cao X, Cui Y, Li X, et al. Genistein inhibits lung cancer cell stem-like characteristics by modulating MnSOD and FoxM1 expression. Oncol Lett. 2020;20(3):2506–15.
124. Hsieh PL, Liao YW, Hsieh CW, Chen PN, Yu CC. Soy isoflavone genistein impedes cancer stemness and mesenchymal transition in head and neck cancer through activating miR-34a/RTCB axis. Nutrients. 2020;12(7):1924.
125. Sanaei M, Kavoosi F, Atashpour S, Haghighat S. Effects of genistein and synergistic action in combination with tamoxifen on the HepG2 human hepatocellular carcinoma cell line. Asian Pac J Cancer Prev. 2017;18(9):2381–5.
126. Hussein AM, El-Sheikh SM, Darwish ZE, Hussein KA, Gaafar AI. Effect of genistein and oxaliplatin on cancer stem cells in oral squamous cell carcinoma: an experimental study. Alexandria Dent J. 2018;43(1):117–23.
127. Montales MT, Simmen RC, Ferreira ES, Neves VA, Simmen FA. Metformin and soybean-derived bioactive molecules attenuate the expansion of stem cell-like epithelial subpopulation and confer apoptotic sensitivity in human colon cancer cells. Genes Nutr. 2015;10(6):49.
128. Xue JP, Wang G, Zhao ZB, Wang Q, Shi Y. Synergistic cytotoxic effect of genistein and doxorubicin on drug-resistant human breast cancer MCF-7/Adr cells. Oncol Rep. 2014;32(4):1647–53.
129. Kashyap D, Mittal S, Sak K, Singhal P, Tuli HS. Molecular mechanisms of action of quercetin in cancer: recent advances. Tumour Biol. 2016;37(10):12927–39.
130. Zhou W, Kallifatidis G, Baumann B, Rausch V, Mattern J, Gladkich J, et al. Dietary polyphenol quercetin targets pancreatic cancer stem cells. Int J Oncol. 2010;37(3):551–61.
131. Lu KT, Wang BY, Chi WY, Chang-Chien J, Yang JJ, Lee HT, et al. Ovatodiolide inhibits breast cancer stem/progenitor cells through SMURF2-mediated downregulation of Hsp27. Toxins. 2016;8(5):127.
132. Yasuda K, Hirohashi Y, Mariya T, Murai A, Tabuchi Y, Kuroda T, et al. Phosphorylation of HSF1 at serine 326 residue is related to the maintenance of gynecologic cancer stem cells through expression of HSP27. Oncotarget. 2017;8(19):31540–53.
133. Wei L, Liu TT, Wang HH, Hong HM, Yu AL, Feng HP, et al. Hsp27 participates in the maintenance of breast cancer stem cells through regulation of epithelial-mesenchymal transition and nuclear factor-κB. Breast Cancer Res. 2011;13(5):R101.
134. Lee CH, Hong HM, Chang YY, Chang WW. Inhibition of heat shock protein (Hsp) 27 potentiates the suppressive effect of Hsp90 inhibitors in targeting breast cancer stem-like cells. Biochimie. 2012;94(6):1382–9.
135. Lee CH, Wu YT, Hsieh HC, Yu Y, Yu AL, Chang WW. Epidermal growth factor/heat shock protein 27 pathway regulates vasculogenic mimicry activity of breast cancer stem/progenitor cells. Biochimie. 2014;104:117–26.
136. Li S, Zhao Q, Wang B, Yuan S, Wang X, Li K. Quercetin reversed MDR in breast cancer cells through down-regulating P-gp expression and eliminating cancer stem cells mediated by YB-1 nuclear translocation. Phytother Res. 2018;32(8):1530–6.

137. To K, Fotovati A, Reipas KM, Law JH, Hu K, Wang J, et al. Y-box binding protein-1 induces the expression of CD44 and CD49f leading to enhanced self-renewal, mammosphere growth, and drug resistance. Cancer Res. 2010;70(7):2840–51.
138. Chang WW, Hu FW, Yu CC, Wang HH, Feng HP, Lan C, et al. Quercetin in elimination of tumor initiating stem-like and mesenchymal transformation property in head and neck cancer. Head Neck. 2013;35(3):413–9.
139. Mojsin M, Vicentic JM, Schwirtlich M, Topalovic V, Stevanovic M. Quercetin reduces pluripotency, migration and adhesion of human teratocarcinoma cell line NT2/D1 by inhibiting Wnt/β-catenin signaling. Food Funct. 2014;5(10):2564–73.
140. Lin YS, Tsai PH, Kandaswami CC, Cheng CH, Ke FC, Lee PP, et al. Effects of dietary flavonoids, luteolin, and quercetin on the reversal of epithelial-mesenchymal transition in A431 epidermal cancer cells. Cancer Sci. 2011;102(10):1829–39.
141. Tsai PH, Cheng CH, Lin CY, Huang YT, Lee LT, Kandaswami CC, et al. Dietary flavonoids luteolin and quercetin suppressed cancer stem cell properties and metastatic potential of isolated prostate cancer cells. Anticancer Res. 2016;36(12):6367–80.
142. Atashpour S, Fouladdel S, Movahhed TK, Barzegar E, Ghahremani MH, Ostad SN, et al. Quercetin induces cell cycle arrest and apoptosis in CD133(+) cancer stem cells of human colorectal HT29 cancer cell line and enhances anticancer effects of doxorubicin. Iran J Basic Med Sci. 2015;18(7):635–43.
143. Chen SF, Nieh S, Jao SW, Liu CL, Wu CH, Chang YC, et al. Quercetin suppresses drug-resistant spheres via the p38 MAPK-Hsp27 apoptotic pathway in oral cancer cells. PLoS One. 2012;7(11):e49275.
144. Mao J, Yang H, Cui T, Pan P, Kabir N, Chen D, et al. Combined treatment with sorafenib and silibinin synergistically targets both HCC cells and cancer stem cells by enhanced inhibition of the phosphorylation of STAT3/ERK/AKT. Eur J Pharmacol. 2018;832:39–49.
145. Vue B, Chen QH. The potential of flavonolignans in prostate cancer management. Curr Med Chem. 2016;23(34):3925–50.
146. Bosch-Barrera J, Queralt B, Menendez JA. Targeting STAT3 with silibinin to improve cancer therapeutics. Cancer Treat Rev. 2017;58:61–9.
147. Jahanafrooz Z, Motamed N, Rinner B, Mokhtarzadeh A, Baradaran B. Silibinin to improve cancer therapeutic, as an apoptotic inducer, autophagy modulator, cell cycle inhibitor, and microRNAs regulator. Life Sci. 2018;213:236–47.
148. Mateen S, Raina K, Agarwal R. Chemopreventive and anti-cancer efficacy of silibinin against growth and progression of lung cancer. Nutr cancer. 2013;65 Suppl 1(01):3–11.
149. Liakopoulou C, Kazazis C, Vallianou NG. Silimarin and cancer. Anticancer Agents Med Chem. 2018;18(14):1970–4.
150. Wang JY, Chang CC, Chiang CC, Chen WM, Hung SC. Silibinin suppresses the maintenance of colorectal cancer stem-like cells by inhibiting PP2A/AKT/mTOR pathways. J Cell Biochem. 2012;113(5):1733–43.
151. Kumar S, Raina K, Agarwal C, Agarwal R. Silibinin strongly inhibits the growth kinetics of colon cancer stem cell-enriched spheroids by modulating interleukin 4/6-mediated survival signals. Oncotarget. 2014;5(13):4972–89.
152. Sameri S, Saidijam M, Bahreini F, Najafi R. Cancer chemopreventive activities of silibinin on colorectal cancer through regulation of E-cadherin/β-catenin pathway. Nutr Cancer. 2020:1–11. https://doi.org/10.1080/01635581.2020.1800764.
153. Khakinezhad Tehrani F, Ranji N, Kouhkan F, Hosseinzadeh S. Apoptosis induction and proliferation inhibition by silibinin encapsulated in nanoparticles in MIA PaCa-2 cancer cells and deregulation of some miRNAs. Iran J Basic Med Sci. 2020;23(4):469–82.
154. Patel S, Waghela B, Shah K, Vaidya F, Mirza S, Patel S, et al. Silibinin, a natural blend in polytherapy formulation for targeting Cd44v6 expressing colon cancer stem cells. Sci Rep. 2018;8(1):16985.

155. Erdogan S, Doganlar O, Doganlar ZB, Serttas R, Turkekul K, Dibirdik I, et al. The flavonoid apigenin reduces prostate cancer CD44(+) stem cell survival and migration through PI3K/Akt/NF-κB signaling. Life Sci. 2016;162:77–86.
156. Ketkaew Y, Osathanon T, Pavasant P, Sooampon S. Apigenin inhibited hypoxia induced stem cell marker expression in a head and neck squamous cell carcinoma cell line. Arch Oral Biol. 2017;74:69–74.
157. Tang AQ, Cao XC, Tian L, He L, Liu F. Apigenin inhibits the self-renewal capacity of human ovarian cancer SKOV3-derived sphere-forming cells. Mol Med Rep. 2015;11(3):2221–6.
158. Yan X, Qi M, Li P, Zhan Y, Shao H. Apigenin in cancer therapy: anti-cancer effects and mechanisms of action. Cell Biosci. 2017;7:50.
159. Cao X, Liu L, Yuan Q, Li X, Cui Y, Ren K, et al. Isovitexin reduces carcinogenicity and stemness in hepatic carcinoma stem-like cells by modulating MnSOD and FoxM1. J Exp Clin Cancer Res. 2019;38(1):264.
160. Xu C, Cao X, Cao X, Liu L, Qiu Y, Li X, et al. Isovitexin inhibits stemness and induces apoptosis in hepatocellular carcinoma SK-Hep-1 spheroids by upregulating miR-34a expression. Anticancer Agents Med Chem. 2020;20(14):1654–63.
161. Liang X, Xu C, Cao X, Wang W. Isovitexin suppresses cancer stemness property and induces apoptosis of osteosarcoma cells by disruption of The DNMT1/miR-34a/Bcl-2 axis. Cancer Manag Res. 2019;11:8923–36.
162. Guo M, Wang M, Zhang X, Deng H, Wang ZY. Broussoflavonol B restricts growth of ER-negative breast cancer stem-like cells. Anticancer Res. 2013;33(5):1873–9.
163. Jeong JH, Ryu JH. Broussoflavonol B from broussonetia kazinoki siebold exerts anti-pancreatic cancer activity through downregulating FoxM1. Molecules (Basel, Switzerland). 2328;25(10):2020.
164. Guo Y, Zhang X, Meng J, Wang ZY. An anticancer agent icaritin induces sustained activation of the extracellular signal-regulated kinase (ERK) pathway and inhibits growth of breast cancer cells. Eur J Pharmacol. 2011;658(2-3):114–22.
165. Chen M, Turhan AG, Ding H, Lin Q, Meng K, Jiang X. Targeting BCR-ABL+ stem/progenitor cells and BCR-ABL-T315I mutant cells by effective inhibition of the BCR-ABL-Tyr177-GRB2 complex. Oncotarget. 2017;8(27):43662–77.
166. Liu S, Guo Y, Wang J, Zhu H, Han Y, Jin M, et al. A novel anticancer agent SNG1153 inhibits growth of lung cancer stem/progenitor cells. Oncotarget. 2016;7(29):45158–70.
167. Han K, Lang T, Zhang Z, Zhang Y, Sun Y, Shen Z, et al. Luteolin attenuates Wnt signaling via upregulation of FZD6 to suppress prostate cancer stemness revealed by comparative proteomics. Sci Rep. 2018;8(1):8537.
168. Wang L, Guo H, Yang L, Dong L, Lin C, Zhang J, et al. Morusin inhibits human cervical cancer stem cell growth and migration through attenuation of NF-κB activity and apoptosis induction. Mol Cell Biochem. 2013;379(1-2):7–18.
169. Lee HJ, da Lyu H, Koo U, Nam KW, Hong SS, Kim KO, et al. Protection of prenylated flavonoids from Mori Cortex Radicis (Moraceae) against nitric oxide-induced cell death in neuroblastoma SH-SY5Y cells. Arch Pharm Res. 2012;35(1):163–70.
170. Dat NT, Binh PT, Quynh LTP, Van Minh C, Huong HT, Lee JJ. Cytotoxic prenylated flavonoids from Morus alba. Fitoterapia. 2010;81(8):1224–7.
171. Guo H, Liu C, Yang L, Dong L, Wang L, Wang Q, et al. Morusin inhibits glioblastoma stem cell growth in vitro and in vivo through stemness attenuation, adipocyte transdifferentiation, and apoptosis induction. Mol Carcinog. 2016;55(1):77–89.
172. Chen C, Xu ZH, Wang L. [The effect of morusin on stemness phenotype of laryngeal cancer stem cell]. Sichuan Da Xue Xue Bao Yi Xue Ban. 2020;51(5):650–7.
173. Gong Q, Cao X, Cao J, Yang X, Zeng W. Casticin suppresses the carcinogenesis of small cell lung cancer H446 cells through activation of AMPK/FoxO3a signaling. Oncol Rep. 2018;40(3):1401–10.
174. Liu J, Yang J, Hou Y, Zhu Z, He J, Zhao H, et al. Casticin inhibits nasopharyngeal carcinoma growth by targeting phosphoinositide 3-kinase. Cancer Cell Int. 2019;19:348.

175. He G, Cao X, He M, Sheng X, Wu Y, Ai X. Casticin inhibits self-renewal of liver cancer stem cells from the MHCC97 cell line. Oncol Lett. 2014;7(6):2023–8.
176. Zhao D, Yao C, Chen X, Xia H, Zhang L, Liu H, et al. The fruits of Maclura pomifera extracts inhibits glioma stem-like cell growth and invasion. Neurochem Res. 2013;38(10):2105–13.
177. Liao WY, Liaw CC, Huang YC, Han HY, Hsu HW, Hwang SM, et al. Cyclohexylmethyl flavonoids suppress propagation of breast cancer stem cells via downregulation of NANOG. Evidence-based Complem Altern Med. 2013;2013:170261.
178. Peiffer DS, Ma E, Wyatt D, Albain KS, Osipo C. DAXX-inducing phytoestrogens inhibit ER+ tumor initiating cells and delay tumor development. NPJ Breast Cancer. 2020;6:37.
179. Kang Q, Gong J, Wang M, Wang Q, Chen F, Cheng KW. 6-C-(E-Phenylethenyl)naringenin attenuates the stemness of hepatocellular carcinoma cells by suppressing Wnt/β-catenin signaling. J Agric Food Chem. 2019;67(50):13939–47.
180. Song L, Chen X, Wang P, Gao S, Qu C, Liu L. Effects of baicalein on pancreatic cancer stem cells via modulation of sonic Hedgehog pathway. Acta Biochim Biophys Sin. 2018;50 (6):586–96.
181. Wu R, Murali R, Kabe Y, French SW, Chiang YM, Liu S, et al. Baicalein targets GTPase-mediated autophagy to eliminate liver tumor-initiating stem cell-like cells resistant to mTORC1 inhibition. Hepatology (Baltimore, MD). 2018;68(5):1726–40.
182. Koh SY, Moon JY, Unno T, Cho SK. Baicalein suppresses stem cell-like characteristics in radio- and chemoresistant MDA-MB-231 human breast cancer cells through up-regulation of IFIT2. Nutrients. 2019;11(3):624.
183. Lin MG, Liu LP, Li CY, Zhang M, Chen Y, Qin J, et al. Scutellaria extract decreases the proportion of side population cells in a myeloma cell line by down-regulating the expression of ABCG2 protein. Asian Pac J Cancer Prev. 2013;14(12):7179–86.
184. Cao D, Zhu GY, Lu Y, Yang A, Chen D, Huang HJ, et al. Luteolin suppresses epithelial-mesenchymal transition and migration of triple-negative breast cancer cells by inhibiting YAP/TAZ activity. Biomed Pharmacother. 2020;129:110462.
185. Cai X, Ye T, Liu C, Lu W, Lu M, Zhang J, et al. Luteolin induced G2 phase cell cycle arrest and apoptosis on non-small cell lung cancer cells. Toxicol In Vitro. 2011;25(7):1385–91.
186. Dia VP, Pangloli P. Epithelial-to-mesenchymal transition in paclitaxel-resistant ovarian cancer cells is downregulated by luteolin. J Cell Physiol. 2017;232(2):391–401.
187. Choi EM, Lee YS. Luteolin suppresses IL-1beta-induced cytokines and MMPs production via p38 MAPK, JNK, NF-kappaB and AP-1 activation in human synovial sarcoma cell line, SW982. Food Chem Toxicol. 2010;48(10):2607–11.
188. Chian S, Thapa R, Chi Z, Wang XJ, Tang X. Luteolin inhibits the Nrf2 signaling pathway and tumor growth in vivo. Biochem Biophys Res Commun. 2014;447(4):602–8.
189. Rao PS, Satelli A, Moridani M, Jenkins M, Rao US. Luteolin induces apoptosis in multidrug resistant cancer cells without affecting the drug transporter function: involvement of cell line-specific apoptotic mechanisms. Int J Cancer. 2012;130(11):2703–14.
190. Davies AH, Reipas K, Hu K, Berns R, Firmino N, Stratford AL, et al. Inhibition of RSK with the novel small-molecule inhibitor LJI308 overcomes chemoresistance by eliminating cancer stem cells. Oncotarget. 2015;6(24):20570–7.
191. Tu DG, Lin WT, Yu CC, Lee SS, Peng CY, Lin T, et al. Chemotherapeutic effects of luteolin on radio-sensitivity enhancement and interleukin-6/signal transducer and activator of transcription 3 signaling repression of oral cancer stem cells. J Formos Med Assoc. 2016;115 (12):1032–8.
192. Huynh DL, Kwon T, Zhang JJ, Sharma N, Gera M, Ghosh M, et al. Wogonin suppresses stem cell-like traits of CD133 positive osteosarcoma cell via inhibiting matrix metallopeptidase-9 expression. BMC Complement Altern Med. 2017;17(1):304.
193. Huynh DL, Sharma N, Kumar Singh A, Singh Sodhi S, Zhang JJ, Mongre RK, et al. Anti-tumor activity of wogonin, an extract from Scutellaria baicalensis, through regulating different signaling pathways. Chin J Nat Med. 2017;15(1):15–40.

194. Koh H, Sun HN, Xing Z, Liu R, Chandimali N, Kwon T, et al. Wogonin influences osteosarcoma stem cell stemness through ROS-dependent signaling. In Vivo (Athens, Greece). 2020;34(3):1077–84.
195. Wang X, Chang Y, Gao M, Zhang F. Wogonoside attenuates cutaneous squamous cell carcinoma by reducing epithelial-mesenchymal transition/invasion and cancer stem-like cell property. OncoTargets Ther. 2020;13:10097–109.
196. Soltanian S, Riahirad H, Pabarja A, Karimzadeh MR, Saeidi KJB. Kaempferol and docetaxel diminish side population and down-regulate some cancer stem cell markers in breast cancer cell line MCF-7. Biocell. 2017;41(2&3):33.
197. Khaw AK, Yong JW, Kalthur G, Hande MP. Genistein induces growth arrest and suppresses telomerase activity in brain tumor cells. Genes Chromosomes Cancer. 2012;51(10):961–74.
198. Ozturk SA, Alp E, Yar Saglam AS, Konac E, Menevse ES. The effects of thymoquinone and genistein treatment on telomerase activity, apoptosis, angiogenesis, and survival in thyroid cancer cell lines. J Cancer Res Ther. 2018;14(2):328–34.
199. Selvakumar P, Badgeley A, Murphy P, Anwar H, Sharma U, Lawrence K, et al. Flavonoids and other polyphenols act as epigenetic modifiers in breast cancer. Nutrients. 2020;12(3):761.
200. Izzo S, Naponelli V, Bettuzzi S. Flavonoids as epigenetic modulators for prostate cancer prevention. Nutrients. 2020;12(4):1010.
201. Zhang Z, Zhou L, Xie N, Nice EC, Zhang T, Cui Y, et al. Overcoming cancer therapeutic bottleneck by drug repurposing. Signal Transduct Targeted Ther. 2020;5(1):113.
202. Jefferson WN, Williams CJ. Circulating levels of genistein in the neonate, apart from dose and route, predict future adverse female reproductive outcomes. Reprod Toxicol (Elmsford, NY). 2011;31(3):272–9.
203. Motlekar N, Khan MA, Youan BBC. Preparation and characterization of genistein containing poly (ethylene glycol) microparticles. J Appl Plym Sci. 2006;101(3):2070–8.
204. Nwaeburu CC, Abukiwan A, Zhao Z, Herr I. Quercetin-induced miR-200b-3p regulates the mode of self-renewing divisions in pancreatic cancer. Mol Cancer. 2017;16(1):23.
205. Cao L, Yang Y, Ye Z, Lin B, Zeng J, Li C, et al. Quercetin-3-methyl ether suppresses human breast cancer stem cell formation by inhibiting the Notch1 and PI3K/Akt signaling pathways. Int J Mol Med. 2018;42(3):1625–36.
206. Shen X, Si Y, Wang Z, Wang J, Guo Y, Zhang X. Quercetin inhibits the growth of human gastric cancer stem cells by inducing mitochondrial-dependent apoptosis through the inhibition of PI3K/Akt signaling. Int J Mol Med. 2016;38(2):619–26.
207. Hoca M, Becer E, Kabadayı H, Yücecan S, Vatansever HS. The effect of resveratrol and quercetin on epithelial-mesenchymal transition in pancreatic cancer stem cell. Nutr Cancer. 2020;72(7):1231–42.
208. Wang R, Yang L, Li S, Ye D, Yang L, Liu Q, et al. Quercetin inhibits breast cancer stem cells via downregulation of aldehyde dehydrogenase 1A1 (ALDH1A1), chemokine receptor type 4 (CXCR4), Mucin 1 (MUC1), and epithelial cell adhesion molecule (EpCAM). Med Sci Monit. 2018;24:412–20.
209. Erdogan S, Turkekul K, Dibirdik I, Doganlar O, Doganlar ZB, Bilir A, et al. Midkine downregulation increases the efficacy of quercetin on prostate cancer stem cell survival and migration through PI3K/AKT and MAPK/ERK pathway. Biomed Pharmacother. 2018;107:793–805.
210. Appari M, Babu KR, Kaczorowski A, Gross W, Herr I. Sulforaphane, quercetin and catechins complement each other in elimination of advanced pancreatic cancer by miR-let-7 induction and K-ras inhibition. Int J Oncol. 2014;45(4):1391–400.
211. Li Y, Wang Z, Jin J, Zhu SX, He GQ, Li SH, et al. Quercetin pretreatment enhances the radiosensitivity of colon cancer cells by targeting Notch-1 pathway. Biochem Biophys Res Commun. 2020;523(4):947–53.

212. Srivastava RK, Tang SN, Zhu W, Meeker D, Shankar S. Sulforaphane synergizes with quercetin to inhibit self-renewal capacity of pancreatic cancer stem cells. Front Biosci (Elite Edition). 2011;3:515–28.
213. Kim B, Jung N, Lee S, Sohng JK, Jung HJ. Apigenin inhibits cancer stem cell-like phenotypes in human glioblastoma cells via suppression of c-Met signaling. Phytother Res. 2016;30 (11):1833–40.
214. Li YW, Xu J, Zhu GY, Huang ZJ, Lu Y, Li XQ, et al. Apigenin suppresses the stem cell-like properties of triple-negative breast cancer cells by inhibiting YAP/TAZ activity. Cell Death Dis. 2018;4:105.
215. Liu F, Cao X, Liu Z, Guo H, Ren K, Quan M, et al. Casticin suppresses self-renewal and invasion of lung cancer stem-like cells from A549 cells through down-regulation of pAkt. Acta Biochim Biophys Sin. 2014;46(1):15–21.

Non-flavonoids Targeting Cancer Stem Cells: A Promising Therapeutic Avenue for Cancer Treatment

8

Faizan Uddin and Mehboob Hoque

Abstract

Despite the concerted efforts in pursuit of developing effective therapy, the human race has merely succeeded in its fight against cancer. The limited success in this battle against cancer may be attributed to the development of resistance to the available therapeutic regimens, frequent recurrence, metastasis, tumor heterogeneity, and immune evasion. The sub-populated cancer stem cells (CSCs) are often held responsible for cancer relapse, therapy resistance, and metastasis. The stemness and tumorigenicity of CSCs are regulated by various pathways such as Wnt/β-catenin, hedgehog, PI3K-AKT, JAK-STAT, TGF-β, and notch signaling. Various therapeutic agents targeting CSCs are now being considered for the treatment of various malignancies. However, conventional therapies are associated with various side effects. Therefore, current therapeutic approaches are witnessing a paradigm shift towards natural compounds. To this end, dietary polyphenols are considered promising drug candidates for their both preventive as well as therapeutic properties. In this chapter, the non-flavonoid polyphenols are discussed in the context of their ability to target CSCs and their role in attenuation of fundamental pathways involved in the maintenance of CSCs such as Wnt/β-catenin, hedgehog, notch, and induction of programmed cell death pathways has been explored. The overview of this chapter will help the oncologist to devise more efficacious combinatorial therapies, utilizing naturally occurring non-flavonoid polyphenols and their derivatives along with

F. Uddin
Epigenetics Research Laboratory, National Institute of Immunology, New Delhi, India

M. Hoque (✉)
Applied Biochemistry Laboratory, Department of Biological Sciences, Aliah University, Kolkata, India
e-mail: m_hoque@aliah.ac.in

S. Tabrez, M. Imran Khan (eds.), *Polyphenols-based Nanotherapeutics for Cancer Management*, https://doi.org/10.1007/978-981-16-4935-6_8

chemotherapeutic drugs, which will offer the advantage of eliminating both the CSCs and other malignant cells in the heterogeneous tumor mass as a multi-pronged approach. The traditional knowledge of phytomedicines along with the current advancements of molecular and precision medicine and suitable delivery system hold a great promise to combat cancer and exterminate it from the root.

Keywords

Cancer stem cells · Cancer therapeutics · Dedifferentiation · Metastasis · Non-flavonoid polyphenols · Phytomedicine · Stemness

Abbreviations

ABCG2	ATP binding cassette transporters
ALDH1	Aldehyde dehydrogenase 1
AML	Acute myeloid leukemia
APC	Adenomatous polyposis coli
BCSCs	Breast cancer stem cells
cAMP-PKA	Cyclic-AMP dependent protein kinase A
CAPE	Caffeic acid phenethyl ester
CK-1α	Casein Kinase 1α
CSCs	Cancer stem cells
ECM	Extracellular matrix
EMT	Epithelial to mesenchymal transition
EpCAM	Epithelial cell adhesion molecule
FAK	Focal adhesion kinase
GLI	Glioma-associated oncogenic TF
GSCs	Glioblastoma stem cells
GSK-3β	Glycogen synthase kinase 3β
Hes1	Hairy enhancer of split
Hh	Hedgehog
HIF-1α	Hypoxia inducible factor 1α
IKK	Inhibitor of κB kinase
IκBs	Inhibitor of κB proteins
JAK	Janus-activated kinase
LRP 5/6	Low density lipoprotein 5/6
M3OMG	Methyl-3-O-methyl gallate
MMPs	Matrix metalloproteases
mTOR	Mammalian target of rapamycin
NF-κB	Nuclear factor kappa-light-chain-enhancer of activated B cells
NICD	Notch intracellular domain
NIK	NF-κB-inducing kinase
NSCCs	Non-stem cancer cells
PI3K/AKT	Phosphoinositide-3-kinase-AKT

Ptch	Patched transmembrane receptor
PTEN	Phosphatase and tensin homolog
ROS	Reactive oxygen species
SMO	Smoothened TF
STAT	Signal transducer and activator of transcription
SUFU	Suppressor of Fused
TCF	T-cell factor
TFs	Transcription factors
TGF-β	Transformation growth factor β
VEGF	Vascular endothelial growth factor

8.1 Introduction

The human body has an inherent ability to overcome physiological insults and initiate homeostasis. However, when the balance between the repair and regulatory mechanisms is disturbed, it can culminate into genetic aberrations leading to the malignant transformation of healthy cells, commonly termed cancer. Collective evidence suggests that cancer is a chronic disease that is manifested across several stages of dysregulation of genes involved in the development and cell turnover [1, 2]. Several factors such as genetic variations, epigenetic modifications, stress, unhealthy diet, sedentary lifestyles, prolonged inflammation due to reactive oxygen species (ROS), and metabolic disorders have been identified to increase the risk associated with the oncogenesis [3]. Among the many factors that lead to cancer malignancies, environmental cues play a significant role in the progression of cancer.

Despite remarkable advances in understanding the molecular basis of cancer and the development of new regimens for diagnosis and treatment, only limited success has been achieved in terms of the long-term survival rate of patients. Such compromised success in the battle against cancer is due to the development of resistance to chemo-radiotherapies, frequent recurrence, metastasis, heterogeneity, and avoidance of immune surveillance. Recent evidence suggests that cancer stem cells (CSCs) possess inherent characteristics that can cause cancer relapse, therapy resistance, metastasis, and the ability to generate new tumors [4, 5].

Most conventional therapies for cancer treatment can target only differentiated tumor cells without impacting the CSCs. The widely practiced cancer chemotherapeutics are largely associated with various adverse effects on healthy cells and reemergence of cancer after a period of latency, especially in children [6, 7].

Moreover, during treatment, some of the cancer cells undergo selective pressure and become highly resistant to chemo or radiation therapy [8, 9]. Also, non-stem cancer cells (NSCCs) have been demonstrated to dedifferentiate into CSCs by activating the expression of pluripotency-related transcription factors (TFs) such as Oct4 and Sox2 [10]. In this context, the incomplete elimination of CSCs by various traditional therapies jeopardizes the efficacy of treatment. Currently, available chemotherapies including monoclonal antibodies, kinase inhibitors, and other targeted therapies are reported to elevate other medical conditions in patients such as cardiomyopathy, congestive heart failure, and coronary artery disease. Surgery has also been explored as a radical approach in the removal of cancerous tissues but is limited to tackle solid tumors where the disease burden is low. But it is not a viable option in the case of small cell carcinomas, non-solid malignancies such as myeloma or leukemia, and when cancer has metastasized to several distal sites that can not be surgically removed.

Since cancer progression is characterized by the aberrant activation of embryonic developmental pathways in CSCs, their selective inhibition has been proposed as a promising strategy for effective treatment [11, 12]. Therefore, there is a pressing need to identify chemical compounds that can specifically target the CSCs with little or no effect on the healthy tissues. Pertinently, researchers have shifted back their focus on naturally available compounds as alternative therapies with negligible or no side effects and high effectiveness against various forms of cancer. Biocompatibility, lower or no adverse effects and universal availability make natural compounds a better choice for next-generation therapeutics for cancer treatment and prevention. Epidemiological studies reveal that consumption of fruits and vegetables lowers the risk of cancer suggesting the chemopreventive role of dietary compounds. This chapter highlights the current development in non-flavonoid dietary polyphenols as potential drug candidates for targeting CSCs. The first section of this chapter describes the various pathways involved in the maintenance of the stemness of CSCs. The later section emphasizes the non-flavonoid dietary polyphenols having the potential to target key signaling pathways in CSCs.

8.2 Cancer Stem Cells

Within the tumor mass, there is vast heterogeneity among the cancer cells and a small proportion of undifferentiated cells feature an aggressive phenotype with enhanced self-renewal capacity and invasive potential [13]. This rare population has been termed as CSCs and represents the most resilient malignant cell type that is often implicated in cancer relapse [4, 14]. The CSCs were first identified in 1994 in human acute myeloid leukemia (AML) and since then have been reported in a wide variety of solid tumors [15, 16]. By undergoing asymmetric division each CSC can generate a single differentiated malignant cell and a CSC [17]. This helps the tumors to retain infinite stemness as well as propagate and multiply. However, in certain tumors, NSCCs can undergo dedifferentiation to acquire CSCs-like phenotype, associated with high tumorigenic potential [18]. This emerging evidence has challenged the notion of a unidirectional hierarchy of CSCs generation and differentiation and thus has offered novel insights into the complex origin of CSCs. The classical and the updated views on the CSC hierarchy are depicted in Fig. 8.1.

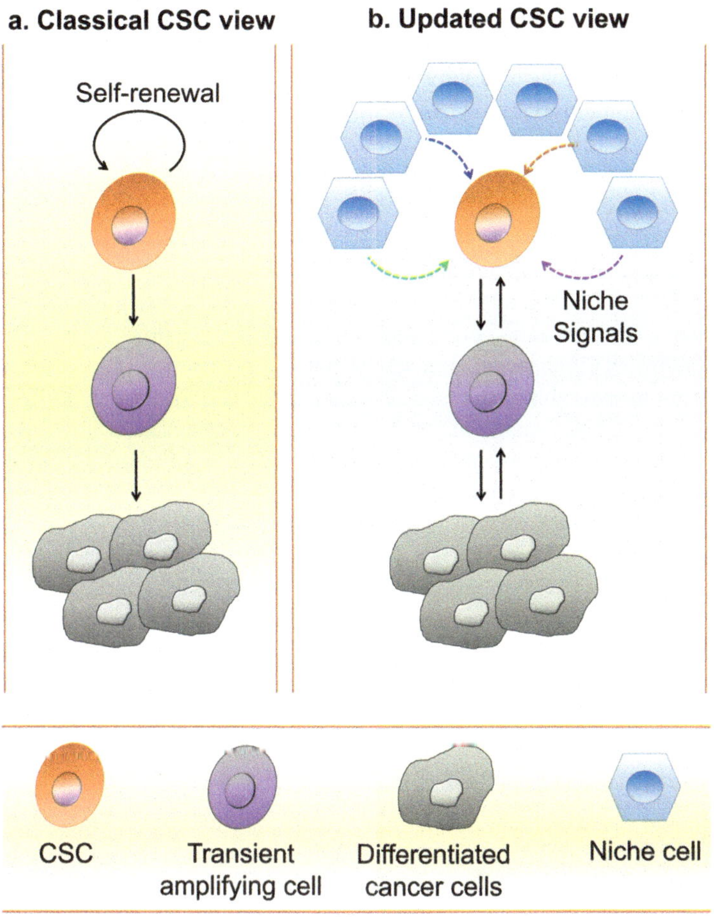

Fig. 8.1 CSC hierarchy showing the classical and updated views. (**a**) The classical view represents a canonical hardwired cellular hierarchy where rare and quiescent CSCs are mainly defined by intrinsic properties. The CSCs undergo an asymmetric cell division giving rise to one stem cell ensuring its self-renewal and one transient amplifying (TA) cell which further divides rapidly and undergoes differentiation. (**b**) According to the updated view, the CSCs are not necessarily rare or quiescent and are regulated by niche signals. The TA cells, as well as the differentiated cells, can be reprogrammed back into stem cells by the niche signals

8.2.1 Characteristics of CSCs

CSCs can arise from the malignant transformation of stem cells harboring the increased burden of mutation or differentiated tumor cells that have transitioned into pluripotent type via abrupt expression of TFs that are active during embryonic development [19, 20]. The expression of Nanog is upregulated in CSCs across multiple cancer types and has been reported to regulate the expression of various embryonic signature genes such as KLF4, Oct4, and Sox2 [21]. This peculiar transcriptional profile enables CSCs to acquire characteristic features of embryonic stem cells such as self-renewability and multipotency. The upregulation of stemness genes enables the CSCs to readily proliferate and resist the toxic effects of radiation and drugs commonly used in the treatment of cancer [21, 22]. CSCs reside in a hypoxic and nutrient deficient environment and are thus hard to be eliminated [23]. As the CSCs multiply and differentiate, they generate spheroid clumps of aggregated cells and some of which enter into the circulation to invade the distant sites [24].

CSCs adopt several strategies to sustain themselves, such as differential expression of drug efflux pumps, activation of DNA repair machinery to overcome damaging effects of radiation, inhibition of apoptosis, slow doubling rate, and upregulation of embryonic transcriptional programs to proliferate [12, 25, 26]. Owing to their ability to maintain a quiescent state for long periods, CSCs can overcome the DNA damage induced in various therapies and avoid apoptotic cell death. Apart from this, inactivating mutations in p53 disable the DNA damage sensing machinery in the malignant cells and allow them to proliferate. Another strategy deployed by CSCs to propagate tumors is to evade apoptosis. The ratio between pro-apoptotic protein Bax and anti-apoptotic Bcl-2 determines the cell fate and it is altered in CSCs to promote their survival [27]. In several studies elevated levels of basal autophagy have been correlated to enhance the survival of CSCs [28–30]. Emerging studies have indicated the involvement of key signaling pathways in maintaining the stemness of CSCs and the associated metastasis [31]. Some of the major pathways in CSCs biology include Wnt/β-catenin, Hedgehog, PI3K/AKT, and Notch signaling pathways [16, 32–34]. The various pathways involved in regulating the stemness and differentiation of CSCs are depicted in Fig. 8.2.

8.2.2 CSCs Biomarkers

Over the years, the expression of numerous cell surface proteins has been specifically associated with a stem cell-like population in the vastly heterogeneous tumor mass in different cancer types [35]. Therefore, the presence of cell surface markers has been utilized as the first-hand approach to identify the multipotent CSCs among the malignant cells, wherein the leukemic stem cells were first characterized as $CD34^{+}/CD38^{-}$ in AML [15, 16, 36]. CSCs feature distinct profiles of cell surface receptors and exhibit dynamic changes in their expression that can represent various stages of cancer progression [13, 37]. The expression of various biomarkers of CSCs, such as aldehyde dehydrogenase 1 (ALDH1) in colorectal cancer and epithelial cell adhesion molecule (EpCAM) in hepatic CSCs, has been reported to positively correlate with mTOR signaling [38]. Breast cancer stem cells (BCSCs) are characterized by $CD44^{+}/CD24^{-}/ALDH1^{+}$ cells [33, 39]. Expression of CD44 and ALDH1 on the surface of CSCs has been correlated to their stemness and confers upon them a distinctive ability of invasive expansion [33, 40, 41]. Also, CSCs exhibiting multidrug resistance have been found to express CD133 that facilitates epithelial to mesenchymal transition (EMT) of cancer cells via activation of PI3K-

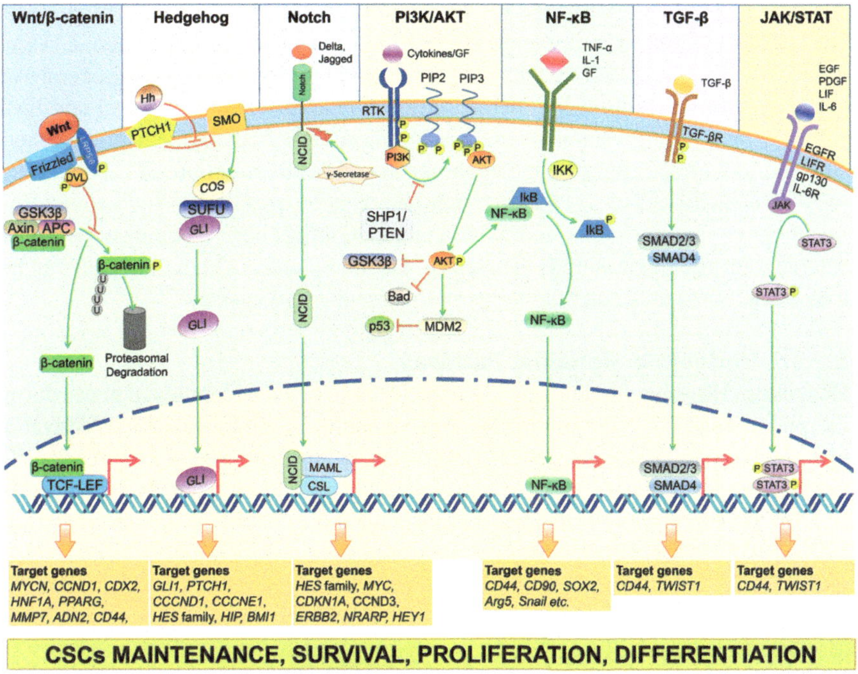

Fig. 8.2 Pathways regulating CSC development. The Wnt/β-catenin, hedgehog, notch, PI3K/AKT, NK-κB, TGF-β, and JAK/STAT signaling pathways are associated with the development of stemness features of CSCs including EMT, cell proliferation, migration, invasion, and tumorigenesis. The target genes of these pathways play important roles in the maintenance, survival, proliferation, and differentiation of CSCs

AKT and ERK signaling pathway [12, 42, 43]. Likewise, $CD133^+$ CSCs in sarcomas are highly resilient towards chemo-radiotherapy [21].

8.2.3 Pathways Regulating CSCs

8.2.3.1 Wnt/β-catenin Signaling Pathway

In normal cells, the free cytoplasmic level of β-catenin is kept in check by ubiquitin-mediated proteasomal degradation. In this process, β-catenin is associated with factors such as Axin and adenomatous polyposis coli (APC) and gets phosphorylated by the activity of glycogen synthase kinase 3β (GSK-3β) and Casein Kinase 1α (CK-1α). The phosphorylated form of β-catenin is then ubiquitinylated and targeted by E3 ligase β-TrCP for subsequent degradation [44]. However, in cancer cells, the Wnt/β-catenin pathway is abruptly activated in the presence of extracellular Wnt ligands which can bind Frizzled and low-density lipoprotein (LRP5/6) receptors and enables the organization of Frizzled-Dishevelled and LRP-Axin-FRAT complex [31]. The de novo generated complex facilitates the inactivation of the destructive complex comprising GSK-3β by promoting its phosphorylation. As a result, β-catenin is stabilized and eventually accumulates in the nuclei, wherein it gets associated with the T-cell factor (TCF) and activates the expression of several Wnt inducible genes including Myc which promotes cancer cell self-renewal and EMT [33, 45, 46]. Wnt/β-catenin signaling has been reported to mediate epigenetic silencing of surface adhesion molecules such as E-cadherin in breast cancer tissues [47]. Mechanistically, E-cadherin inhibits cancer metastasis by sequestering membrane-bound β-catenin and its downregulation has been recognized as a characteristic feature of EMT [33]. Therefore, the Wnt/β-catenin signaling pathway has long been touted as a potential target in the treatment of cancer.

8.2.3.2 Hedgehog Signaling Pathway

Hedgehog (Hh) signaling induces the expression of key developmental genes during morphogenesis and relies on the paracrine signaling by Hh ligands for its activation [48]. The activity of these genes is strictly regulated by their temporal expression and helps to maintain pluripotency in stem and progenitor cells, whereas dysregulation of Hh signaling has been reported to constitute 25% of human malignant transformations [49, 50]. The major components of the Hh signaling pathway consist of tumor-suppressive Patched transmembrane receptors (Ptch 1 and 2), a Frizzled class G-protein coupled receptor termed as Smoothened (SMO), and glioma-associated oncogenic (GLI) TF. In the absence of Hh ligands, Ptch receptors are localized on the cilia and inhibit the translocation of SMO at the cilia to suppress Hh signaling by a mechanism yet to be fully understood [51]. However, emerging data suggest that Ptch regulates the activity of SMO by lowering the concentration of small molecules such as sterol and cholesterol in the cytoplasm. At the same time, GLI is suppressed by the binding of a transcriptional co-repressor, Suppressor of Fused (SUFU) to the full-length GLI, subsequently phosphorylated by cyclic-AMP dependent protein kinase A (cAMP-PKA), and undergoes proteolytic cleavage by β-TrCP. The resultant truncated form of GLI (GLI-R) acts as a transcriptional repressor and is translocated into the nuclei to suppress the promoters of target genes. Apart from this, Ptch has been reported to arrest the cell cycle by sequestering the cyclin B1-CDK1 complex.

However, the binding of Hh ligands at the outer domain of Ptch causes it to oligomerize and undergo endosomal degradation. Ptch inhibition is followed by the relocalization of SMO to the cilia and the phosphorylation of its C-terminal domain by a variety of kinases. Activated SMO then mediates the rescue of GLI from the repressive SUFU complex and its translocation into the nuclei. Consequently, the expression of various GLI-regulated oncogenes such as *N-myc, Foxm1, VEGFA, Cyclin D1,* anti-apoptotic gene *Bcl-2*, cell cycle regulators (*CCND2, CCNE1*), and positive regulators of the Wnt signaling pathway is upregulated [51]. Expression of GLI downstream target genes is crucial for promoting the survival and renewal of CSCs [52]. Aberrant activation of many of these genes has been implicated in several aspects of carcinogenesis such as EMT, angiogenesis, and metastasis. In CSCs, Hh signaling has also been reported to enhance the expression of pluripotency markers SOX2 and OCT4 [53]. Acquisition of the stemness factors has a key role in facilitating EMT of cancer cells and enables them to regenerate and increase the propensity of spheroid formation [54].

8.2.3.3 Notch Signaling Pathway

Though notch signaling has a fundamental role to play in stem cell renewal and cellular differentiation, its hyperactivation has been observed in several cancer types [55]. During notch signaling activation, notch transmembrane receptors (Notch 1-4) on one cell are bound by the notch ligands from an adjacent cell [56]. As a result, the proteolytic activity of γ-secretase is induced which mediates the cleavage of notch intracellular domain (NICD). Subsequently, the NICD is translocated into the nuclei to promote the transcription of its target genes cyclin D1 and hairy enhancer of split (Hes1). Since notch signaling is also involved in the development of mammary glands, its deregulation has been implicated in breast cancer and several other solid tumors [57, 58]. Pertinently, CSCs in renal cell carcinoma and breast cancers have been characterized by marked upregulation of notch receptors and their expression has been correlated with enhanced chemoresistance and self-renewal capacity of CSCs [57, 59].

8.2.3.4 PI3K/AKT/mTOR Signaling Pathway

Hyperactivation of phosphoinositide-3-kinase-AKT (PI3K/AKT) and mammalian target of rapamycin (mTOR) signaling has been observed in a variety of solid tumors and blood malignancies [38]. The heterodimeric class 1A PI3K complex consists of a regulatory (p85α/β, p55α/γ, p50α) and a catalytic subunit (p110α/β/γ), which is activated by the binding of the regulatory subunit to an activated receptor tyrosine kinases. Alternatively, the catalytic subunits (p110α/γ) can also be activated by direct interaction with RAS or GTPase-mediated activation of p110β. Activated PI3K complex is recruited at the plasma membrane and the signaling is commenced with the conversion of phosphoinositide $PI(4,5)P_2$ into its phosphorylated second messenger $PI(3,4,5)P_3$ and its derivative dephosphorylated form $PI(3,4)P_2$. The secondary messenger serves as effector molecules that are recognized by the phosphoinositide-binding domains of serine/threonine kinases such as AKT and subsequently regulate the activity of downstream targets such as GSK-3β, forkhead box O, and mTOR complexes (mTORC1 and 2) [60].

In the normal developmental context, PI3K mediated phosphoinositide signaling regulates the proliferation of cells and its activity is modulated by negative feedback loops comprising lipid phosphatases such as phosphatase and tensin homolog (PTEN). By mediating dephosphorylation of both $PI(3,4,5)P_3$ and $PI(3,4)P_2$, PTEN act as a tumor suppressor and downregulates PI3K/AKT signaling. Activation of ribosomal S3 kinase by mTORC1 also serves to limit PI3K activity as a regulatory mechanism. However, the activating mutations in the catalytic subunit of PI3Kα render it to be active constitutively and have been observed in multiple cancer types. PI3Kα variant H1047R has been found to induce the dedifferentiation of tumor cells into CSCs and enhance their stemness properties [60]. In luminal breast cancer cells, the repression of mTOR inhibitors serves as an intrinsic mechanism of the altered mTOR signaling. Recently, comparative analysis of genome-wide methylation patterns between CSCs and NSCCs has revealed that genes related to PI3K signaling are indeed hypomethylated in CSCs thus exhibiting a positive correlation with the hyperactivation of PI3K/AKT signaling in CSCs [61]. Also, the activity of drug efflux pumps such as ATP binding cassette transporters (ABCG2) in CSCs is augmented by AKT-mediated regulation. In various sarcoma cell lines, the upregulated PI3K/AKT signaling was found to be essential for the expression of Nanog in $CD133^+$ CSCs and resulted in high resistance to doxorubicin and radiation therapy [21]. In gastric adenocarcinoma, inhibiting the activity of PI3K was found to reduce the expression of CD44 in CSCs, along with significant downregulation of mesenchymal trans-differentiation marker Slug. The data suggest that upregulation of CSCs-markers is critical for the enhanced tumor initiation ability of CSCs. Altogether, the activation of PI3K/AKT/mTOR signaling endows the CSCs to proliferate while exhibiting resistance to chemotherapeutic drugs [22].

So far, multiple studies have demonstrated a complex network of cross-talk between PI3K and other dysregulated signaling pathways in cancer cells [60]. As GSK-3β can phosphorylate MYC and prime it for degradation, the activation of oncogenic PI3K signaling has an opposing effect and tends to stabilize MYC by promoting degradation of GSK-3β. AKT-mediated degradation of GSK-3β also preserves the activity of β-catenin, leading to the upregulation of its downstream effector NODAL, which further promotes TGF-β signaling in CSCs. Suppression of GSK-3β activity also helps to stabilize Snai1 [44, 62]. The enhanced stabilization of β-catenin and Snai1 is indispensable for upregulating the expression of CD44 and maintenance of stem cell-like features of cancer cells [63, 64]. Furthermore, PI3K/AKT signaling has been reported to promote the stemness of malignant cells via the CXCR4-STAT3 pathway by upregulating the expression of the chemokine receptor CXCR4. Therefore, PI3K/AKT signaling act in unison with several other pathways that facilitate cancer metastasis and therapeutic relapse. The targeting of PI3K signaling in CSCs has been suggested to synergize the cytotoxic effects of chemotherapeutic drugs and can help to improve their overall efficiency in curing malignancies.

8.2.3.5 NF-κB Signaling Pathway

Enhanced inflammation is of paramount importance to modulate the tumor microenvironment and involves the constitutive activation of nuclear factor kappa-light-chain-enhancer of activated B cells (NF-κB) signaling. The upregulated NF-κB pathway in cancer cells has been found to promote the expression of genes involved in cell proliferation, inhibition of programmed cell death, and metastasis [65, 66]. NF-κB family includes the TFs such as RelA (p65), RelB, and proto-oncogene c-rel that are activated by canonical and non-canonical signaling by the proteolytic cleavage of p105 and p100, respectively [67]. During a steady-state, the inactive RelA/RelB complexes are bound by the inhibitor of κB proteins (IκBs) and localized in the cytosol. Various stimuli such as developmental signal, LPS, and pro-inflammatory cytokines (TNF-α, IL-1) are known to trigger the activation of the NF-κB signaling pathway. The activation of NF-κB by canonical pathway requires the phosphorylation and proteasomal degradation of IκBα by the activity of the inhibitor of κB kinase complex (IKK). Degradation of IκBα results in the nuclear translocation of p65-p50 heterodimers and transcriptional activation of genes such as IL-6, cyclin D1, and anti-apoptotic factors. In the non-canonical pathway, the activation of the RelB-p100 complex is mediated by the activity of NF-κB-inducing kinase (NIK). NIK-induced activation of IKKα dimers facilitates the phosphorylation and cleavage of p100 into p52, and the subsequent accumulation of RelB-p52 dimers into the nuclei to regulate transcription of downstream effector genes.

The activity of NF-κB is modulated by negative feedback mechanisms involving regulators such as A20 and IκBα. However, its aberrant activation in solid tumors and hematological malignancies has been linked with the amplification of positive regulators such as IKKs and c-rel. Besides this, the loss of negative regulators has also been observed in various cancer types. In B-cell lymphomas, the loss of inhibitory factor p100 due to rearrangement and overproduction of p52 were found to activate non-canonical signaling pathways, whereas mono-allelic deletions of IκBα have been reported in glioblastomas to upregulate canonical signaling. Various other mechanisms have also been found to mediate the oncogenic activation of NF-κB signaling such as enhanced expression of receptor activator of NF-κB ligand (RANKL) in BCSCs and upregulation of osteopontin in hepatocellular carcinoma stem cells [65, 68].

In malignant tissues, the aberrant activation of the NF-κB pathway has been demonstrated to promote cell survival and proliferation by upregulating the expression of anti-apoptotic proteins (cIAPs, XIAP, Bcl-2, and Bcl-xL) and positive regulators of the cell cycle (cyclin D1, cyclin E, and c-Myc). Moreover, NF-κB induced expression of pro inflammatory cytokines (IL-1, IL-6. TNF-α, COX-2, and iNOS) further aggravates the tumor microenvironment that supports the growth and proliferation of CSCs [65, 69]. Overproduction of cytokines such as IL-6 by the NF-κB pathway also tends to activate the oncogenic genes along the IL-6/STAT3 axis in hepatocellular carcinomas. In ovarian cancer, the oncogenic attributes of NF-κB signaling have been further exhibited in maintaining the stemness of $CD133^+$/$CD44^+$ CSCs by upregulating the expression of pluripotency factors such as Nanog and Sox2 [70]. Likewise, NF-κB induced STAT3 activation has been found to regulate the expression of KLF4 and NKX3.1 in CSCs of prostate cancers [65]. Besides this, NF-κB also facilitates the stabilization of IL-6 mRNAs by downregulating the expression of let-7, a miRNA targeting IL-6, in Lin-28 dependent manner [69].

NF-κB signaling also contributes to EMT by facilitating the remodeling of extracellular matrix (ECM) via the expression of vimentin, vascular endothelial growth factor (VEGF), and matrix metalloproteases (MMPs) [67, 69]. ECM not only serves in imparting structural stability but also helps to sequester growth factors, angiogenic factors, and cytokines. During cancer invasion, ECM is degraded by the activity of endopeptidases such as MMPs and subsequently alters the tissue microenvironment that becomes permissible for EMT [71]. Additionally, MMPs promote angiogenesis by facilitating the mobilization of endothelial cells and helps the tumors to acquire an invasive phenotype. Both MMP2 and MMP9 have been reported to be upregulated during angiogenesis and are highly expressed at the tumor-stromal interface. Apart from this, MMP9 has also been implicated in cleaving the IL-2α receptor on the surface of T cells and thus inhibits their proliferation in response to IL-2 signaling. Other biological roles of MMPs include degradation of E-cadherin, modulation of signaling pathways by altering the availability of signaling molecules and their surface receptors [71].

8.2.3.6 TGF-β Signaling Pathway

Transformation growth factor β (TGF-β) family cytokines are ubiquitously secreted in the extracellular milieu by mammalian cells and have been found to possess both tumor-suppressive and proliferative properties depending upon the cellular context [72]. In normal epithelial and premalignant cells, TGF-β1 induces cell cycle arrest at the G1/S checkpoint by upregulating the expression of p15, p21, and p27, which then impair the interaction of various cyclins with cyclin-dependent kinases. Also, the cytostatic functions of TGF-β1 are mediated by inhibiting the expression of c-MYC. However, aberrant TGF-β signaling in several cancer types has been found to promote EMT by activation of ERK, MAPK, and PI3K-AKT signaling pathways [73]. Signaling cascade initiated with the binding of TGF-β at its receptor TGFβRII results in its auto-phosphorylation and subsequent phosphorylation of TGFβRI at Tyr residues. Consequently, ShcA is activated to mediate the assembly of the ShcA/Grb2/Sos complex that is required for the induction of genes along the Ras-MEK-Erk axis. ERK activation leads to the phosphorylation of SMAD1, 2, and 3 and marks them for proteasomal degradation in the cytoplasm thereby abolishing the tumor-suppressive function of SMAD complexes. Also, the TGF-β induced interaction of TGFβRI with TGFβRII has been found to trigger the activation of AKT regulatory subunit p85 and signal transduction via the PI3K-AKT pathway. The altered gene expression due to SMAD- and non-SMAD-mediated pathways are characterized by upregulation of TFs such as Zeb1 and 2, MMPs, Snail, and Slug. These TFs are known to negatively regulate the expression of E-cadherin in cancer cells and confers enhanced invasive capacity upon the malignant cells to undergo EMT. [74].

Apart from the induction of metastasis, TGF-β signaling has recently been demonstrated to promote the dedifferentiation of NSCCs into a more primitive CSC-like phenotype [75]. In colorectal cancer patients, the heterogeneous tumor mass consists of $CD44^-$ NSCCs with very low tumorigenic potential and $CD44^+$ CSCs with high reconstitution ability. Furthermore, $CD44^+$ cells were characterized by marked upregulation of TGF-β signaling genes along with high expression of pluripotency TFs such as OCT4, SOX2, and NANOG. Interestingly, stimulation of $CD44^-$ NSCCs with TGF-β enabled them to gain the expression of CSC-specific marker CD44 and exhibited high tumorigenic potential upon subsequent transplantation in immuno-deficient mice. These results were recapitulated by ectopic expression of TWIST1 in $CD44^-$ cells thereby suggesting that the dedifferentiation process was mediated by TGF-β induced activation of TWIST1 in $CD44^-$ NSCCs. In the tumor microenvironment, excessive local secretion of TGF-β by infiltrating macrophages and fibroblasts, surrounding mesenchymal cells as well as autocrine production by cancer cells has been correlated with worse prognosis and facilitates metastasis.

Similar observations have been made in basal breast cancer patients wherein TGF-β signaling-driven dedifferentiation of $CD44^{-}$ NSCCs into $CD44^{+}$ CSCs has a profound role in cancer progression [76]. The $CD44^{hi}$ basal breast cancer cells have been reported to have higher tumor-initiating capacity compared to luminal breast cancer cells which are mostly $CD44^{lo}$. The difference in tumorigenic potential between the basal and luminal breast cancer cells is further reflected by the evidence that $CD44^{lo}$ basal breast cancer cells are more efficient in generating $CD44^{+}$ CSCs than their luminal counterparts. The underlying differences were mediated by the differential expression of ZEB1 and ZEB2 in TGF-β dependent manner. The chromatin at *Zeb1* promoter in $CD44^{-}$ luminal breast cancer cells was found in a repressed state (enriched for H3K27-me3), whereas in basal breast cancer cells it was characterized by bivalent histone modifications of H3K4-me3 and H3K27-me3, indicative of its poised state. The stimulation of basal breast cancer cells with TGF-β enabled the transition of the ZEB1 promoter from the poised to an active state by the removal of H3K27-me3. Active *Zeb1* transcription was found to be essential for inhibiting the transcription of tumor-suppressive MIR200 family miRNAs and the subsequent acquisition of stemness properties by the transformed cells. Therefore, differential expression of *Zeb1* in basal breast cancer cells was found to be essential for modulating the plasticity between $CD44^{lo/-}$ NSCCs and $CD44^{hi}$ CSCs.

8.2.3.7 JAK/STAT Signaling Pathway

The binding of the IL-6 family cytokines to IL-6 receptor-α is known to trigger the activation of receptor-associated Janus-activated kinases (JAK) that are ubiquitously expressed in mammalian cells. The kinase domain in JAK family proteins (JAK1, JAK2, and TYK2) subsequently induces the phosphorylation of signal transducer and activator of transcription (STAT) family TFs at tyrosine-705 to constitute the JAK/STAT signaling pathway. The acetylation of active STAT3 at lysine-685 in the SH2 domain enables its dimerization and subsequent translocation into the nucleus through importin-β1, where it serves to activate the downstream effector genes. However, the elevated expression of IL-6 has been demonstrated to facilitate the aberrant activation of the JAK/STAT signaling pathway in several tumors such as renal cell carcinoma, myxoid liposarcoma, breast, prostate, and gastrointestinal cancers [77–79]. Dysregulated JAK/STAT signaling in malignant cells can be attributed to factors such as non-receptor tyrosine kinase PYK2 mediated enhanced phosphorylation of STAT3 in TNBC, constitutive activation of STAT3 due to the loss of SMAD4 in pancreatic cancer, and the enrichment of SMYD3/RNAPII complex at the JAK1 and JAK2 promoters in colon cancer. Also, the concerted activity of non-canonical TGF-β1 signaling and activated STAT3 has been implicated in the induction of EMT [78, 80]

The accumulating evidence suggests that IL-6/JAK2/STAT3 axis contributes to the tumorigenesis by transcriptional activation of pluripotency genes such as Nanog and Oct4 in CSCs, promoting EMT via upregulation of TFs such as SNAI1, ZEB1,

TWIST-1, and JUNB, and enhancing the motility of malignant cells by activating focal adhesion kinase (FAK) [78]. Also, active STAT3 signaling has been found to enhance stemness by inducing the expression of *c-Myc* via upregulation of PIM-1. Furthermore in breast cancer cells, the active STAT3 associates with estrogen receptor and induces the expression of LIV1, which then inactivates GSK-3β to stabilize Snail. Apart from inducing the expression of EMT-related TFs, STAT3 also promotes cell proliferation of stromal fibroblasts by inhibiting the expression of CDKIs (p16 and p21) in AUF1-dependent manner and thus boosting the secretion of TGF-β1 from the fibroblast in the tumor microenvironment. In prostate cancer, STAT3 has been reported to stabilize the hypoxia-inducible factor 1α (HIF-1α) by indulging in direct physical interaction with HIF-1α and thus preventing its degradation by the proteasomal machinery. The ensuing STAT3-HIF-1α complex is subsequently recruited at the promoters of Twist-1 and VEGF to propagate cancer metastasis. STAT3/HIF-1α signaling has also been implicated in the SOX2 mediated expression of Slug.

The induction of JAK2/STAT3 signaling via oncostatin M is crucial for the generation of CSCs [79]. CD44 is closely associated with STAT3 in breast and colorectal cancer wherein the CD44-acetylated STAT3 complex is readily translocated into the nuclei to promote the expression of stemness genes such as c-Myc, Oct4, and Sox2. In basal-like breast cancer cell line MDA-MB-231, the induction of JAK/STAT3 signaling via autocrine production of IL-6 by NSCCs was found to facilitate their dedifferentiation into highly tumorigenic CSCs via upregulation of stemness marker OCT-4 [81]. The production of OCT-4 enabled NSCCs to acquire characteristic properties of CSCs with increased capacity of mammosphere formation. The observations also suggest that there exists a state of equilibrium between the number of CSCs and NSCCs within the tumor mass. In an in vitro analysis of MCF-7-derived mammospheres, genes involved in JAK/STAT signaling (*JAK3, STAT5A*, and *CCND2*) are hypomethylated corresponding to their upregulation in $CD44^+$ CSCs compared to NSCCs [82]. Therefore, modulation of the epigenetic landscape can explain in part the dysregulation of the JAK-STAT signaling pathway in CSCs. Moreover, aberrant activation of JAK/STAT signaling in CSCs isolated from myxoid liposarcoma has been found to correlate with their resistance to chemotherapy and ability to generate sarcospheres [77]. However, impairment of JAK/STAT3 signaling led to a reduction in the size of sarcospheres and overcome drug resistance. Interestingly, phosphorylated STAT3 was also found to interact with a component of the SWI/SNF chromatin remodeling complex thereby underscoring the notion that active STAT3-mediated epigenetic reprogramming can be vital for the generation and maintenance of CSCs.

8.2.3.8 Hypoxia-Mediated Modulation of the Tumor Microenvironment

Tumor hypoxia helps the cancer cells to evade ROS-mediated cell death and thrive in a low oxygen environment [83]. Under hypoxic conditions, HIF-1α is markedly stabilized in the tumor cells by the activity of TGF-β1 and is crucial for promoting angiogenesis by upregulating the expression of VEGF [84, 85]. Hypoxia-associated angiogenesis is a characteristic feature of cancer metastasis and correlates with the higher degree of cell migration during hypoxia [86, 87, 88]. Furthermore, HIF-α has been demonstrated to enhance the expression of pluripotency inducing TFs such as OCT4, KLF4, and SOX2 [89] and helps to maintain CSCs population in the tumor mass [90, 91]. The overall changes in the tumor microenvironment facilitate the progression to an aggressive phenotype that becomes highly resistant to radiation or chemotherapy and results in a poor outcome of treatment [92].

8.3 Therapeutic Targeting of CSCs

The CSCs function is regulated by various factors including transcription factors, drug efflux pumps, cell surface CSCs specific biomarkers, and intracellular signaling pathways as discussed in the previous sections. Besides, the CSCs microenvironment also regulates the CSCs self-renewal, differentiation, angiogenesis and promotes invasion and metastasis [16]. These regulating factors of CSCs are the essential targets for the development of novel therapeutics based on small molecules, vaccines, antibodies, and cellular therapy. Four major strategies have been developed to eradicate CSCs in recent years that include targeting CSCs specific surface markers, intervening key signaling pathways, selectively inhibiting drug efflux transporters (ABC transporters), and ameliorating the CSC microenvironment [16, 93].

8.4 Non-flavonoids Targeting CSCs

In recent times, bioactive phytochemicals have emerged as vital resources in the prevention and treatment of cancer by either delaying the cancer cell invasion or their specific elimination ([94, 95]). Owing to the ready availability and safer metabolic processing of bioactive compounds in the plant-based diet, several phytochemicals have been hailed as a suitable alternative in cancer treatment since these compounds exhibit no cytotoxicity to healthy primary cells [96]. Interestingly, many phytochemicals have been recognized to exhibit anticancer properties by targeting CSCs. Dietary polyphenols in particular have been demonstrated to reduce the number of CSCs thereby inhibiting the underlying tumorigenesis [95, 97]. These compounds have been demonstrated to mediate their salubrious effects by modulating a broad spectrum of signaling pathways that are dysregulated in CSCs and aid in the arrest of cancer progression. Many of these compounds have the promising ability to alter the tumor microenvironment by modulating the expression of inflammatory signals, growth factors, and drug transporters [94, 95, 98, 99].

The polyphenols comprise a large number of heterogeneous organic compounds characterized by the presence of phenyl ring(s) and one/or more hydroxyl substituents [100]. Among the dietary polyphenols, majority comprises the flavonoids or non-flavonoids. The non-flavonoid polyphenols are further subdivided into phenolic acids, stilbenes, lignans, tannins, and diferuloylmethane [100, 101]. Several non-flavonoids have been reported to exhibit anticancer properties as well as inhibit the self-renewal and survival of CSCs in various forms of cancer. Additionally, recent studies suggest that some non-flavonoids can also enhance the anti-CSC therapy by sensitizing them to conventional therapies. The non-flavonoids mostly regulate CSCs or eliminate them by targeting various signaling pathways involved in maintaining the stemness of the CSCs. Though the exact mechanisms by which non-flavonoids regulate CSCs remain elusive, they have been shown to inhibit self-renewal, stemness, and EMT, induce cell cycle arrest, apoptosis, and autophagy, and target various CSCs pathways such as Wnt/β-catenin, hedgehog, notch, PI3K/AKT, NF-κB, and JAK/STAT signaling pathways (Table 8.1). Various non-flavonoids rendering the regulation of CSCs growth and maintenance by targeting these signaling pathways are discussed in the following sections.

8.4.1 Phenolic Acid

The phenolic acids, mainly the hydroxybenzoic and hydroxycinnamic acids represent most of the non-flavonoids that have shown potent anticancer activities in several in vitro as well as in vivo studies [98, 101].

8.4.1.1 Hydroxybenzoic Acid

Various forms of hydroxybenzoic acid derivatives such as gallic acid, ellagic acid, protocatechuic acid, syringic acid, and vanillic acid have been reported to display anticancer properties [98, 99, 102, 148]. Among these gallic acid, methyl-3-O-methyl gallate, and ellagic acids have also been reported to target and inhibit CSCs.

Gallic Acid

Gallic acid (3,4,5-trihydroxy benzoic acid), widely present in various plant-based food sources such as *Rubus, Fragaria* (Rosaceae), and *Vaccinium* (Ericaceae) genera, tea (*Camellia sinensis L.*), grapes (*Vitis vinifera L.*), and sumac (*Rhus coriaria L.*) exhibit protective and therapeutic activities against various forms of cancer [102, 149, 150]. Gallic acid has been demonstrated to inhibit the CSCs of the prostatosphere in DU145 prostate cancer cells [102]. It showed inhibitory activity in cancer cell proliferation, self-renewal, and prostatosphere formation by inhibiting the NF-κB signaling pathway.

Methyl-3-O-methyl Gallate

The methyl-3-O-methyl gallate (M3OMG), is a non-flavonoid, the esterified derivative of gallic acid isolated from an evergreen shrub, the Chilean lantern tree (*Crinodendron hookerianum*), and rhizomatous perennial herb *Peltiphyllum peltatum*, used as food and in traditional medicine [102, 151]. The M3OMG has shown greater potential inhibiting the CSC-enriched prostatosphere formation in DU145 prostate cancer cells than gallic acids [102]. It effectively inhibits CSCs self-renewal and proliferation by inhibiting the NF-κB signaling pathway.

Table 8.1 Non-flavonoid polyphenols with anti-CSC activity

Non-flavonoid class and subclass of	Dietary polyphenols	Structure	Source	Cancer type	Cell line/Model	Conclusions	References
Phenolic acid -Hyroxybenzoic acid	Gallic acid	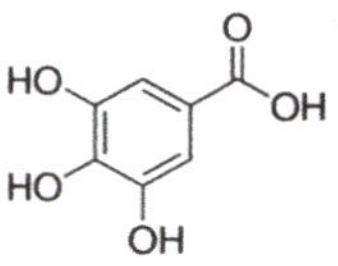	*Rubus, Fragaria* (Rosaceae) and *Vaccinium* (Ericaceae) genera; tea (*Camellia sinensis* L.); grapes (*Vitis vinifera L.*) and sumac (*Rhus coriaria L.*)	Prostate cancer	DU145 prostate cancer cells	Inhibition of CSCs in prostatosphere by downregulating NF-kB signaling pathway	[102]
	Methyl-3-O-methyl gallate	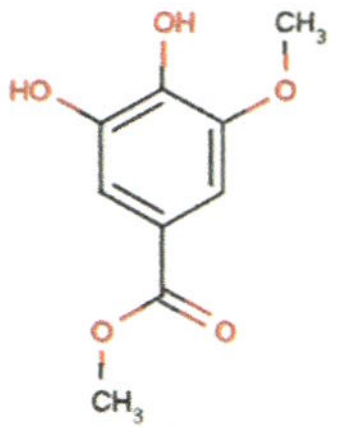	Umbrella plant (*Peltiphyllum peltatum*); Chilean lantern tree (*Crinodendron hookerianum*)	Prostate cancer	DU145 prostate cancer cells	Inhibition of CSCs in prostatosphere by downregulating NF-kB signaling pathway	[102]
	Ellagic acid	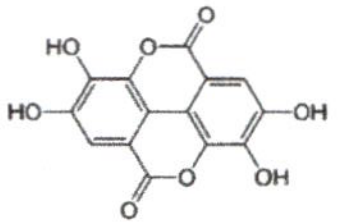	Pomegranate (*Punica granatum*), persimmon (*Diospyros*), berries (*Rubus, Fragaria*	Breast cancer	MDA-MB-23 and BT-549 breast cancer cell lines; in vivo xenograft mice model	Decrease in number and size of mammospheres; Downregulation of β-catenin pathway by interruption of the ACTN4/β-catenin	[103]

(continued)

Table 8.1 (continued)

Non-flavonoid class and subclass of	Dietary polyphenols	Structure	Source	Cancer type	Cell line/Model	Conclusions	References
			Rosaceae), nuts (*Juglans*, *Prunus*)			interaction; Inhibition of CSCs-related metastasis	
				Colon cancer	Caco-2 human colon cancer cell line; Patient-derived primary tumor	Downregulation of ALDH1	[104]
				Colon cancer	HCT116 human colon cancer cell line; Patient-derived primary tumor	Downregulation of the CSC markers, CD133, CD44, DLK1, Notch1, and Wnt/ β-catenin signaling pathways; Suppression of self-renewal capacity	[105]
- Hydroxycinnamic acid	Caffeic acid	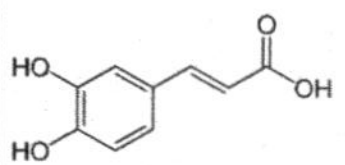	Coffee (*Coffea Arabica*), wheat (*Triticum*), quinoa (*Chenopodium quinoa*), barley (*Hordeum vulgare*), corn (*Zea mays*), oat	Breast cancer, Hepatocellular carcinoma	MDA-MB-231 breast cancer cells; MHCC97H Hepatocellular carcinoma cells; In vivo xenograft BALB/c nude mice	Inhibition of TGFβ-SMAD2 signal pathway mediated by microRNA-148a	[106]

			(*Avena sativa*), rye (*Secale cereal*), rice (*Oryza sativa*), thyme (*Thymus vulgaris*), oregano (*Origanum vulgare*), *Sorghum,* propolis, some fruits, and vegetables	Colorectal cancer	HCT116 human colon cancer cell line; in vivo xenograft mice model	Suppression of self-renewal capacity, stem-like characteristics and migratory capacity; Downregulation of PI3K/AKT signaling pathway	[107]
	Caffeic acid phenethyl ester	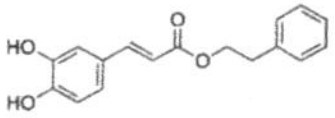	Propolis, a honeybee-derived natural product	Breast cancer	MDA-MB-231 breast cancer cells; xenograft nude mice	Inhibition of self-renewal and progenitor formation.	[108]
	Chlorogenic acid	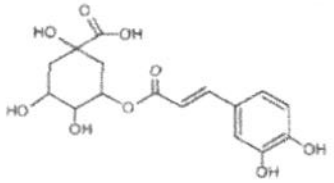	*Eucommia ulmoides, honeysuckle,* and coffee (*Coffea Arabica*)	Lung cancer	Lu 65 and Lu 135 cells derived from lung cancer tissue; A549 cells adenocarcinoma cells	Upregulation of p38 MAP signaling pathway; Downregulation of stem cell markers: NANOG, POU5F1, and SOX2	[109]
	p-coumaric acid	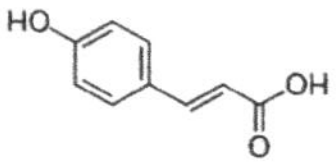	Bamboo grass (*Sasa quelpaertensis)*	Colon cancer	HT29 and HCT116 cell lines; In vivo xenograft	Downregulation of Wnt/β-catenin signaling and HIF-1α signaling; Blocking the	[110]

(continued)

Table 8.1 (continued)

Non-flavonoid class and subclass of	Dietary polyphenols	Structure	Source	Cancer type	Cell line/Model	Conclusions	References
					BALB/c nude mice	expression of stem cell markers—DLK1, Notch1, and Sox-2	
Stilbenes	Resveratrol	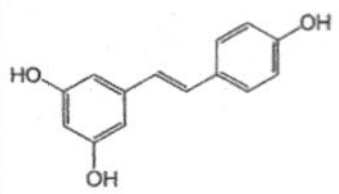	Grapes (*Vitis vinifera*), peanuts (*Arachis hypogaea*), berries (*Rubus, Fragaria* Rosaceae), and red wine	Pancreatic cancer	Human pancreatic CSCs ($CD133^+$, $CD44^+$, $CD24^+$, ESA^+) in NOD/SCID mice; CSCs derived from $Kras^{G12D}$ transgenic mice and human pancreatic tumor	Inhibition of self-renewal capacity; Inhibition of pluripotency maintaining factors; Inhibition of migration and invasion; Inhibition of EMT	[111]
				Breast cancer	Cancer stem-like cells (CD24−/CD44+/ESA+) isolated from ER+ and ER− breast cancer cell lines.	Inhibition of fatty acid synthase	[112]
				Head and neck cancer (HNC)	CD44+ HNC cells; HNC-Tumor Initiating Cells;	Reduced self-renewal property, stemness, and EMT	([113],)

				Leukemia	Human promyeloblastic leukemia KG-1a cells	Sensitizes to cytokine-induced killer cell-mediated cytolysis	[114]
				Breast cancer	MDA-MB-231-Luc-D3H2LN cells orthotopically inoculated on female SCID mice	Upregulation of Argonaute 2 causing increased expression of tumor-suppressive miRNAs, miR-16,—141, -143, and -200c	[115]
				Acute myeloid leukemia	HL-60 human acute myeloid leukemia cells; Patient-derived samples	Downregulation of IL-6-stimulated Sonic Hedgehog Signaling	[116]
				Glioblastoma	Patient-derived Glioma Stem Cell (GSCs) cultures; and Intracranial xenograft models of GSCs in BALB/cAJcl-nu/nu mice	Upregulation of p53/p21 pathway by inhibiting Nanog Loss of stemness by suppressing Nanog	[117]
				Breast cancer	MCF7 and SUM159 breast cancer cell lines; NOD/SCID mice	Induction of autophagy via suppressing Wnt/β-catenin signaling pathway	[118]

(continued)

Table 8.1 (continued)

Non-flavonoid class and subclass of	Dietary polyphenols	Structure	Source	Cancer type	Cell line/Model	Conclusions	References
				Glioblastoma	GSCs derived from Human glioblastoma tissue	Inhibition of Sirtuin-2	[119]
				Ovarian cancer	A2780 human ovarian cancer cells	Induction of apoptosis; ROS generation; and Loss of self-renewal capacity	[120]
				Colon cancer	Colorectal CSCs induced from colon cancer cell line HCT116	Cell cycle arrest in the G0/G1 phase; and Induction of apoptosis	[121]
				Lung cancer	A549 lung cancer cell line; In vivo BALB/c nude mice xenograft	Augments tumor necrosis factor-related apoptosis-inducing ligand (TRAIL)-mediated cytotoxicity	[122]
				Colon cancer	HCT116 colon cancer cell line; in vivo $APC^{Min}/^{+}$ mice	Downregulation of Wnt/β-catenin signaling; Induction of apoptosis	[123]
				Glioblastoma multiform	U87 glioma cells; Patient-derived GBM stem-like cell;	Inhibition of GSCs growth and infiltration via AKT deactivation and p53 induction	[124]

					in vivo xenografts in mice model		
				Glioblastoma multiforme	Human glioblastoma tissue-derived glioma stem cells from patients.	Decreased cell proliferation; Increased cell mortality; and Decreased cell motility via Wnt signaling and EMT pathway mediators.	[125]
				Cervical cancer	HeLa cell lines	Induction of apoptosis	[126]
				Osteosarcoma	Human osteosarcoma cell lines—MNNG/HOS, MG-63, and Osteoblast line hFOB1.19.	Decreased cytokines synthesis; Inhibition of JAK2/STAT3 signaling	[127]
				Glioblastoma	LN18 and U87 glioblastoma cells; U87 xenograft models	GSCs inhibition by EMT suppression via regulating Smad-dependent signaling	[128]
				Colorectal cancer	Human Colorectal cancer cell lines: HCT116, SW480, and RKO	Downregulation of TNF-β/TNF-βR-induced EMT via suppression of NF-κB and focal adhesion kinase (FAK)	[129]

(continued)

Table 8.1 (continued)

Non-flavonoid class and subclass of	Dietary polyphenols	Structure	Source	Cancer type	Cell line/Model	Conclusions	References
				Pancreatic cancer	MiaPaCa-2 pancreatic cancer cell lines and KPC mouse models of pancreatic ductal adenocarcinoma (PDA)	Reverses the stemness induced by gemcitabine by targeting SREBP1	[130]
				Gastric cancer	Patient tissue-derived gastric cancer-derived mesenchymal stem cells	Restriction of cell mobility; Suppression of EMT by inactivating the Wnt/β-catenin signaling; Inhibition of metastasis	[131]
				Renal cancer	ACHN and 786-O derived renal carcinoma stem cells	Downregulation of Sonic Hedgehog Signaling	[132]
Lignan	Eucommicin A	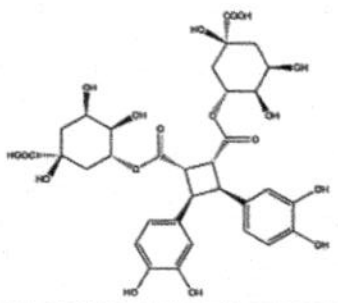	Du-zhong tea *(Eucommia ulmoides)*	-	Induced CSC-like (iCSCL) model cells	Abrogates sphere formation and self-renewal ability	[133]

Tannin	Ellagitannins (Urolithin A)	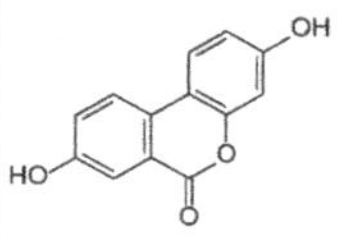	Pomegranate (*Punica granatum*), walnuts (*Juglans*)	Colon cancer	Caco-2 cells and patient-derived primary tumor cells	Inhibition of the number and size of colonospheres and ALDH1 activity	[104]
	Tannic acid	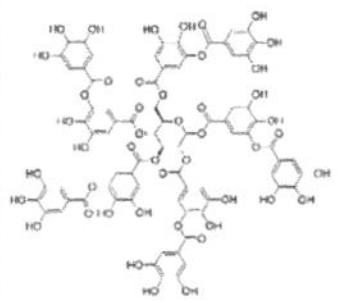	Found in a wide range of plants, including fruits, green and black teas, nuts, and grains	Breast cancer	MCF7, T47D, MDA-MB-231 breast cancer cells; In vivo xenograft Balb/c nude mice	Inhibition of mammosphere formation and ALDH1; Inhibition of NF-κB-pathway and EMT.	[134]
	Corilagin	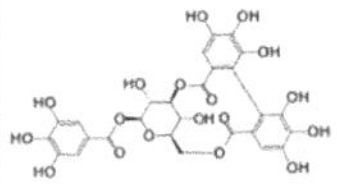	Longan, *Lumnitzera racemose, Terminalia catappa L, Phyllanthus sp.*	Glioblastoma	U251 glioblastoma (stem-like) cells	Induction of cell cycle arrest; Inhibition of NF-κB pathway	[135]
Diferuloylmethane	Curcumin	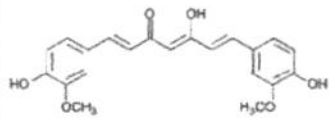	Turmeric (*Curcuma longa*)	Breast cancer	MCF-7 and Sum159 breast cancer cell lines	Inhibition self-renewal, ALDH1, and Wnt signaling	[136]
				Colon cancer	HCT116 and HT29 colon cancer cell lines; in vivo APC^{Min} $^{+/-}$ mice colorectal adenomas	Augmented the effect of Dasatinib; Decreased level of CSCs specific markers: CD44, CD166 EpCAM, ALDH1	[137]
				Glioblastoma	Cells obtained from glioblastoma	Induction of autophagy;	[138]

(continued)

Table 8.1 (continued)

Non-flavonoid class and subclass of	Dietary polyphenols	Structure	Source	Cancer type	Cell line/Model	Conclusions	References
					patient resected samples		
				Breast cancer	MCF-7 breast CSCs	Inhibition of β-catenin nuclear translocation, increased E-cadherin/β-catenin, suppress EMT and migration of BCSCs.	[139]
				Colon cancer	HCT116 colorectal cancer cell line	Augmented the effect of 5-FU; Decreased level of CSC-specific markers: CD133, CD44, ALDH1	[140]
				Lung cancer	A549 and H2170 lung cancer cell lines	Augmented the effect of cisplatin; Decreased migration capacity and self-renewal; Cell cycle regulation	[141]
				Lung cancer	A549 and H1299 lung cancer cell lines	Inhibition of Wnt/β-catenin and Sonic Hedgehog Pathways	[142]
				Breast cancer	MCF-7 breast cancer cells	Cell cycle arrest; Inhibition of hypoxia-inducible factor-1	[143]

				Thyroid cancer	Papillary thyroid cancer cell lines: BCPAP and TPC-1	Augmented the effect of cisplatin; Suppression of JAK/STAT3 pathway; Induction of apoptosis	[144]
Others	6-Shogaol	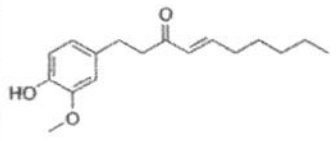	Dry ginger (*Zingiber officinale*)	Breast cancer	MCF-7 and MDA-MB-231 cell lines	Modulation of Notch Signaling Pathway and Induction of Autophagy	[145]
	Rottlerin	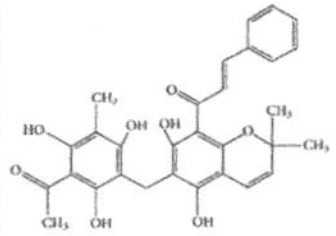	Asian Kamala plant (*Mallotus philippensis*)	Pancreatic cancer	Human pancreatic CSCs ($CD44^+/CD24^+/ESA^+$)	Induction of autophagy; Induction of apoptosis via inhibition of PI3K/AKT/mTOR pathway and activation of caspase	[29]
				Breast cancer	Primary tumor-derived human breast CSCs [$CD44^{(+)}/CD24^{(-/low)}$]	Induction of autophagy and apoptosis via activating several pathways such as via AMPK pathway activation and proteasome inhibition	[146]
				Prostate cancer	Patient-derived prostate cancer cells	Induction of autophagy and apoptosis via PI3K/AKT/mTOR signaling pathway	[147]

Ellagic Acid

Ellagic acid (2,3,7,8-tetrahydroxy-chromeno[5,4,3-cde]chromene-5,10-dione, C14H6O8) is a polyphenol dietary non-flavonoid found in numerous fruits and vegetables such as pomegranate (*Punica granatum*), persimmon (*Diospyros*), berries (*Rubus, Fragaria* Rosaceae), and nuts (*Juglans, Prunus*) [99, 152]. Ellagic acid shows anti-proliferative activity in vitro as well as in vivo cancer models of various origins such as skin, breast, colon, and esophageal cancer by inducing cell cycle arrest and apoptosis, inhibiting metastasis and angiogenesis [103, 152]. Moreover, it is a strong antioxidant, plays important role in DNA maintenance, prevents genomic instability, and also prevents cancer initiation and progression [152]. Owing to the strong anticancer activity, ellagic acid has been further investigated for its anti-CSC potential. [103] have reported that ellagic acid treatment reduced the number and size of CSCs-generated mammospheres derived from breast cancer cell lines MDA-MB-23 and BT-549, as well as in the xenograft mice model. It also effectively inhibited the CSCs metastasis. Ellagic acid controls CSCs by downregulating both the nuclear and cytoplasmic β-catenin in the AKT/GSK-3β signaling pathway. Moreover, the ellagic acid treatment also decreased the expression levels of Nanog, c-Myc, Oct-4, Survivin, Cyclin D1, Snail, ZEB1, and Slug in breast CSCs. It directly targets the breast cancer cell motile apparatus ACTN4 that promotes breast cancer tumorigenesis and inhibits CSCs metastasis [103]. In another study, [105] demonstrated that walnut phenolic extract containing ellagic acid and gallic had high inhibitory potential in CSCs derived from colon cancer cell line HCT116 as well as CSCs isolated from primary tumors by promoting cell differentiation and inhibiting the CSC markers, CD133, CD44, DLK1, Notch1, and Wnt/β-catenin signaling pathways. This study also showed that the combination of ellagic acid and gallic acid was more efficient than the individual compounds [105]. Further studies on Caco-2 human colon cancer cell line and primary tumor-derived CSCs revealed that a mixture of gut microbiota-derived metabolites urolithins and ellagic acid inhibit the development and growth of colonospheres by suppressing ALDH expressing cell population of CSCs [104].

8.4.1.2 Hydroxycinnamic Acid

The hydroxycinnamic acid derivatives—caffeic acid, chlorogenic acid, ferulic acid, p-coumaric acid, and sinapic acid have been reported to exhibit inhibitory activities against CSCs in various cancer types [98, 106, 108–110].

Caffeic Acid

Caffeic acid (3,4-dihydroxycinnamic acid), the main hydroxycinnamic acid derivative in the human diet, is commonly found in coffee (*Coffea Arabica*), wheat (*Triticum*), quinoa (*Chenopodium quinoa*), barley (*Hordeum vulgare*), corn (*Zea mays*), oat (*Avena sativa*), rye (*Secale cereal*), rice (*Oryza sativa*), thyme (*Thymus vulgaris*), oregano (*Origanum vulgare*), *Sorghum,* some fruits, and vegetables [153]. Caffeic acid has numerous pharmaceutical importance including antioxidants, antiviral, anti-inflammatory, immunomodulatory, and anticancer activities. The caffeic acid has shown potential as an important chemopreventive as well as a therapeutic agent against various forms of cancer [106, 107, 153]. Recent studies showed the prospective role of caffeic acid in maintaining CSCs and their possible mechanism of action. [106] demonstrated that caffeic acid attenuated various CSCs-like properties of breast cancer and colon cancer in vitro and in vivo. Treatment with caffeic acid reduced the expression level of CSCs surface markers CD44, EpCAM, ALDH-1, Oct-4, BMI-1, and Lin-28B and also suppressed the formation of mammospheres. As a mechanism, the caffeic acid inhibits the CSCs-like properties via miRNA-148a-mediated inhibition of the TGFβ-SMAD2 signaling pathway. In another recent study, caffeic acid has been demonstrated to effectively suppress the self-renewal, stemness, and migration of $CD44^+$ and $CD133^+$ colorectal CSCs in vitro and in vivo via inhibition of the PI3K/AKT signaling pathway [107].

Caffeic Acid Phenethyl Ester

Caffeic acid phenethyl ester (CAPE) is one of the major biologically active constituents of propolis, a honeybee-derived product with numerous medicinal values [108, 154]. CAPE has been reported to display a wide range of biological activities, including antioxidant, antibacterial, antiviral, anti-inflammatory, and anti-cancer activities. It exerts the anticancer effect by various mechanisms including inhibition of DNA synthesis, induction of apoptosis, and interfering with various signaling pathways [155]. CAPE has been shown to inhibit self-renewal and progenitor formation in breast CSCs in vitro and in vivo [108]. CD44 levels were decreased after treatment with CAPE.

Chlorogenic Acid

Chlorogenic acid, a dietary non-flavonoid, is formed by quinic acid and caffeic acid, is commonly found in foods, cosmetics, and medicines, and is one of the active constituents in many traditional Chinese medicines such as *Eucommia ulmoides, honeysuckle,* and coffee (*Coffea Arabica*) [156]. Chlorogenic acid has shown a wide range of biological activities including antioxidant, anti-inflammatory, cardioprotective, and anticancer activities (Abd [157]). Moreover, it showed the ability to effectively chemosensitize various cancer cells that cause suppression of cancer growth via various signaling pathways. The chlorogenic acid has been reported to regulate CSCs by downregulating the expression of stem cell markers NANOG, POU5F1, and SOX2 in lung cancer A549 cells [109].

p-coumaric Acid

The p-coumaric acid, a type of hydroxycinnamic acid, is largely found in edible plants like cereal bran, peanuts, tomatoes, carrots and is reported to exhibit anti-mutagenic and anticancer activity [158]. Studies also demonstrated that p-coumaric acid is an able inhibitor of CSCs growth. [110] showed that the leaf extract of *Sasa quelpaertensis* and its two bioactive compounds p-coumaric acid and tricin exert an anti-CSC effect in $CD133^+CD44^+$ cells isolated from colon cancer HT29 and HCT116 cell lines. The p-coumaric acid was found to suppress self-renewal and decreased the number and size of spheres by inhibiting the β-catenin signaling pathway. However, the extract containing p-coumaric acid and tricin was found to be much more effective in controlling CSCs characteristics. Further, the extract also enhanced cell differentiation by upregulating CK20 and inhibiting several stem cell markers such as DLK1, Notch1, and Sox-2. Besides, the extract also inhibits tumor growth in the xenograft model by downregulating stem cell markers via β-catenin and HIF-1α signaling pathways.

8.4.2 Stilbenes

Stilbenes are the relatively small group of non-flavonoids containing 1,2-diphenylethylene backbone having classical C6–C2–C6 structures with two hydroxyl groups on one ring and one on the other [159, 160]. They are found in various edible plants such as grapevine, berries, and peanuts. They occur as aglycones or glycosides and protect against bacterial, mold, or fungal invasion. Besides, they also protect against many chronic diseases such as cancer, cardiovascular, and neurodegenerative diseases. Resveratrol is the most extensively studied stilbene due to its wide range of biological activities.

8.4.2.1 Resveratrol

Resveratrol (3,4,5-trihydroxystilbene) is the most well-known stilbene that exists in both *cis-* and *trans-* isomeric forms, commonly found in fruits like grapes (*Vitis vinifera*), peanuts (*Arachis hypogaea*), berries (*Rubus, Fragaria* Rosaceae), and red wine [99, 161]. Several studies have revealed the anti-inflammatory, antioxidant, anti-atherosclerotic, and anti-neoplastic properties of resveratrol owing to its ability for modulating the gene regulatory mechanisms and signaling pathways in various cell types [162–164]. Resveratrol is one non-flavonoid that has been extensively studied for therapeutic potential against various forms of cancer as well as CSCs [99, 165]. Accumulating literature suggests effective preventive as well as therapeutic activities of resveratrol against CSCs of various types as described in Table 8.1.

Resveratrol was found to reduce the viability of SUM159 and MCF-7 breast cancer cells as well as the number of $ALDH1^+$ breast CSCs by inducing the expression of autophagic genes LC3-II, Beclin-I, and Atg7 [118]. Consistently, a higher number of autophagosomes were formed in the treated cells and the inhibitory effects were also reproduced in the tumor xenograft model in SCID mice. Resveratrol administration was found effective to prevent the growth of secondary tumors and significantly reduced the size of mammospheres. As the Wnt/β-catenin pathway has a major role to play in maintaining CSCs, the expression of β-catenin and cyclin D1 was downregulated in BCSCs upon resveratrol treatment. The data highlights the antitumor potential of resveratrol in eliminating CSCs via a multipronged approach constituting induction of autophagy and concordant inhibition of the Wnt/β-catenin pathway.

In another study, [112] demonstrated that resveratrol treatment caused the reduction of cell viability and mammosphere formation and induction apoptosis in $CD24^-/CD44^+/ESA^+$ cancer stem-like cells isolated from both ER^+ and ER^- breast cancer cell lines. This activity of resveratrol is accompanied by downregulation of fatty acid synthase (FAS) gene resulting in reduced lipid synthesis and upregulation of DAPK2 and BNIP3 pro-apoptotic genes [112]. The intraperitoneal administration of resveratrol and its methylated analog, pterostilbene, in SCID mice, was able to suppress the tumor formation by inhibiting the invasion and proliferation of cancer cells [115]. These effects were mediated by specific depletion of BCSCs in the cancerous tissues, leading to a drastic reduction in the size and numbers of mammospheres. As a mechanism, treatment of breast cancer cells with resveratrol induced the expression of tumor-suppressive miRNAs such as miR-16, miR-141, miR-143, and miR-200c, and RNAi activity was further supplemented by enhanced expression of Argonaute2, a key component of miRNA machinery. Studies on human pancreatic CSCs showed that resveratrol controls the growth and development of pancreatic cancer and self-renewal of pancreatic CSCs in $Kras^{G12D}$ mice [111]. As a mechanism, resveratrol treatment caused induction of apoptosis, inhibition of Nanog, Sox-2, c-Myc, and Oct-4 required for maintaining CSCs pluripotency, inhibition of drug resistance gene ABCG2, inhibition of CSCs migration and invasion, and EMT. In AML, resveratrol was found to target IL-6 and decrease sonic hedgehog signaling pathway and Gli-1 nuclear translocation, thus reversing the proliferation and stemness of AML-derived CSCs [116]. In a more recent study, [132] showed that resveratrol inhibited proliferation and sphere formation and induced apoptosis in renal CSCs by targeting the sonic hedgehog signaling pathway [132].

Resveratrol inhibits the self-renewal as well as the tumor-initiating capacity of glioblastoma stem cells (GSCs) by suppressing Nanog via proteasome degradation and activating the p53/p21 pathway [117]. Another study showed that resveratrol blocked GSC proliferation and induced necrosis at a higher dose by targeting SIRT2 [119]. Moreover, resveratrol inhibits the proliferation, sphere formation, and invasion of U87 glioma and patient-derived GSCs via AKT deactivation and p53 induction [124]. Resveratrol shows a significant effect on the Wnt pathway as it is evident from the modulation of c-Myc and β-catenin genes in patient-derived GSCs [125]. It has also been shown to inhibit the EMT in GSCs by downregulating Snail and Twist1. A recent study showed that resveratrol suppresses EMT-induced self-renewal of GSCs and stem cell markers Bmi1 and Sox2 by regulating SMAD-dependent signaling [128].

Resveratrol was also shown to inhibit stemness by generating intracellular ROS in CSCs derived from A2780 ovarian cancer cells [120]. Resveratrol also inhibits JAK2/STAT3 signaling pathway to suppress osteosarcoma stem cell proliferation and tumor-inducing capacity [127]. In a study with colon cancer-derived CSCs, resveratrol was found to downregulate TNF-β/TNF-βR-induced EMT via suppression of NF-κB and FAK, and regulate CSCs growth and infiltration [129]. Recently, a study with gastric cancer-derived mesenchymal stem cells, demonstrated that resveratrol restricted the metastasis and reverses the EMT progression by inactivating the Wnt/β-catenin signaling pathway [131].

8.4.3 Lignan

Lignans are the non-flavonoids characterized by the presence of two propylbenzene units (C6-C3) found in legumes, seeds, and vegetables. Flaxseed lignans have been reported to exhibit preventive as well as therapeutic activity against cancer specifically breast cancer [166, 167].

8.4.3.1 Eucommicin A

Eucommicin A (3,4,3',4'-tetrahydroxy-β-truxinic acid) is a type of lignan isolated from a small tree *Eucommia ulmoides* native to China. The aqueous extract of *E. ulmoides* is a popular drink in China and Japan and is commonly known as Du-zhong tea [133]. Several chemical constituents of *E. ulmoides* have been identified to possess important biological functions including anti-hypertensive, anti-inflammatory, anti-bacterial, neuroprotective, and anticancer activity. Eucommicin A was isolated from the leaves of *E. ulmoides* that shows anti-CSC activity by inhibiting self-renewal and sphere formation [133].

8.4.4 Tannin

Tannins are the non-flavonoids representing a group of water-soluble polyphenols. Hydrolyzable tannins are mostly found as a complex with alkaloids, polysaccharides, or proteins and are categorized into two major groups—gallotannins and ellagitannins [168]. The ellagitannins, tannic acids, and corilagin have been reported to provide preventive as well as therapeutic activities against cancer including CSCs [134, 135, 169–171].

8.4.4.1 Ellagitannins (Urolithin A)

Ellagitannins are polymeric ellagic acids, found in pomegranate (*Punica granatum*), walnuts (*Juglans*), and berries. Similar to ellagic acid, the ellagitannins have shown important biological effects including prevention against various diseases like cancer, diabetes, cardiovascular diseases, and neurodegenerative diseases [172]. However, the ellagic acid as well as ellagitannins have poor absorption and are extensively metabolized into urolithins which represent a potent bioactive compound. Urolithin A (3,8-dihydroxyurolithin) is the most representative compound of all urolithins that have demonstrated a significant preventive and therapeutic role in certain cancers including colorectal and prostate cancers [173]. However, there is a dearth of evidence showing the preventive role of urolithin A on CSCs. A study on human colon cancer cell line Caco-2 and primary tumor-derived CSCs showed that a mixture of urolithin A (85%), Urolithin C (10%), and ellagic acid (5%) efficiently inhibit the development and growth of colonospheres by suppressing ALDH expressing cell population of CSCs [104].

8.4.4.2 Tannic Acid

Tannic acid is a type of tannin that consists of numerous phenolic rings found in a wide range of plants, including fruits, green and black teas, nuts, and grains. It is a strong antioxidant that has shown potential in inducing apoptosis and restrict the growth of various forms of cancers [169, 174]. Moreover, it has also shown an inhibitory role in breast cancer angiogenesis. Anti-CSCs role of tannic acid has also been evaluated in breast cancer MCF-7, T47D, MDA-MB-231 cells, and in vivo xenograft Balb/c nude mice model. It has been found that tannic acid treatment inhibits mammosphere formation and ALDH1 activity. Tannic acid inhibits the NF-κB signaling and prevents EMT in CSCs, and thus it may be considered as a promising therapy for eliminating CSCs.

8.4.4.3 Corilagin

Corilagin (β-1-O-galloyl-3,6-(R)-hexahydroxydiphenoyl-d-glucose) is a type of tannin widely found in several medicinal plants including Longan, *Lumnitzera racemose, Terminalia catappa L*, and *Phyllanthus* species [175]. It possesses several biological and pharmaceutical properties such as anti-microbial, anti-diabetic, anti-inflammatory, hepato-protective, anti-hypertensive, and anticancer activities. Corilagin selectively targets cancer cells by inducing apoptosis and autophagy while leaving the healthy cells unaffected [176]. Inhibitory effect of corilagin has also been reported in U251 GSCs proliferation by inducing cell cycle arrest and modulating the NF-κB signaling pathway [135].

8.4.5 Diferuloylmethane

Another type of non-flavonoid polyphenols, the diferuloylmethane contain two hydroxyl-substituted aromatic rings linked by an aliphatic chain containing carbonyl groups. Curcumin, an important diferuloylmethane is a bright yellow compound abundant in *Curcuma longa* (turmeric) with various medicinal activities [99]. It has been reported to exhibit anticancer activity against various forms of cancers.

8.4.5.1 Curcumin

Curcumin is one of the most studied non-flavonoid compounds that shows anticancer activity by targeting various cell survival pathways. It has also been demonstrated to exhibit antitumor properties by eliminating CSCs (Table 8.1). In thyroid cancers, the constitutive activation of the JAK/STAT pathway has been reported to drive the proliferation of cancer cells by upregulation of cyclin D1 and anti-apoptotic genes along with concomitant downregulation of CDKIs. The presence of $ALDH^{+}/CD44^{+}$ CSCs in thyroid tumors allows them to sustain long-lasting invasive potential. However, inhibition of JAK2 phosphorylation by curcumin has been reported to impair the activation of the JAK2/STAT3 pathway in thyroid cancer cells [144]. Furthermore, the treatment with curcumin decreased the expression of *Sox2* and *c-Myc* in CSCs, thereby reducing the size and frequency of thyrospheres. As STAT3 phosphorylation can help the cancer cells to evade apoptosis by increasing the expression of anti-apoptotic factors, such as Bcl2, Bcl-xL, and XIAPs, its inactivation by curcumin led to the induction of apoptosis in CSCs. Interestingly, curcumin was found to enhance the sensitivity of malignant cells towards cisplatin-induced apoptosis by elevating ROS-mediated oxidative stress. Besides the induction of apoptosis, curcumin treatment also led to the upregulation of CDKIs such as p21 and p27 and thus induced cell cycle arrest at the G0/G1 phase of the cell cycle.

The antitumor properties of curcumin have also been demonstrated via downregulation of pluripotency inducing genes such as *Oct4*, *Nanog*, and *Sox2* in BCSCs [177]. Decrease in expression of the stemness genes significantly inhibited mammosphere formation in serum-free culture of MCF-7 and MDA-MB-231 cells and a corresponding reduction in the number of $CD44^+/CD24^-$ CSCs. The observations suggest that curcumin treatment can prevent the proliferation and differentiation of CSCs. The therapeutic effects of curcumin were further amplified by its ability to decrease the expression of EMT network genes such as *Vimentin*, *Fibronectin*, and *β-catenin* and increase in the mRNA levels of *E-cadherin*. The resultant loss of the mesenchymal-like state of CSCs drastically impaired their invasive capacity and metastatic potential.

Recently, $CD44^+/CD24^-$ CSCs isolated from the MCF-7 breast cancer cell line was found to be highly susceptible to early apoptosis and cell cycle arrest at the G2/M phase upon curcumin treatment [143]. The effects were found to be more pronounced in CSCs as compared to NSCCs under hypoxic conditions. The cytotoxic attributes of curcumin were mediated by the downregulation of HIF-2α and aryl hydrocarbon receptor nuclear translocator (ARNT), wherein the latter is required for activation of the HIF-1 complex. The accumulating evidence indicates that curcumin can mediate its antitumor effects by simultaneous targeting of several pathways that are dysregulated in CSCs.

8.4.6 Others

8.4.6.1 6-Shogaol

6-Shogaol, a dehydrated derivative of gingerol isolated from dried ginger (*Zingiber officinale*), has also been demonstrated to arrest the growth of cancer cells and initiate programmed cell death in a wide variety of tumors [145, 178, 179]. Another interesting attribute of 6-shogaol is its anti-inflammatory action as it can downregulate the expression of NF-κB in breast cancer cells [180]. In another study, Bawadood et al. have reported the anti-proliferative activity of 6-shogaol against breast cancer cells by downregulating the notch signaling pathway [181]. It also causes cell cycle arrest at the G2/M phase and induces apoptosis. In another study, 6-shagaol effectively inhibited the proliferation of breast cancer spheroids containing $CD44^+CD24^{-/low}$ CSCs via γ-secretase mediated downregulation of notch signaling pathway [145].

8.4.6.2 Rottlerin

Rottlerin is a non-flavonoid isolated from the Asian Kamala plant *Mallotus philippinensis* that exhibits several pharmacological and medicinal properties [182]. It has been used as an inhibitor of protein kinase C-δ (PKC-δ). The rottlerin has been shown to possess antitumor activity inhibiting cell proliferation, metastasis, and invasion. It also induces apoptosis through mitochondrial membrane depolarization and induces starvation response leading to autophagy. In a study with human pancreatic CSCs, rottlerin has been shown to induce autophagy followed by apoptosis via inhibition of PI3K/AKT/mTOR pathway [29]. Similarly, induction of autophagy via activation of AMPK pathway and apoptosis via inhibition PI3K/AKT/mTOR pathway were found to be induced by rottlerin treatment in human breast as well as prostate CSCs [146, 147]

8.5 Conclusion and Prospects

CSCs are responsible for the development of resistance against conventional cancer therapy, including radiotherapy as well as chemotherapy, and cause metastasis and relapses. Elimination of CSCs by targeting them is now being considered as a potential remedy for anticancer therapy. However, therapies targeting CSCs suffer from many hurdles, importantly the lack of well-characterized CSC markers for specific types of tumor and the presence of some common signaling pathways as in the normal stem cell. This makes it difficult to use all the CSCs regulating factors as a therapeutic target. Therefore, the identification of CSC-specific markers would offer the development of novel strategies to target CSCs and restrict cancer progression. Natural bioactive compounds provide many advantages in preventing cancer progression by targeting CSCs, such as low toxicity, availability in diet, and their potential to directly or indirectly target self-renewal pathways of CSCs. Among the natural compounds, numerous non-flavonoid polyphenols have been shown to eradicate and sensitize CSCs of various cancer types by modulating several signaling pathways. Though considerable efforts are being made to incorporate non-flavonoids in supplementing the existing treatment therapies, their limited bioavailability and lack of knowledge of the required dosage has emerged as a major hurdle to utilize their full potential in targeting CSCs. Strategies need to be developed to overcome these issues and improve their bioavailability at an optimal dose. Chemical modification of the dietary non-flavonoids may enhance their stability, and their strategic delivery could enhance their bioavailability and efficiency. Moreover, several non-flavonoids have been found to increase the sensitivity of drug-resistant CSCs to the available drugs/therapies thereby enhancing their efficacy in cancer treatment. Surely, the combination of non-flavonoids with conventional chemotherapeutics would increase their efficiency in a synergistic manner. Nevertheless, further studies are required to comprehend the mechanisms underlying the anti-CSCs efficacy of non-flavonoids and develop strategies to evaluate their effectiveness in clinical trials before translating them as drugs in clinics.

References

1. Paduch R. Theories of cancer origin. Eur J Cancer Prev. 2015;24(1):57–67. https://doi.org/10.1097/CEJ.0000000000000024.
2. Tabassum DP, Polyak K. Tumorigenesis: it takes a village. Nat Rev Cancer. 2015;15(8):473–83. https://doi.org/10.1038/nrc3971.
3. Sloan FA, Gelband H. Cancer control opportunities in low- and middle-income countries. Washington, DC: National Academies Press; 2007.
4. Batlle E, Clevers H. Cancer stem cells revisited. Nat Med. 2017;23(10):1124–34. https://doi.org/10.1038/nm.4409.
5. Yang L, Shi P, Zhao G, Xu J, Peng W, Zhang J, Zhang G, Wang X, Dong Z, Chen F, Cui H. Targeting cancer stem cell pathways for cancer therapy, vol. 5. Berlin: Springer; 2020a.
6. Bowers DC, Nathan PC, Constine L, Woodman C, Bhatia S, Keller K, Bashore L. Subsequent neoplasms of the CNS among survivors of childhood cancer: a systematic review. Lancet Oncol. 2013;14(8):e321–8. https://doi.org/10.1016/S1470-2045(13)70107-4.
7. Naujokat C, Steinhart R. Salinomycin as a drug for targeting human cancer stem cells. J Biomed Biotechnol. 2012;2012:44–6. https://doi.org/10.1155/2012/950658.
8. Dean M, Fojo T, Bates S. Tumour stem cells and drug resistance. Nat Rev Cancer. 2005;5(4):275–84. https://doi.org/10.1038/nrc1590.
9. Lu B, Morrison R, Schleicher SM, Sun Y, Niermann KJ, Kim S, Spratt DE, Chung CH. Targeting the mechanisms of resistance to chemotherapy and radiotherapy with the cancer stem cell hypothesis. J Oncol. 2011;2011 https://doi.org/10.1155/2011/941876.
10. Chaffer CL, Brueckmann I, Scheel C, Kaestli AJ, Wiggins PA, Rodrigues LO, Brooks M, Reinhardt F, Suc Y, Polyak K, Arendt LM, Kuperwasser C, Bierie B, Weinberg RA. Normal and neoplastic nonstem cells can spontaneously convert to a stem-like state. Proc Natl Acad Sci U S A. 2011;108(19):7950–5. https://doi.org/10.1073/pnas.1102454108.
11. Iqbal W, Alkarim S, AlHejin A, Mukhtar H, Saini KS. Targeting signal transduction pathways of cancer stem cells for therapeutic opportunities of metastasis. Oncotarget. 2016;7(46):76337–53. https://doi.org/10.18632/oncotarget.10942.
12. Lytle NK, Barber AG, Reya T. Stem cell fate in cancer growth, progression and therapy resistance. Nat Rev Cancer. 2018;18(11):669–80. https://doi.org/10.1038/s41568-018-0056-x.
13. de Beça FF, Caetano P, Gerhard R, Alvarenga CA, Gomes M, Paredes J, Schmitt F. Cancer stem cells markers CD44, CD24 and ALDH1 in breast cancer special histological types. J Clin Pathol. 2013;66:91–19. https://doi.org/10.1136/jclinpath-2012-201169.
14. Jordan, CT, Monica LG, Noble M. Cancer stem cells. 2006;355(12):1253–61.
15. Lapidot T, Sirard C, Vormoor J, Murdoch B, Hoang T, Caceres-Cortes J, Minden M, Paterson B, Caligiuri MA, Dick JE. A cell initiating human acute myeloid leukaemia after transplantation into SCID mice. Nature. 1994;367(6464):645–8. https://doi.org/10.1038/367645a0.
16. Yang L, Shi P, Zhao G, Xu J, Peng W, Zhang J, Zhang G, Wang X, Dong Z, Chen F, Cui H. Targeting cancer stem cell pathways for cancer therapy. Signal Transduct Targeted Ther. 2020b;5(1):8. https://doi.org/10.1038/s41392-020-0110-5.
17. Yoo YD, Kwon YT. Molecular mechanisms controlling asymmetric and symmetric self-renewal of cancer stem cells. J Anal Sci Technol. 2015;6(1) https://doi.org/10.1186/s40543-015-0071-4.
18. Friedmann-Morvinski D, Verma IM. Dedifferentiation and reprogramming: origins of cancer stem cells. EMBO Rep. 2014;15(3):244–53. https://doi.org/10.1002/embr.201338254.
19. Aponte PM, Caicedo A. Stemness in cancer: stem cells, cancer stem cells, and their microenvironment. Stem Cells Int. 2017, 2017; https://doi.org/10.1155/2017/5619472.
20. Gupta PB, Fillmore CM, Jiang G, Shapira SD, Tao K, Kuperwasser C, Lander ES. Stochastic state transitions give rise to phenotypic equilibrium in populations of cancer cells. Cell. 2011;146(4):633–44. https://doi.org/10.1016/j.cell.2011.07.026.

21. Yoon C, Lu J, Yi BC, Chang KK, Celeste Simon M, Ryeom S, Yoon SS. PI3K/Akt pathway and nanog maintain cancer stem cells in sarcomas. Oncogene. 2021;10(1) https://doi.org/10.1038/s41389-020-00300-z.
22. Deng J, Bai X, Feng X, Ni J, Beretov J, Graham P, Li Y. Inhibition of PI3K/Akt/MTOR signaling pathway alleviates ovarian cancer chemoresistance through reversing epithelial-mesenchymal transition and decreasing cancer stem cell marker expression. BMC Cancer. 2019;19(1):1–12. https://doi.org/10.1186/s12885-019-5824-9.
23. Prager BC, Xie Q, Bao S, Rich JN. Cancer stem cells: the architects of the tumor ecosystem. Cell Stem Cell. 2019;24(1):41–53. https://doi.org/10.1016/j.stem.2018.12.009.
24. Juan S, Beatriz P, Garcia-Leon MJ, Rangel L, Goetz JG, Chaffer CL. The complexities of metastasis. Cancer. 2019;11(10):1–21. https://doi.org/10.3390/cancers11101575.
25. Eyler CE, Rich JN. Survival of the fittest: cancer stem cells in therapeutic resistance and angiogenesis. J Clin Oncol. 2008;26(17):2839–45. https://doi.org/10.1200/JCO.2007.15.1829.
26. Shukla S, Ohnuma S, Ambudkar SV. Improving cancer chemotherapy with modulators of ABC drug transporters. Curr Drug Targets. 2011;12(5):621–30. https://doi.org/10.2174/138945011795378540.
27. Safa AR. Resistance to cell death and its modulation in cancer stem cells. Crit Rev Oncog. 2016;21(3–4):203–19. https://doi.org/10.1615/CritRevOncog.2016016976.
28. Lock R, Debnath J. Ras, autophagy and glycolysis. Cell Cycle. 2011;10(10):1516–7. https://doi.org/10.4161/cc.10.10.15434.
29. Singh BN, Kumar D, Shankar S, Srivastava RK. Rottlerin induces autophagy which leads to apoptotic cell death through inhibition of PI3K/Akt/MTOR pathway in human pancreatic cancer stem cells. Biochem Pharmacol. 2012;84(9):1154–63. https://doi.org/10.1016/j.bcp.2012.08.007.
30. Yang ZJ, Chee CE, Huang S, Sinicrope FA. The role of autophagy in cancer: therapeutic implications. Mol Cancer Ther. 2011;10(9):1533–41. https://doi.org/10.1158/1535-7163.MCT-11-0047.
31. Clara JA, Monge C, Yang Y, Takebe N. Targeting signalling pathways and the immune microenvironment of cancer stem cells — a clinical update. Nat Rev Clin Oncol. 2020;17(4):204–32. https://doi.org/10.1038/s41571-019-0293-2.
32. Curtin JC, Lorenzi MV. Erratum: drug discovery approaches to target WNT signaling in cancer stem cells. Oncotarget. 2018;9(78):34856. https://doi.org/10.18632/oncotarget.26220.
33. Li J, Zhou BP. Activation of β-catenin and Akt pathways by twist are critical for the maintenance of EMT associated cancer stem cell-like characters. BMC Cancer. 2011;11:49.
34. Roma J, Almazán-Moga A, De Toledo JS, Gallego S. Notch, Wnt, and hedgehog pathways in rhabdomyosarcoma: from single pathways to an integrated network. Sarcoma. 2012;2012 https://doi.org/10.1155/2012/695603.
35. Nguyen LV, Vanner R, Dirks P, Eaves CJ. Cancer stem cells: an evolving concept. Nat Rev Cancer. 2012;12(2):133–43. https://doi.org/10.1038/nrc3184.
36. Bonnet D, Dick JE. Human acute myeloid leukemia is organized as a hierarchy that originates from a primitive hematopoietic cell. Nat Med. 1997;3(7):730–7. https://doi.org/10.1038/nm0797-730.
37. Tsang JYS, Huang YH, Luo MH, Ni YB, Chan SK, Lui PCW, Yu AMC, Tan PH, Tse GM. Cancer stem cell markers are associated with adverse biomarker profiles and molecular subtypes of breast cancer. Breast Cancer Res Treat. 2012;136(2):407–17. https://doi.org/10.1007/s10549-012-2271-6.
38. Xia P, Xiao-yan X. PI3K/Akt/MTOR signaling pathway in cancer stem cells: from basic research to clinical application. Am J Cancer Res. 2015;5(5):1602–9.
39. Ma F, Li H, Wang H, Shi X, Fan Y, Ding X, Lin C, Zhan Q, Qian H, Binghe X. Enriched CD44+/CD24- population drives the aggressive phenotypes presented in triple-negative breast cancer (TNBC). Cancer Lett. 2014;353(2):153–9.

40. Kim RJ, Park JR, Roh KJ, Ram Choi A, Kim SR, Kim PH, Yu JH, Lee JW, Ahn SH, Gong G, Hwang JW, Kang KS, Kong G, Sheen YY, Nam JS. High aldehyde dehydrogenase activity enhances stem cell features in breast cancer cells by activating hypoxia-inducible factor-2α. Cancer Lett. 2013a;333(1):18–31.
41. Su J, Wu S, Wu H, Li L, Guo T. CD44 is functionally crucial for driving lung cancer stem cells metastasis through Wnt/β-catenin-FoxM1-twist signaling. Mol Carcinog. 2016;55 (12):1962–73. https://doi.org/10.1002/mc.22443.
42. Ashrafizadeh M, Zarrabi A, Hushmandi K, Kalantari M, Mohammadinejad R, Javaheri T, Sethi G. Association of the epithelial–mesenchymal transition (EMT) with cisplatin resistance. Int J Mol Sci. 2020;21(11):1–46. https://doi.org/10.3390/ijms21114002.
43. Ding Q, Miyazaki Y, Tsukasa K, Matsubara S, Yoshimitsu M, Takao S. CD133 Facilitates epithelial-mesenchymal transition through interaction with the ERK pathway in pancreatic cancer metastasis. Mol Cancer. 2014;13(1):1–11. https://doi.org/10.1186/1476-4598-13-15.
44. Liu C, Li Y, Semenov M, Han C, Baeg G-H, Tan Y, Zhang Z, Lin X, He X. Control of β-catenin phosphorylation/degradation by a dual-kinase mechanism. Cell. 2002;108 (6):837–47. https://doi.org/10.1016/S0092-8674(02)00685-2.
45. Chang YW, Ying Jhen S, Hsiao M, Wei KC, Lin WH, Liang CL, Chen SC, Lee JL. Diverse targets of β-catenin during the epithelial-mesenchymal transition define cancer stem cells and predict disease relapse. Cancer Res. 2015;75(16):3398–410.
46. Macdonald BT, Tamai K, He X. Developmental cell review Wnt/b-catenin signaling: components, mechanisms, and diseases. Dev Cell. 2009;17:9–26.
47. Prasad CP, Mirza S, Sharma G, Prashad R, DattaGupta S, Rath G, Ralhan R. Epigenetic alterations of CDH1 and APC genes: relationship with activation of Wnt/β-catenin pathway in invasive ductal carcinoma of breast. Life Sci. 2008;83(9–10):318–25.
48. Qi X, Li X. Mechanistic insights into the generation and transduction of hedgehog signaling. Trends Biochem Sci. 2020;45(5):397–410. https://doi.org/10.1016/j.tibs.2020.01.006.
49. Dandawate PR, Subramaniam D, Jensen RA, Anant S. Targeting cancer stem cells and signaling pathways by phytochemicals: novel approach for breast cancer therapy. Semin Cancer Biol. 2016;40–41:192–208. https://doi.org/10.1016/j.semcancer.2016.09.001
50. Monkkonen T, Lewis MT. New paradigms for the hedgehog signaling network in mammary gland development and breast cancer. Biochim Biophys Acta. 2017;1868(1):315–32. https://doi.org/10.1016/j.bbcan.2017.06.003.
51. Skoda AM, Simovic D, Karin V, Kardum V, Vranic S, Serman L. The role of the hedgehog signaling pathway in cancer: a comprehensive review. Bosnian J Basic Med Sci. 2018;18 (1):8–20. https://doi.org/10.17305/bjbms.2018.2756.
52. Du WZ, Feng Y, Wang XF, Piao XY, Cui YQ, Chen LC, Lei XH, Xu S, Liu X, Wang HB, Li XF, Yang DB, Sun Y, Zhao ZF, Jiang T, Li YL, Jiang CL. Curcumin suppresses malignant glioma cells growth and induces apoptosis by inhibition of SHH/GLI1 signaling pathway in vitro and vivo. CNS Neurosci Ther. 2013;19(12):926–36. https://doi.org/10.1111/cns.12163.
53. Zhou M, Hou Y, Yang G, Zhang H, Gang T, Du YE, Wen S, Xu L, Tang X, Tang S, Yang L, Cui X, Liu M. LncRNA-Hh strengthen cancer stem cells generation in twist-positive breast cancer via activation of hedgehog signaling pathway. Stem Cells. 2016;34(1):55–66.
54. Koury J, Zhong L, Hao J. Targeting signaling pathways in cancer stem cells for cancer treatment. Stem Cells Int. 2017;2017:1–10. https://doi.org/10.1155/2017/2925869.
55. Xiao W, Gao Z, Duan Y, Yuan W, Yang K. Notch signaling plays a crucial role in cancer stem-like cells maintaining stemness and mediating chemotaxis in renal cell carcinoma. J Exp Clin Cancer Res. 2017;36(1):1–13. https://doi.org/10.1186/s13046-017-0507-3.
56. Miele L. Notch signaling. Clin Cancer Res. 2006;12(4):1074–9. https://doi.org/10.1158/1078-0432.CCR-05-2570.
57. BeLow MK, Osipo C. Notch signaling in breast cancer: a role in drug resistance. Cell. 2020;9 (10):1–19. https://doi.org/10.3390/cells9102204.

58. Dontu G, Jackson KW, McNicholas E, Kawamura MJ, Abdallah WM, Wicha MS. Role of notch signaling in cell-fate determination of human mammary stem/progenitor cells. Breast Cancer Res. 2004;6(6) https://doi.org/10.1186/bcr920.
59. Pal D, Kolluru V, Chandrasekaran B, Baby BV, Aman M, Suman S, Sirimulla S, Sanders MA, Alatassi H, Ankem MK, Damodaran C. Targeting aberrant expression of Notch-1 in ALDH + cancer stem cells in breast cancer. Mol Carcinog. 2017;56(3):1127–36. https://doi.org/10.1002/mc.22579.
60. Madsen RR. PI3K in stemness regulation: from development to cancer. Biochem Soc Transl. 2020;48(1):301–15. https://doi.org/10.1042/BST20190778.
61. Oo AKK, Calle AS, Nair N, Mahmud H, Vaidyanath A, Yamauchi J, Khayrani AC, Du J, Alam MJ, Seno A, Mizutani A, Murakami H, Iwasaki Y, Chen L, Kasai T, Seno M. Up-regulation of PI 3-kinases and the activation of PI3K-Akt signaling pathway in cancer stem-like cells through DNA hypomethylation mediated by the cancer microenvironment. Trans Oncol. 2018;11(3):653–63. https://doi.org/10.1016/j.tranon.2018.03.001.
62. Zhou BP, Deng J, Xia W, Xu J, Li YM, Gunduz M, Hung MC. Dual regulation of snail by GSK-3β-mediated phosphorylation in control of epithelial-mesenchymal transition. Nat Cell Biol. 2004;6(10):931–40. https://doi.org/10.1038/ncb1173.
63. Cheng GZ, Chan J, Wang Q, Zhang W, Sun CD, Wang LH. Twist transcriptionally up-regulates AKT2 in breast cancer cells leading to increased migration, invasion, and resistance to paclitaxel. Cancer Res. 2007;67(5):1979–87. https://doi.org/10.1158/0008-5472.CAN-06-1479.
64. Kurrey NK, Jalgaonkar SP, Joglekar AV, Ghanate AD, Chaskar PD, Doiphode RY, Bapat SA. Snail and slug mediate radioresistance and chemoresistance by antagonizing P53-mediated apoptosis and acquiring a stem-like phenotype in ovarian cancer cells. Stem Cells. 2009;27(9):2059–68.
65. Rinkenbaugh A, Baldwin A. The NF-KB pathway and cancer stem cells. Cells. 2016;5(2):16. https://doi.org/10.3390/cells5020016.
66. Zakaria N, Yusoff NM, Zakaria Z, Widera D, Yahaya BH. Inhibition of NF-KB signaling reduces the stemness characteristics of lung cancer stem cells. Front Oncol. 2018;8(May) https://doi.org/10.3389/fonc.2018.00166.
67. Brücher BLDM, Lang F, Jamall IS. NF- κB signaling and crosstalk during carcinogenesis. 4open. 2019;2:13. https://doi.org/10.1051/fopen/2019010.
68. Gomes I, de Almeida BP, Dâmaso S, Mansinho A, Correia I, Henriques S, Cruz-Duarte R, Vilhais G, Félix P, Alves P, Corredeira P, Barbosa-Morais NL, Costa L, Casimiro S. Expression of receptor activator of NFkB (RANK) drives stemness and resistance to therapy in ER+HER2- breast cancer. Oncotarget. 2020;11(19):1714–28.
69. Kaltschmidt C, Banz-Jansen C, Benhidjeb T, Beshay M, Förster C, Greiner J, Hamelmann E, Jorch N, Mertzlufft F, Pfitzenmaier J, Simon M, Esch JSA, Vordemvenne T, Wähnert D, Weissinger F, Wilkens L, Kaltschmidt B. A role for NF-KB in organ specific cancer and cancer stem cells. Cancer. 2019;11(5)
70. House CD, Jordan E, Hernandez L, Ozaki M, James JM, Kim M, Kruhlak MJ, Batchelor E, Elloumi F, Cam MC, Annunziata CM. NFκB promotes ovarian tumorigenesis via classical pathways that support proliferative cancer cells and alternative pathways that support ALDH + cancer stem–like cells. Cancer Res. 2017;77(24):6927–40. https://doi.org/10.1158/0008-5472.CAN-17-0366.
71. Sternlicht, Mark D., and Zena Werb. How m atrix m etalloproteinases. 2001:463–516. https://doi.org/10.1146/annurev.cellbio.17.1.463.
72. Liu S, Chen S, Zeng J. TGF-β signaling: a complex role in tumorigenesis (review). Mol Med Rep. 2017;17(1):699–704. https://doi.org/10.3892/mmr.2017.7970.
73. Papageorgis P. TGF β signaling in tumor initiation, epithelial-to-mesenchymal transition, and metastasis. J Oncol. 2015;2015:1–15. https://doi.org/10.1155/2015/587193.
74. Daniele V, Simeone P, Frank J, Trerotola M, Anna G, Loredana C, Andrea T, Claudia B, Isabelle F, Gaballo A, Saverio A, Michel S, Michele M. Translating epithelial mesenchymal

transition markers into the clinic: novel insights from proteomics. EuPA Open Proteom. 2016;10:31–41. https://doi.org/10.1016/j.euprot.2016.01.003.
75. Nakano M, Kikushige Y, Miyawaki K, Kunisaki Y, Mizuno S, Takenaka K, Tamura S, Okumura Y, Ito M, Ariyama H, Kusaba H, Nakamura M, Maeda T, Baba E, Akashi K. Dedifferentiation process driven by TGF-beta signaling enhances stem cell properties in human colorectal cancer. Oncogene. 2019;38(6):780–93. https://doi.org/10.1038/s41388-018-0480-0.
76. Chaffer CL, Marjanovic ND, Lee T, Bell G, Kleer CG, Reinhardt F, D'Alessio AC, Young RA, Weinberg RA. XPoised chromatin at the ZEB1 promoter enables breast cancer cell plasticity and enhances tumorigenicity. Cell. 2013;154(1):61. https://doi.org/10.1016/j.cell.2013.06.005.
77. Dolatabadi S, Jonasson E, Lindén M, Fereydouni B, Bäcksten K, Nilsson M, Martner A, Forootan A, Fagman H, Landberg G, Åman P, Ståhlberg A. JAK–STAT signalling controls cancer stem cell properties including chemotherapy resistance in myxoid liposarcoma. Int J Cancer. 2019;145(2):435–49. https://doi.org/10.1002/ijc.32123.
78. Jin W. Role of JAK/STAT3 signaling in the regulation of metastasis, the transition of cancer stem cells, and chemoresistance of cancer by epithelial–mesenchymal transition. Cell. 2020;9(1):217. https://doi.org/10.3390/cells9010217.
79. Junk DJ, Bryson BL, Smigiel JM, Parameswaran N, Bartel CA, Jackson MW. Oncostatin M promotes cancer cell plasticity through cooperative STAT3-SMAD3 signaling. Oncogene. 2017;36(28):4001–13. https://doi.org/10.1038/onc.2017.33.
80. Khera L, Vinik Y, Maina F, Lev S. The AXL-PYK2-PKCα axis as a nexus of stemness circuits in TNBC. Life Sci Alliance. 2021;4(6):e202000985. https://doi.org/10.26508/lsa.202000985.
81. Kim SY, Kang JW, Song X, Kim BK, Yoo YD, Kwon YT, Lee YJ. Role of the IL-6-JAK1-STAT3-Oct-4 pathway in the conversion of non-stem cancer cells into cancer stem-like cells. Cell Signal. 2013b;25(4):961–9. https://doi.org/10.1016/j.cellsig.2013.01.007.
82. Hernández-Vargas H, Ouzounova M, Le Calvez-Kelm F, Lambert M-P, McKay-Chopin S, Tavtigian SV, Puisieux A, Matar C, Herceg Z. Methylome analysis reveals Jak-STAT pathway deregulation in putative breast cancer stem cells. Epigenetics. 2011;6(4):428–39. https://doi.org/10.4161/epi.6.4.14515.
83. Keith B, Celeste Simon M. Hypoxia-inducible factors, stem cells, and cancer. Cell. 2007;129(3):465–72. https://doi.org/10.1016/j.cell.2007.04.019.
84. Benckert C, Jonas S, Cramer T, Von Marschall Z, Schäfer G, Peters M, Wagner K, Radke C, Wiedenmann B, Neuhaus P, Höcker M, Rosewicz S. Transforming growth factor B1 stimulates vascular endothelial growth factor gene transcription in human cholangiocellular carcinoma cells. Cancer Res. 2003;63(5):1083–92.
85. Sánchez-Elsner T, Botella LM, Velasco B, Angel C, Attisano L, Bernabéu C. Synergistic cooperation between hypoxia and transforming growth factor-β pathways on human vascular endothelial growth factor gene expression. J Biol Chem. 2001;276(42):38527–35. https://doi.org/10.1074/jbc.M104536200.
86. Bergers G, Benjamin LE. Tumorigenesis and the angiogenic switch. Nat Rev Cancer. 2003;3(6):401–10. https://doi.org/10.1038/nrc1093.
87. Das B, Tsuchida R, Malkin D, Koren G, Baruchel S, Yeger H. Hypoxia enhances tumor stemness by increasing the invasive and tumorigenic side population fraction. Stem Cells. 2008;26(7):1818–30. https://doi.org/10.1634/stemcells.2007-0724.
88. Nejad E, Asieh SN, Rostami A, Sistani A, Shojaeifar S, Esparvarinha M, Nedaeinia R, Javanmard SH, Taherian M, Ahmadlou M, Salehi R, Sadeghi B, Manian M. The role of hypoxia in the tumor microenvironment and development of cancer stem cell: a novel approach to developing treatment. Cancer Cell Int. 2021;21(1):1–26. https://doi.org/10.1186/s12935-020-01719-5.
89. Choi YJ, Heo K, Park HS, Yang KM, Jeong MH. The resveratrol analog HS-1793 enhances radiosensitivity of mouse-derived breast cancer cells under hypoxic conditions. Int J Oncol. 2016;49(4):1479–88. https://doi.org/10.3892/ijo.2016.3647.

90. Li Z, Bao S, Wu Q, Wang H, Eyler C, Sathornsumetee S, Shi Q, Cao Y, Lathia J, McLendon RE, Hjelmeland AB, Rich JN. Hypoxia-inducible factors regulate tumorigenic capacity of glioma stem cells. Cancer Cell. 2009;15(6):501–13. https://doi.org/10.1016/j.ccr.2009.03.018.
91. Schwab LP, Peacock DL, Majumdar D, Ingels JF, Jensen LC, Smith KD, Cushing RC, Seagroves TN. Hypoxia-inducible factor 1α promotes primary tumor growth and tumor-initiating cell activity in breast cancer. Breast Cancer Res. 2012;14(1):R6. https://doi.org/10.1186/bcr3087.
92. Vaupel P. The role of hypoxia-induced factors in tumor progression. Oncologist. 2004;9 (S5):10–7. https://doi.org/10.1634/theoncologist.9-90005-10.
93. Chen K, Huang Y-h, Chen J-l. Understanding and targeting cancer stem cells: therapeutic implications and challenges. Acta Pharmacol Sin. 2013;34(6):732–40. https://doi.org/10.1038/aps.2013.27.
94. Dayem AA, Choi HY, Yang GM, Kim K, Saha SK, Cho SG. The anti-cancer effect of polyphenols against breast cancer and cancer stem cells: molecular mechanisms. Nutrients. 2016;8(9) https://doi.org/10.3390/nu8090581.
95. Liskova A, Kubatka P, Samec M, Zubor P, Mlyncek M, Bielik T, Samuel SM, Zulli A, Kwon TK, Büsselberg D. Dietary phytochemicals targeting cancer stem cells. Molecules. 2019;24 (5):1–20. https://doi.org/10.3390/molecules24050899.
96. Wu CH, Hong BH, Ho CT, Yen GC. Targeting cancer stem cells in breast cancer: potential anticancer properties of 6-shogaol and pterostilbene. J Agric Food Chem. 2015;63 (9):2432–41. https://doi.org/10.1021/acs.jafc.5b00002.
97. Gu HF, Mao XY, Min D. Prevention of breast cancer by dietary polyphenols—role of cancer stem cells. Crit Rev Food Sci Nutr. 2020;60(5):810–25. https://doi.org/10.1080/10408398.2018.1551778.
98. Abotaleb M, Liskova A, Kubatka P, Büsselberg D. Therapeutic potential of plant phenolic acids in the treatment of cancer. Biomolecules. 2020;10(2):1–23. https://doi.org/10.3390/biom10020221.
99. Cianciosi D, Varela-Lopez A, Forbes-Hernandez TY, Gasparrini M, Afrin S, Reboredo-Rodriguez P, Zhang JJJ, Quiles JL, Nabavi SF, Battino M, Giampieri F. Targeting molecular pathways in cancer stem cells by natural bioactive compounds. Pharmacol Res. 2018;135 (August):150–65. https://doi.org/10.1016/j.phrs.2018.08.006.
100. Han X, Shen T, Lou H. Dietary polyphenols and their biological significance. Int J Mol Sci. 2007;8(9):950–88. https://doi.org/10.3390/i8090950.
101. Singla RK, Dubey AK, Garg A, Sharma RK, Fiorino M, Ameen SM, Haddad MA, Al-Hiary M. Natural polyphenols: chemical classification, definition of classes, subcategories, and structures. J AOAC Int. 2019;102(5):1397–400. https://doi.org/10.5740/jaoacint.19-0133.
102. Civenni G, Iodice MG, Nabavi SF, Habtemariam S, Nabavi SM, Catapano CV, Daglia M. Gallic acid and methyl-3-O-methyl gallate: a comparative study on their effects on prostate cancer stem cells. RSC Adv. 2015;5(78):63800–6. https://doi.org/10.1039/c5ra07988h.
103. Wang N, Wang Q, Tang H, Zhang F, Zheng Y, Wang S, Zhang J, Wang Z, Xie X. Direct inhibition of ACTN4 by ellagic acid limits breast cancer metastasis via regulation of β-catenin stabilization in cancer stem cells. J Exp Clin Cancer Res. 2017;36(1):172. https://doi.org/10.1186/s13046-017-0635-9.
104. Núñez-Sánchez MÁ, Karmokar A, González-Sarrías A, García-Villalba R, Tomás-Barberán FA, García-Conesa MT, Brown K, Espín JC. In vivo relevant mixed urolithins and ellagic acid inhibit phenotypic and molecular colon cancer stem cell features: a new potentiality for ellagitannin metabolites against cancer. Food Chem Toxicol. 2016;92:8–16. https://doi.org/10.1016/j.fct.2016.03.011.
105. Lee J, Kim YS, Lee JH, Heo SC, Lee KL, Choi SW, Kim Y. Walnut Phenolic extract and its bioactive compounds suppress colon cancer cell growth by regulating colon cancer stemness. Nutrients. 2016;8(7):1–14. https://doi.org/10.3390/nu8070439.
106. Li Y, Jiang F, Chen L, Yang Y, Cao S, Ye Y, Wang X, Juan M, Li Z, Li L. Blockage of TGFβ-SMAD2 by demethylation-activated MiR-148a is involved in caffeic acid-induced

inhibition of cancer stem cell-like properties in vitro and in vivo. FEBS Open Biol. 2015;5:466–75.
107. Park S-R, Kim S-R, Hong I-S, Lee H-Y. A novel therapeutic approach for colorectal cancer stem cells: blocking the PI3K/Akt signaling axis with caffeic acid. Front Cell Dev Biol. 2020;8 https://doi.org/10.3389/fcell.2020.585987.
108. Omene CO, Wu J, Frenkel K. Caffeic acid phenethyl ester (CAPE) derived from propolis, a honeybee product, inhibits growth of breast cancer stem cells. Invest New Drugs. 2012;30 (4):1279–88. https://doi.org/10.1007/s10637-011-9667-8.
109. Yamagata K, Izawa Y, Onodera D, Tagami M. Chlorogenic acid regulates apoptosis and stem cell marker-related gene expression in A549 human lung cancer cells. Mol Cell Biochem. 2018;441(1–2):9–19. https://doi.org/10.1007/s11010-017-3171-1.
110. Min SJ, Lim JY, Kim HR, Kim SJ, Kim Y. Sasa quelpaertensis leaf extract inhibits colon cancer by regulating cancer cell stemness in vitro and in vivo. Int J Mol Sci. 2015;16 (5):9976–97. https://doi.org/10.3390/ijms16059976.
111. Shankar S, Nall D, Tang SN, Meeker D, Passarini J, Sharma J, Srivastava RK. Resveratrol inhibits pancreatic cancer stem cell characteristics in human and KrasG12D transgenic mice by inhibiting pluripotency maintaining factors and epithelial-mesenchymal transition. PLoS One. 2011;6(1) https://doi.org/10.1371/journal.pone.0016530.
112. Pandey PR, Okuda H, Watabe M, Pai SK, Liu W, Kobayashi A, Xing F, Fukuda K, Hirota S, Sugai T, Wakabayashi G, Koeda K, Kashiwaba M, Suzuki K, Chiba T, Endo M, Fujioka T, Tanji S, Mo YY, Cao D, Wilber AC, Watabe K. Resveratrol suppresses growth of cancer stem-like cells by inhibiting fatty acid synthase. Breast Cancer Res Treat. 2011;130(2):387–98. https://doi.org/10.1007/s10549-010-1300-6.
113. Hu FW, Tsai LL, Yu CH, Chen PN, Chou MY, Cheng Chia Y. Impairment of tumor-initiating stem-like property and reversal of epithelial-mesenchymal transdifferentiation in head and neck cancer by resveratrol treatment. Mol Nutr Food Res. 2012a;56(8):1247–58.
114. Hu L, Cao D, Li Y, He Y, Guo K. Resveratrol sensitized leukemia stem cell-like KG-1a cells to cytokine-induced killer cells-mediated cytolysis through NKG2D ligands and TRAIL receptors. Cancer Biol Ther. 2012b;13(7):516–26. https://doi.org/10.4161/cbt.19601.
115. Hagiwara K, Kosaka N, Yoshioka Y, Takahashi RU, Takeshita F, Ochiya T. Stilbene derivatives promote Ago2-dependent tumour-suppressive MicroRNA activity. Sci Rep. 2012;2:1–9. https://doi.org/10.1038/srep00314.
116. Su YC, Li SC, Wu YC, Wang LM, Chao KSC, Liao HF. Resveratrol downregulates interleukin-6-stimulated sonic hedgehog signaling in human acute myeloid leukemia. Evidence-Based Complement Altern Med. 2013;2013 https://doi.org/10.1155/2013/547430.
117. Sato A, Okada M, Shibuya K, Watanabe E, Seino S, Suzuki K, Narita Y, Shibui S, Kayama T, Kitanaka C. Resveratrol promotes proteasome-dependent degradation of nanog via P53 activation and induces differentiation of glioma stem cells. Stem Cell Res. 2013;11 (1):601–10. https://doi.org/10.1016/j.scr.2013.04.004.
118. Fu Y, Chang H, Peng X, Bai Q, Yi L, Zhou Y, Zhu J, Mi M. Resveratrol Inhibits breast cancer stem-like cells and induces autophagy via suppressing Wnt/β-catenin signaling pathway. PLoS One. 2014;9(7)
119. Sayd S, Thirant C, El-Habr EA, Lipecka J, Dubois LG, Bogeas A, Tahiri-Jouti N, Chneiweiss H, Junier MP. Sirtuin-2 activity is required for glioma stem cell proliferation arrest but not necrosis induced by resveratrol. Stem Cell Rev Rep. 2014;10(1):103–13. https://doi.org/10.1007/s12015-013-9465-0.
120. Seino M, Okada M, Shibuya K, Seino S, Suzuki S, Takeda H, Ohta T, Kurachi H, Kitanaka C. Differential contribution of ROS to resveratrol-induced cell death and loss of self-renewal capacity of ovarian cancer stem cells. Anticancer Res. 2015;35(1):85–96.
121. Yang J, Liu J, Lyu X, Fei S. [Resveratrol inhibits cell proliferation and up-regulates mica/b expression in human colon cancer stem cells]. Xi Bao Yu Fen Zi Mian Yi Xue Za Zhi. 2015a;31(7):889–893.

122. Yang Y, Xu H, Huang W, Ding M, Xiao J, Yang D, Li H, Liu XY, Liang C. Targeting lung cancer stem-like cells with TRAIL gene armed oncolytic adenovirus. J Cell Mol Med. 2015b;19(5):915–23. https://doi.org/10.1111/jcmm.12397.
123. Reddivari L, Charepalli V, Radhakrishnan S, Vadde R, Elias RJ, Lambert JD, Vanamala JKP. Grape compounds suppress colon cancer stem cells in vitro and in a rodent model of colon carcinogenesis. BMC Complement Altern Med. 2016;16(1):1–12. https://doi.org/10.1186/s12906-016-1254-2.
124. Clark PA, Bhattacharya S, Elmayan A, Darjatmoko SR, Thuro BA, Yan MB, Van Ginkel PR, Polans AS, Kuo JS. Resveratrol targeting of AKT and P53 in glioblastoma and glioblastoma stem-like cells to suppress growth and infiltration. J Neurosurg. 2017;126(5):1448–60. https://doi.org/10.3171/2016.1.JNS152077.
125. Cilibrasi C, Riva G, Romano G, Cadamuro M, Bazzoni R, Butta V, Paoletta L, Dalpra L, Strazzabosco M, Lavitrano M, Giovannoni R, Bentivegna A. Resveratrol impairs glioma stem cells proliferation and motility by modulating the wnt signaling pathway. PLoS One. 2017;12(1):1–20. https://doi.org/10.1371/journal.pone.0169854.
126. Ruíz G, Valencia-González HA, León-Galicia I, García-Villa E, García-Carrancá A, Gariglio P. Inhibition of RAD51 by SiRNA and resveratrol sensitizes cancer stem cells derived from hela cell cultures to apoptosis. Stem Cells Int. 2018;2018 https://doi.org/10.1155/2018/2493869.
127. Peng L, Jiang D. Resveratrol eliminates cancer stem cells of osteosarcoma by STAT3 pathway inhibition. PLoS One. 2018;13(10):1–13. https://doi.org/10.1371/journal.pone.0205918.
128. Song Y, Chen Y, Li Y, Lyu X, Cui J, Cheng Y, Zheng T, Zhao L, Zhao G. Resveratrol suppresses epithelial-mesenchymal transition in GBM by regulating smad-dependent signaling. BioMed Res Int. 2019;2019 https://doi.org/10.1155/2019/1321973.
129. Buhrmann C, Yazdi M, Popper B, Kunnumakkara AB, Aggarwal BB, Shakibaei M. Induction of the epithelial-to-mesenchymal transition of human colorectal cancer by human TNF-β (lymphotoxin) and its reversal by resveratrol. Nutrients. 2019;11(3)
130. Zhou C, Qian W, Ma J, Liang C, Jiang Z, Yan B, Li J, Duan W, Sun L, Cao J, Wang F, Wu F, Wu Z, Ma Q, Li X. Resveratrol enhances the chemotherapeutic response and reverses the stemness induced by gemcitabine in pancreatic cancer cells via targeting SREBP1. Cell Prolif. 2019;52(1):1–12. https://doi.org/10.1111/cpr.12514.
131. Yin L, Zhang R, Hu Y, Li W, Wang M, Liang Z, Sun Z, Ji R, Xu W, Qian H. Gastric-cancer-derived mesenchymal stem cells: a promising target for resveratrol in the suppression of gastric cancer metastasis. Hum Cell. 2020;33(3):652–62. https://doi.org/10.1007/s13577-020-00339-5.
132. Sun H, Zhang T, Liu R, Cao W, Zhang Z, Liu Z, Qian W, Wang D, Yu D, Zhong C. Resveratrol inhibition of renal cancer stem cell characteristics and modulation of the sonic hedgehog pathway. Nutr Cancer. 2020:1–11. https://doi.org/10.1080/01635581.2020.1784966.
133. Fujiwara A, Nishi M, Yoshida S, Hasegawa M, Yasuma C, Ryo A, Suzuki Y. Eucommicin A, a β-truxinate lignan from eucommia ulmoides, is a selective inhibitor of cancer stem cells. Phytochemistry. 2016;122:139–45. https://doi.org/10.1016/j.phytochem.2015.11.017.
134. Kim D-A, Choi HS, Ryu E-S, Ko J, Shin H-S, Lee J-M, Chung H, Jun E, Eok-Soo O, Kang D-H. Tannic acid attenuates the formation of cancer stem cells by inhibiting NF-KB-mediated phenotype transition of breast cancer cells. Am J Cancer Res. 2019;9(8):1664–81.
135. Yang W-T, Li G-H, Li Z-Y, Feng S, Liu X-Q, Han G-K, Zhang H, Qin X-Y, Zhang R, Nie Q-M, Jin F. Effect of corilagin on the proliferation and NF- κ B in U251 glioblastoma cells and U251 glioblastoma stem-like cells. Evid Based Complement Alternat Med. 2016;2016:1–9. https://doi.org/10.1155/2016/1418309.
136. Kakarala M, Brenner DE, Korkaya H, Cheng C, Tazi K, Ginestier C, Liu S, Dontu G, Wicha MS. Targeting breast stem cells with the cancer preventive compounds curcumin and piperine. Breast Cancer Res Treat. 2010;122(3):777–85. https://doi.org/10.1007/s10549-009-0612-x.

137. Nautiyal J, Kanwar SS, Yu Y, Majumdar APN. Combination of dasatinib and curcumin eliminates chemo-resistant colon cancer cells. J Mol Signal. 2011;6(1):7. https://doi.org/10.1186/1750-2187-6-7.
138. Zhuang W, Long L, Zheng B, Ji W, Yang N, Zhang Q, Liang Z. Curcumin promotes differentiation of glioma-initiating cells by inducing autophagy. Cancer Sci. 2012;103(4):684–90. https://doi.org/10.1111/j.1349-7006.2011.02198.x.
139. Mukherjee S, Mazumdar M, Chakraborty S, Manna A, Saha S, Khan P, Bhattacharjee P, Guha D, Adhikary A, Mukhjerjee S, Das T. Curcumin inhibits breast cancer stem cell migration by amplifying the E-cadherin/β-catenin negative feedback loop. Stem Cell Res Ther. 2014;5(5):116. https://doi.org/10.1186/scrt506.
140. Shakibaei M, Buhrmann C, Kraehe P, Shayan P, Lueders C, Goel A. Curcumin chemosensitizes 5-fluorouracil resistant MMR-deficient human colon cancer cells in high density cultures. PLoS One. 2014;9(1):1–12. https://doi.org/10.1371/journal.pone.0085397.
141. Baharuddin P, Satar N, Fakiruddin KS, Zakaria N, Lim MN, Yusoff NM, Zakaria Z, Yahaya BH. Curcumin improves the efficacy of cisplatin by targeting cancer stem-like cells through P21 and cyclin D1-mediated tumour cell inhibition in non-small cell lung cancer cell lines. Oncol Rep. 2016;35(1):13–25. https://doi.org/10.3892/or.2015.4371.
142. Zhu JY, Xue Y, Chen Y, Jiang Y, Wang SJ, Li Y, Wang XQ, Yu M, Zhu MM, Ma X, Huang C, Wu R, Xie CF, Li XT, Geng SS, Wu JS, Zhong CY, Han HY. Curcumin suppresses lung cancer stem cells via inhibiting Wnt/β-catenin and sonic hedgehog pathways. Phytother Res. 2017;31(4):680–8.
143. Sarighieh MA, Montazeri V, Shadboorestan A, Ghahremani MH, Ostad SN. The inhibitory effect of curcumin on hypoxia inducer factors (Hifs) as a regulatory factor in the growth of tumor cells in breast cancer stem-like cells. Drug Res. 2020;70(11):512–8. https://doi.org/10.1055/a-1201-2602.
144. Khan AQ, Ahmed EI, Elareer N, Fathima H, Prabhu KS, Siveen KS, Kulinski M, Azizi F, Dermime S, Ahmad A, Steinhoff M, Uddin S. Curcumin-mediated apoptotic cell death in papillary thyroid cancer and cancer stem-like cells through targeting of the JAK/STAT3 signaling pathway. Int J Mol Sci. 2020;21(2) https://doi.org/10.3390/ijms21020438.
145. Ray A, Vasudevan S, Sengupta S. 6-shogaol inhibits breast cancer cells and stem cell-like spheroids by modulation of notch signaling pathway and induction of autophagic cell death. Plos One. 2015;10(9):e0137614. https://doi.org/10.1371/journal.pone.0137614.
146. Kumar D, Shankar S, Srivastava RK. Rottlerin-induced autophagy leads to the apoptosis in breast cancer stem cells: molecular mechanisms. Mol Cancer. 2013;12(1):1–15. https://doi.org/10.1186/1476-4598-12-171.
147. Kumar D, Shankar S, Srivastava RK. Rottlerin induces autophagy and apoptosis in prostate cancer stem cells via PI3K/Akt/MTOR signaling pathway. Cancer Lett. 2014;343(2):179–89. https://doi.org/10.1016/j.canlet.2013.10.003.
148. Khorsandi K, Kianmehr Z, Hosseinmardi Z, Hosseinzadeh R. Anti-cancer effect of gallic acid in presence of low level laser irradiation: ROS production and induction of apoptosis and ferroptosis. Cancer Cell Int. 2020;20(1):1–14. https://doi.org/10.1186/s12935-020-1100-y.
149. Badhani B, Sharma N, Kakkar R. Gallic acid: a versatile antioxidant with promising therapeutic and industrial applications. RSC Adv. 2015;5(35):27540–57. https://doi.org/10.1039/C5RA01911G.
150. Verma S, Singh A, Mishra A. Gallic acid: molecular rival of cancer. Environ Toxicol Pharmacol. 2013;35(3):473–85. https://doi.org/10.1016/j.etap.2013.02.011.
151. Habtemariam S. Methyl-3- O -methyl gallate and gallic acid from the leaves of peltiphyllum peltatum: isolation and comparative antioxidant, prooxidant, and cytotoxic effects in neuronal cells. J Med Food. 2011;14(11):1412–8. https://doi.org/10.1089/jmf.2010.0257.
152. Derosa G, Maffioli P, Sahebkar A. Ellagic acid and its role in chronic diseases. Adv Exp Med Biol. 2016;928:473–9.

153. Espíndola KMM, Ferreira RG, Narvaez LEM, Rosario ACRS, da Silva AHM, Silva AGB, Vieira APO, Monteiro MC. Chemical and pharmacological aspects of caffeic acid and its activity in hepatocarcinoma. Front Oncol. 2019;9 https://doi.org/10.3389/fonc.2019.00541.
154. Yordanov Y. Caffeic acid phenethyl ester (CAPE): cornerstone pharmacological studies and drug delivery systems. Pharmacia. 2019;66(4):223–31. https://doi.org/10.3897/pharmacia.66.e38571.
155. Olgierd B, Kamila Ż, Anna B, Emilia M. The pluripotent activities of caffeic acid phenethyl ester. Molecules. 2021;26(5):1335. https://doi.org/10.3390/molecules26051335.
156. Wang L, Hongwu D, Chen P. Chlorogenic acid inhibits the proliferation of human lung cancer A549 cell lines by targeting annexin A2 in vitro and in vivo. Biomed Pharmacother. 2020;131:110673. https://doi.org/10.1016/j.biopha.2020.110673.
157. Elrazik A, Nesma A, El-Mesery M, El-Karef A, Eissa LA, El Gayar AM. Chlorogenic acid potentiates antitumor effect of doxorubicin through upregulation of death receptors in solid ehrlich carcinoma model in mice. Egypt J Basic Appl Sci. 2019;6(1):158–72. https://doi.org/10.1080/2314808X.2019.1682331.
158. Rosa L, Jordão N, da Costa Pereira Soares N, DeMesquita J, Monteiro M, Teodoro A. Pharmacokinetic, antiproliferative and apoptotic effects of phenolic acids in human colon adenocarcinoma cells using in vitro and in silico approaches. Molecules. 2018;23(10):2569. https://doi.org/10.3390/molecules23102569.
159. Khawand E, Toni AC, Valls J, Richard T, Krisa S. A review of dietary stilbenes: sources and bioavailability. Phytochem Rev. 2018;17(5):1007–29. https://doi.org/10.1007/s11101-018-9578-9.
160. Martinez KB, Mackert JD, McIntosh MK. Polyphenols and intestinal health. In: Nutrition and functional foods for healthy aging. Amsterdam: Elsevier; 2017. p. 191–210.
161. Burns J, Yokota T, Ashihara H, Lean MEJ, Crozier A. Plant foods and herbal sources of resveratrol. J Agric Food Chem. 2002;50(11):3337–40. https://doi.org/10.1021/jf0112973.
162. Alayev A, Yang S, Snyder R, Berger SM, Yu J, Holz M. Resveratrol prevents rapamycin-induced upregulation of autophagy and selectively induces apoptosis in TSC2-deficient cells. Cell Cycle. 2014;13(3):371–82. https://doi.org/10.4161/cc.27355.
163. Harikumar KB, Kunnumakkara AB, Sethi G, Diagaradjane P, Anand P, Pandey MK, Gelovani J, Krishnan S, Guha S, Aggarwal BB. Resveratrol, a multitargeted agent, can enhance antitumor activity of gemcitabine in vitro and in orthotopic mouse model of human pancreatic cancer. Int J Cancer. 2010;127 https://doi.org/10.1002/ijc.25041.
164. Vergara D, Simeone P, Toraldo D, Del Boccio P, Vergaro V, Leporatti S, Pieragostino D, Tinelli A, De Domenico S, Alberti S, Urbani A, Salzet M, Santino A, Maffia M. Resveratrol downregulates Akt/GSK and ERK signalling pathways in OVCAR-3 ovarian cancer cells. Mol Biosyst. 2012;8(4):1078–87. https://doi.org/10.1039/c2mb05486h.
165. Bhaskara VK, Mittal B, Mysorekar VV, Amaresh N, Simal-Gandara J. Resveratrol, cancer and cancer stem cells: a review on past to future. Curr Res Food Sci. 2020;3(August):284–95. https://doi.org/10.1016/j.crfs.2020.10.004.
166. Calado A, Neves PM, Santos T, Ravasco P. The effect of flaxseed in breast cancer: a literature review. Front Nutr. 2018;5(February):1–7. https://doi.org/10.3389/fnut.2018.00004.
167. De S, Franklyn S, Alcorn J. Flaxseed lignans as important dietary polyphenols for cancer prevention and treatment: chemistry, pharmacokinetics, and molecular targets. Pharmaceuticals. 2019;12(2):21–38. https://doi.org/10.3390/ph12020068.
168. Jourdes M, Pouységu L, Deffieux D, Teissedre P-L, Quideau S. Hydrolyzable tannins: gallotannins and ellagitannins. In: Natural products. Berlin: Springer; 2013. p. 1975–2010.
169. Baer-Dubowska W, Szaefer H, Majchrzak-Celińska A, Krajka-Kuźniak V. Tannic acid: specific form of tannins in cancer chemoprevention and therapy-old and new applications. Curr Pharmacol Rep. 2020;6(2):28–37. https://doi.org/10.1007/s40495-020-00211-y.
170. Ismail T, Calcabrini C, Diaz AR, Fimognari C, Turrini E, Catanzaro E, Akhtar S, Sestili P. Ellagitannins in cancer chemoprevention and therapy. Toxins. 2016;8(5):1–22. https://doi.org/10.3390/toxins8050151.

171. Jia L, Zho J, Zhao H, Yanjin H, Lv M, Zhao N, Zheng Z, Lu Y, Ming Y, Yinhua Y. Corilagin sensitizes epithelial ovarian cancer to chemotherapy by inhibiting snail-glycolysis pathways. Oncol Rep. 2017;38(4):2464–70.
172. Espín JC, Larrosa M, García-Conesa MT, Tomás-Barberán F. Biological significance of urolithins, the gut microbial ellagic acid-derived metabolites: the evidence so far. Evid Based Complement Alternat Med. 2013;2013:1–15. https://doi.org/10.1155/2013/270418.
173. Cásedas G, Les F, Choya-Foces C, Hugo M, López V. The metabolite urolithin-a ameliorates oxidative stress in neuro-2a cells, becoming a potential neuroprotective agent. Antioxidants. 2020;9(2):177. https://doi.org/10.3390/antiox9020177.
174. Nagesh PKB, Chowdhury P, Hatami E, Jain S, Dan N, Kashyap VK, Chauhan SC, Jaggi M, Yallapu MM. Tannic acid inhibits lipid metabolism and induce ROS in prostate cancer cells. Sci Rep. 2020;10(1):980. https://doi.org/10.1038/s41598-020-57932-9.
175. Hwang ST, Yang MH, Kumar AP, Sethi G, Ahn KS. Corilagin represses epithelial to mesenchymal transition process through modulating Wnt/β-catenin signaling cascade. Biomolecules. 2020;10(10):1406. https://doi.org/10.3390/biom10101406.
176. Tong Y, Zhang G, Yang L, Xu J, Yuan J, Zhang B, Hu T, Song G. Corilagin inhibits breast cancer growth via reactive oxygen species-dependent apoptosis and autophagy. J Cell Mol Med. 2018;22(8):3795–807. https://doi.org/10.1111/jcmm.13647.
177. Hu C, Li M, Guo T, Wang S, Huang W, Yang K, Liao Z, Wang J, Zhang F, Wang H. Anti-metastasis activity of curcumin against breast cancer via the inhibition of stem cell-like properties and EMT. Phytomedicine. 2019;58 https://doi.org/10.1016/j.phymed.2018.11.001.
178. Chen CY, Liu TZ, Liu YW, Tseng WC, Liu RH, Lu FJ, Lin YS, Kuo SH, Chen CH. 6-Shogaol (alkanone from ginger) induces apoptotic cell death of human hepatoma P53 mutant mahlavu subline via an oxidative stress-mediated caspase-dependent mechanism. J Agric Food Chem. 2007;55(3):948–54. https://doi.org/10.1021/jf0624594.
179. Hung JYU, Hsu YAL, Te Li C, Ko YC, Ni WC, Huang MS, Kuo PL. 6-Shogaol, an active constituent of dietary ginger, induces autophagy by inhibiting the AKT/MTOR pathway in human non-small cell lung cancer A549 cells. J Agric Food Chem. 2009;57(20):9809–16. https://doi.org/10.1021/jf902315e.
180. Ling H, Yang H, Tan SH, Chui WK, Chew EH. 6-Shogaol, an active constituent of ginger, inhibits breast cancer cell invasion by reducing matrix metalloproteinase-9 expression via blockade of nuclear factor-KB activation. Br J Pharmacol. 2010;161(8):1763–77.
181. Bawadood AS, Al-Abbasi FA, Anwar F, El-Halawany AM, Al-Abd AM. 6-Shogaol suppresses the growth of breast cancer cells by inducing apoptosis and suppressing autophagy via targeting notch signaling pathway. Biomed Pharmacother. 2020;128:110302. https://doi.org/10.1016/j.biopha.2020.110302.
182. Lee T-H, Chen J-L, Liu P-S, Tsai M-M, Wang S-J, Hsieh H-L. Rottlerin, a natural polyphenol compound, inhibits upregulation of matrix metalloproteinase-9 and brain astrocytic migration by reducing PKC-δ-dependent ROS signal. J Neuroinflammation. 2020;17(1):177. https://doi.org/10.1186/s12974-020-01859-5.

Polyphenols and Nutrition: Nanotherapeutic and Immunomodulatory Implications in Cancer

9

Fauzia A. Sherwani

Abstract

Polyphenols are plant-based compounds and natural products which, increasingly, have been gaining traction due to their diverse roles as therapeutics, food supplements, and preservatives. Despite their occurrence only in plants, polyphenols are increasingly finding their use in various foods—seafood, meats, and plant products—to enhance their flavor, texture, shelf-life, and overall quality. As therapeutics, polyphenols have been shown to possess antioxidant and anti-inflammatory properties. As a result, they have been used as therapeutic and/or treatment agents directly and/or in combination with other compounds for the treatment of many cancers, metabolic diseases, neurodegenerative diseases, and inflammation. Oxidation is a phenomenon characterized by the loss of oxygen leading to oxidative stress which can compromise the detoxifying capabilities of biological systems. Oxidative stress has been implicated in the damage/disruption of DNA function including DNA-repair mechanism, cellular structure, lipid membrane bilayer, and protein-folding. Maintaining an equilibrium between cell death and cell survival is necessary for an organism to remain healthy—increased cell death can lead to tissue deterioration while increased cell survival can lead to cancer. Polyphenols, the most abundant antioxidants and anti-inflammatory agents in human diets, play important therapeutic roles in oxidative stress by terminating the oxidation chain reactions to retain cell viability, function, and molecular signaling pathways. In this chapter, the author explores the following three areas: (1) Polyphenols and their role in nutrition, (2) Nutrition focusing on fish and other seafood-based diets enhanced with polyphenols, and (3) Role of polyphenols as immune/chemotherapeutic agents in cancer treatment and prevention.

F. A. Sherwani (✉)
Department of Zoology, Women's College, Aligarh Muslim University, Aligarh, India

S. Tabrez, M. Imran Khan (eds.), *Polyphenols-based Nanotherapeutics for Cancer Management*, https://doi.org/10.1007/978-981-16-4935-6_9

Keywords

Polyphenols · Nutrition · Oxidation · Antioxidant · Anti-inflammatory · Cancer

9.1 Introduction

Polyphenols occur naturally as organic compounds in almost all plants, their products, and plant-based diets [1–3]. They possess a phenolic structure which comprises of several hydroxyl groups (–OH) attached to aromatic benzenoid ring representing the phenyl group ($-C_6H_5$). Being moderately water-soluble and with a molecular weight of 500–8000 Da, polyphenols are small enough compounds which can diffuse into the lipid bilayer of the cell membrane to establish themselves into intercellular spaces and remain intact upon senescence or the death of cell, tissue, organ, or organism. Because of this property, polyphenols have traditionally been used as dyes, especially in the context of the Indian subcontinent [4]. The properties of polyphenols were no secret in the non-nutritional industry—fabric dyeing—but their importance in nutrition is becoming more evident only now. For example, tannins, a type of polyphenol, have been used for centuries for processing leather—tanning—a process that involves treating the raw hide to convert it into leather and, in the process, possibly coloring it too [5]. Polyphenols have opened the door for sustainable green chemistry and environmental chemistry as part of which the chemical processes in various industries have become plant-based, resource-efficient, less polluting, and more environment-friendly [6].

Polyphenols have been shown to possess antioxidant and anti-inflammatory properties which can help to reduce the risks of various diseases especially obesity, Type 2 diabetes, cardiovascular diseases (CVDs), neurodegenerative diseases, cancers, and inflammation as illustrated in Fig. 9.1 [7–11]. Oxidation is a process that results in the production of oxidants, free radicals, or reactive oxygen species (ROS) which can be detrimental to the cell and cellular processes [10–12]. Polyphenols primarily function as antioxidants which inhibit oxidation and free radical formation. Antioxidants, such as polyphenols, can minimize or terminate these chain reactions of ROS which can compromise vital cellular components and functions, increasing the risk of various metabolic diseases [13]. Inflammation can be at the root of many chronic illnesses. Depending upon the food, amount, ripeness, farming practices, transportation, storage, and preparedness, polyphenols can be present in specific amounts. Polyphenols, when consumed as part of a plant-based diet provide the maximum health benefits; however, when overconsumed especially as supplements and/or isolated compounds, have been shown to cause harmful effects such as inhibition of iron absorption, especially nonheme iron, and interference with thyroid hormone biosynthesis [14]. The lack of regulation across the world has led to overhyped claims of the health benefits of polyphenols encouraging overconsumption of these compounds which can be detrimental to human health at increased and harmful doses especially in patients dealing with neurodegenerative diseases and can compromise kidneys and thyroid hormone levels [14].

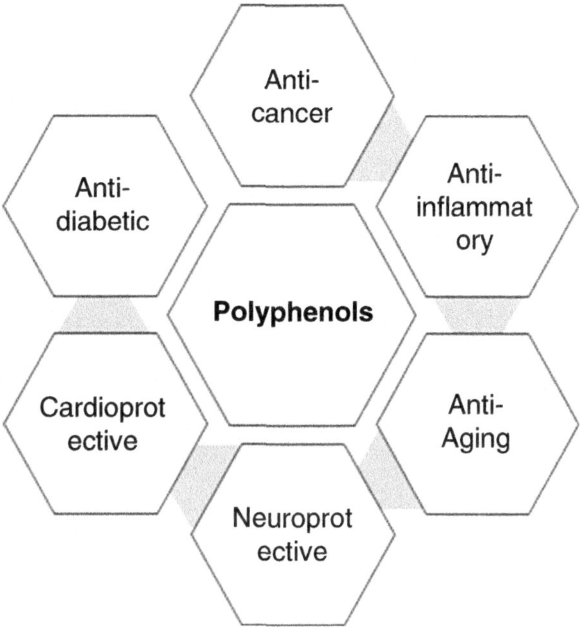

Fig. 9.1 Biological properties of polyphenols in humans

Classification and characterization of polyphenols continue to be a matter of confusion due to their variable origin, structure, and function. Due to the differences in biochemical processes within cells, a consensus on the exact classification—classes, subclasses, groups, subgroups, and types—of some polyphenols and flavonoids has not been possible, at least not yet. Increasingly, polyphenols are categorized into four main classes namely, (1) flavonoids, (2) phenolic acids, (3) stilbenes, and (4) lignans as illustrated in Fig. 9.2 [15–17]. Together, phenolic acids, stilbenes, and lignans are referred to as non-flavonoids. For detailed information, please refer to Phenol-Explorer, "the first comprehensive database on phenol content in foods [which] contains more than 35,000 content values for 500 different polyphenols in over 400 foods" [18].

Flavonoids are the most common class of polyphenols, occurring abundantly and naturally in plants. Despite the lack of consensus, depending upon their chemical structure, especially the position of aromatic rings (C-ring), flavonoids are typically classified into six subclasses namely, (1) flavones (olives, hot peppers, celery, parsley, oregano), (2) flavanols (apples, apricot, grapes, chocolate, cocoa, tea), (3) flavanones (citrus fruits, red peppers, mint, peppermint, parsley, chamomile), (4) flavonols (apples, grapes, berries, plums, raisins, onions, tomatoes, tea), (5) anthocyanins (berries, pomegranate, black currant), and (6) isoflavones (grapes, legumes), as illustrated in Fig. 9.3 [19]. Phenolic acids occur abundantly in nature and are divided into two subclasses namely, (1) hydroxycinnamic acid (apple, citrus fruits, berries, pear, spinach, coffee, tea) and (2) hydroxybenzoic acid (grapes, pomegranate, berries) [19–21]. A general classification of polyphenols is presented in Fig. 9.4.

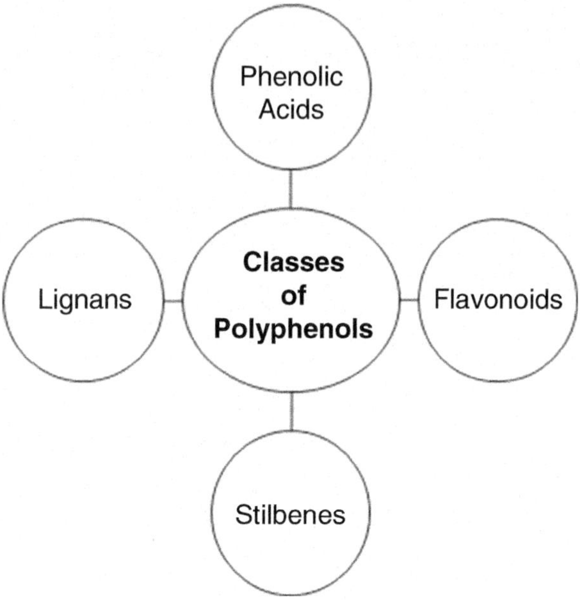

Fig. 9.2 Classes of polyphenols

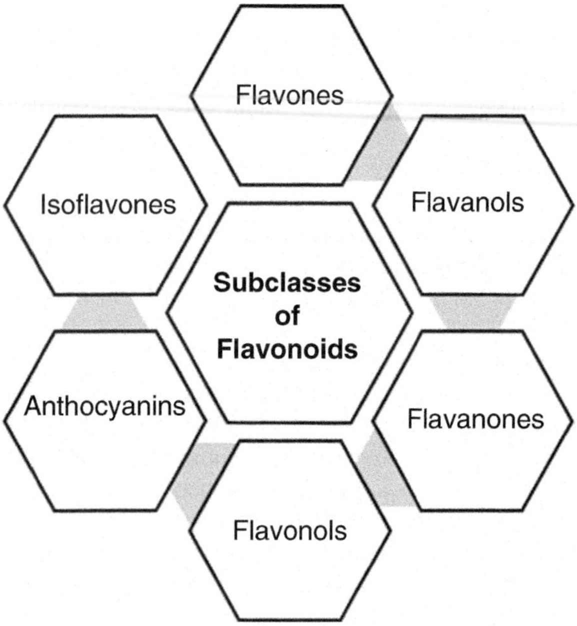

Fig. 9.3 Subclasses of flavonoids

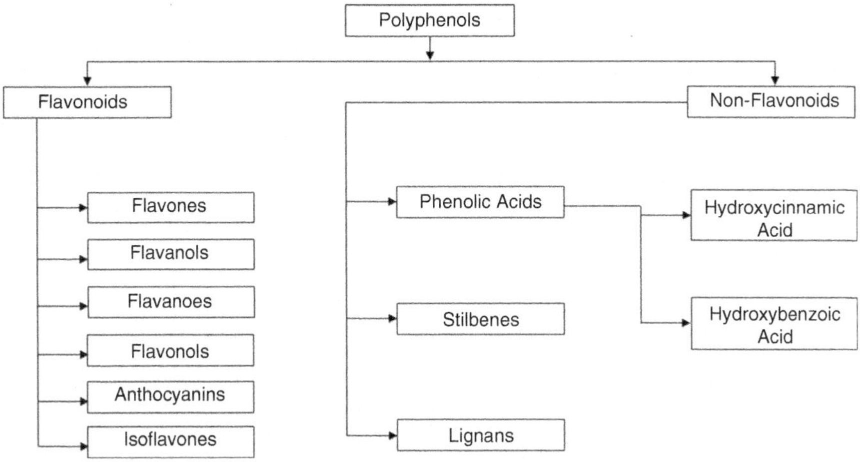

Fig. 9.4 General classification of polyphenols

9.2 Polyphenols and Nutrition

To understand nutrition and nutrients is to understand both human health and human suffering—the cycle of life and death. A whole-person approach, focusing on a healthy body and a healthy mind, can address the disease at the cellular level, comprehend the reason(s) behind it, and help in curing the disease instead of just treating the symptoms—a common approach in modern medicine. Understanding disease etiology can help in identifying the cause of the disease and suffering. Maintaining a healthy lifestyle by using a nutritious diet in combination with physical activity can help in reducing morbidity and mortality. Many factors—socioeconomic, political, and infrastructural—can create barriers for access to healthy and nutritious foods, especially for vulnerable and marginalized individuals, families, and communities.

Like all animals, humans require nutrition for sustenance. Food that humans consume throughout their lifetimes undergoes various biochemical processes to release energy captured in the form of adenosine triphosphate (ATP) which, in turn, is utilized for various metabolic pathways [21]. The biochemical processes that result due to nutritional interactions can determine how specific foods and diet interact with the body to affect health and illness. Ill bodies are the most vulnerable causing morbidity and mortality. Understanding nutrition and the interactions of various foods during various biochemical pathways can lead to positive outcomes and help to improve overall human health. Nutrition consists of nutrients which are classified as (1) macronutrients, (2) micronutrients, and (3) non-nutrients [22]. Macronutrients such as proteins, carbohydrates, and fats are consumed in abundant amounts and used in maintaining bodily structure and functions. Micronutrients, comprising of vitamins and minerals, occur naturally within the body while others must be supplemented or produced in the presence of sunlight (e.g., vitamin D). Non-nutrients or bio-actives such as polyphenols originate from plants and plant-based foods [22]. Polyphenols possess antioxidant and anti-inflammatory properties which offer potential health benefits and therapeutic capabilities against several diseases including cancers [7–13, 22].

Nutrition and diet play important roles in developing a healthy body with capabilities for fighting diseases. Non-nutrients are neither stored in the body nor do they contribute directly to the nutritional needs of the body; however, they help in managing cellular stress and trauma. These non-nutrients are commonly identified with such terms as polyphenols, bio-actives, antioxidants, phytonutrients, among several others. Plant-sourced diets can be nutritionally healthier than animal-sourced diets as they pack necessary all kinds of nutrients—macronutrients, micronutrients, and non-nutrients [22]. In the last few decades, non-nutrients have continued to generate increased interest among nutritionists, biochemists, physiologists, oncologists, and individuals interested in living a healthier lifestyle. Polyphenols are prevalent in plant-based foods in variable quantities, especially in fruits, vegetables, teas, and coffee. Increasingly, polyphenols are being used in other foods as additives, enhancers, preservatives, or consumed directly as supplements. They are also being added to fish feed in aquaculture to improve flavor, texture, smell, and overall quality. The antioxidant and anti-inflammatory properties of polyphenols have implications in chronic diseases such as cancers, metabolic, degenerative, and CVDs [7–13, 22].

Obesity is fast becoming a global epidemic, affecting both high-income (developed) and low-income (developing) countries with high impact rates in both rural and urban settings [23]. It is especially challenging for those who have chronic conditions and are disabled as a result thereof. Because of the sedentary lifestyle due to industrialization, mechanization, processed foods, and high calorie diets, obesity has become highly prevalent in all cultures [23]. The rural poor are the most vulnerable as they lack access to nutritious food choices due to socioeconomic and infrastructural barriers. Obese individuals have a higher risk of developing Type 2 diabetes. Despite being a largely preventable disease, some individuals and populations are more prone to developing Type 2 diabetes than others due to genetic susceptibility, lifestyle choices, ethnicity, culture, and environment [24]. Due to a lack of infrastructure, the rural poor lack safe and regular access to healthcare providers and healthcare facilities. The urban poor, on the other hand, do not have safe, easy, and affordable access to exercise and other physical activity options. Cultural barriers compromise the health of one gender (female) more than the other (male), with transgender individuals facing unprecedented obstacles in seeking and receiving healthcare [25]. For example, in certain cultures, girls, women, and transgender individuals are either not allowed, or discouraged, or feel unsafe while exercising or performing physical activity outside their homes, especially at certain times of the day/night. Likewise, nutrition, calories, and choice of foods are also barriers that contribute to lifestyle choices and affect different genders differently [26].

A sedentary lifestyle can be anathema to healthy living. Excess body fat specifically around the waistline, hypertension, elevated levels of blood glucose (insulin resistance), cholesterol, and triglycerides among others are contributory risk factors for metabolic syndrome [27]. Consuming an agrarian diet full of red meats and carbohydrates when a vast majority of individuals are not even involved in the agrarian practices is a recipe for disaster. Research shows that consuming red meats, processed foods, refined grains, and concentrated sugars are detrimental to health and healthy living [28]. Despite the advances in the understanding of health, disease, nutrition, and biochemical pathways, individuals continue to consume an animal-based diet with devastating health consequences for themselves, families, community—putting an extra burden on the community and the system [29].

Metabolism is a 24/7 process where carbohydrates, proteins, and fats present in foods are regularly broken down in the presence of enzymes and other specific proteins to release energy for consumption within cells [28, 29]. Some of these compounds are produced in one cell/tissue/organ and transported for use in another. Sometimes, the metabolic process can become disrupted leading to compromised pathways which, in turn, leads to metabolic disorders [28–30]. Metabolic disorders can be classified into: (1) common metabolic disorders (CMD) or (2) inherited metabolic disorders (IMD) [31]. Type 2 Diabetes is the most CMD, which can also be inherited but it is more of a lifestyle-oriented (environmental) disease. The IMDs, also known as inborn errors of metabolism (IEM), on the other hand, are typically inherited from both parents [30]. Examples of IMDs include Hurler syndrome, Tay-Sachs disease, Gaucher disease, Krabbe disease, galactosemia, glycogen storage diseases, mitochondrial disorders, metal metabolism disorders, hemochromatosis, organic acidemias, and urea cycle disorders, among others. Symptoms associated with IMDs include poor appetite, lethargy, abdominal pain, vomiting, stunted growth, seizures, and developmental delay—cognitive and physical [32]. These symptoms may be a result of malnutrition, consuming certain types of foods, beverages, medications, and dehydration. Most of the symptoms are present at birth, especially if the mother is malnourished and the child is born with low birth weight, while others appear after many years of living and, in both cases, can be detected through routine biomarker screening [33].

Malnutrition can lead to metabolic syndrome which includes disorders like obesity, Type 2 diabetes, organ failure, CVDs, and cancers [28–30, 34]. Malnutrition can also be a consequence of cancer as the appetite of the patient becomes increasingly compromised leading-up to cancer, during cancer treatments (radiotherapy, chemotherapy, or immunotherapy), surgery (partial or complete removal of tumor/cancer), and recovery [35]. Cancer patients struggle to consume enough calories necessary to regain vital body functions and be healthy individuals again, if/when they have access to healthy and nutritious foods [35]. On the other hand, those with lack of access to healthy and nutritious foods, whether due to socioeconomic, healthcare, or infrastructural vulnerabilities, often, become nutritionally compromised and succumb to malnutrition, increased recovery challenges, and death. Several risk factors for CVDs have been identified and prominent among them are obesity, Type 2 diabetes, hypertension, hypercholesterolemia, and dyslipidemia. A plant-based diet has been shown to be more effective in mitigating the risks and prevalence of obesity, Type 2 diabetes, hypertension, CVDs, and cancers [36].

Exposure to, or lack of, specific foods and nutrition can indicate cancer risk in life across gender, age, and culture. Despite the advances in the understanding of metabolic disorders, IMDs, nutrition, exercise, and lifestyle choices, their relationship with cancers remains a paradox. Even with the recent progress made in the treatment and management of cancers, the mortality rate remains incredibly high. Morbidity, quality of life (QOL), and mortality can be improved through lifestyle choices and environmental changes for better outcomes [37]. For example, the risk of lung cancer can be lowered significantly through smoking cessation and decreased tobacco chewing consumption [37]. The relationship between nutrition, diet, and cancer (prevention) needs to be extrapolated.

To understand the relationships between nutrition, diet, lifestyle choices, environmental factors, and the risk for cancer and other chronic diseases, the International Agency for Research on Cancer (IARC) of the World Health Organization (WHO) sponsored a prospective, longitudinal (15 years), and multinational (10 countries) study—European Prospective Investigation into Cancer and Nutrition (EPIC) study (http://epic.iarc.fr) [38]. As part of the EPIC study, researchers investigated 521,000 participants for nutritional epidemiology, genetic analyses, and lifestyle investigations. The EPIC study focused on the following six research areas: (1) Mediterranean diet and health, (2) Genetic predisposition to lung cancer, (3) Abdominal adiposity and mortality, (4) Alcohol and cancer incidence, (5) Vitamin D and colorectal cancer, and (6) Biomarkers for early detection of HPV-driven oropharyngeal cancer [38]. The findings showed a significant association between diet and cancers. For example, a diet rich in red meats and processed meats showed an increased risk of gastric cancers, while a diet rich in fish, dietary fiber, vitamin D, and calcium showed a decreased risk of colorectal cancer [38, 39].

9.3 Polyphenols: Role in Aquaculture

Polyphenols, increasingly, are being used as natural food additives, preservatives, and flavoring agents for enhancing food quality, taste, and safeguarding measures against food spoilage [14, 40]. Such foods include seafood, especially fish, fish products, and fish feed. Foods like seafood, meats, fresh fruits, and vegetables undergo spoilage—microbiological, environmental, and chemical—during handling (processing, packaging, and transportation) and storage [41]. Compromised food quality (nutrition, rancidity, color, and texture) is a major problem that the food industry must address as it can lead to spoilage, disease outbreaks, illnesses, recalls, brand damage, and public relations nightmare. These issues can lead to low customer satisfaction and confidence, reduced bottom line, and potential lawsuits. To overcome these problems and increase the nutritional value of foods, naturally occurring polyphenols, as opposed to synthetic additives and preservatives, are increasingly being preferred and used in various food items at all stages of culture, growth, harvesting, processing, and preservation [40, 41].

Polyphenols are safe and commonly used as additives in enhancing fish feed during aquaculture [41]. Fish farming, as part of aquaculture, utilizes strategic approaches to enhance the quality and quantity of fish. Proximity within limited spaces can cause increased oxidative stress among fish which can lead to immune-suppressed behavior and increased mortality [42]. As compared to hormones, vitamins, antibiotics, and probiotics, which have been used successfully in aquaculture, the use of polyphenols is a recent phenomenon. Naturally occurring and plant-based, polyphenols present negligible side effects while enhancing the antioxidant and anti-inflammatory properties of fish and other organisms raised via aquaculture—thus enhancing their quality and value [14, 43, 44]. In addition to enhancing the quality of fish, the use of polyphenols instead of chemical compounds can improve food quality, safety, and productivity [14, 43, 44].

9.3.1 Polyphenols and Oxidation

Oxidation is a chemical phenomenon during which atoms lose electrons and become oxidized [45]. During reduction, atoms gain electrons and become reduced. Oxidation occurs in tandem with reduction (redox reaction) during which one species (reductant or reducing agent) loses electrons and becomes oxidized while the other (oxidant or oxidizing agent) gains electrons and becomes reduced [45]. During the breakdown of glucose in cellular respiration, redox reactions are the main source of energy which is captured in the form of ATP when electrons move from higher energy states to lower energy states. Oxidation can be triggered by reactive molecular species (RMS)—oxidants and free radicals (peroxides), heat, light, ionizing radiation, and metals generated or consumed as part of food or food production [46].

Overproduction of RMS or free radicals, which typically occurs in the form of reactive oxygen species (ROS) and reactive nitrogen species (RNS)—ROS/RNS—along with reactive sulfur species (RSS) and reactive carbon species (RCS), can cause cell senescence, aging, compromised immune functions, cancers, and death [47, 48]. Quenching access ROS/RNS and other RMS are of the essence in minimizing senescence. A higher-than-normal concentration of RMS can trigger lipid oxidation, causing rancidity, degradation, compromised quality, texture, flavor, and smell of food. In the nutrition sector, lipid oxidation and ensuing rancidity are major concerns which can lead to losses in bottom line and brand equity. Many natural supplements like polyphenols are increasingly being used as antioxidants and anti-inflammatory supplements to enhance cell function, maintain oxidation equilibrium, and retain food quality [13, 14, 43, 44]. Polyphenols also help in minimizing oxidative onslaught on regulatory mechanisms and signaling pathways within cells helping in delaying senescence, aging, and death [43, 44].

Lipid oxidation is a complex phenomenon which can compromise the quality of all foods, especially those rich in unsaturated fats and polyunsaturated fatty acids (PUFA) [49]. Briefly defined, lipid oxidation is the degradation of PUFA mediated by free radicals. As regulators of lipid metabolism, PUFA have been shown to possess anticancer and anti-inflammatory properties. Whether on land or sea, animals can sense stress before capture, slaughter, or killing which can lead to a cascade of metabolic pathways resulting in (over)production of RMS. Cells have an endogenous ability to quench normal oxidant production, maintain physiologic redox potential, while preserving the inherent ability to detoxify RMS [43, 44, 49].

Lipid oxidation in fish occurs at a higher rate because fish lipids are highly unsaturated, and, hence, spoil faster than meats [49, 50]. Brain, being rich in lipid content and consuming a higher level of oxygen is highly susceptible to lipid oxidation [50, 51]. Cholesterol—a type of lipid (sterol)—is an important component of all cell membranes in animal cells and is hydrophobic in nature. Oxidation, a normal physiological process, can be detrimental to the health of cholesterol cells if overproduction of oxidized cholesterol is triggered by the body creating ripe conditions for a perfect lipid oxidation storm [10–12, 45]. Upon oxidation, when cholesterol becomes oxidized and lines the inner arterial walls, it can cause many health issues including CVDs such as atherosclerosis in humans and animals [52].

9.4 Polyphenols and Human Health: Implications in Cancer Treatment and Prevention

Polyphenols have been found to be associated with many health benefits [13, 14, 21, 53]. Although, a lack of polyphenols in a diet has not been shown to result in any specific disease, regular consumption of polyphenols, especially in their natural state, has been shown to be linked with a reduced risk of several chronic or non-communicable diseases (NCDs) [14]. Chronic diseases or NCDs are those diseases which are not contracted from one person to the other (noninfectious and non-transmissible) [14]. There is a long list of NCDs but commonly prevalent among them are: (1) Cancers (lung, breast, prostate, colorectal, melanoma, endometrial, leukemia, pancreas), (2) Autoimmune diseases or AID [HIV-AIDS, rheumatoid arthritis, Type 1 diabetes, inflammatory bowel disease (IBD), psoriasis, and multiple sclerosis (MS), Guillain-Barre syndrome], (3) Metabolic syndrome (obesity, diabetes, liver cirrhosis), (4) CVDs, often considered a part of metabolic syndrome, they typically have their own category (coronary artery disease or CAD, hypertension, atherosclerosis, stroke, myocardial infection or heart attack, heart failure, cardiomyopathy), (5) Chronic respiratory diseases (COPD, asthma, cystic fibrosis, black lung), and (6) Neurodegenerative diseases (Alzheimer's, Parkinson's, Huntington's, brain tumors) [12, 14].

Polyphenols have low absorption and low bioavailability in their natural state which continue to be problematic for their stability and lipid oxidation prevention [14, 21, 54, 55]. Polyphenols are absorbed poorly and breakdown rather easily in the presence of common elements/signals like oxygen, light, and heat. The way polyphenols are consumed determines their effectiveness. The effectiveness of polyphenols is directly proportional to the method of consumption—raw, steamed, boiled, cooked on open-flame, or fried [14, 54, 55]. Antioxidant and anti-inflammatory effects of polyphenols falls on the spectrum of the cooking method with raw consumption of polyphenols offering the highest value while fried ones offering the lowest. But all foods, plants, and plant products cannot be consumed raw—they are usually consumed cooked, boiled, steamed, and increasingly processed. Unfortunately, with food processing, polyphenols lose their effectiveness significantly [14, 54, 55]. So, the concentration of polyphenols in foods and supplements needs to be enhanced to make them effective and beneficial. Because their natural taste is mostly bitter, other ingredients are often added to foods and beverages during processing to reduce bitterness and improve taste which can compromise their effectiveness.

9.4.1 Global Burden of Cancer

Cancer is a chronic disease. According to the National Cancer Institute [56], "cancer is the name given to a collection of related diseases. In all types of cancer, some of the body's cells begin to divide without stopping and spread into surrounding tissues." Globally, cancer is the second biggest cause of death (9.56 million), right behind CVDs (17.79 million), annually [57]. The incidence of cancer is directly proportional to age. The annual number of deaths from cancer in children 5–14 years old is at a staggering more than 62,000 [57]. In people aged 15–49 years old, the deaths from cancers increase to 1.05 million annually [57]. In people belonging to the 50–69 years old category, cancers are the cause of death at an annual rate of 3.96 million [57]. For people 70 years old and older, the annual number of deaths are reported to be 4.53 million [57]. Among men, the top-5 occurring cancers are lung, liver, stomach, colorectal, and prostate while, among women, they are breast, lung, colorectal, cervical, and stomach [58].

Cancer causing cells and tumor cells have the capacity to undergo uncontrolled division, increase their numbers rather quickly, damage healthy cells and tissue in their vicinity or the microenvironment [59–61]. It is important to distinguish between cancer and tumor even though the two terms are closely related and, often, used interchangeably. Cancer is a disease in which the cells can divide uncontrollably almost anywhere in the body. Tumor, on the other hand, is a growth that occurs uncontrollably in organs, muscles, or bones [12, 14]. Cancers may be localized, or they may metastasize throughout the host body. Cancers metastasize throughout the body through the blood and lymphatic systems by avoiding detection from the robust defense mechanisms of the immune system—"hiding" from the immune system [62]. When localized, they affect the cells, tissues, and organ (s) surrounding the cancerous cells. When metastasized, especially if they enter the bone marrow (leukemia and lymphoma), cancers can compromise the immune response by blocking or compromising the genesis of new blood cells [62].

9.4.2 Immune Response in Cancer

The immune system has the innate ability to recognize healthy and unhealthy cells [63]. The healthy cells are the normal cells which form, divide, and die regularly—normal lifecycle. The unhealthy cells are comprised of dead and dying cells which do not receive/follow the cell signal(s) correctly. As a result, these unhealthy cells continue to live beyond when they should be dying/dead and, in the process, becoming cancerous and causing cancers and tumors. The unhealthy cells may also be those which have been attacked/infected by invading pathogens causing disease, infection, or injury. The role of the immune system is to prevent or reduce infection from invading pathogens [63, 64]. The immune system comprises of a complex network of proteins, cells, tissues, and organs which detect and safeguard against any insults or assaults on the body—disease, infection, and injury. The function of the immune system is to help the body cope effectively by scavenging invading pathogens with minimal damage to the host cells and tissues. This coordinated task is accomplished via a complex regulatory system of cytokines, protein–protein interactions, and enzymatic reactions which function efficiently as the cells work toward maintaining a state of cellular equilibrium (homeostasis) with least damage [64]. Sometimes, cancer cells, tumor cells, and even healthy cells as part of the tumor microenvironment can escape detection by the immune system by producing different immune suppressive cytokines and manipulating certain regulatory pathways [64, 65].

9.4.2.1 Leukocytes: Role and Function in Immune Response

White blood cells or leukocytes are the first line of defense of the body. Leukocytes constantly look for pathogens and, upon finding them, multiply in numbers and alert other cells to perform accordingly to build a robust defense mechanism leading to the destruction or neutralization of the pathogen [65]. There are two main types of leukocytes namely, (1) phagocytes and (2) lymphocytes. The function of phagocytes is to surround a pathogen by their plasma membrane, break it down, and engulf it—phagocytosis. Phagocytes also help the system by consuming/removing dead or dying cells. Based upon their functions, different types of phagocytes have been identified which include macrophages, monocytes, neutrophils, and mast cells [65]. Macrophages defend against invading pathogens and digest dead and dying cells. Acting as antigen presenting cells (APCs), macrophages play an important role in immune response by presenting some portions of the pathogen (antigens) and triggering antibody formation/stimulation following pathogen disintegration and/or digestion [65].

Lymphocytes are the memory cells of the body responsible for generating protective immune responses against pathogens. Their function is to memorize the previous pathogens and remember them if they return or the same infection happens again to provide an appropriate response [65]. Lymphocytes are created in the bone marrow. Those that remain in the bone marrow are designated as bone marrow lymphocytes or B lymphocytes (B cells), while others that migrate to the thymus are referred to as thymus lymphocytes or T lymphocytes (T cells) [66, 67]. The role of B cells is to detect the antigens, produce antibodies, and alert the T cells of any imminent danger from invading pathogens or infections—protecting against disease. Whereas the role of T cells is to disintegrate and destroy the body's dead and dying cells and remove cell debris and alert other lymphocytes. The "memory" characteristic of lymphocytes (both B cells and T cells) is utilized in developing vaccines which trigger immunity by mimicking the pathogen when it presents itself again [66, 67].

9.4.3 Polyphenols and Inflammation

Cytokines are low molecular weight signaling molecules which help in intercellular communication. During the immune response, cytokines are produced by leukocytes (interleukins) and lymphocytes (lymphokines) on demand depending upon the need of the cell to ward off infection. Cytokines play important immunoregulatory and immunomodulatory roles in cell signaling during normal, developmental, and pathological situations [68]. Immunoregulatory role of cytokines can be characterized by the general and natural regulation of immune response(s) such as production of antibodies (humoral regulators). Immunomodulatory, on the other hand, involves modifying or changing the body's immune system (response) by using certain compounds (drugs, stimulants) by upregulating or downregulating certain proteins. Immunosuppressive drugs, commonly used in solid organ transplants, utilize the immunomodulating principle. Immunomodulating drugs are increasingly being used as part of therapeutic and treatment options in various cancers. Natural products like polyphenols are strong modulators of inflammatory response that reduce inflammation and relieve pain [68].

Proinflammatory biomarkers play a negative role in cell function causing inflammation, worsening disease condition, and compromising healing. Anti-inflammatory biomarkers, on the other hand, help in reducing inflammation and stimulating healing. If the equilibrium between proinflammatory and anti-inflammatory cytokines is disturbed, inflammation and diseases including cancers can occur [68]. Interleukins are a group of cytokines which play an important role in inflammatory response and immunity. Proinflammatory biomarkers commonly associated with pain and trauma include interleukin 1 beta (IL-1β), IL-6, IL-12, IL-18, tumor necrosis factor alpha (TNF-α), interferon gamma (IFNγ), and granulocyte-macrophage colony-stimulating factor (GM-CSF) [68]. Many nonsteroidal anti-inflammatory drugs (NSAIDs) are available in the market both over the counter (OTC) and via prescription. Polyphenols, on the other hand, are a group of naturally occurring plant-based compounds that possess potent anti-inflammatory and antioxidant properties and have shown promise in regulating metabolism and cellular functions and combatting inflammation and disease.

Inflammation and the resulting inflammatory response can cause oxidative stress which, in turn, can compromise the antioxidant capability of cells and tissues leading to overaccumulation of free radicals [68]. Free radicals such as ROS can interact with various entities such as proteins, fatty acids, and free fatty acids (FFAs) in the membrane lipid bilayer causing loss of cellular integrity, function(s), and ultimately death [68]. Oxidative stress is defined as the imbalance between the production of RMS (oxidants and free radicals, such as ROS) and the body's ability to quench or detoxify their excess within cells and tissues [13, 14, 47, 48, 68]. The oxygen-containing free radicals (ROS) possess odd number of electrons which makes them highly reactive with other molecules. The abnormal production and accumulation of ROS can be detrimental to the cellular structure and function and lead to chronic inflammation [10, 47, 48, 68]. Hence, these reactive byproducts must be scavenged regularly to detoxify the cell environment, repair cell damage, and maintain cellular integrity. During disease, infection, and injury, the body's immune response is triggered, and the immune cells called macrophages patrol and defend the body against such pathogenic onslaughts. The free radicals, produced by macrophages while fighting disease, infection, and injury, can cause damage to healthy cells while triggering inflammation [40, 68, 69]. Oxidative stress can be a trigger or result of inflammation—a cause of many NCDs including cancers.

Polyphenols play an important role in controlling oxidation and inflammation. Given their antioxidant and anti-inflammatory capabilities, polyphenols can react with free radicals like ROS, RNS, RSS, and RCS (mostly ROS and RNS) to terminate chain reaction(s) to preserve cell structure and function while maintaining cell viability [40, 47, 48, 68, 69]. Abnormal production and nonoptimal removal (quenching or detoxification) of free radicals during oxidation can trigger inflammation or inflammatory response within cells or tissues due to disease, infection, or injury. The inflammatory response can also be triggered by heat, ionizing radiation, metal toxicity, and trauma. The inflammatory response leads to a cascading effect during which (injured) cells synthesize and secrete biochemicals such as proinflammatory cytokines which cause cellular insults including inflammation, pain, and chronic diseases including cancers [40, 64, 65, 68].

9.5 Discussion

Polyphenols are all the rage in nutrition and cancer biology these days because of their nutritional and therapeutic benefits. Evidence exists that polyphenols can lower the risk of many chronic diseases including certain cancers and can be used as therapeutic and treatment agents [64, 65, 68–70]. Many studies have shown that a plant-based diet consisting of fruits and vegetables with high polyphenolic content can be effective in reducing the risk of various types of cancers [7–14, 22, 36]. The anticancer efficacy of polyphenols is associated with their antioxidant, anti-inflammatory, and anticarcinogenic properties. Tumor cells and cancers spread by evading the body's immune response, reprograming metabolic pathways, and avoiding programmed cell death (apoptosis) [62]. For cancer to grow and metastasize, cancerous cells must undergo repeated angiogenesis and develop and retain cell signaling capabilities within a robust and self-sustaining microenvironment [59–61, 64, 65]. Polyphenols, acting as antioxidant, anti-inflammatory, and carcinogenic agents, influence regulatory pathways leading to blocking cancer initiation and progression [43, 44, 64, 68]. Cancer cells contribute to, and thrive upon, the imbalance between cell division and cell death. When certain cells do not receive or cannot process the death signal, they remain intact and continue to live beyond their span thus becoming cancerous. Polyphenols have been found to enhance apoptosis of cancer cells [43, 44, 47, 48, 62, 68].

Significant data are accumulating in favor of polyphenols as being the golden molecule(s) which could be the panacea for all ills [17, 22]. The move toward pharmaceutical formulation has been slow even though there has been significant growth in other industries, especially nutraceuticals. Polyphenols have established a strong foothold in nutrition (additives, enhancers, food supplements, preservatives), natural products, and cosmetic industries [7, 13, 22]. Given the tremendous promise that polyphenols present in preventing and treating cancer, it is important that we move toward consuming mostly a plant-based diet enriched with fruits, vegetables, whole grains, legumes, pulses, seeds, and nuts [34–39, 61, 64].

Lung cancer is the most common cancer worldwide and different polyphenols have shown promising results in anticancer activities [69–71]. Breast cancer is the most common among women worldwide. Polyphenols have been shown to have antimetabolic effects on breast cancer cells (highly dependent upon glucose) and inhibit breast cancer metastasis [72–74]. Polyphenols may also act by blocking the hormonal biomarkers of breast cancer such as the estrogen receptor (ER) and progesterone receptor (PR) [74]. Many studies are underway but more short-term and longitudinal studies are needed for studying the health effects and benefits of polyphenols in patients with breast cancer and their healthy controls. Polyphenols, extracted from green tea, have been shown to possess anticancer properties and help in the treatment and prevention of prostate cancer (globally, the most common cancer among men) through the cell signaling pathway [75, 76].

Evidence about the health benefits of polyphenols has been derived mostly from laboratory-based (in vitro or in vivo) and observational studies and limited clinical studies [77–79]. Most clinical results from these studies are significant and promising but there has not been much consensus on the optimum concentration of polyphenols that individuals can consume. The bioavailability of polyphenols continues to be problematic in determining compounding concentrations. It does not help much that polyphenols are not properly regulated, with manufacturers making tall and deceptive claims and selling supplements with high overages. Polyphenols at higher concentrations can be injurious to the health of the consumer [40]. Several studies of different polyphenolic compounds in varying concentrations in both cancer and tumor cell lines, as well as animal models of cancers (lung, breast, prostate, colon, gastric, cervical), have revealed significant, promising, and reproducible results [54, 69, 70, 73–76].

Polyphenols can be consumed as part of a natural plant-based diet, additives in non-plant-based diets such as seafood, especially fish, or natural food supplements. Polyphenols play important roles as protective, preventive, and therapeutic agents while utilizing their antioxidant, anti-inflammatory, and anticarcinogenic properties in combatting cancer and other chronic diseases. Due to their low absorption and low bioavailability, their formulation as drugs continues to be a limiting factor in the pharmaceutical industry. Several polyphenols have shown slow, steady, and significant progress in the pharmaceutical industry. Polyphenols like epigallocatechin gallate (EGCG), lycopene, resveratrol, curcumin, and oleuropein have been shown to help in lowering the risk of breast cancer [80]. These polyphenols possess antitumor activities and play important roles in signaling pathways associated with cell survival during breast cancer. Lycopene, curcumin, resveratrol, and EGCG have been shown to exert an antitumor effect in prostate cancer by modulating the inflammatory pathways, inducing apoptosis and cell cycle arrest [80]. Resveratrol, EGCG, and ginkgetin have been effective in lowering the risk of colon cancer and lung cancer treatment has shown promising results with the use of resveratrol, curcumin, and ECGC [80]. Systematic delivery of drugs continues to be problematic due to the low bioavailability of polyphenols. Researchers, nutraceutical formulators, and pharmaceutical manufacturers continue to make progress in developing different matrices for better bioavailability and increased absorption of polyphenols.

9.6 Conclusion

Polyphenols are sought after by consumers for their health benefits and the willing food manufacturers are happy to provide what the market demands. Industries representing nutrition, nutraceuticals, cosmetics, and natural supplements continue to make nutrition and health claims which may or may not be accurate, at least not 100%. False or over-exaggerated claims along with selling supplements with increased concentrations of polyphenols can be detrimental to the health of the consumer—a total opposite of the initial goal—health benefits of polyphenols. Overconsumption can lead to overaccumulation of high levels of polyphenols within the cells, tissues, organs, and organisms. Polyphenols continue to garner the attention of researchers and study results have consistently shown great potential for cancer therapy but more research, followed by clinical trials, is needed to determine their efficiency, efficacy, and safety.

9.7 Limitations and Future Perspectives

Given their immense potential and promise, why have polyphenols not made deeper inroads into the pharmaceutical industry? The answer(s) may lie in a myriad of factors and may offer insights into the limitations. To reap the health benefits, the main goal is to deliver a bioactive form of polyphenols which can induce the desired response systematically. Unfortunately, in vivo and clinical studies have consistently shown that polyphenols have low absorption and low bioavailability which makes them challenging pharmaceutical moieties or compounds for drug development. Regulation of polyphenols continues to lag the progress in research and consumption and is not as tightly regulated as the pharmaceuticals. The United States Food and Drug Administration (FDA), the European Food Safety Authority (EFSA), and the

Food and Agriculture Organization (FAO) of the World Health Organization (WHO) have loose regulations on natural products and food supplements such as polyphenols which is a major safety concern, especially for patients dealing with cancers, tumors, and other chronic diseases. So, researchers and consumers must tread with caution.

The current research and knowledge discussed in this chapter present the possibilities of future research in several areas of polyphenol and have implications in their development as therapeutic agents for cancer treatment and prevention. Despite the promising role of polyphenols in the treatment and prevention of cancer and tumors, their bioavailability and bioabsorption remain major obstacles in their use as mainstream pharmaceuticals. Future research involves investigating the possibility of delivering these therapeutic compounds, potentially via targeted drug-delivery systems, or slow release using nanotechnology or other engineering technologies. Following Hippocrates's proclamation, "let your food be your medicine," it is important to explore further the interactions between polyphenols, food, and cancer. There is a potential for enhancing and supplementing other foods, such as fish, meats, dairy, which are not rich in polyphenols, for effective cancer fighting properties. Clinical studies focusing on the role of polyphenols in cancer treatment and prevention are limited and continue to lag the developments in animal model research and in vitro studies. It is important to conduct more clinical studies to understand the efficacy of polyphenols leading to their use as potential therapeutic agents in the treatment and prevention of cancer.

References

1. Bravo L. Polyphenols: chemistry, dietary sources, metabolism, and nutritional significance. Nutr Rev. 1998;56(11):317–33. https://doi.org/10.1111/j.1753-4887.1998.tb01670.x. PMID: 9838798
2. Manach C, Scalbert A, Morand C, Rémésy C, Jiménez L. Polyphenols: food sources and bioavailability. Am J Clin Nutr. 2004;79(5):727–47.
3. Marranzano M, Rosa RL, Malaguarnera M, Palmeri R, Tessitori M, Barbera AC. Polyphenols: plant sources and food industry applications. Curr Pharm Des. 2018;24(35):4125–30.
4. Dabas D. Polyphenols as colorants. Adv Food Technol Nutr Sci Open J. 2016;SE(2):S1–6. https://doi.org/10.17140/AFTNSOJ-SE-2-101.
5. Auad P, Spier F, Gutterres M. Vegetable tannin composition and its association with the leather tanning effect. Chem Eng Commun. 2020;207(5):722–32. https://doi.org/10.1080/00986445.2019.1618843.
6. Kharissova OV, Kharisov BI, Oliva González CM, Méndez YP, López I. Greener synthesis of chemical compounds and materials. R Soc Open Sci. 2019;6(11):191378. https://doi.org/10.1098/rsos.191378.
7. Ambriz-Pérez DL, Leyva-López N, Gutierrez-Grijalva EP, Heredia JB, Yildiz F. Phenolic compounds: natural alternative in inflammation treatment. A review. Cogent Food Agric. 2016;2:1. https://doi.org/10.1080/23311932.2015.1131412.
8. Sobhani M, Farzaei MH, Kiani S, Khodarahmi R. Immunomodulatory; anti-inflammatory/antioxidant effects of polyphenols: a comparative review on the parental compounds and their metabolites. Food Rev Int. 2020; https://doi.org/10.1080/87559129.2020.1717523.

9. Hussain T, Tan B, Yin Y, Blachier F, Tossou MC, Rahu N. Oxidative stress and inflammation: What polyphenols can do for us? Oxid Med Cell Longev. 2016;2016:7432797. https://doi.org/10.1155/2016/7432797.
10. Magrone T, Magrone M, Russo MA, Jirillo E. Recent advances on the anti-inflammatory and antioxidant properties of red grape polyphenols: in vitro and in vivo studies. Antioxidants (Basel). 2019;9(1):35. https://doi.org/10.3390/antiox9010035.
11. Perez-Jimenez J, Neveu V, Vos F, Scalbert A. Identification of the 100 richest dietary sources of polyphenols: an application of the phenol-explorer database. Eur J Clin Nutr. 2010;64(Suppl. 3):S112–20. https://doi.org/10.1038/ejcn.2010.221.
12. McCord JM. The evolution of free radicals and oxidative stress. Am J Med. 2000;108(8):652–9. https://doi.org/10.1016/s0002-9343(00)00412-5.
13. Del Rio D, Rodriguez-Mateos A, Spencer JP, et al. Dietary (poly)phenolics in human health: structures, bioavailability, and evidence of protective effects against chronic diseases. Antioxid Redox Signal. 2013;18:1818–92.
14. Cory H, Passarelli S, Szeto J, Tamez M, Mattei J. The role of polyphenols in human health and food systems: a mini review. Front Nutr. 2018;5:87. https://doi.org/10.3389/fnut.2018.00087.
15. Tsao R. Chemistry and biochemistry of dietary polyphenols. Nutrients. 2010;2(12):1231–46. https://doi.org/10.3390/nu2121231.
16. Durazzo A, Lucarini M, Souto EB, et al. Polyphenols: a concise overview on the chemistry, occurrence, and human health. Phytother Res. 2019;33:2221–43. https://doi.org/10.1002/ptr.6419.
17. Scalbert A, Williamson G. Dietary intake and bioavailability of polyphenols. J Nutr. 2000;130(8):2073S–85S. https://doi.org/10.1093/jn/130.8.2073S.
18. Phenol-Explorer. Phenol-Explorer: an online comprehensive database on polyphenol contents in foods; 2010. Available at http://www.phenol-explorer.eu
19. Tangney CC, Rasmussen HE. Polyphenols, inflammation, and cardiovascular disease. Curr Atheroscler Rep. 2013;15(5) https://doi.org/10.1007/s11883-013-0324-x.
20. Hanhineva K, Törrönen R, Bondia-Pons I, et al. Impact of dietary polyphenols on carbohydrate metabolism. Int J Mol Sci. 2010;11(4):1365–402. https://doi.org/10.3390/ijms11041365.
21. Amiot MJ, Riva C, Vinet A. Effects of dietary polyphenols on metabolic syndrome features in humans: a systematic review. Obes Rev. 2016;17(7):573––86.
22. Williamson G. The role of polyphenols in modern nutrition. Nutr Bull. 2017;42(3):226–35. https://doi.org/10.1111/nbu.12278.
23. Bleich SN, Cutler D, Murray C, Adams A. Why is the developed world obese? Annu Rev Publ Health. 2008;29(1):273–95.
24. Kolb H, Martin S. Environmental/lifestyle factors in the pathogenesis and prevention of type 2 diabetes. BMC Med. 2017;15(1):131. https://doi.org/10.1186/s12916-017-0901-x.
25. Safer JD, Coleman E, Feldman J, et al. Barriers to healthcare for transgender individuals. Curr Opin Endocrinol Diabetes Obes. 2016;23(2):168–71. https://doi.org/10.1097/MED.0000000000000227.
26. Corella D, Coltell O, Portolés O, et al. A guide to applying the sex-gender perspective to nutritional genomics. Nutrients. 2018;11(1):4. https://doi.org/10.3390/nu11010004.
27. Rochlani Y, Pothineni NV, Kovelamudi S, Mehta JL. Metabolic syndrome: pathophysiology, management, and modulation by natural compounds. Ther Adv Cardiovasc Dis. 2017;11(8):215–25. https://doi.org/10.1177/1753944717711379.
28. McCracken E, Monaghan M. Sreenivasan S. Pathophysiology of the metabolic syndrome. Clin Dermatol. 2018;36(1):14–20. https://doi.org/10.1016/j.clindermatol.2017.09.004. Epub 2017 Sep 8. PMID: 29241747
29. Larsson SC, Wolk A. Meat consumption and risk of colorectal cancer: a meta-analysis of prospective studies. Int J Cancer. 2006;119(11):2657–64. https://doi.org/10.1002/ijc.22170.
30. Aguilar-Salinas CA, Viveros-Ruiz T. Recent advances in managing/understanding the metabolic syndrome. F1000Res. 2019;8:F1000 Faculty Rev-370. https://doi.org/10.12688/f1000research.17122.1.

31. Bower A, Imbard A, Benoist JF, Pichard S, Rigal O, Baud O, Schiff M. Diagnostic contribution of metabolic workup for neonatal inherited metabolic disorders in the absence of expanded newborn screening. Sci Rep. 2019;9(1):14098. https://doi.org/10.1038/s41598-019-50518-0. PMID: 31575911; PMCID: PMC6773867
32. Boyer SW, Barclay LJ, Burrage LC. Inherited metabolic disorders: aspects of chronic nutrition management. Nutr Clin Pract. 2015;30(4):502–10. https://doi.org/10.1177/0884533615586201.
33. Agana M, Frueh J, Kamboj M, Patel DR, Kanungo S. Common metabolic disorder (inborn errors of metabolism) concerns in primary care practice. Ann Transl Med. 2018;6(24):469. https://doi.org/10.21037/atm.2018.12.34.
34. Ravasco P. Nutrition in cancer patients. J Clin Med. 2019;8(8):1211. https://doi.org/10.3390/jcm8081211.
35. Coa KI, Epstein JB, Ettinger D, et al. The impact of cancer treatment on the diets and food preferences of patients receiving outpatient treatment. Nutr Cancer. 2015;67(2):339–53. https://doi.org/10.1080/01635581.2015.990577.
36. Catany Ritter A, Egger AS, Machacek J, Aspalter R. Impact of elimination or reduction of dietary animal proteins on cancer progression and survival: protocol of an online pilot cohort study. JMIR Res Protoc. 2016;5(3):e157. https://doi.org/10.2196/resprot.5804.
37. Jassem J. Tobacco smoking after diagnosis of cancer: clinical aspects. Transl Lung Cancer Res. 2019;8(Suppl 1):S50–8. https://doi.org/10.21037/tlcr.2019.04.01.
38. The European Prospective Investigation into Cancer and Nutrition (EPIC) study [Internet]. Highlights. 2021. Available from: https://epic.iarc.fr/. Cited 15 Jan 2021.
39. Bradbury KE, Appleby PN, Key TJ. Fruit, vegetable, and fiber intake in relation to cancer risk: findings from the European Prospective Investigation into Cancer and Nutrition (EPIC). Am J Clin Nutr. 2014;100(1):394S–8S. https://doi.org/10.3945/ajcn.113.071357.
40. Silva RFM, Pogačnik L. Polyphenols from food and natural products: neuroprotection and safety. Antioxidants (Basel). 2020;9(1):61. https://doi.org/10.3390/antiox9010061.
41. Mei J, Ma X, Xie J. Review on natural preservatives for extending fish shelf life. Foods. 2019;8(10):490. https://doi.org/10.3390/foods8100490.
42. Balasch JC, Tort L. Netting the stress responses in fish. Front Endocrinol (Lausanne). 2019;10:62. https://doi.org/10.3389/fendo.2019.00062.
43. Oniszczuk T, Oniszczuk A, Gondek E, Guz L, Puk K, Kocira A, et al. Active polyphenolic compounds, nutrient contents and antioxidant capacity of extruded fish feed containing purple coneflower (Echinacea purpurea (L.) Moench.). Saudi J Biol Sci. 2019;26(1):24–30. https://doi.org/10.1016/j.sjbs.2016.11.013. Epub 2016 Nov 22. PMID: 30622403; PMCID: PMC6318779
44. Maqsood S, Benjakul S, Shahidi F. Emerging role of phenolic compounds as natural food additives in fish and fish products. Crit Rev Food Sci Nutr. 2013;53(2):162–79. https://doi.org/10.1080/10408398.2010.518775. PMID: 23072531
45. Forman HJ, Ursini F, Maiorino M. An overview of mechanisms of redox signaling. J Mol Cell Cardiol. 2014;73:2–9. https://doi.org/10.1016/j.yjmcc.2014.01.018. Epub 2014 Feb 8. PMID: 24512843; PMCID: PMC4048798
46. Hannukainen JC, Lautamäki R, Mari A, Pärkkä JP, Bucci M, Guzzardi MA, et al. Elevated glucose oxidation, reduced insulin secretion, and a fatty heart may be protective adaptions in ischemic CAD. J Clin Endocrinol Metab. 2016;101(7):2701–10. https://doi.org/10.1210/jc.2015-4091. Epub 2016 Apr 5. PMID: 27045985; PMCID: PMC4929844
47. Wölfle U, Seelinger G, Bauer G, Meinke MC, Lademann J, Schempp CM. Reactive molecule species and antioxidative mechanisms in normal skin and skin aging. Skin Pharmacol Physiol. 2014;27(6):316–32. https://doi.org/10.1159/000360092.
48. Bild W, Ciobica A, Padurariu M, Bild V. The interdependence of the reactive species of oxygen, nitrogen, and carbon. J Physiol Biochem. 2013;69(1):147–54. https://doi.org/10.1007/s13105-012-0162-2. Epub 2012 Mar 29. PMID: 22456998
49. Gaschler MM, Stockwell BR. Lipid peroxidation in cell death. Biochem Biophys Res Commun. 2017;482(3):419–25. https://doi.org/10.1016/j.bbrc.2016.10.086.

50. Li H, Zhou X, Gao P, et al. Inhibition of lipid oxidation in foods and feeds and hydroxyl radical-treated fish erythrocytes: A comparative study of Ginkgo biloba leaves extracts and synthetic antioxidants. Anim Nutr. 2016;2(3):234–41. https://doi.org/10.1016/j.aninu.2016.04.007.
51. Ehsani A, Jasour MS. Improvement of lipid stability of refrigerated rainbow trout (Oncorhynchus mykiss) fillets by pre-storage α-tocopherol acetate dipping treatment. Vet Res Forum. 2012;3(4):269–73.
52. Gamba P, Staurenghi E, Testa G, Giannelli S, Sottero B, Leonarduzzi G. A crosstalk between brain cholesterol oxidation and glucose metabolism in Alzheimer's disease. Front Neurosci. 2019;13:556. https://doi.org/10.3389/fnins.2019.00556.
53. Leri M, Scuto M, Ontario ML, et al. Healthy effects of plant polyphenols: molecular mechanisms. Int J Mol Sci. 2020;21(4):1250. https://doi.org/10.3390/ijms21041250.
54. Brglez Mojzer E, Knez Hrnčič M, Škerget M, Knez Ž, Bren U. Polyphenols: Extraction methods, antioxidative action, bioavailability and anticarcinogenic effects. Molecules. 2016;21(7):901. https://doi.org/10.3390/molecules21070901.
55. Lorenzo JM, Mousavi-Khaneghah A, Gavahian M, Marszałek K, Eş I, Munekata PES, et al. Understanding the potential benefits of thyme and its derived products for food industry and consumer health: from extraction of value-added compounds to the evaluation of bioaccessibility, bioavailability, anti-inflammatory, and antimicrobial activities. Crit Rev Food Sci Nutr. 2019;59(18):2879–95. https://doi.org/10.1080/10408398.2018.1477730.
56. National Cancer Institute [Internet]. What is cancer? Available from: https://www.cancer.gov/about-cancer/understanding/what-is-cancer. Cited 15 Jan 2021.
57. Global Burden of Disease [Internet]. Global burden of disease (GBD). Available from: http://www.healthdata.org/gbd/2019. Cited 15 Jan 2021.
58. Cancer – World Health Organization [Internet]. Cancer. Available from: https://www.who.int/news-room/fact-sheets/detail/cancer. Cited 15 Jan 2021.
59. Ferlay J, Soerjomataram I, Dikshit R, Eser S, Mathers C, Rebelo M, Parkin DM, Forman D, Bray F. Cancer incidence and mortality worldwide: sources, methods and major patterns in GLOBOCAN 2012. Int J Cancer. 2015;136(5):E359–86. https://doi.org/10.1002/ijc.29210.
60. Wei Y, Wu B, Jiang W, Yin T, Jia X, Basu S, Yang G, Hu M. Revolving door action of breast cancer resistance protein (BCRP) facilitates or controls the efflux of flavone glucuronides from UGT1A9-overexpressing HeLa cells. Mol Pharm. 2013;10(5):1736–50.
61. Afshari K, Haddadi NS, Haj-Mirzaian A, Farzaei MH, Rohani MM, Akramian F, et al. Natural flavonoids for the prevention of colon cancer: a comprehensive review of preclinical and clinical studies. J Cell Physiol. 2019;234:21519–46. https://doi.org/10.1002/jcp.28777.
62. Messerschmidt JL, Prendergast GC, Messerschmidt GL. How cancers escape immune destruction and mechanisms of action for the new significantly active immune therapies: helping nonimmunologists decipher recent advances. Oncologist. 2016;21(2):233–43. https://doi.org/10.1634/theoncologist.2015-0282.
63. Gonzalez H, Hagerling C, Werb Z. Roles of the immune system in cancer: from tumor initiation to metastatic progression. Genes Dev. 2018;32(19–20):1267–84. https://doi.org/10.1101/gad.314617.118.
64. Soldati L, Di Renzo L, Jirillo E, Ascierto PA, Marincola FM, De Lorenzo A. The influence of diet on anti-cancer immune responsiveness. J Transl Med. 2018;16(1):75. https://doi.org/10.1186/s12967-018-1448-0.
65. Malech HL, Deleo FR, Quinn MT. The role of neutrophils in the immune system: an overview. Methods Mol Biol. 2014;1124:3–10. https://doi.org/10.1007/978-1-62703-845-4_1.
66. Crotty S. A brief history of T cell help to B cells. Nat Rev Immunol. 2015;15(3):185–9. https://doi.org/10.1038/nri3803.
67. Petersone L, Edner NM, Ovcinnikovs V, et al. T cell/B cell collaboration and autoimmunity: an intimate relationship. Front Immunol. 2018;9:1941. https://doi.org/10.3389/fimmu.2018.01941.
68. Yahfoufi N, Alsadi N, Jambi M, Matar C. The immunomodulatory and anti-inflammatory role of polyphenols. Nutrients. 2018;10(11):1618. https://doi.org/10.3390/nu10111618.

69. Niedzwiecki A, Roomi MW, Kalinovsky T, Rath M. Anticancer efficacy of polyphenols and their combinations. Nutrients. 2016;8(9):552. https://doi.org/10.3390/nu8090552.
70. Sak K. Cytotoxicity of dietary flavonoids on different human cancer types. Pharmacogn Rev. 2014;8(16):122–46. https://doi.org/10.4103/0973-7847.134247.
71. Zhou Y, Zheng J, Li Y, et al. Natural polyphenols for prevention and treatment of cancer. Nutrients. 2016;8(8):515. https://doi.org/10.3390/nu8080515.
72. Keating E, Martel F. Antimetabolic effects of polyphenols in breast cancer cells: focus on glucose uptake and metabolism. Front Nutr. 2018;5:25. https://doi.org/10.3389/fnut.2018.00025.
73. Avtanski D, Poretsky L. Phyto-polyphenols as potential inhibitors of breast cancer metastasis. Mol Med. 2018;24:29. https://doi.org/10.1186/s10020-018-0032-7.
74. Losada-Echeberría M, Herranz-López M, Micol V, Barrajón-Catalán E. Polyphenols as promising drugs against main breast cancer signatures. Antioxidants (Basel). 2017;6(4):88. https://doi.org/10.3390/antiox6040088.
75. Costea T, Nagy P, Ganea C, Szöllősi J, Mocanu MM. Molecular mechanisms and bioavailability of polyphenols in prostate cancer. Int J Mol Sci. 2019;20(5):1062. https://doi.org/10.3390/ijms20051062.
76. Miyata Y, Shida Y, Hakariya T, Sakai H. Anti-cancer effects of green tea polyphenols against prostate cancer. Molecules. 2019;24(1):193. https://doi.org/10.3390/molecules24010193.
77. Godos J, Vitale M, Micek A, Ray S, Martini D, Del Rio D, Riccardi G, Galvano F, Grosso G. Dietary polyphenol intake, blood pressure, and hypertension: a systematic review and meta-analysis of observational studies. Antioxidants. 2019;8:152. https://doi.org/10.3390/antiox8060152.
78. Rienks J, Barbaresko J, Nöthlings U. Association of polyphenol biomarkers with cardiovascular disease and mortality risk: a systematic review and meta-analysis of observational studies. Nutrients. 2017;9:415.
79. Fraga CG, Croft KD, Kennedy DO, Tomás-Barberán FA. The effects of polyphenols and other bioactives on human health. Food Funct. 2019;10:514–28. https://doi.org/10.1039/C8FO01997E.
80. Briguglio G, Costa C, Pollicino M, Giambò F, Catania S, Fenga C. Polyphenols in cancer prevention: new insights (Review). Int J Funct Nutr. 2020;1:9. https://doi.org/10.3892/ijfn.2020.9.

Nanoparticulate Systems for Encapsulation of Polyphenols 10

Nazia Khan, Mohammad Imran Khan, Shams Tabrez,
Mohd Faiyaz Khan, and Mohd Ibrahim Khan

Abstract

Researchers are continuously searching for various sources that could provide new promising molecules for therapeutic purposes. Nature, is one source that abundantly provides a basis for the exploration of these beneficial molecules. A class of compounds that has attracted the attention of biomedical and pharmaceutical scientists are polyphenols. Polyphenols are specifically preferred for their unique medicinal and therapeutic properties. They are generally categorised as secondary metabolites, and are predominantly employed for their antioxidant, anti-inflammatory, anticancer, cardioprotective, and antibacterial properties. Various forms of polyphenolic compounds are present in nature, and based on

N. Khan (✉)
Department of Pharmaceutics, School of Pharmaceutical Education and Research, New Delhi, India

M. I. Khan
Department of Biochemistry, Faculty of Science, King Abdulaziz University, Jeddah, Kingdom of Saudi Arabia
e-mail: mikhan@kau.edu.sa

S. Tabrez
King Fahd Medical Research Center, King Abdulaziz University, Jeddah, Kingdom of Saudi Arabia
e-mail: stabrez@kau.edu.sa

M. F. Khan
Department of Clinical Pharmacy, College of Pharmacy, Prince Sattam Bin Abdulaziz University, Al-Kharj, Kingdom of Saudi Arabia
e-mail: moh.khan@psau.edu.sa

M. I. Khan
Department of Pharmaceutical Sciences, Sam Higginbottom University of Agriculture, Technology & Sciences, Allahabad, India
e-mail: mohd.ibrahim.khan@shiats.edu.in

S. Tabrez, M. Imran Khan (eds.), *Polyphenols-based Nanotherapeutics for Cancer Management*, https://doi.org/10.1007/978-981-16-4935-6_10

chemical structure and origin; they are categorized into different classes and subclasses. Although polyphenols have abundant medicinal properties but their use is greatly limited mainly due to low aqueous solubility and they are prone to environmental degradation, upon exposure to heat, moisture, and atmospheric stress. Polymeric and lipid nanoparticles are increasingly used for the encapsulation of polyphenols as they prove to be an exceptional source for drug delivery, which not only enhances their aqueous solubility and bioavailability but also protects them from various types of environmental degradation. In this chapter, the classification of polyphenols is discussed briefly along with their encapsulation in different nanoparticulate systems.

Keywords

Bioavailability · Nanoparticles · Natural and synthetic polymers · Polyphenols · Solubility

10.1 Introduction

Among the various groups of phytochemicals present in nature, polyphenols are one class that are abundantly present in the plant kingdom with not less than 10,000, unlike compounds. Polyphenols, as secondary metabolites, play various essential roles in plants, such as fortification against ultraviolet radiation, protection from exorbitant growth of reactive oxygen species, prevention from the development of pathogens and stresses due to various environmental factors. Apart from these, involvement in the physiological functions for good growth of the plants, lignification, and pigmentation are a few of the other functions of polyphenols [1]. The biological properties of these compounds primarily include anticancer, antibacterial, antioxidant, anti-inflammatory, and cardioprotective. Polyphenols such as resveratrol, grape seed proanthocyanidins, green tea polyphenols, curcumin, silymarin quercetin, genistein, and luteolin have been found to have potential anticancer properties [2]. However, the probable use of the polyphenolic compounds in humans is particularly restricted by several factors, the most common being its insoluble nature, i.e., insolubility, impermeability, fast release, low bioavailability, and ability to be influenced by various environmental factors (heat, temperature, moisture, etc.).

10.2 Classification of Polyphenols

Classification of polyphenols can be attained specifically based on their varied chemical structures. The extent of oxidation, hydroxylation, glycosylation, and methylation in the chemical compositions of polyphenols are commonly diversified. A simplified form of classification of polyphenols is shown in Fig. 10.1. Flavonoids, phenolic acids, and non-flavonoids are the main classes of polyphenols, while subclasses of non-flavonoids include lignans, tannins, stilbenoids, and

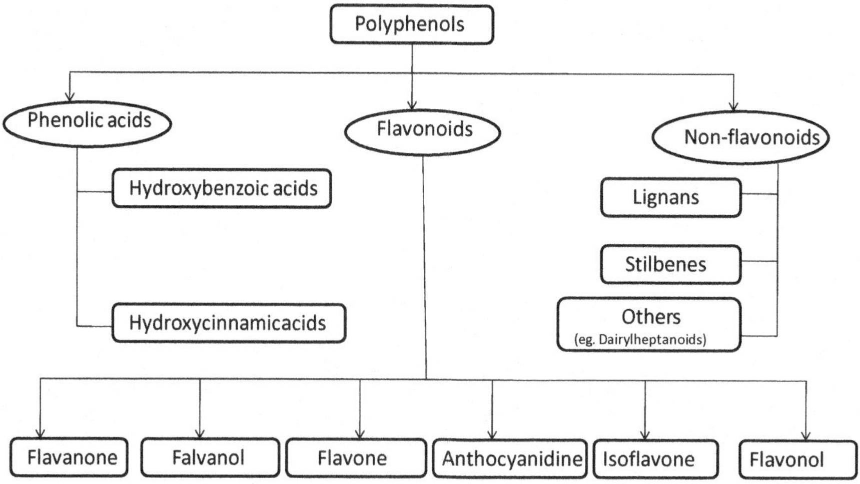

Fig. 10.1 Diagrammatic representation of the classification of polyphenols

diarylheptanoids. Contrary to these, anthraquinones and polyphenolic amides are the other subclasses of non-flavonoids that are less common [3].

Flavonoids are estimated to be two-thirds of all the polyphenolics in our diet. Their chemical structure fundamentally comprises of two aromatic rings bonded with three carbons that are generally present in an oxygenated heterocyclic ring. Depending on the types of variations in the heterocyclic rings, they are further classified into flavonols, flavanones, flavanols, flavones, isoflavonoids, and anthocyanidins. In plant-based food, the two most common phenolics present are flavones and flavonols [4].

Phenolic acids and their hydroxybenzoic acid and hydrocinnamic acid classes comprise one-third of the nutritional polyphenols. In plants, these polyphenols are present in both free and bound forms. Compounds like ellagic acid, protocatechuic acid, *p*- hydroxybenzoic acid, gallic acid, and vanillic acid are the derivatives of hydroxybenzoic acid, whereas *p*-coumaric acid, ferulic acid, caffeic acid, and sinapic acid are the derivatives of hydrocinnamic acid [3, 5, 6].

Characterization of non-flavonoids is as discussed earlier. Tannins, a subclass of non-flavonoids, are considered to be high molecular weight polyphenols. A unique feature of tannins is their ability to form cross-linked bonds within molecules like carbohydrates and proteins, which distinguishes them from other subclasses of non-flavonoid polyphenols [7]. They are composed of both hydrolyzable and non-hydrolyzable or condensed tannins. Hydrolyzable tannins are esters of gallotannins, gallic acids, ellagitannins, and ellagic acid. In contrast, non-hydrolyzable or condensed tannins are also known as proanthocyanidins, are basically formed by the condensation of flavans, and do not possess a sugar moiety [3].

Another subclass of non-flavonoid polyphenols are natural stilbenes, which have 1,2-diphenylethylene nucleus in their chemical skeleton. Not less than 400 natural stilbenes are known. Still, due to less expression of stilbene synthase, a key enzyme engaged in the biosynthesis of stilbene, they are present in a very limited group of heterogeneous plant families. Resveratrol, a stilbene, is a potent anticancer agent and has shown chemopreventive actions [2]. Wang et al. [8] formulated and characterized resveratrol-cyclodextrin complex encapsulated within biodegradable poly lactic glutamic acid (PLGA) nanoparticles. The inhalable nanoparticles were developed for the treatment of non-small cell lung cancer. The formulation was found to possess enhanced cytotoxicity and apoptosis due to increased cellular uptake and was able to retain its antioxidant action.

Lignan is the type of non-flavonoid polyphenols which are obtained from phenylalanine. Some of the common forms of lignans include enterodiol, matairesinol enterolignans, secoisolariciresinol, lariciresinol, and enterolactone [3, 9]. Another class of non-flavonoid polyphenols is diarylheptanoids which, as the name suggests, consists of two aromatic rings (aryl groups) linked with a seven carbon chain. Broadly, they can be categorized into two types, i.e., linear cyclic diarylheptanoids (curcuminoids), for example, curcumin and cyclic diarylheptanoids like myricanone [3].

10.3 Nanoparticulate Systems for Encapsulation and Delivery of Polyphenolic Compounds

Low solubility leads to low bioavailability; therefore, to enhance the bioavailability of the polyphenolic compounds, they are frequently formulated using carrier systems. The different forms of carrier systems provide various advantages to polyphenols, such as prevention from its degradation caused by different environmental factors, increased biocompatibility, and the ability to avert the possible interactions with other bodily components. Among the various forms of carrier systems used in the fabrication and encapsulation of polyphenols, nanoparticulate systems are the most demonstrated ones. They are an excellent source for the development and encapsulation of polyphenolic compounds with improved solubility and bioavailability.

10.3.1 Polymeric Nanoparticles (Nanocapsules and Nanospheres)

Though polyphenols are broadly researched for their numerous medical benefits, their use is often limited due to insolubility, leading to low bioavailability and impermeability, as discussed earlier. Over recent years, polymeric nanoparticles have gained significant interest owing to their small (nano) size and excellent entrapment and encapsulation efficiencies.

Nanocarrier systems or nanomaterials are basically defined as particle sizes having a diameter in the range of 1–1000 nm as a minimum in one dimension [10]. Encapsulation in nanomaterials or nanoencapsulation is chiefly termed as a packaging technology of active pharmaceutical ingredient (API) in solid, liquid, or gaseous form (active or core) encapsulated within a secondary matter (matrix) for the formation of nanocapsules [11]. Other than nanocapsules, nanospheres can also be produced but with a slightly different approach, where the API is uniformly dispersed within the matrix system. The release process of the API from the matrix system generally occurs due to diffusion of the core or by trigger responses like pH, osmotic pressure, enzymatic activity, etc., leading to a controlled and targeted delivery at the required site [3]. Some of the basic advantages of encapsulation of drugs in polymeric nanoparticles are their ability to encapsulate or entrap hydrophilic and lipophilic drugs, ability to release the drug in a sustained or controlled manner upon administration, targeted delivery of drugs, protection of the active moieties against degradation due to several environmental factors, and last but not the least enhancing the bioavailability and the therapeutic index of the active moiety.

A number of natural as well as synthetic polymers are increasingly used for the development of polyphenol loaded nanoparticles, natural polymeric materials like chitosan, collagen, gelatin, albumin, sodium alginate are employed for the development of nanoparticles [12]. Palacio et al. [13] formulated succinyl-chitosan nanoparticles of three polyphenols, viz., propyl gallate, epigallocatechin-3-gallate, and gallic acid; each with different hydroxyl groups and molecular weights, and studied the possible interactions between them. The nanoparticles were developed using the ionic cross-linking technique, and from the results, it was observed that gallic acid showed the highest encapsulation efficiency among the three polyphenolic compounds. Quiroz-Reyes et al. [14] developed and characterized cocoa-derived polyphenolic extract gelatin nanoparticles. The study was performed using cocoa, because it is a major and good source of antioxidants. The aim of the study was to preserve the bioactive compound's antiradical activity. The polyphenolic extract loaded nanoparticles were developed by employing the nanoprecipitation technique, and average size nanoparticles ranging from 120 to 250 nm sizes were achieved.

A number of advantages are presented by the use of these polymers, which are that the properties of these polymers allow them to biodegrade (reabsorbed or eliminated) from the human system once the active constituent(s) are released and absorbed in the biological fluids. They are biocompatible with reduced toxicity and readily adhere to the targeted area, which leads to enhanced penetration and residence time of API. However, some disadvantages linked with the use of natural polymers are that they are sometimes complicated; requiring expensive processes for extraction, complex in nature, and variability can be seen to a great extent when produced from animal sources [15]. Synthetic polymers often used are polylactic acid, polyglycolic acid, PLGA, and polyvinyl alcohol.

Ahmad *et al.* [16] developed PLGA nanoparticles encapsulated with polyphenolic extracts from *Callistemon Citrinus* and berberine for the treatment of three breast cancer cell lines namely MCF-7 (less invasive), MCF 10A (moderately invasive), and MDA-MB 231 (extremely invasive). The polyphenolic loaded nanoparticles were prepared using the nanoprecipitation technique with polyvinyl alcohol as a stabilizer. Polyphenolic extracts of *Callistemon Citrinus* and berberine were encapsulated within nanoparticles individually and in combination, and the results showed that in both cases, a two-fold increase in anticancer activity. Singh *et al.* [17] fabricated catechin loaded polylactic acid-polyethylene glycol nanoparticles for their controlled delivery and studied their stability and antioxidant potential. With the use of the double emulsion solvent evaporation method, the formulation was developed, and 95% encapsulation efficiency of catechin within nanoparticles was observed. The polyethylene glycol coating on the surface of catechin nanoparticles not only protected it from gastrointestinal enzymatic activity but also improved the free radical inhibition potential. With the use of synthetic polymers for the fabrication of nanoparticles, following advantages are provided, a high degree of mechanical and chemical stability, alleviate modifications, lesser protein binding, reduced variation between the batches, which ultimately leads to enhanced reproducibility, good biodegradability, and enhanced biocompatibility. On the other hand, a few disadvantages include their capacity to aggregate toxic monomers, the association of residual material to them, and degradation processes that are toxic in nature [3, 18].

10.3.2 Lipid Nanoparticles

Phenolic compounds other than polymeric nanoparticles are also frequently encapsulated in lipid nanoparticles like solid lipid nanoparticles (SLNs), nanostructured lipid carriers (NLCs), nanoemulsions, liposomes, lipid-polymer hybrid nanoparticles, and ethosomes. In this chapter, we have discussed SLN and NLC in detail.

10.3.2.1 Solid Lipid Nanoparticles (SLNs)

SLNs are generally used for the development of controlled release systems for the compound where the mobility needs to be low and that is possible especially when it is encapsulated in one or more solid state. SLNs are generally the lipid-based carrier systems where the ratio of lipid usually varies between 0.1% (w/w) and 30% w/w and remains in a solid state at the room and body temperatures. The process by which SLNs are prepared basically employs dispersion of the lipid in a suitable aqueous medium and stabilized with the use of an appropriate surfactant (0.5% w/w–5% w/w) which basically performs the function of covering up the solid core of lipidic nanoparticles. Ionic, nonionic, and neutral types of surfactants, i.e., all the three forms can be used in the SLNs development process, and selection should be made depending upon the properties of the API, targeted areas, and their possible interactions with the lipid, API, and other components to be used in the formulation development process. A variety of physiological lipids can be employed in the fabrication of SLNs like sterols, glycerides, partial glycerides, waxes, and fatty acids [19].

A number of techniques are available for the development of SLNs, namely solvent emulsification method, high-pressure homogenization, solvent injection method, micro-emulsion technique, double emulsion method, and ultrasonication method. The probable reasons or, in other words, the advantages for encapsulation of polyphenolic compounds in SLNs are their ability to release the drug in a controlled/ sustained manner, targeting of the drugs, hydrophilic and lipophilic compounds can be incorporated, undergo sterilization processes without affecting their stability, labile compounds are least affected from chemical degradation, biocompatible and biodegradable in nature and scaling-up of the process is possible. Conversely, some disadvantages or rather problems that can be encountered while formulating SLNs are difficulty in drug incorporation in the final product due to high water content, which is typically between 70% and 99.9%, loading of the drug is relatively low due to their crystalline configuration and expulsion of the drug may occur during storage due to changes in the crystallization process [19, 20]. While encapsulating phytophenols, one issue that needs to be sincerely addressed is the molecule's solubility in the lipid matrices. For instance, Quercetin, a plant-based flavonoid, has good solubility when solubilized in oil phases; however, during the formulation process, it exhibited amphiphilic behavior since it distributed itself at the oil/tensioactive interface. Wang *et al.* [21] developed and delivered solid lipid nanoparticles of curcumin for the treatment of non-small cell lung cancer. The formulated SLN-curcumin was delivered in a targeting manner to lung and xenografts. The encapsulation of curcumin in SLN overcame its major drawbacks like low bioavailability, in vivo fast metabolism, and low dispersity. On A459 cells, the SLN-curcumin displayed about five folds enhanced anticancer activity and was found to have inhibition effects on tumors leading to its application medically on a lung cancer cure.

10.3.2.2 Nanostructured Lipid Carriers (NLCs)

NLCs are sometimes referred to second-generation SLN because they somewhat overcome the latter's disadvantages. They can be basically described as lipid nanoparticles that are formed by blending spatially dissimilar lipids collectively. As compared to other lipid nanoparticles, drugs can be firmly immobilized when encapsulated within NLCs and also coalescing of particles can be prevented due to their solid matrix. With SLN, the expulsion of the drug may sometimes occur due to β modification; however, this may not be seen with NLCs, where chances of drug expulsion are very less due to strong immobilization. NLCs are better formulated where organic solvents need not be incorporated during the formulation process [22]. NLCs loaded with polyphenolic active caffeic acid (hydrophilic) were developed by Coc *et al.* [23]. The aim of the authors was to formulate the NLC, which can effectively encapsulate hydrophilic polyphenolic compounds. Different ratios of surfactants and lipids were mixed together, formulated, and studied for the encapsulation of caffeic acid using high-pressure homogenization technique. Physical characteristics of the developed formulation were evaluated, and from the results, it was concluded that caffeic acid can be effectively encapsulated within NLC and can be utilized in different food and cosmetic sectors. Pimentel-Moral *et al.* [24]

developed NLC of polyphenol enriched extracts (quercetin and anthocyanins.) of *Hibiscus sabdariffa* and performed optimization using the multi-response surface methodology. The nanostructured lipid nanoparticles were developed using a pressurized liquid extraction process and were characterized for various physico-chemical parameters.

10.4 Conclusion

Polyphenols are the phytoconstituents, abundantly present in the plant kingdom. Classification of polyphenols is a complex phenomenon and based on their chemical structures, they can be invariably classified. Flavonoids, phenolic acids, and non-flavonoids are the major classes of polyphenols with their respective subclasses. Polyphenols are insoluble in nature with low permeability and bioavailability. To overcome their major drawbacks, they are frequently incorporated in polymeric and lipid nanoparticles. The incorporation of polyphenols in the nanoparticulate system allows them to offer increased solubility, permeability, and bioavailability. Nanoparticles containing polyphenols are relatively less toxic and more easily tolerated in the human system.

References

1. Krstić L, González-García MJ, Diebold Y. Ocular delivery of polyphenols: meeting the unmet needs. Molecules. 2021;26(2):370.
2. Sirerol JA, Rodríguez ML, Mena S, Asensi MA, Estrela JM, Ortega AL. Role of natural stilbenes in the prevention of cancer. Oxid Med Cell Longev. 2016;2016:3128951.
3. Rambaran TF. Nanopolyphenols: a review of their encapsulation and anti-diabetic effects. SN Appl Sci. 2020;2(8):1–26.
4. Puupponen-Pimiä R, Nohynek L, Meier C, Kähkönen M, Heinonen M, Hopia A, Oksman-Caldentey KM. Antimicrobial properties of phenolic compounds from berries. J Appl Microbiol. 2001;90(4):494–507.
5. Zadernowski R, Naczk M, Nesterowicz J. Phenolic acid profiles in some small berries. J Agric Food Chem. 2005;53(6):2118–24.
6. Lee J, Dossett M, Finn CE. Rubus fruit phenolic research: the good, the bad, and the confusing. Food Chem. 2012;130(4):785–96.
7. Fraga-Corral M, García-Oliveira P, Pereira AG, Lourenço-Lopes C, Jimenez-Lopez C, Prieto MA, Simal-Gandara J. Technological application of tannin-based extracts. Molecules. 2020;25 (3):614.
8. Wang X, Parvathaneni V, Shukla SK, Kulkarni NS, Muth A, Kunda NK, Gupta V. Inhalable resveratrol-cyclodextrin complex loaded biodegradable nanoparticles for enhanced efficacy against non-small cell lung cancer. Int J Biol Macromol. 2020;164:638–50.
9. Durazzo A, Lucarini M, Camilli E, Marconi S, Gabrielli P, Lisciani S, Gambelli L, Aguzzi A, Novellino E, Santini A, Turrini A. Dietary lignans: definition, description and research trends in databases development. Molecules. 2018;23(12):3251.
10. Jeevanandam J, Barhoum A, Chan YS, Dufresne A, Danquah MK. Review on nanoparticles and nanostructured materials: history, sources, toxicity and regulations. Beilstein J Nanotechnol. 2018;9(1):1050–74.

11. Augustin MA, Hemar Y. Nano-and micro-structured assemblies for encapsulation of food ingredients. Chem Soc Rev. 2009;38(4):902–12.
12. Khan N, Khanna K, Bhatnagar A, Ahmad FJ, Ali A, Chitosan coated PLGA. nanoparticles amplify the ocular hypotensive effect of forskolin: Statistical design, characterization and in vivo studies. Int J Biol Macromol. 2018;116:648–63.
13. Palacio J, Monsalve Y, Ramírez-Rodríguez F, López B. Study of encapsulation of polyphenols on succinyl-chitosan nanoparticles. J Drug Deliv Sci Technol. 2020;57:101610.
14. Quiroz-Reyes CN, Ronquillo-de Jesús E, Duran-Caballero NE, Aguilar-Méndez MÁ. Development and characterization of gelatin nanoparticles loaded with a cocoa-derived polyphenolic extract. Fruits. 2014;69(6):481–9.
15. Anwunobi AP, Emeje MO. Recent applications of natural polymers in nanodrug delivery. J Nanomed Nanotechnol. 2011;S4(002) https://doi.org/10.4172/2157-7439.S4-002.
16. Ahmed R, Tariq M, Ahmad IS, Fouly H, Hasan A, Kushad M. Poly (lactic-co-glycolic acid) nanoparticles loaded with *Callistemon citrinus* phenolics exhibited anticancer properties against three breast cancer cell lines. J Food Qual. 2019;2019:2638481.
17. Singh NA, Mandal AK, Khan ZA. Fabrication of PLA-PEG nanoparticles as delivery systems for improved stability and controlled release of catechin. J Nanomater. 2017;2017:6907149.
18. Muhamad II, Selvakumaran S, Lazim NA. Designing polymeric nanoparticles for targeted drug delivery system. Nanomedicine. 2014;287:287.
19. Borges A, Freitas VD, Mateus N, Fernandes I, Oliveira J. Solid lipid nanoparticles as carriers of natural phenolic compounds. Antioxidants. 2020;9(10):998.
20. Ghasemiyeh P, Mohammadi-Samani S. Solid lipid nanoparticles and nanostructured lipid carriers as novel drug delivery systems: applications, advantages and disadvantages. Res Pharm Sci. 2018;13(4):288.
21. Wang P, Zhang L, Peng H, Li Y, Xiong J, Xu Z. The formulation and delivery of curcumin with solid lipid nanoparticles for the treatment of on non-small cell lung cancer both in vitro and in vivo. Mater Sci Eng C. 2013;33(8):4802–8.
22. Bhise K, Kashaw SK, Sau S, Iyer AK. Nanostructured lipid carriers employing polyphenols as promising anticancer agents: quality by design (QbD) approach. Int J Pharm. 2017;526 (1–2):506–15.
23. Coc LM, Lacatusu I, Badea N, Barbinta-Patrascu ME, Meghea A. Effective lipid nanocarriers based on linseed oil for delivery of natural polyphenolic active. J Nanomater. 2021;2021:8853941.
24. Pimentel-Moral S, Teixeira MC, Fernandes AR, Borrás-Linares I, Arráez-Román D, Martínez-Férez A, Segura-Carretero A, Souto EB. Polyphenols-enriched Hibiscus sabdariffa extract-loaded nanostructured lipid carriers (NLC): Optimization by multi-response surface methodology. J Drug Deliv Sci Technol. 2019;49:660–7.

Polyphenols-Enhanced Functionality Via Nanotechnology Approaches

11

Mulham Alfatama, Kifayat Ullah Shah, and Asif Nawaz

Abstract

Nanotechnology is an emerging technique, implementing widely in various fields of sciences, including pharmaceutical design, delivery, and targeting of drugs. The small size and flexibility to tune their physicochemical properties render them high biocompatibility and diverse functionality. Polyphenols have been extensively researched and demonstrated essential characteristics such as antimicrobial, antidiabetic, antioxidant, and anticancer activities. However, mere use of these molecules is encountered with several challenges including poor stability, solubility, and bioavailability that limited their applications and usefulness. To circumvent these limitations and to enhance polyphenols' applications as therapeutics, drug delivery system-based nanotechnology is envisaged to pose a promising strategy. The main objective of this chapter is to highlight the recent advancement in polyphenols-based nanotechnology for pharmaceutical applications. The focus will be on the most studied molecules including quercetin, resveratrol, epigallocatechin-3-gallate, and curcumin.

Keywords

Nanotechnology · Polyphenols · Antioxidant · Quercetin · Resveratrol · Gallic acid · Curcumin

M. Alfatama (✉)
Faculty of Pharmacy, Universiti Sultan Zainal Abidin, Besut, Malaysia
e-mail: mulham@unisza.edu.my

K. U. Shah · A. Nawaz
Department of Pharmaceutics, Faculty of Pharmacy, Gomal University, Dera Ismail Khan, Pakistan

S. Tabrez, M. Imran Khan (eds.), *Polyphenols-based Nanotherapeutics for Cancer Management*, https://doi.org/10.1007/978-981-16-4935-6_11

11.1 Introduction

Polyphenols exhibit one of the most widely and extensively distributed groups of natural compounds in the vegetable kingdom. Until the present, more than 8000 diverse polyphenolic compounds have been identified. Phenolic molecules comprise of single or multiple aromatic rings with at least one hydroxyl group and can be classified into phenolic acids, flavonoids, stilbenes, and lignans (Fig. 11.1).

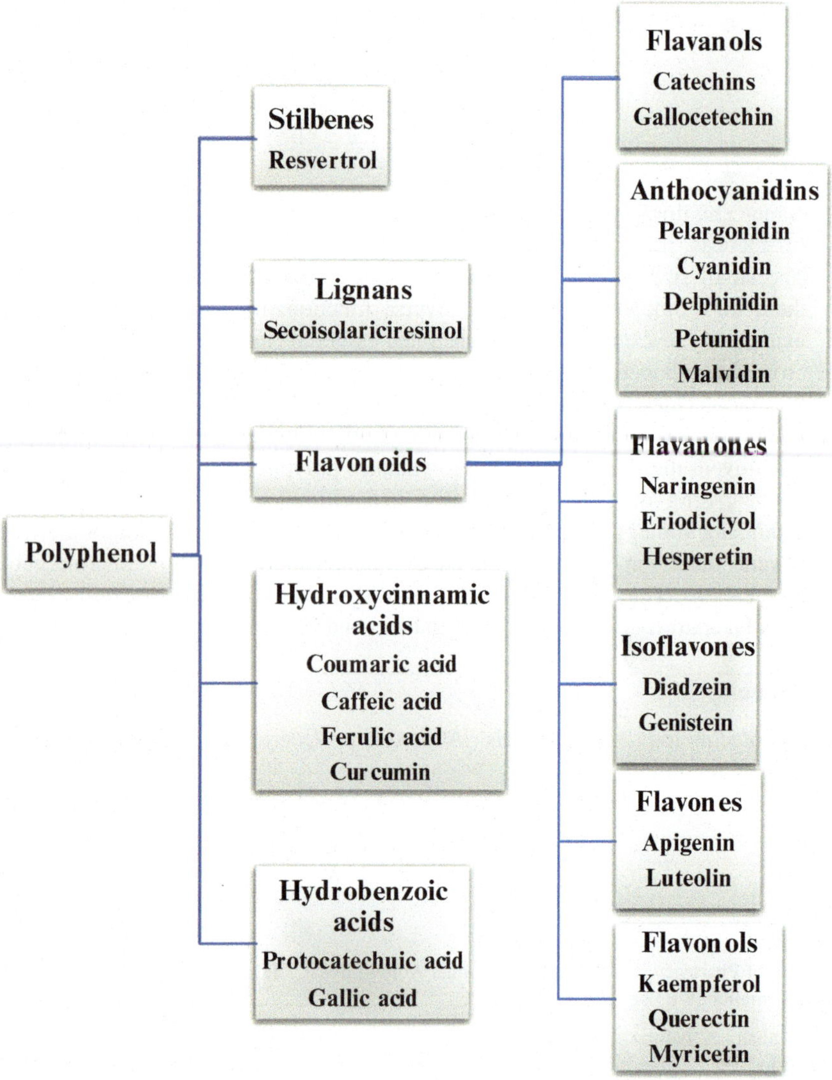

Fig. 11.1 Classifications of polyphenols

Polyphenols refer to a group of secondary metabolites including various subgroups of phenolic compounds with phenolic structural features [1]. These pervading phytochemicals are envisaged to have a fundamental function in the reproduction and growth, appearance, and the plant defense mechanism against parasites, predators, and pathogens [2]. This class of molecules is widely available in vegetables, fruits, olives, cereals, dry legumes, beverages (such as coffee, tea, chocolate wine, and beer), and other natural products. These compounds are demonstrated to improve the health and are estimated to be highly abundant in the diet with the daily average intake of 1 g.

Numerous biological attributes have been reported for polyphenols such as antidiabetic, anti-inflammatory, antioxidant, and antimicrobial effects [3, 4]. Despite the unique advantages of dietary polyphenols that were reported in numerous research studies, certain constraints like stability, bioavailability, and metabolic transformation under physiological conditions limit the application of polyphenols as a therapeutic agent [5]. These variabilities are mediated by various factors that reduce the capability of the compounds to endow their effects in target sites due to their poor bioavailability in humans [6]. While polyphenol's bioavailability is highly impacted by the intrinsic physicochemical characteristics such as solubility, stability at low pH, and size of the molecule, some of the major limitations including intrinsic variation like rate of elimination, gut microbiota, and formulation excipients of polyphenols are of high concern [7, 8]. To circumvent these limitations, particular approaches of prodrug and nanoencapsulation have been attempted. The synthesis of polyphenol nanoparticles (NPs) to promote the bioavailability is an emerging area of research. The small size of NPs allows penetration through cells and tissues to the target site and releasing the payload in a sustained manner. Different types of NPs have been suggested to encapsulate polyphenols such as dendrimers, lipid-based NPs and polymeric nanomaterials. The compositions and preparation techniques of these nanoparticulate enable modification of the physicochemical attributes of polyphenols. The focus of this chapter is therefore to display the recent studies of polyphenol nanosystems with emphasis on their characteristics and advantages.

11.2 Polyphenol-based Nanotechnology

The application of nanotechnology-based systems to encapsulate bioactive natural products like polyphenols offers many advantages in the interaction with the biological environment; protection against degradation; enhancement of absorption, retention time, bioavailability; control delivery of these compounds and improvement of intracellular penetration [9]. Liposomes, micelles, and NPs have been synthesized as nanocarriers for polyphenol delivery, evidencing significant improvement in the rate of dissolution and absorption as well as the bioavailability. Moreover, certain nanosystems confer resistance to the undesired liver metabolism, maintaining therapeutic concentrations of polyphenols in the blood circulation for an extended period of time compared to free ones [10]. Therefore, polyphenol NPs are able to overcome the in vivo-associated limitations [11]. However, nanoencapsulation of polyphenols is correlated with some concerns regarding the solubility, varying structures, and high oxidation in basic conditions [12]. Thus, it is essential to consider these impairing alterations of polyphenol compounds while designing the nanosystem. There are numerous materials used in nanoformulations and many methods to synthesis different types of nanocarriers. The following section will serve to explore the most widely used preparation methods of polyphenol NPs.

11.3 Synthesis of Polyphenol Nanoparticles

Various methods are being developed for the synthesis and enhancement of the activity of polyphenol NPs (Fig. 11.2).

11.3.1 Coacervation Technique

Coacervation is one of the simplest techniques for nanocarriers synthesis. Its fundamental principle is by the formation of coacervate phase of polyelectrolyte mixture and deposition of active materials within the newly formed matrix. The number of polymers involved determines the complexity of coacervation process. The nature of biopolymers complex and strength of interactions are influenced by many factors such as concentration, ionic strength, pH, and biopolymers types and ratio. The electrostatic attraction between oppositely charged moieties is the main driving force

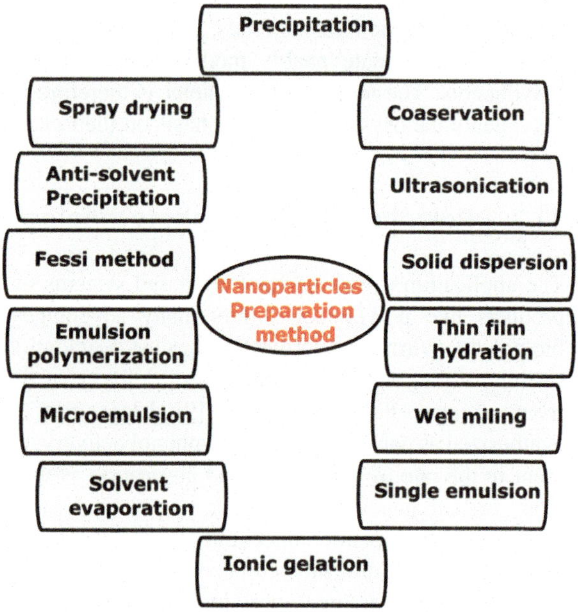

Fig. 11.2 Methods for the synthesis of polyphenol nanoparticles

of coacervation. Moreover, hydrophobic interactions and hydrogen bonding affect complex coacervation inversely. The functional efficiency of the formulated NPs relies on the surface characteristics and chemical nature of the biopolymer shell, where the nanoencapsulation capability is directly proportional to the surface charge [13]. The size range obtained via coacervation method is between 100 to 600 nm, where the technique of drying holds a great role. Chitosan and alginate are examples of oppositely charged polymers commonly used in coacervation, in addition to acacia gum and gelatin [14]. The tendency of chitosan to solubilize in an acid medium is hindered by alginate that is insoluble in low pH. Deladino et al., have employed these polyelectrolytes to successfully encapsulate polyphenolic extract that is composed of flavonoids such as chlorogenic acid, caffeoyl derivatives, quercetin, kaempferol, rutin, and dicaffeoylquinic acid [15].

11.3.2 Nanoprecipitation Method/Solvent Displacement

Solvent displacement includes polymer precipitation from an organic solution and dispersing of a solvent in an aqueous phase with/without the help of stabilizer (Fig. 11.3). Polymers, polyphenol, and/or hydrophilic surface-active agents are dissolved in a semi-polar aqueous miscible solvent such as ethanol or acetone. The solution is then passed into an aqueous solution enclosing surfactant under magnetic stirring. NPs are formed spontaneously as a result of a rapid solvent diffusion. Then, the solvent is evaporated under low pressure from the suspension. The size of the formed particles is strongly influenced by the addition rate of the organic phase into the aqueous medium. It was reported that particle size and encapsulation efficiency could be reduced upon increasing the rate of mixing of the two phases [16]. Moreover, the yield and drug release were demonstrated to be effectively tuned by controlling preparation parameters. In addition, appropriate polymer concentration in the organic phase was essential to enable the production of reduced particle size

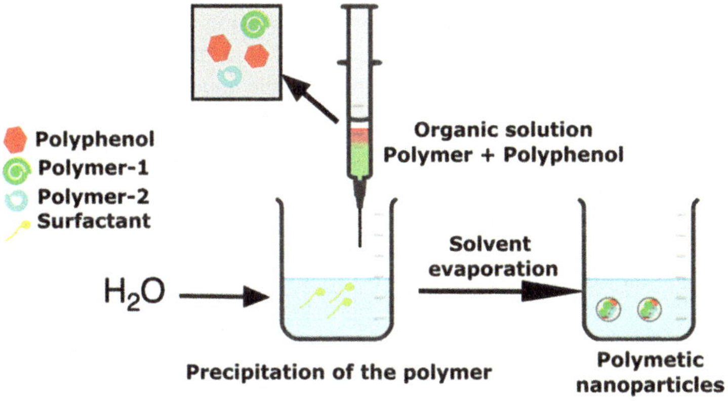

Fig. 11.3 Schematic illustration of the nanoprecipitation method

via restriction of a specific range of polymer to drug ratio [17]. Nanoparticle synthesis via precipitation is well-suited for most of the sparingly soluble compounds.

11.3.3 Solvent Evaporation

Solvent evaporation was the first technique proposed to prepare polymeric NPs from a preformed polymer. This method involves the preparation of an oil-in-water (o/w) emulsion to produce nanospheres [18, 19]. Firstly, the organic phase of polymer dissolved in polar organic solvent is prepared while the active ingredient (polyphenol) is incorporated by dispersion or dissolution. Chloroform and dichloromethane have been widely used in the past, but due to their toxicity, ethyl acetate has been used instead, which exhibits a safer toxicological profile for biomedical applications [20, 21].

An aqueous phase comprises of a surfactant, such as polyvinyl acetate (PVA), which has been commonly prepared. The organic solution is emulsified in the aqueous medium with the presence of surfactant, followed by processing via ultrasonication or high-speed homogenization, leading to dispersion of nanodroplets [22]. A suspension of NPs is formed upon polymer solvent evaporation. The evaporation process takes place under either low pressure or continuous magnetic stirring at room temperature. The solidified NPs after solvent removal can be washed and centrifugally collected, followed by freeze-drying for long-term storage. This method allows the formation of nanospheres [23].

11.3.4 Spray Drying Method

Spray drying method is a well-established technique that is widely utilized in the pharmaceutical industry for converting drug suspension to powder. Pressure nozzle and rotary atomizers mediate the production of fine droplets via vibrating mesh technology. Briefly, polyphenol is suspended in the aqueous polymer solution with the help of an emulsifier (Tween 80) and filtered through 0.45μm syringe filter before spray drying to prevent nozzle blockage. The resultant suspension is then sprayed at a range of outlet temperature ranging between 30 and 80 °C and specific flow rate and pressure. Millions of homogenized droplets are formed as a result of air pressure or vibration of mesh caused by the piezoelectric actuator that is mediated by controllable ultrasonic frequency (i.e., 60 KHz). The droplets are then dried by the hot air and directed to an electrostatic particle collector comprising of cylindrical electrode (anode) and grounded star electrode (cathode) to be collected as a fine powder [13].

11.4 Nanoparticles of Selected Polyphenol Compounds

Polyphenols possess several hydroxyl groups in the aromatic rings and are the basic components of tea leaves including flavanones, flavanols, catechins, glycosides, phenolic acids, and the aglycones from vegetable pigments [24]. These compounds are classified into different categories based on the number of phenolic rings they have and the structural linkage that connect them together [25, 26]. The polyphenol's strong antioxidant property is mediated by free radicals elimination or metals chelation with redox characteristics [27–29]. Nevertheless, the instabilities of polyphenols caused by their poor bioavailability limit the biological activity in vivo [30]. The abundance of hydroxyl groups of benzene rings renders them react readily through autooxidation, epimerization, alkylation, and esterification, resulting in reduced stability of these molecules. Thus, they may display low oral efficiency and poor biological activity. The antioxidant activity of polyphenol is reduced when they are placed in $pH > 7$, similar to the human intestine where the pH is alkaline [31–33]. Hence, nanoencapsulation was proposed as an alternative approach to overcome these limitations and endow protection and stability to polyphenols. Many authors have attempted to formulate nanopolyphenols from nontoxic materials such as Pluronic F127® [34] and biodegradable materials like chitosan [35] and PLGA-PEG [36].

11.5 Quercetin (QT) Nanoparticles

Quercetin is a flavonoid found in various fruits and vegetables like lingonberry, cranberry, and onion bulbs. It presents mostly in the leaves as glycosides or aglycones (3-position or/and 4′-position) where the highest sugar group is glucose, although rhamnose and lactose can be bound also with QT phenolic groups. QT is among dietary flavonoids with huge health applications including anticancer, cardiovascular guarding, antiviral, anti-allergy, anti-ulcer, anti-inflammatory, anti-infective and immunomodulatory attributes [37, 38]. It has also been demonstrated to induce epithelial cells and fibroblasts proliferation as well as angiogenesis [39]. Moreover, QT can be a potential agent for wound healing if the water solubility and skin penetration properties could be overcome [40–42]. QT-loaded NPs have been evidenced to enhance topical delivery in vitro and in vitro, hence, it can be an alternative approach for effective and safer topical delivery [43]. These NPs enable better shelf-life and controlled drug release, a pivotal requirement for the prolonged process of wound healing (Fig. 11.4) [44].

Incorporation of QT into hydrophilic food bases encounters major challenges including poor aqueous solubility, low physicochemical stability, and relatively short shelf-life [45]. On the other hand, the high rates of first pass metabolism of these compounds lead to only 5.3% being unchanged thus the bioavailability and biological activity are significantly reduced. Therefore, various delivery systems are proposed to encapsulate QT to improve the physicochemical stability in food products and bioavailability in the human body [46].

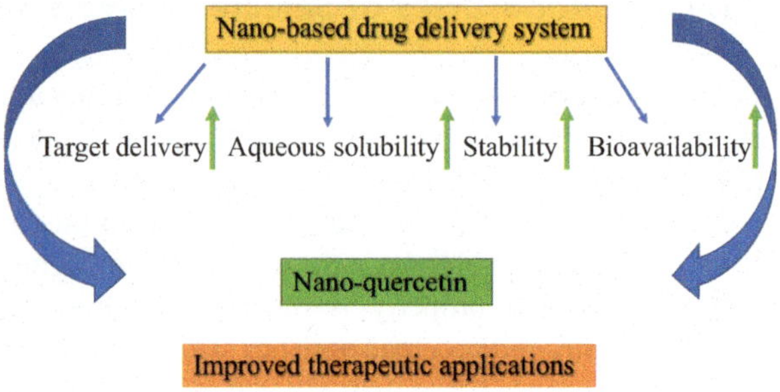

Fig. 11.4 Applications of nanotechnology-based quercetin

Extracts-based plant or their derived substances such as flavonoids were widely known for their anti-inflammatory properties mediated by controlling IL-1β, transcription factors, cytokines, and role in migration of transendothelial [44]. Saha et al., have demonstrated the ability of Dolichos biflorus L. (Fabaceae) seed extract in hindering the CaOx crystal nephrolithiasis in rats [47]. In this setting, QT, a well-recognized flavonoid derived from this seed extract, possesses health beneficial properties such as antibacterial, antioxidant, anticarcinogenic, hepato-protective and anti-inflammatory effects [48]. QT has been evidenced to suppress the synthesis of proinflammatory cytokines and stimulate anti-inflammatory cytokines production [49]. However, the reduced bioavailability and water solubility of crude extract hinder QT to reach pharmacological threshold concentration after oral administration to display local anti-inflammatory activity, hence, limiting the therapeutic effects and clinical applications.

The combined antioxidant and anti-inflammatory properties of QT can reduce cell death and stimulate neurons viability in many neurodegenerative conditions, slowing the disease progression [50]. In Alzheimer's disease, in particularity, QT demonstrated the ability to decrease protein oxidation, neuronal cell death, and lipid peroxidation caused by the disease [51]. Furthermore, QT was manifested to hamper the aggregation of amyloid-beta peptide Aβ, the highly neurotoxic species in amyloid cascade, illustrating its substantial potential as antiaging and neuroprotector agent [51].

Several nanoencapsulation strategies have been introduced with this regard including halloysite nanotubes [52], silica NPs [53], chitin-glucan- aldehyde-QT conjugate [54], albumin nano-assemblies [55], and PLGA NPs [56] (Fig. 11.5). Nanosystems have received much interest for the delivery of drugs, genes, proteins, and nucleic acids. Drug delivery-based nanocarriers enabled commercial and ameliorated therapeutic application of highly bioactive compounds with poor solubility to be transported selectively and release the payload at the site of action. Accordingly, the nanocarrier should protect the encapsulant from being lost, interacting with other molecules in the blood circulation, or premature release at wrong site as well. Therefore, the nanomatrix must also comply with the properties of the payload and the target site. Table 11.1 represents the recent nano-based QT and their characterizations.

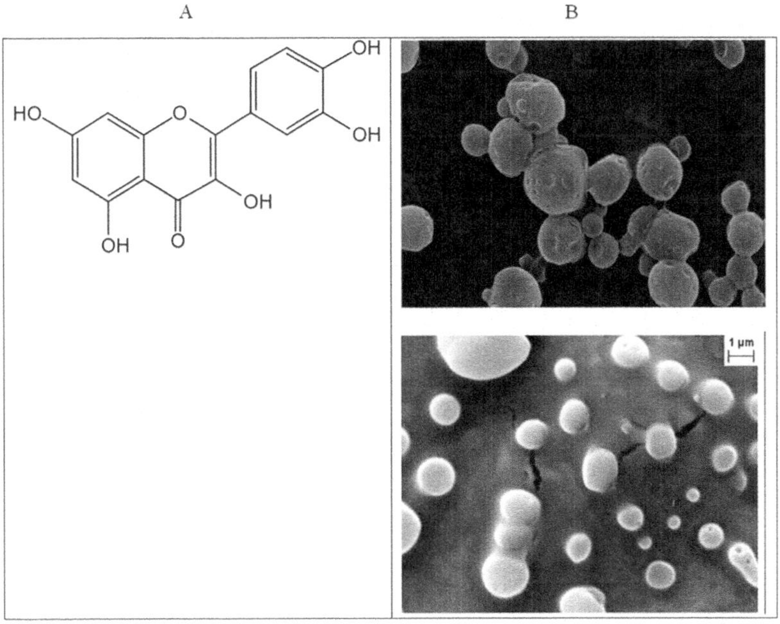

Fig. 11.5 Quercetin chemical structure (**a**) and the images of scanning electron microscope (SEM) of resveratrol PLGA nanoparticles (**b**) [56]

11.6 Epigallocatechin-3-gallate (EGCG) Nanoparticles

Polyphenols are found amply in food plants as naturally occurring compounds. They are emerging high interest to be introduced in pharmaceutical products and functional foods owing to their potential health benefits. EGCG is the most plentiful and biologically active polyphenolic compound found in green tea. The estimated amount of catechins in one brewed cup of green tea is about 200–300 mg or 50–80% of EGCG. It possesses a strong antioxidant property that could be used as health-promoting and therapeutic approach as well as prevention of cancer and other chronic diseases. Moreover, due to its potent anti-inflammatory, ability to reduce cholesterol level and glucose metabolism homeostasis and T-cell immunity, EGCG poses a potential therapeutic candidate for the management of various diseases such as diabetes, cardiovascular diseases, neurodegenerative, arthritis, obesity and autoimmune diseases [67]. Figure 11.6 demonstrates a summary of the properties and limitations of EGCG.

Tea is the most popular and widely consumed around the globe. Lately, polyphenols-based green tea has gained great attention due to its potent health benefits such as anticancer, antidiabetic and anti-inflammatory [68]. The main polyphenolic constituent of green tea is gallic acid ester of EGCG, has been broadly investigated for its biological attributes including anti-HIV, DNA protective effects,

Table 11.1 Quercetin nanoparticles

Nanocarrier composition	Method	PS (nm)	PDI	ZP (mV)	EE (%)	Formulation remarks	Refs.
Chitosan NP	Ionic gelation	361.70 ± 9.72	0.12 ± 0.003	NR	90.00 ± 3.30	QT NPs-enabled significant enhancement of wound healing through regulation of growth factors and cytokines that play an important role in inflammatory and wound healing proliferative phases	[57]
Chitosan-lecithin NP	Electrostatic interactions	240.81 ± 10.82	>0.24	+38.90 ± 1.60	98.31 ± 0.01%	The NPs have efficiently removed the ABTS and DPPH radicals via similar mechanism to free QT. Also, they displayed antimicrobial property and absence of any cytotoxicity against (L-929 and PBMC) normal cells	[58]
Niosomes of tween 80/span 80, and tween 60/span 60 PEG 400, 1500, and 10,000, propylene glycol (PG), glycerol, and cholesterol	Thin-layer hydration	92.00–415.00	NR	NR	48.30–78.90	The nanosystem was stable in terms of PS and EE for 30 days in a cold environment	[59]

Lipid NPs functionalized with transferrin, cetyl palmitate Tween 80	Hot homogenization technique followed by sonication	200.00	>0.20	−30.00	80.00–90.00	The NPs were nontoxic and safe for central nervous system applications, specifically, for Alzheimer's disease because of their ability to suppress the aggregation of amyloid-beta	[60]
Casein NPs	Coacervation	200.00	>0.26	−15.20	82.90	Oral bioavailability of casein NPs was around 37% which is equivalent to nine-fold more than flavonoid solution consumed orally	[61]
Silica NPs	Acidification and pressurize of rice husk	82.00	NR	NR	45.00	The NPs of QT have significantly decreased the growth rate and colony development of MCF-7 cells and cell vitality via stimulating apoptosis and halting the cell cycle greater than QT solution.	[53]
QT-capped gold NPs (AuNPs)	Reduction of AuCl4 using sodium citrate as the reducing agent.	>100.00	NR	−54.80	79.00	The antioxidant activity of AuNP was significantly improved compared to QT solution. Different concentrations of both NPs and free QT were nontoxic against L929	[62]

(continued)

Table 11.1 (continued)

Nanocarrier composition	Method	PS (nm)	PDI	ZP (mV)	EE (%)	Formulation remarks	Refs.
						fibroblast cells. The NPs demonstrated a great anti-fungal property against A. fumigatus that isolated from aspergillosis' patients	
Almond gum, a novel biological macromolecule, and tween 80 as stabilizers and shellac as core material	Antisolvent precipitation	135.00	0.25	NR	97.70	The encapsulated QT exhibited higher antioxidant attribute and absorption tendency compared to the mere use of QT solution	[63]
Fe3+, QT, and poly (vinyl pyrrolidone) (PVP)	One pot synthesis strategy	23.00	NR	Neutral at pH 5 Negative at pH 7	45.80	The NPs showed efficient antioxidation activity and photothermal property	[64]
Liquid crystalline NPs of monoolein and poloxamer 407	Ultrasonication	210.00–268.70	0.16–0.42	−14.60 to 22.30	97.60–99.40	The NPs of QT could pose a potent candidate to treat asthma by inhibiting the production of the main inflammatory cytokines involved in the development of asthma	[65]
Starch NPs	Nanoprecipitation	91.20–246.50	0.27–0.67	NR	44.00–49.00	The antioxidant property was improved. The release of QT followed Fickian diffusion	[66]

CS Chitosan, *NR* not reported, *PP* polyphenol, *PS* particle size, PDI polydispersity index, *ZP* Zeta potential, *EE* encapsulation efficiency

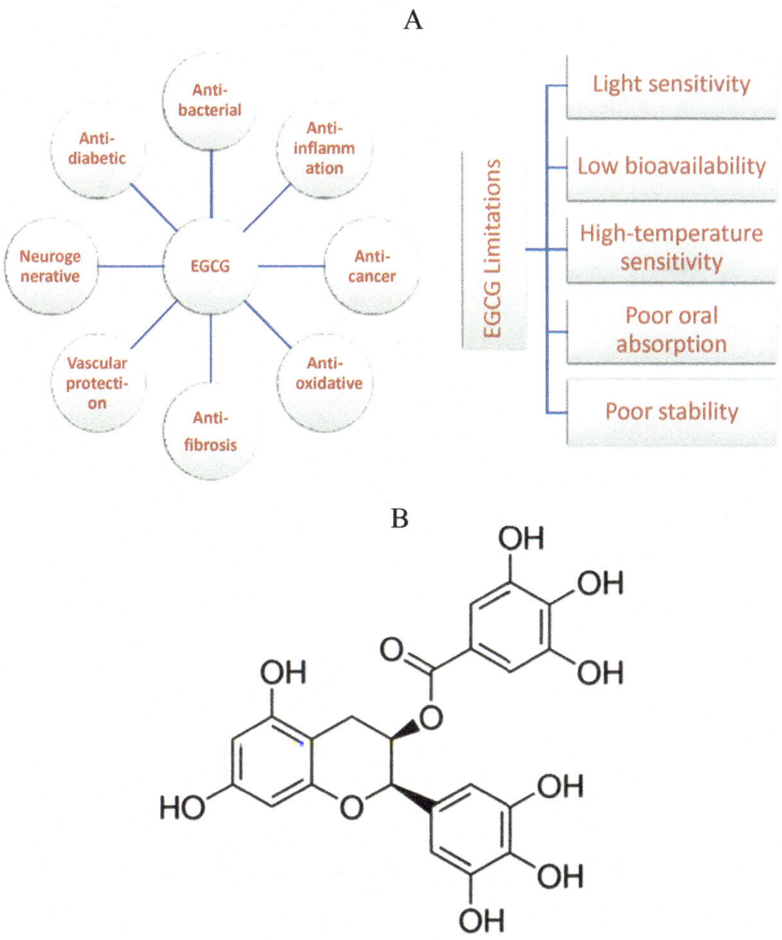

Fig. 11.6 Summary of EGCG properties and limitations (**a**) and its chemical structure (**b**)

neuroprotective and anticancer effect against a vast range of human cancer cell lines [69]. The potent anticancer activity is mediated by inducing apoptosis, regulating several cell signaling proteins linked with tumor proliferation, angiogenesis, and invasion. The bioactive catechin extracted from green tea demonstrated a strong cytotoxic effect on breast cancer cells like MDA-MB-468 and MDA-MB-231 [70]. EGCG has also been found to restrain tumor proliferation via suppressing the release of factor-alpha of tumor necrosis. Therefore, it is envisaged that EGCG could endow cytotoxic effect against pre- and malignant cells while sparing healthy normal tissue. The potential anticancer property of this compound has been examined in vitro utilizing many cancer cell lines originated from breast, liver, colon, cervix and ovary, whereas limited studies have been investigated in living models, owing to its rapid decomposition, short half-life, poor lipo-solubility and bioavailability

[68]. Furthermore, introducing EGCG to neutral or alkaline medium renders it unstable followed by decomposition in the human gastrointestinal tract (GIT). The hydroxyl groups present on the catechin molecule phenol rings are readily deprotonated leading to rapid degradation. This poor stability in addition to the low membrane permeability and intestinal transporter-mediated efflux endow sub-optimal systemic delivery and poor oral bioavailability of EGCG, disregarding its high-water solubility. Attempts have been made to enhance the physiological stability including peracetate methylation protection, sulfate protection of hydroxyl functions and glucuronidation, nevertheless, the in vivo EGCG biological activity was hindered [71]. Table 11.2 represents the recent nano-based EGCG and their characterizations.

11.7 Curcumin Nanoparticles

Curcumin (1,7-bis-(4-hydroxy-3-methoxy-phenyl)-hepta-1, 6-diene-3,5-dione) is a hydrophobic yellow plant-origin alkaloid obtained from the rhizome of *Curcuma longa* and has been applied extensively in traditional medicine and food industry since its discovery. Recent studies have demonstrated that curcumin is not only functional in health reinforcement, anti-inflammation, antiaging and antioxidation [80], it is also well-documented to possess a great anticancer activity against certain types including breast cancer [81], gastric cancer [82] and rectal cancer [83, 84]. Nevertheless, the low oral bioavailability, high hydrophobicity and inherent physicochemical instability have limited the applications of curcumin in food and pharmaceutical industries, where mass production is hindered [85]. Curcumin possesses a heavily double-bonded structure comprised of phenolic hydroxyl and carbonyl groups that are readily reactive leading to destabilization of its structure. Also, the presence of some metal ions can render curcumin structure destabilized. Figure 11.7 demonstrates a summary of the properties and limitations of curcumin.

Lately, the application of natural substances such as curcumin suggested as an effective and alternative strategy for neurological and neurodegenerative diseases. Curcumin has been utilized for numerous nutritional benefits and it is widely used for medicinal and dietary properties in India and China [86]. In addition to the pleiotropic therapeutic effects, curcumin is also able to bypass the blood-brain barrier (BBB), endowing it as a potential therapeutic agent for various nervous system diseases [87]. Moreover, curcumin possesses massive benefits for the management of more diseases such as cystic fibrosis, hyperglycemia, hypertension and malaria [88]. On account of pleiotropic effects of curcumin towards the nervous system, it may exhibit a potential neuroprotective candidate to manage various illnesses. The neuroinflammatory effects of turmeric in illnesses including Alzheimer's disease, multiple sclerosis and Parkinson's disease have been reported in many experimental researches and clinical studies [89].

In spite of the incredible pharmacological attributes of curcumin, poor body fluid stability, high metabolism rate, quick clearance and insufficient absorption in the GIT have hindered its clinical uses. Even though extensive clinical trials of curcumin

Table 11.2 Epigallocatechin-3-gallate nanoparticles

Nanocarrier composition	Method	Size (nm)	PDI	Zeta potential (mV)	EE (%)	Formulation remarks	Refs.
N-succinyl chitosan (CS), TPP NPs	Ionic-crosslinking	244.40–307.00	NR	14.70–18.70	60.80–65.10	The smallest particle size was obtained at 6:1 ratio of CS:TPP with invert relationship to the amount of PP used. ZP was not affected by the PP amount while EE increased proportionally to the PP amount	[72]
Gelatin and CS	Complex coacervation	265.60 ± 2.30	0.25 ± 0.01	26.80 ± 1.80	NR	When drug and NPs were compared to the decorated NPs, the last demonstrated superior anticancer property and apoptotic propensity as a result of improved bioavailability and extended circulation time in the blood	[73]
PEGylated-PLGA NPs	Double emulsion	169.00	<0.10	−23.30 ± 5.30	95.00	The number and intensity of epileptic episodes were reduced significantly after the consumption of the NPs compared to the free drug. This was advocated by the reduction of neuronal death based on	[74]

(continued)

Table 11.2 (continued)

Nanocarrier composition	Method	Size (nm)	PDI	Zeta potential (mV)	EE (%)	Formulation remarks	Refs.
						immunohistochemistry and neurotoxicity tests	
EGCG-loaded solid lipid NPs of cocoa butter	Hot homogenization	108.00–122.00	0.10–0.15	−56.70 to −52.90	68.50	The stability of EGCG-based food grade loaded solid lipid NPs was improved during storage and at neutral pH conditions	[67]
Hordein NPs of barley flour.	Liquid-liquid dispersion	160.00 ± 10.00	0.30 ± 0.02	20.70 ± 0.40	91.20	The pH was the key to determine the stability of EGCG-hordein NPs	[75]
pH-responsive quaternary CS NPs	Electrostatic interaction	191.80–208.50	NR	27.60–29.30	42.40–46.10	The encapsulated EGCG was protected from the decomposition and the NPs facilitated the permeation across epithelia caco-2 cell monolayer. In addition, the antibacterial, antioxidant, and enzyme inhibitory properties were increased	[76]
Modified debranched starch NPs	Etherification reaction	50.00–100.00	NR	−26	84.40	NPs showed controlled release of EGCG into simulated gastric and intestinal fluids	[77]
An EGCG-loaded zein particle-	Solvent evaporation	69.40 ± 2.40	0.14 ± 0.02	−26.50 ± 0.30	52.10	Highly stable properties, less EGCG released and	[78]

stabilized double loaded o/w Pickering emulsion						increased bioaccessibility of prepared emulsion	
Poly(lactic-co-glycolic acid) and Pluronic® F127 based NPs	Emulsion/solvent evaporation	100.00	≤0.10	NR	86.00	EGCS-loaded NPs inhibit the formation of rotenone-induced ROS. Also, the disruption of mitochondrial membrane and fragmentation in the nerve cells was avoided	[36]
CS-PEG-folate-Fe (III) complexes	Coordination complexes from Fe (III) ions and blends of modified CS with polyethylene glycol and folic acid.	200.00	0.20	NR	60.0	The release of EGCG from the NPs followed a controlled manner with no burst release. This pattern followed Korsmeyer-Peppas model, suggesting the presence of interactions between the polymer matrix and EGCG	[79]

TPP Tripolyphosphate, *CS* chitosan, *PP* polyphenol, *PS* particle size, *PDI* polydispersity index, *ZP* Zeta potential, *EE* encapsulation efficiency, *NR* not reported

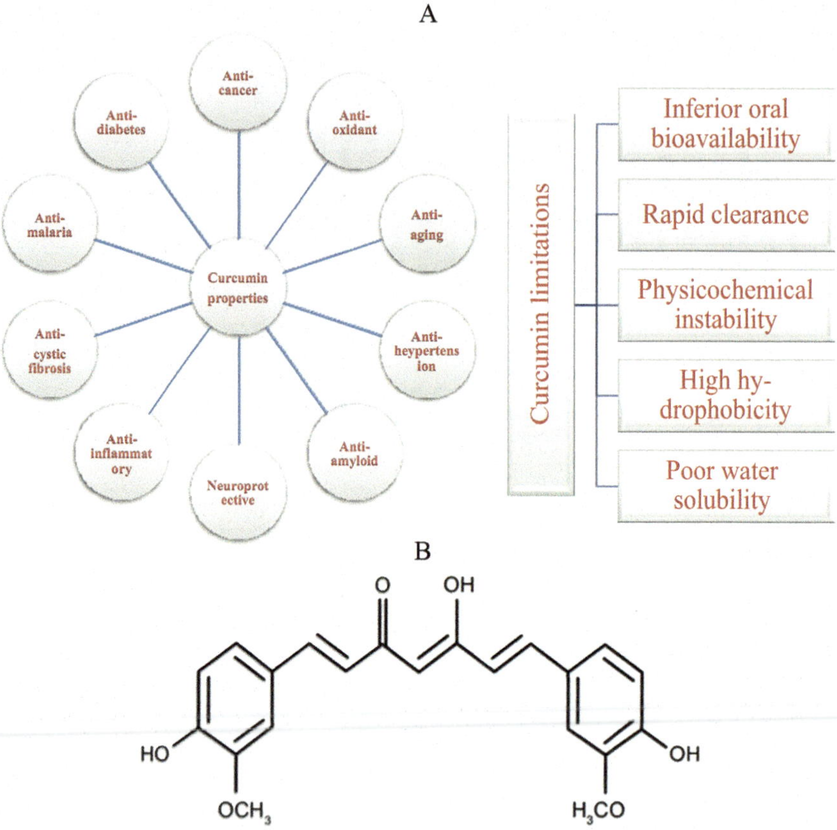

Fig. 11.7 Summary of curcumin properties and limitations (**a**) and its chemical structure (**b**)

has been conducted, curcumin-based drug for clinical application has yet to be approved [90]. Nonetheless, many strategies including application of combination molecules such as quercetin, piperine or silibinin, curcumin analogs, complexation with phospholipids, proteins or polysaccharides and curcumin bio-conjugates with alanine or curcumin oil have been experimented to improve the bioavailability and solubility [91]. Despite the success of the abovementioned approaches to promote stability to some extent, most of the curcumin formulations are unable to provide complete protection and they eventually undergo high metabolism and rapid clearance. Additionally, such tactics do not offer an efficient approach for curcumin targeting specific site of action.

Nanoencapsulation of curcumin has been emerged as an effective approach delivery system to overcome these obstacles. Specifically, protein NPs such as egg white protein [92], kafirin [93], and wheat gliadin [94] have displayed a great potential as carrier delivery owing to their high nutritional value, biocompatibility, inherent biodegradability and nontoxicity. In recent decades, scientists have examined the important properties of many nanoformulations that can be employed in drug delivery and site-targeted possibilities. Impressively, NPs have been emerged as a novel delivery system to confer improved aqueous solubility and enhanced bioavailability of therapeutic compounds like curcumin. It has been evidenced that loading curcumin into NPs substantially prevents enzymatic and pH degradation and improves chemical stability as well as prolongs circulation in the body [95]. Consequently, plentiful nanomaterial formulations have been proposed to improve curcumin characteristics. Nanoformulation strategies may comprise stabilizers, lipid/liposomes, conjugates/polymer conjugates, micelles, NPs and nano/micro/hydrogels [96].

Aforementioned studies highlighted the importance of tumeric nanoformulations in the enhancement of the bioavailability and efficacy in vitro and in vivo. Nevertheless, more research is required to study the efficacy and toxicity of curcumin nanocarriers in a large sample of patients. Moreover, adjuvant therapy with curcumin NPs enables dose reduction of the main drug and hence, reducing the toxicity-associated while maintaining the therapeutic effects. Even though decorated NPs exhibit efficient targeting, the large surface area and reduced size may lead to aggregation of the particles and reduced drug loading [97]. Aggregation pattern and mechanical attributes influence the toxicity of the NPs that related to the method of synthesis and purification. Thus, additional studies are prerequisite to formulate toxic-free tumeric NPs. Toxicity concerns of NPs in drug delivery systems include excitotoxicity, neuroinflammation, allergic responses and DNA damage. Therefore, biodegradability and biocompatibility of nanoformulation should be precisely investigated. Table 11.3 summarizes the recent literature regarding the various applications of curcumin NPs.

11.8 Resveratrol Nanoparticles

Resveratrol is a natural phytoalexin that belongs to polyphenols and made by plants as a protection tool from external harmful entities [107]. This polyphenol has been extracted from 12 families among 31 genus and 72 plant species such as blueberries, grapes, berries, peanuts and chocolate [108]. With regard to the physicochemical properties, the molecular weight of resveratrol is at 228.2 g/mol and melting point in the range of 253 and 255 °C [109]. In addition, its partition coefficient (log $P_{o/w}$) in 1-octanol/water is at 3.1, indicating the hydrophobicity nature and hence solubility in apolar solvents. The resveratrol functional groups, especially the three hydroxyl groups attached to the aromatic rings, render its ability for further modulations, resulting in various derivatives, where pterostilbene is the most well-known. Moreover, resveratrol is confined, since two isomers are available for this compound, namely, trans- (the identified active form of resveratrol) and cis-resveratrol that confer it prone to auto-oxidation and light-prompt isomerization [110]. In addition, resveratrol stability is mainly regarded to the pH value of the solution. Pharmacokinetically, it rapidly metabolizes into sulfate and glucuronide conjugates to end up with a short half-life (8–14 min) in blood circulation.

Table 11.3 Examples of curcumin nanoparticles

Nanocarrier composition	Method	Size (nm)	PDI	Zeta potential (mV)	EE (%)	Formulation remarks	Refs.
Zein/carboxymethyl dextrinNPs	Antisolvent precipitation	212.00	>0.20	−25.00	85.50	The photothermal stability and antioxidant activity of curcumin were significantly enhanced and curcumin release in simulated gastrointestinal fluids was significantly reduced	[98]
Curcumin NPs	Complexation	386.20 ± 7.32	0.16 ± 0.03	30.40 ± 1.11	79.50	The release of curcumin was sustained in simulated gastric medium. The stability of the NPs was enhanced at a pH range of 3–9, salt range of 0–100, and temperature range of 30–60 °C	[99]
Soybean protein isolate and fucoidan NPs	Electrostatic interaction under acidic and neutral conditions	236.60	NR	NR	>95.00	The NPs exhibited improved dispersion stability and salt and heat resistance	[100]
Nanoporous starch aerogels	Hydrogel and alcogel formation	66.00	NR	NR	NR	The NPs enabled significant improvement of curcumin bioaccessibility by 173-fold higher than the free curcumin	[101]
Chitosan, trypolyphosphate, natrium alginate and	Reinforcement ionic gelation	272.90	0.49	12.05	86.08–91.41	Curcumin NPs showed a great stability in simulated	[102]

calcium chloride NPs						gastric and intestinal mediums	
Saponin-coated curcumin NPs	pH-driven method	48.80 ± 0.90–223.50 ± 38.30	0.17 ± 0.03–0.42 ± 0.03	−31.92 ± 0.45 to −17.40 ± 1.34	44.10 ± 7.10–93.20 ± 3.90	The bioavailability was 8.9-fold higher compared to curcumin solution using Sprague Dawley rats	[103]
Caseinate-zein-polysaccharide nanocomplex	Complexation	160.00–210.00	0.27.00	<−30.00	80.00	The NPs showed promising results to be an oral delivery system for lipophilic-based nutrients	[104]
Chitosan-coated solid lipid NPs	High shear homogenization and ultrasonication technique	451.80 ± 19.62	0.44 ± 0.02	−26.33 ± 1.92	100.00	The NPs showed improved oral bioavailability compared to free curcumin	[105]
Pectin-coated sodium caseinate/zein NPs		112.00 ± 5.90–201.50 ± 8.60	0.15 ± 0.01–0.18 ± 0.01	−42.50 ± 1.60 to - 47.1 ± 1.7	61.60 ± 5.60–920.00 ± 5.00	The antioxidant property of curcumin NPs was significantly improved and the release profile was prolonged in simulated gastric and intestinal mediums	[106]

PS Particle size, *PDI* polydispersity index, *ZP* Zeta potential, *EE* encapsulation efficiency, *NR* not reported

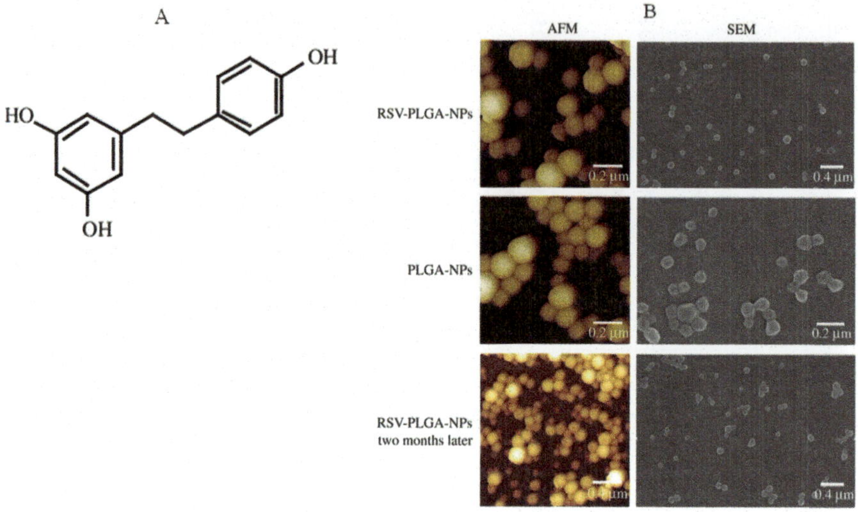

Fig. 11.8 Resveratrol chemical structure (**a**) and the images of AFM and SEM of resveratrol PLGA nanoparticles (**b**) [56]

Resveratrol-based nanotechnology can be formulated from polymers, with biocompatible, biodegradable, and nontoxic attributes. These nanocarriers are categorized with regard to their origin into naturally occurring polymers like polysaccharides (e.g., alginate, chitosan, Arabic gum) and proteins (e.g., albumin, silk, zein, gelatin) and synthetic-based polymers such as poly (lactic acid) (PLA), poly (lactic-co-glycolic acid) (PLGA), poly (acrylic acid)- poly (methacrylic acid), and poly (ε-caprolactone) (PCL). Polymeric nanospheres can be formed when the payload (resveratrol) is solubilized or dispersed in the polymeric matrix, while nanocapsules are produced when the payload is located in an inner core confined by a polymeric matrix [111]. Polymeric NPs can be synthesized by various methods such as electrostatic interaction of polymers, coacervation, ionic gelation solvent evaporation, self-assembly emulsion and desolvation [111, 112]. Polymers are characterized by the ability to deliver the encapsulant to the target site through modifying the nanoparticle compositions to control their behavior in biological mediums in response to different stimuli conditions. Hence, polymeric NPs design is synthesized based on therapeutic application, administration route, and target site. Figure 11.8 represents the chemical structure, AFM and SEM images of resveratrol NPs.

Food grade proteins have been widely used for resveratrol nanoencapsulation to improve the aqueous solubility, chemical stability and bioavailability [113]. Various proteins have been investigated in this regard including bovine serum albumin [113], gelatin [114], zein [115], and gliadin [116]. Zein displays unique properties such as low cost, high abundance and great solubility in concentrated aqueous ethanol solutions. Moreover, it possesses low water solubility which enables a simple synthesis of resveratrol NPs via antisolvent precipitation method with high encapsulation efficiency [117].

11.9 Conclusion

Polyphenols are therapeutic agents with potent characteristics synthesized by plants and some marine organisms, and display elegant combination of biological, chemical, and physiological activities. Nonetheless, their limited solubility, stability and poor bioavailability have to be addressed in order to fully exploit their vast applications in human health. The development of polyphenol nanoparticles displayed an effective means to overcome these limitations and endow stability of the incorporated compounds. Most frequently encapsulated polyphenols are quercetin, epigallocatechin, curcumin and resveratrol. Nanocarriers synthesized from different materials such as alginate, chitosan, gelatin, protein, zein, or cyclodextrins are typically used as nanovehicle. These nanosystems protect polyphenols from environmental stimuli such as thermal and oxidation decomposition, while maintaining the beneficial bioactivity thereby contributing to prolong the shelf-life of bioactive ingredients. Moreover, nanocarriers are also able to modulate the physicochemical characteristics of the original compound, control the release at the target site and elevate the bioavailability of the polyphenolic substances. Further development must be carried out to investigate the pharmacokinetics and pharmacodynamics of phenolic compounds to be translated into clinical settings.

References

1. Rambaran TF. Nanopolyphenols: a review of their encapsulation and anti-diabetic effects. SN Appl Sci. 2020;2(8):1–26.
2. Tsao R. Chemistry and biochemistry of dietary polyphenols. Nutrients. 2010;2(12):1231–46.
3. Campbell TF, McKenzie J, Murray J, Delgoda R, Bowen-Forbes CS. *Rubus rosifolius* varieties as antioxidant and potential chemopreventive agents. J Funct Foods. 2017;37:49–57.
4. Den Hartogh DJ, Tsiani E. Antidiabetic properties of naringenin: a citrus fruit polyphenol. Biomol Ther. 2019;9(3):99.
5. Upputuri RTP, Kulandaivelu K, Mandal AKA. Nanotechnology-based approach for enhanced bioavailability and stability of tea polyphenols—a review. Stud Nat Prod Chem. 2016;50:399–410.
6. Bohn T. Dietary factors affecting polyphenol bioavailability. Nutr Rev. 2014;72(7):429–52.
7. Oracz J, Nebesny E, Zyzelewicz D, Budryn G, Luzak B. Bioavailability and metabolism of selected cocoa bioactive compounds: a comprehensive review. Crit Rev Food Sci Nutr. 2020;60(12):1947–85.
8. Aguirre A, Borneo R. Improving bioavailability of polyphenols using nanodelivery systems based on food polymers. In: Polyphenols in plants. Amsterdam: Elsevier; 2019. p. 59–65.
9. Santos AC, Pereira I, Pereira-Silva M, Ferreira L, Caldas M, Collado-González M, et al. Nanotechnology-based formulations for resveratrol delivery: effects on resveratrol in vivo bioavailability and bioactivity. Colloids Surfaces B Biointerfaces. 2019;180:127–40.
10. Tsai Y-M, Chien C-F, Lin L-C, Tsai T-H. Curcumin and its nano-formulation: the kinetics of tissue distribution and blood–brain barrier penetration. Int J Pharm. 2011;416(1):331–8.

11. Khushnud T, Mousa SA. Potential role of naturally derived polyphenols and their nanotechnology delivery in cancer. Mol Biotechnol. 2013;55(1):78–86.
12. Nair HB, Sung B, Yadav VR, Kannappan R, Chaturvedi MM, Aggarwal BB. Delivery of antiinflammatory nutraceuticals by nanoparticles for the prevention and treatment of cancer. Biochem Pharmacol. 2010;80(12):1833–43.
13. Fang Z, Bhandari B. Encapsulation of polyphenols–a review. Trends Food Sci Technol. 2010;21(10):510–23.
14. Choukaife H, Doolaanea AA, Alfatama M. Alginate nanoformulation: influence of process and selected variables. Pharmaceuticals. 2020;13(11):335.
15. Deladino L, Anbinder PS, Navarro AS, Martino MN. Encapsulation of natural antioxidants extracted from Ilex paraguariensis. Carbohydr Polym. 2008;71(1):126–34.
16. Fessi H, Puisieux F, Devissaguet JP, Ammoury N, Benita S. Nanocapsule formation by interfacial polymer deposition following solvent displacement. Int J Pharm [Internet]. 1989;55(1):R1–4. Available from: http://www.sciencedirect.com/science/article/pii/0378517389902810
17. Pal SL, Jana U, Manna PK, Mohanta GP, Manavalan R. Nanoparticle: an overview of preparation and characterization. J Appl Pharm Sci. 2011;1(6):228–34.
18. Vieira R, Souto SB, Sánchez-López E, López Machado A, Severino P, Jose S, et al. Sugar-lowering drugs for type 2 diabetes mellitus and metabolic syndrome—review of classical and new compounds: part-I. Pharmaceuticals. 2019;12(4):152.
19. Jose S, Sowmya S, Cinu TA, Aleykutty NA, Thomas S, Souto EB. Surface modified PLGA nanoparticles for brain targeting of Bacoside-a. Eur J Pharm Sci. 2014;63:29–35.
20. Bohrey S, Chourasiya V, Pandey A. Polymeric nanoparticles containing diazepam: preparation, optimization, characterization, in-vitro drug release and release kinetic study. Nano Converg. 2016;3(1):1–7.
21. Christine V, Ponchel G. Polymer nanoparticles for nanomedicines. A guide for their design. Anticancer Res. 2017;37:1544.
22. Sharma N, Madan P, Lin S. Effect of process and formulation variables on the preparation of parenteral paclitaxel-loaded biodegradable polymeric nanoparticles: a co-surfactant study. Asian J Pharm Sci. 2016;11(3):404–16.
23. Szczęch M, Szczepanowicz K. Polymeric core-shell nanoparticles prepared by spontaneous emulsification solvent evaporation and functionalized by the layer-by-layer method. Nano. 2020;10(3):496.
24. Manach C, Scalbert A, Morand C, Rémésy C, Jiménez L. Polyphenols: food sources and bioavailability. Am J Clin Nutr. 2004;79(5):727–47.
25. Cutrim CS, Cortez MAS. A review on polyphenols: classification, beneficial effects and their application in dairy products. Int J Dairy Technol. 2018;71(3):564–78.
26. Tsimogiannis D, Oreopoulou V. Classification of phenolic compounds in plants. In: Polyphenols in plants. Amsterdam: Elsevier; 2019. p. 263–84.
27. Grzesik M, Naparło K, Bartosz G, Sadowska-Bartosz I. Antioxidant properties of catechins: comparison with other antioxidants. Food Chem. 2018;241:480–92.
28. Della Pelle F, Scroccarello A, Sergi M, Mascini M, Del Carlo M, Compagnone D. Simple and rapid silver nanoparticles based antioxidant capacity assays: reactivity study for phenolic compounds. Food Chem. 2018;256:342–9.
29. Della Pelle F, Compagnone D. Nanomaterial-based sensing and biosensing of phenolic compounds and related antioxidant capacity in food. Sensors. 2018;18(2):462.
30. Tang D-W, Yu S-H, Ho Y-C, Huang B-Q, Tsai G-J, Hsieh H-Y, et al. Characterization of tea catechins-loaded nanoparticles prepared from chitosan and an edible polypeptide. Food Hydrocoll. 2013;30(1):33–41.
31. Khalifa I, Zhu W, Li K, Li C. Polyphenols of mulberry fruits as multifaceted compounds: compositions, metabolism, health benefits, and stability—a structural review. J Funct Foods. 2018;40:28–43.

32. Xiao J. Stability of dietary polyphenols: It's never too late to mend? Food Chem Toxicol. 2018;119:3–5.
33. Deng J, Yang H, Capanoglu E, Cao H, Xiao J. Technological aspects and stability of polyphenols. In: Polyphenols: properties, recovery, and applications. Amsterdam: Elsevier; 2018. p. 295–323.
34. Sánchez-Giraldo V, Monsalve Y, Palacio J, Mendivil-Perez M, Sierra L, Velez-Pardo C, et al. Role of a novel (−)-epigallocatechin-3-gallate delivery system on the prevention against oxidative stress damage in vitro and in vivo model of Parkinson's disease. J Drug Deliv Sci Technol. 2020;55:101466.
35. Liang J, Yan H, Puligundla P, Gao X, Zhou Y, Wan X. Applications of chitosan nanoparticles to enhance absorption and bioavailability of tea polyphenols: a review. Food Hydrocoll. 2017;69:286–92.
36. Hoyos-Ceballos GP, Sánchez-Giraldo V, Mendivil-Perez M, Jimenez-Del-Rio M, Sierra-Garcia L, Vélez-Pardo C, et al. Design of epigallocatechin gallate loaded PLGA/PF127 nanoparticles and their effect upon an oxidative stress model. J Drug Deliv Sci Technol. 2018;48:152–60.
37. Mehrbod P, Abdalla MA, Fotouhi F, Heidarzadeh M, Aro AO, Eloff JN, et al. Immunomodulatory properties of quercetin-3-O-α-L-rhamnopyranoside from Rapanea melanophloeos against influenza a virus. BMC Complement Altern Med. 2018;18(1):1–10.
38. Prakash O, Singh R, Singh N, Verma N, Mahapatra DK, Kumar S, et al. Exploring the potentials of quercetin and kaempferol combinations along with regular antibiotics for the effective management of methicillin-resistant Staphylococcus aureus (MRSA). RRJ Micro Virol. 2018;8:6–9.
39. Gopalakrishnan A, Ram M, Kumawat S, Tandan SK, Kumar D. Quercetin accelerated cutaneous wound healing in rats by increasing levels of VEGF and TGF-β1. Indian J Exp Biol. 2016;54:187–95.
40. Koohpayma H, Goudarzi I, Salmani ME, Abrari K, Lashkarbolouki T. The effect of quercetin on skin wound healing in dexamethasone-treated rats. J Arak Univ Med Sci. 2015;18(9):66–73.
41. Frenzel M, Steffen-Heins A. Impact of quercetin and fish oil encapsulation on bilayer membrane and oxidation stability of liposomes. Food Chem. 2015;185:48–57.
42. Bose S, Du Y, Takhistov P, Michniak-Kohn B. Formulation optimization and topical delivery of quercetin from solid lipid based nanosystems. Int J Pharm. 2013;441(1–2):56–66.
43. Shegokar R, Müller RH. Nanocrystals: industrially feasible multifunctional formulation technology for poorly soluble actives. Int J Pharm. 2010;399(1–2):129–39.
44. Alexis F, Pridgen E, Molnar LK, Farokhzad OC. Factors affecting the clearance and biodistribution of polymeric nanoparticles. Mol Pharm. 2008;5(4):505–15.
45. Sharma G, Park J, Sharma AR, Jung J-S, Kim H, Chakraborty C, et al. Methoxy poly (ethylene glycol)-poly (lactide) nanoparticles encapsulating quercetin act as an effective anticancer agent by inducing apoptosis in breast cancer. Pharm Res. 2015;32(2):723–35.
46. Souza MP, Vaz AFM, Costa TB, Cerqueira MA, De Castro CMMB, Vicente AA, et al. Construction of a biocompatible and antioxidant multilayer coating by layer-by-layer assembly of κ-carrageenan and quercetin nanoparticles. Food Bioprocess Technol. 2018;11(5):1050–60.
47. Saha S, Verma RJ. Antinephrolithiatic and antioxidative efficacy of Dolichos biflorus seeds in a lithiasic rat model. Pharm Biol. 2015;53(1):16–30.
48. Materska M. Quercetin and its derivatives: chemical structure and bioactivity-a review. Polish J Food Nutr Sci. 2008;58(4):407–13.
49. Carvalho KMMB, Morais TC, de Melo TS, de Castro Brito GA, de Andrade GM, Rao VS, et al. The natural flavonoid quercetin ameliorates cerulein-induced acute pancreatitis in mice. Biol Pharm Bull. 2010;33(9):1534–9.

50. Zhang ZJ, Cheang LCV, Wang MW, Lee SM-Y. Quercetin exerts a neuroprotective effect through inhibition of the iNOS/NO system and pro-inflammation gene expression in PC12 cells and in zebrafish. Int J Mol Med. 2011;27(2):195–203.
51. Andrade S, Ramalho MJ, Loureiro JA, Pereira M d C. Natural compounds for Alzheimer's disease therapy: a systematic review of preclinical and clinical studies. Int J Mol Sci. 2313;20 (9):2019.
52. Yamina AM, Fizir M, Itatahine A, He H, Dramou P. Preparation of multifunctional PEG-graft-halloysite nanotubes for controlled drug release, tumor cell targeting, and bio-imaging. Colloids Surfaces B Biointerfaces. 2018;170:322–9.
53. Aghapour F, Moghadamnia AA, Nicolini A, Kani SNM, Barari L, Morakabati P, et al. Quercetin conjugated with silica nanoparticles inhibits tumor growth in MCF-7 breast cancer cell lines. Biochem Biophys Res Commun. 2018;500(4):860–5.
54. Singh A, Dutta PK, Kumar H, Kureel AK, Rai AK. Synthesis of chitin-glucan-aldehyde-quercetin conjugate and evaluation of anticancer and antioxidant activities. Carbohydr Polym. 2018;193:99–107.
55. Karimi M, Bahrami S, Ravari SB, Zangabad PS, Mirshekari H, Bozorgomid M, et al. Albumin nanostructures as advanced drug delivery systems. Expert Opin Drug Deliv. 2016;13 (11):1609–23.
56. Wan S, Zhang L, Quan Y, Wei K. Resveratrol-loaded PLGA nanoparticles: enhanced stability, solubility and bioactivity of resveratrol for non-alcoholic fatty liver disease therapy. R Soc Open Sci. 2018;5(11):181457.
57. Choudhary A, Kant V, Jangir BL, Joshi VG. Quercetin loaded chitosan tripolyphosphate nanoparticles accelerated cutaneous wound healing in Wistar rats. Eur J Pharmacol. 2020;880:173172.
58. Valencia MS, da Silva Júnior MF, Júnior FHX, de Oliveira VB, de Oliveira Borba EF, da Silva TG, et al. Bioactivity and cytotoxicity of quercetin-loaded, lecithin-chitosan nanoparticles. Biocatal Agric Biotechnol. 2021;31:101879.
59. Javani R, Hashemi FS, Ghanbarzadeh B, Hamishehkar H. Quercetin-loaded niosomal nanoparticles prepared by the thin-layer hydration method: formulation development, colloidal stability, and structural properties. LWT. 2021;141:110865.
60. Pinheiro RGR, Granja A, Loureiro JA, Pereira MC, Pinheiro M, Neves AR, et al. Quercetin lipid nanoparticles functionalized with transferrin for Alzheimer's disease. Eur J Pharm Sci. 2020;148:105314.
61. Peñalva R, Esparza I, Morales-Gracia J, González-Navarro CJ, Larrañeta E, Irache JM. Casein nanoparticles in combination with 2-hydroxypropyl-β-cyclodextrin improves the oral bioavailability of quercetin. Int J Pharm. 2019;570:118652.
62. Milanezi FG, Meireles LM, de Christo Scherer MM, de Oliveira JP, da Silva AR, de Araujo ML, et al. Antioxidant, antimicrobial and cytotoxic activities of gold nanoparticles capped with quercetin. Saudi Pharm J. 2019;27(7):968–74.
63. Doost AS, Kassozi V, Grootaert C, Claeys M, Dewettinck K, Van Camp J, et al. Self-assembly, functionality, and in-vitro properties of quercetin loaded nanoparticles based on shellac-almond gum biological macromolecules. Int J Biol Macromol. 2019;129:1024–33.
64. Tang S-H, Li R, Tan J, Wang Y, Jiang Z-T. One pot synthesis of water-soluble quercetin derived multifunctional nanoparticles with photothermal and antioxidation capabilities. Colloids Surfaces B Biointerfaces. 2019;183:110429.
65. Yong DOC, Saker SR, Wadhwa R, Chellappan DK, Madheswaran T, Panneerselvam J, et al. Preparation, characterization and in-vitro efficacy of quercetin loaded liquid crystalline nanoparticles for the treatment of asthma. J Drug Deliv Sci Technol. 2019;54:101297.
66. Farrag Y, Ide W, Montero B, Rico M, Rodríguez-Llamazares S, Barral L, et al. Preparation of starch nanoparticles loaded with quercetin using nanoprecipitation technique. Int J Biol Macromol. 2018;114:426–33.
67. Shtay R, Keppler JK, Schrader K, Schwarz K. Encapsulation of (—)-epigallocatechin-3-gallate (EGCG) in solid lipid nanoparticles for food applications. J Food Eng. 2019;244:91–100.

68. Rady I, Mohamed H, Rady M, Siddiqui IA, Mukhtar H. Cancer preventive and therapeutic effects of EGCG, the major polyphenol in green tea. Egypt J Basic Appl Sci. 2018;5(1):1–23.
69. Reygaert WC. Green tea catechins: their use in treating and preventing infectious diseases. Biomed Res Int. 2018;2018:9105261.
70. Hong O, Noh E, Jang H, Lee Y, Lee BK, Jung SH, et al. Epigallocatechin gallate inhibits the growth of MDA-MB-231 breast cancer cells via inactivation of the β-catenin signaling pathway. Oncol Lett. 2017;14(1):441–6.
71. Landis-Piwowar KR, Huo C, Chen DI, Milacic V, Shi G, Chan TH, et al. A novel prodrug of the green tea polyphenol (−)-epigallocatechin-3-gallate as a potential anticancer agent. Cancer Res. 2007;67(9):4303–10.
72. Palacio J, Monsalve Y, Ramírez-Rodríguez F, López B. Study of encapsulation of polyphenols on succinyl-chitosan nanoparticles. J Drug Deliv Sci Technol. 2020;57:101610.
73. Wang R, Huang J, Chen J, Yang M, Wang H, Qiao H, et al. Enhanced anti-colon cancer efficacy of 5-fluorouracil by epigallocatechin-3-gallate co-loaded in wheat germ agglutinin-conjugated nanoparticles. Nanomed Nanotechnol Biol Med. 2019;21:102068.
74. Cano A, Ettcheto M, Espina M, Auladell C, Calpena AC, Folch J, et al. Epigallocatechin-3-gallate loaded PEGylated-PLGA nanoparticles: a new anti-seizure strategy for temporal lobe epilepsy. Nanomed Nanotechnol Biol Med. 2018;14(4):1073–85.
75. He A, Guan X, Song H, Li S, Huang K. Encapsulation of (−)-epigallocatechin-gallate (EGCG) in hordein nanoparticles. Food Biosci. 2020;37:100727.
76. Huang T-W, Ho Y-C, Tsai T-N, Tseng C-L, Lin C, Mi F-L. Enhancement of the permeability and activities of epigallocatechin gallate by quaternary ammonium chitosan/fucoidan nanoparticles. Carbohydr Polym. 2020;242:116312.
77. Liu Q, Cai W, Zhen T, Ji N, Dai L, Xiong L, et al. Preparation of debranched starch nanoparticles by ionic gelation for encapsulation of epigallocatechin gallate. Int J Biol Macromol. 2020;161:481–91.
78. Zhang S, Jiang W, Zhang Z, Zhu Y, Wang L, Fu J. A nanoparticle/oil double epigallocatechin gallate-loaded Pickering emulsion: stable and delivery characteristics. LWT. 2020;130:109369.
79. Echeverri-Cuartas CE, Agudelo NA, Gartner C. Chitosan-PEG-folate-Fe (III) complexes as nanocarriers of epigallocatechin–3–gallate. Int J Biol Macromol. 2020;165:2909–19.
80. Li X-M, Wu Z-Z, Zhang B, Pan Y, Meng R, Chen H-Q. Fabrication of chitosan hydrochloride and carboxymethyl starch complex nanogels as potential delivery vehicles for curcumin. Food Chem. 2019;293:197–203.
81. Hu C, Li M, Guo T, Wang S, Huang W, Yang K, et al. Anti-metastasis activity of curcumin against breast cancer via the inhibition of stem cell-like properties and EMT. Phytomedicine. 2019;58:152740.
82. Remedio LN, dos Santos JWS, Maciel VBV, Yoshida CMP, de Carvalho RA. Characterization of active chitosan films as a vehicle of potassium sorbate or nisin antimicrobial agents. Food Hydrocoll. 2019;87:830–8.
83. Kumar D, Raj V, Verma A, Kumar P, Pandey J. Novel binary grafted chitosan nanocarrier for sustained release of curcumin. Int J Biol Macromol. 2019;131:184–91.
84. Pan Y, Wu Z, Zhang B, Li X-M, Meng R, Chen H-Q, et al. Preparation and characterization of emulsion stabilized by octenyl succinic anhydride-modified dextrin for improving storage stability and curcumin encapsulation. Food Chem. 2019;294:326–32.
85. Pan Y, Li X-M, Meng R, Zhang B. Exploration of the stabilization mechanism and curcumin bioaccessibility of emulsions stabilized by whey protein hydrolysates after succinylation and glycation in different orders. J Agric Food Chem. 2019;68(2):623–32.
86. Wang X-S, Zhang Z-R, Zhang M-M, Sun M-X, Wang W-W, Xie C-L. Neuroprotective properties of curcumin in toxin-base animal models of Parkinson's disease: a systematic experiment literatures review. BMC Complement Altern Med. 2017;17(1):1–10.
87. Maiti P, Dunbar GL. Use of curcumin, a natural polyphenol for targeting molecular pathways in treating age-related neurodegenerative diseases. Int J Mol Sci. 2018;19(6):1637.

88. Yallapu MM, Jaggi M, Chauhan SC. Curcumin nanomedicine: a road to cancer therapeutics. Curr Pharm Des. 2013;19(11):1994–2010.
89. Yavarpour-Bali H, Ghasemi-Kasman M, Pirzadeh M. Curcumin-loaded nanoparticles: a novel therapeutic strategy in treatment of central nervous system disorders. Int J Nanomedicine. 2019;14:4449.
90. Dende C, Meena J, Nagarajan P, Nagaraj VA, Panda AK, Padmanaban G. Nanocurcumin is superior to native curcumin in preventing degenerative changes in experimental cerebral malaria. Sci Rep. 2017;7(1):1–12.
91. Yallapu MM, Nagesh PKB, Jaggi M, Chauhan SC. Therapeutic applications of curcumin nanoformulations. AAPS J. 2015;17(6):1341–56.
92. Chang C, Meikle TG, Su Y, Wang X, Dekiwadia C, Drummond CJ, et al. Encapsulation in egg white protein nanoparticles protects anti-oxidant activity of curcumin. Food Chem. 2019;280:65–72.
93. Li X, Maldonado L, Malmr M, Rouf TB, Hua Y, Kokini J. Development of hollow kafirin-based nanoparticles fabricated through layer-by-layer assembly as delivery vehicles for curcumin. Food Hydrocoll. 2019;96:93–101.
94. Wu W, Kong X, Zhang C, Hua Y, Chen Y. Improving the stability of wheat gliadin nanoparticles–effect of gum arabic addition. Food Hydrocoll. 2018;80:78–87.
95. Szymusiak M, Hu X, Plata PAL, Ciupinski P, Wang ZJ, Liu Y. Bioavailability of curcumin and curcumin glucuronide in the central nervous system of mice after oral delivery of nano-curcumin. Int J Pharm. 2016;511(1):415–23.
96. Ghalandarlaki N, Alizadeh AM, Ashkani-Esfahani S. Nanotechnology-applied curcumin for different diseases therapy. Biomed Res Int. 2014;2014:394264.
97. Kaur IP, Bhandari R, Bhandari S, Kakkar V. Potential of solid lipid nanoparticles in brain targeting. J Control Release. 2008;127(2):97–109.
98. Meng R, Wu Z, Xie Q-T, Cheng J-S, Zhang B. Preparation and characterization of zein/carboxymethyl dextrin nanoparticles to encapsulate curcumin: physicochemical stability, antioxidant activity and controlled release properties. Food Chem. 2021;340:127893.
99. Su Z, Han C, Liu E, Zhang F, Liu B, Meng X. Formation, characterization and application of arginine-modified chitosan/γ-poly glutamic acid nanoparticles as carrier for curcumin. Int J Biol Macromol. 2021;168:215–22.
100. Fan L, Lu Y, Ouyang X, Ling J. Development and characterization of soybean protein isolate and fucoidan nanoparticles for curcumin encapsulation. Int J Biol Macromol. 2021;169:194–205.
101. Ubeyitogullari A, Ciftci ON. A novel and green nanoparticle formation approach to forming low-crystallinity curcumin nanoparticles to improve curcumin's bioaccessibility. Sci Rep. 2019;9(1):1–11.
102. Suryani, Halid NHA, Akib NI, Rahmanpiu, Mutmainnah N. Preparation of curcumin nano-particle by using reinforcement ionic gelation technique. In: AIP Conference Proceedings. Melville, NY: AIP Publishing LLC; 2017. p. 20013.
103. Peng S, Li Z, Zou L, Liu W, Liu C, McClements DJ. Improving curcumin solubility and bioavailability by encapsulation in saponin-coated curcumin nanoparticles prepared using a simple pH-driven loading method. Food Funct. 2018;9(3):1829–39.
104. Chang C, Wang T, Hu Q, Luo Y. Caseinate-zein-polysaccharide complex nanoparticles as potential oral delivery vehicles for curcumin: effect of polysaccharide type and chemical cross-linking. Food Hydrocoll. 2017;72:254–62.
105. Ramalingam P, Yoo SW, Ko YT. Nanodelivery systems based on mucoadhesive polymer coated solid lipid nanoparticles to improve the oral intake of food curcumin. Food Res Int. 2016;84:113–9.
106. Chang C, Wang T, Hu Q, Zhou M, Xue J, Luo Y. Pectin coating improves physicochemical properties of caseinate/zein nanoparticles as oral delivery vehicles for curcumin. Food Hydrocoll. 2017;70:143–51.

107. Kiselev KV. Perspectives for production and application of resveratrol. Appl Microbiol Biotechnol. 2011;90(2):417–25.
108. Gambini J, Inglés M, Olaso G, Lopez-Grueso R, Bonet-Costa V, Gimeno-Mallench L, et al. Properties of resveratrol: in vitro and in vivo studies about metabolism, bioavailability, and biological effects in animal models and humans. Oxidative Med Cell Longev. 2015;2015:837042.
109. Nawaz W, Zhou Z, Deng S, Ma X, Ma X, Li C, et al. Therapeutic versatility of resveratrol derivatives. Nutrients. 2017;9(11):1188.
110. Chen J, Wei N, Lopez-Garcia M, Ambrose D, Lee J, Annelin C, et al. Development and evaluation of resveratrol, vitamin E, and epigallocatechin gallate loaded lipid nanoparticles for skin care applications. Eur J Pharm Biopharm. 2017;117:286–91.
111. Esfanjani AF, Jafari SM. Biopolymer nano-particles and natural nano-carriers for nano-encapsulation of phenolic compounds. Colloids Surfaces B Biointerfaces. 2016;146:532–43.
112. Wei Y, Yang S, Zhang L, Dai L, Tai K, Liu J, et al. Fabrication, characterization and in vitro digestion of food grade complex nanoparticles for co-delivery of resveratrol and coenzyme Q10. Food Hydrocoll. 2020;105:105791.
113. Davidov-Pardo G, McClements DJ. Resveratrol encapsulation: designing delivery systems to overcome solubility, stability and bioavailability issues. Trends Food Sci Technol. 2014;38 (2):88–103.
114. Karthikeyan S, Hoti SL, Prasad NR. Resveratrol loaded gelatin nanoparticles synergistically inhibits cell cycle progression and constitutive NF-kappaB activation, and induces apoptosis in non-small cell lung cancer cells. Biomed Pharmacother. 2015;70:274–82.
115. Penalva R, Esparza I, Larraneta E, González-Navarro CJ, Gamazo C, Irache JM. Zein-based nanoparticles improve the oral bioavailability of resveratrol and its anti-inflammatory effects in a mouse model of endotoxic shock. J Agric Food Chem. 2015;63(23):5603–11.
116. Joye IJ, Davidov-Pardo G, Ludescher RD, McClements DJ. Fluorescence quenching study of resveratrol binding to zein and gliadin: towards a more rational approach to resveratrol encapsulation using water-insoluble proteins. Food Chem. 2015;185:261–7.
117. Huang X, Dai Y, Cai J, Zhong N, Xiao H, McClements DJ, et al. Resveratrol encapsulation in core-shell biopolymer nanoparticles: impact on antioxidant and anticancer activities. Food Hydrocoll. 2017;64:157–65.

Green Nanoparticles: A Hope for Targeted Delivery of Natural Therapeuticals for the Management of Glioblastoma Multiforme (GBM) 12

Ehraz Mehmood Siddiqui, Andleeb Khan, Sidharth Mehan, and Rakesh Sahu

Abstract

Every year, large populations of primary malignant brain tumors are reported, of which approximately 70% are malignant gliomas. Over half of malignant glioma patients are of glioblastoma multiforme (GBM) linked with high mortality rates. The progression of GBM leads through several complicated pathways, which have also been expressed in the recurring segment. Previous researches have shown that various compounds found in edible plants, known colloquially as phytochemicals, can simultaneously influence multiple genetic pathways and can be used to treat GBM as a potential drug agent. Polysaccharides and flavonoids are among the phytochemicals extensively analyzed for their antioxidant, anti-neoplastic, and anti-inflammatory actions. Likewise, a broad detail of phytochemicals that have significant effects on GBM had been provided. Green nanoparticles have the ability to prevent or reverse carcinogenesis by halting or redirecting the start process or stopping the progression phase. Centered on a deep understanding of the intrinsic properties of GBM, such novel methods of drug delivery have demonstrated promise to overcome certain barriers. The BBB obstructs drug distribution to the brain and inhibits the efficacy of both old and new medications at the specified location. Because current GBM treatments are preventative instead of therapeutic, new delivery mechanisms are critical, and

E. M. Siddiqui
Department of Pharmacology, Buddha Institute of Pharmacy, Gorakhpur, India

A. Khan (✉)
Department of Pharmacology and Toxicology, College of Pharmacy, Jazan University, Jazan, Saudi Arabia

S. Mehan · R. Sahu
Neuropharmacology Division, Department of Pharmacology, ISF College of Pharmacy, Moga, India

S. Tabrez, M. Imran Khan (eds.), *Polyphenols-based Nanotherapeutics for Cancer Management*, https://doi.org/10.1007/978-981-16-4935-6_12

nanoparticles will be at the forefront of future initiatives. This chapter discusses the role of natural phytochemicals in enhancing glioblastoma patient expectancy and life expectancy by increasing treatment potential and reducing significant side effects. Furthermore, many novel GBM treatments will use better delivery systems and abandon the current approach of injecting medications and devices directly into the tumor. Nano-biotechnology, especially nanoparticles, contributes significantly to improving the delivery of drugs into carcinoma cells, and many of these technologies can be used in GBM. Finally, this chapter therefore emphasized the potential of natural products and novel drug delivery systems in GBM treatment by regulating multiple cancer pathways, such as toxicity reduction and side effects.

Keywords

Glioblastoma multiforme · Malignant gliomas · Green nanoparticles · Phytochemicals · Blood-brain barrier

Abbreviations

GBM	Glioblastoma multiforme
WHO	World health organization
PDGF	Platelet-derived growth factor
MDM2	Mouse double minute 2
EGFR	Epidermal growth factor receptor
PTEN	Phosphatase and tensin homolog
Wnt	Wingless-related integration site
PI3K	Phosphatidylinositol 3-kinase
AKT/PKB	Protein kinase B
LRP5	Low-density lipoprotein receptor-related protein 5
MMPs	Matrix metalloproteinases
Fz	Frizzled receptor
P56	Transcription factor
IKK	IκB kinase
Nf-kB	Nuclear factor kappa B
ICAM-1	Intercellular adhesion molecule-1
Bcl-2	B cell lymphoma
INK4	Cyclin-dependent kinase inhibitors
IL-8	Interleukin
VEGF	Vascular endothelial growth factor
MAPK	mitogen-activated protein kinase
RelA	Rel Avian Reticuloendotheliosis Viral Oncogene Homolog A
TGF-α	Transforming growth factor-α
Ser473 and Thr308	serine/threonine kinase sites
mTOR	The mechanistic target of rapamycin

TCS1/2	Tuberous sclerosis complex
PTCH	Transmembrane receptor Patched
GLI1	Glioma-associated oncogene
PTCH1	Protein patched homolog 1
PDGF-R	*Platelet-derived growth factor receptors*
QCT	Quercetin
STAT3	Signal transducer and activator of transcription 3
RVT	Resveratrol
BBB	Blood-brain barrier
ROS	Reactive oxygen species
AMPK	Adenosine monophosphate-activated protein kinase
DMBA	Dimethylbenz(a)anthracene
UPA/UPAR	Urokinase receptor
TNF-α	*Tumor Necrosis Factor Alpha*
CCM	Curcumin
BAD	BCL2 Associated Agonist of Cell Death
COX-2	Cyclooxygenase-2
CRS	Chrysin
PPAR	Peroxisome proliferator-activated receptor
ERK	a type of serine/threonine protein kinase
TBK1	TANK-binding kinase 1
MCF-7	Michigan Cancer Foundation-7
NRF-2	Nuclear factor erythroid 2-related factor 2
NADPH	Nicotinamide adenine dinucleotide phosphate
GST	Genistein
BC-A	Biochanin A
EGG	Epigallocatechin gallate
HeLa	Henrietta Lacks
LNCaP	Lymph Node Carcinoma
PARP	Poly (ADP-ribose) polymerase
CDK	Cyclin-dependent kinase
CD	Cluster of Differentiation
LTN	Lentinan
Dectin-1	C-type lectin domain family 7 member A
CR3	Complement receptors 3
NK	Natural killer cells
TH1/2	T helper
DLD	D.L. Dexter
PD-L1	Programmed cell death ligand
RTN	Retinoids
OPBA	Ophiobolin A
ER stress	Endoplasmic Reticulum Stress
ITC	Isothiocyanates
TMZ	Temozolomide
ECM	Extracellular matrix

SKN	Shikonin
DRB	Doxorubicin
NPs	Nanoparticles
SPA	Super-paramagnetic particle adducts
GW	Gliadel Wafers
FDA	Food and Drug Administration
BM	Biomimetic
CLT	Cyclic decapeptide
mAb	Monoclonal antibody
PEBBLEs	Probes encapsulated by biologically localized embedding

12.1 Introduction

The worst and most havoc form of glioma is Glioblastoma multiforme (GBM), which is reported to have emerged from CNS. Cushing was first known when surgery was being performed on a patient with this type of tumor in 1904 [1, 2]. GBM can also be described as a basic, it is a primary brain neoplasm, having phenotypically and a genetically variant group of tumors [3, 4]. Although it is categorized into four types, the most prominent and worst is GBM. According to WHO, gliomas could be of astrocytomas/oligodendrogliomas of lower grade to the astrocytomas/glioblastoma of high grade (GBM) [5, 6]. Elderly peoples and Europeans have a high tendency to get acquired by GBM. Patients suffering from Li-Fraumeni syndrome, neurofibromatosis, Turcot's syndrome are more susceptible to GBM [7, 8]. Likewise, certain environmental factors are related to the development of these lesions.

The etiopathological factors comprise ionizing radiation, smoking, electromagnetic induction, allergy, and viral infections [9, 10]. Maximum of the GBM emerge from primary glioblastoma through multistep tumorigenesis. In contrast, the remaining ones are the secondary neoplasm, which takes about 3–5 years and tends to develop from low-grade tumors (Fig. 12.1). Over-expression of PDGF and alteration in the p53 gene lead to the astrocytomas of lower grade. With the decline of tumor-suppressor genes on chromosomes 9p, 13q, or 19q, these tumors convert into anaplastic astrocytomas [11].

Furthermore, activation of MDM2 and EGFR genes and suppression of the PTEN gene is directly linked with the progression of GBM. Moreover, several other pathways, such as Wnt, PI3K/AKT beta-catenin degradation pathways, and hedgehog pathways, are also linked with the progression of GBM [12]. Surgical excision of the tumor, accompanied by radiotherapy and chemotherapy, are the new therapeutic approaches in GBM [13, 14]. Current research states that different compounds collectively called phytochemicals can effectively target several genetic pathways and are beneficial in cancer extermination as a single drug source [15]. Their various neuroprotective and biological roles, such as anticancer, antioxidant, and anti-

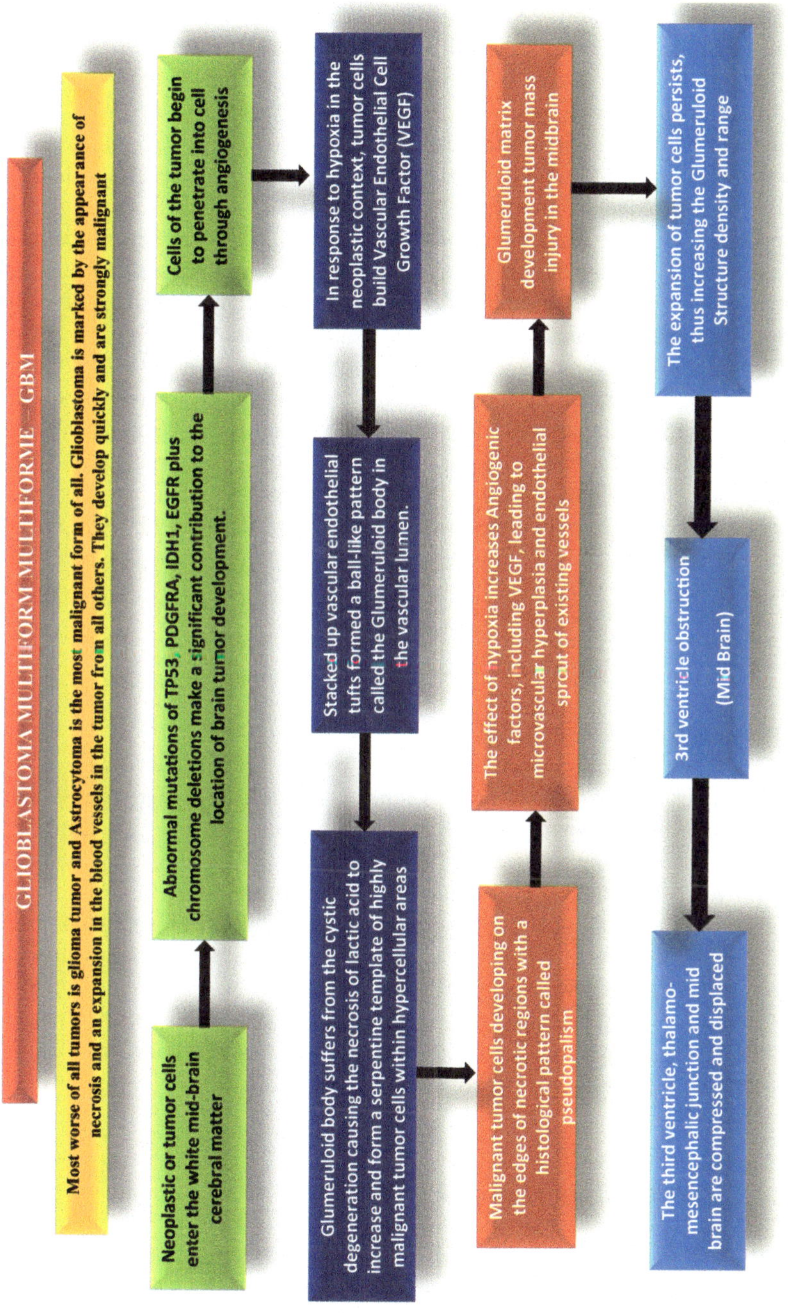

Fig. 12.1 Progression of GBM in human body

inflammatory activities, polysaccharides, and flavonoids, have been widely evaluated for their possible effects [16, 17]. After discovering the antitumor and immunomodulatory and properties, the polysaccharides received a lot of interest in immune pharmacology research [18, 19]. A broad range of bioactive substances has been recognized and listed below for their antioxidant nature and cancer chemopreventive ability.

Our main goal is to explain the importance of certain bioactive substances in improving chemotherapeutic drugs' effectiveness in GBM treatment [20, 21]. Additionally, we also tried to provide the consequences of innovative drug delivery systems for the management of GBM with the molecular mechanism and pathways involved [22, 23]. Nanoparticles are attractive delivery mechanisms for both drug and gene delivery due to their ease of size, shape, and structure adjustment, as well as their loading potential. Increased precision would be possible with these NPs, to improve GBM clinical outcomes. Clinical studies have been conducted or are currently being conducted on various delivery mechanisms, including liposomes, proteins, and gold nanoparticles, demonstrating the promise of such technologies. Nevertheless, the FDA has yet to approve any of the NP formulations for the treatment of GBM. We also tried to emphasize current research progression and provide future perspectives of nano-medicines and nanotechnology by exploring the chemopreventive effects of green nanoparticles in GBM.

12.2 Pathways Involved in GBM

12.2.1 Wnt Nodding in GBM

In embryogenesis, tissue repair, and self-renewal of adult cells, there is an involvement of wingless/Int1 signaling pathways directly or indirectly [24] (Fig. 12.2). They are affected by multiple cancers (breast, colon, glioblastoma, and leukemia) [25]. Wnt ligands (Wnt1, Wnt2, Wnt3a, Wnt5a) are exaggerated in the gliomatic field [26, 27]. The Wnt1 disruption causes the growth of noninvasive glial tumors, while in Wnt3, disruption prevents the formation of tumors in experimental mice [28, 29]. *MMP-2 and GBM invasion were blocked in vitro when Wnt5 was disrupted* [30]. Canonical Wnt/β-catenin-dependent, non-canonical planar cell polarity, and the Wnt/Ca++ route are three Wnt routes that could be described further. We mainly focused on the β-catenin pathway for exploring the GBM [31–33].

12.2.2 β-catenin Degradation in GBM

When Wnt complexes adhere to their receptor on the cell surface (Frizzled receptor), the β-catenin cascade communicates with its protein 5/6 (LRP5/6), which is a co-receptor [34]. Therefore, establishing a matrix that appears to trigger the scaffolding protein in the cytoplasm. On the other hand, the matrix gets to the nucleus,

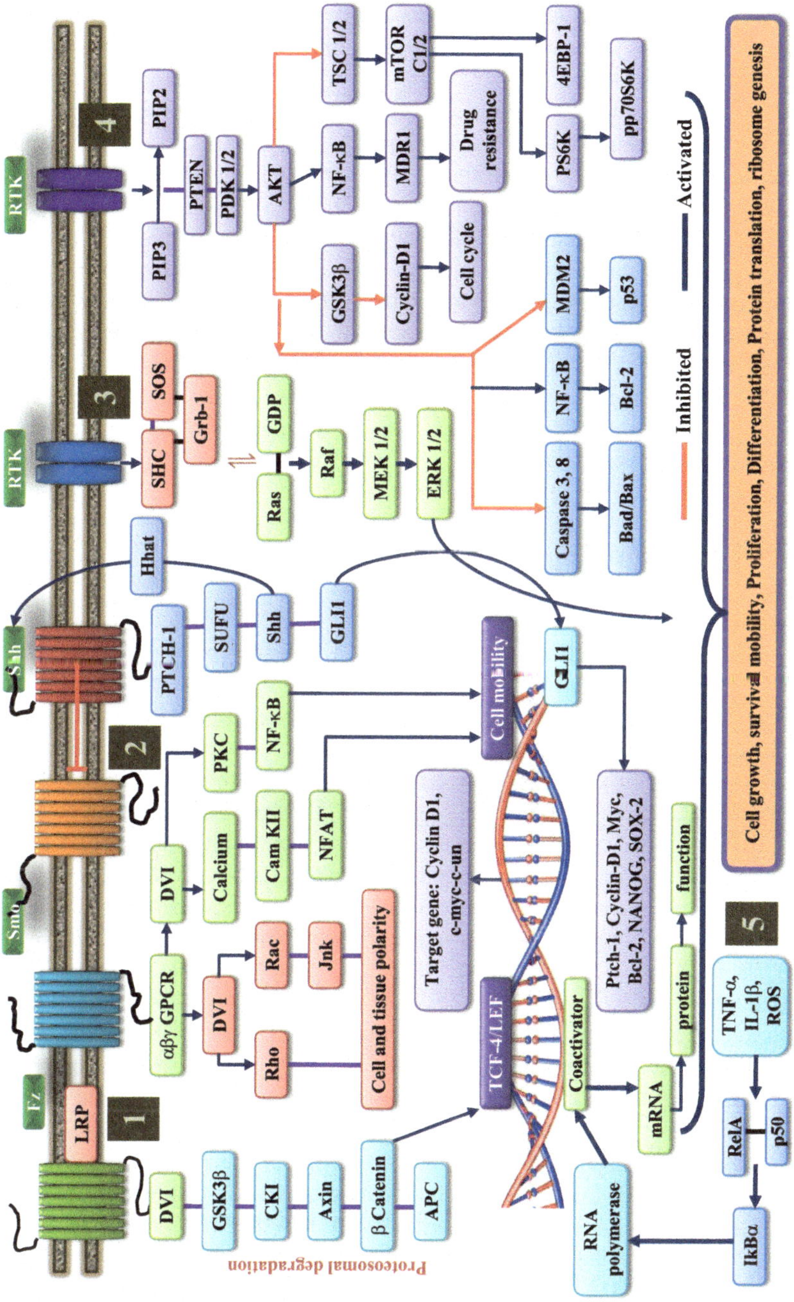

Fig. 12.2 All possible signaling mechanism of GBM

where it interacts with transcription factors, allowing it further to govern the expression of target genes such as MMPs, cyclin, c-Myc [35] (Fig. 12.2).

The C-Myc and cyclin D are liable for cell differentiation, whereas MMPs can enhance glioma cells' ability. The PCP cascade, on either hand, begins through Wnt signaling, which appears to stimulate Fz and triggers mitogen-activated protein kinase. Several Fz and Wnt homologs induce protein kinase-C and calmodulin/calcium-dependent kinase II in the third pathway, the Wnt/Ca++ pathway. The aforementioned signaling systems have been upregulated in GBM, followed by activating a large number of Wnt analogs [36].

Glycogen synthase kinase-3β (GSK-β) attaches to the beta-catenin if Wnt signals are not available. The mechanism persists with the phosphorylation of β-catenin, leading to destruction by the proteasome with diverse factors that affect this pathway [37]. EGFR is triggered by beta-catenin when its interaction with alpha-catenin is interrupted. The blockade of GSK-β blocked the depletion of β-catenin by FRAT-1 thus further promoting the upregulation of GBM invasion and development. From the other side, GBM development is driven by a transcription factor called Lef-11 [38].

12.2.3 NF-κB Signaling in GBM

The primary dimmers found in GBM cells are p65 and P50 (formed from p105) that are directly linked with NF κB [39] (Fig. 12.2). Unless it is being dimerized with a C-terminus transcription factor realm isoform such as p65 or connected with a trans-activating co-regulator, p50 works as an inhibitory protein [40, 41]. Although p65 is often sustained at rest in the cytoplasm, a massive concentration of cytokine and oncogene stimulation arises in cancerous cells, resulting in increased IKK expression and nuclear p65 efflux [42, 43]. As stated, the target of signaling pathways transductions entailed in influencing an enormous span of physiological processes, such as angiogenesis, apoptosis, and cell proliferation, is NF-κB [44, 45].

A study revealed that many gene regulators or modifiers were kindred with cell proliferation and apoptosis, such as intercellular adhesion molecule-1 (ICAM-1), Bcl-xL, Bcl-2, Cyclin D1, and C-Myc [46]. Thus, NF-κB contributes to these genes' expression, causing biological and anti-apoptotic effects [47]. Moreover, NF-κB is progressively manifested in various malignant cancers, such as melanoma, GBM, pancreatic cancer, and prostate cancer [48]. Over the last several years, a lot of research has revealed that modifying associated genetic variables can mediate the creation and propagation of GBM cells via the NF-κB signaling pathway [49]. Neurofibromin-1 and p53 knockdown are two of the most common genetic changes found in GBM, along with amplification of MDM2 and epidermal growth factor receptor, INK4A loss, upregulation of PI3K/Akt, PTEN loss [50]. Several findings have shown that tumorigenic EGFR channels significantly contribute to tumor growth and GBM intrusion, suggesting a crucial role for NF-κB. A receptor-combining protein-1, an ambitious oncogenic activator of NF-κB, tends to amplify MDM2, a particular p53 inhibitor, suggesting a monotonous interaction between p53 and NF-κB [51]. It should be noted that both RIP1 and MDM2 are frequently over-expressed in GBM. EGFR variant has been shown to induce GBM angiogenesis and growth via NF-κB signaling pathway and IL-8, a typical pro-angiogenic gene in contrast. In addition, NF-κB governs the production of VEGF, an essential angiogenesis catalyst [52].

GBM progression and angiogenesis are reliably declined by inhibiting the NF-κB signaling. Several reports have shown that EGFR supports NF-κB via AKT, and this signaling system promotes chemoresistance in GBM cells. In order to enable the transcriptional activation capability of NF-κB, AKT utilizes at least three different mechanisms (IKK α, MAPK, and RelA). This modulation seems to be incorporated into the positive feedback mechanism. Activation of NF-κB further activates Akt as a PI3K negative modulator through downregulation of the PTEN [53, 54]. The protein tyrosine phosphatase (SHP-2) and Gab1 are the key components necessary for the interaction of gene transcription of EGFR with NF-κB through the signaling cascade of PI3K/Akt in GBM cells. The NF-κB/Akt signaling pathway regulates apoptosis, cell proliferation, viability, and malignant (GBM) transformation [55, 56].

Various natural biomolecules and chemical compounds such as sulfasalazine, niclosamide, MG132 (proteasome blocker), BAY117082, and arsenic trioxide have lethal effects on GBM through inhibiting NF-κB [57–59]. These integrated findings reinforce the function of the signaling pathway for NF-κB and provide a reliable explanation for GBM pathogenesis.

12.2.4 PI3/Akt Signaling Pathway

Almost more than 60% of all brain tumors are linked with PI3/Akt signaling pathway. It proceeds with the alteration in some genes that are directly linked with this pathway. These are PIK3CA, EGFR, PIK3R1, and PTEN [60]. PI3/Akt/mTOR pathway is initiated by two of the growth factors like transforming growth factor-α (TGF-α) and epithelial growth factor (EGF) [61]. On cohering with the respective receptors, such as EGFR [62], these get dimerized (hetero/homo), which in turn phosphorylate its intracellular tyrosine kinase domain [63] (Fig. 12.2).

Class I PI3K is the most important pathway for tumorigenesis. It comprises two units, a resistor subunit p85 and a catalytic subunit p110 (α, β, γ). When the process is initiated, tyrosine gets phosphorylated. In turn, EFGR binds to p85. Thus, the p110 subunit gets released [64]. Phosphatidylinositol-3 and 4-bisphosphate (PIP2) gets phosphorylated by the triggered p110 into secondary messenger 5-bisphosphate (PIP3) and phosphatidylinositol-3 and 4 [65]. The PI3K antagonist PTEN reverses the same reaction and vice versa [34]. Consequently, Akt is phosphorylated on its serine/threonine kinase sites (Ser473 and Thr308) with the help of PIP3 that activates the downstream Akt to inner membranes [66]. Many other proteins, such as GSK-3β, are activated by Akt phosphorylation, which further stabilizes β-catenin [67].

PI3/Akt enhances the MMP-2 and MMP-3 activity inside the peripheral cells, encouraging them to infiltrate regular brain tissue [68]. PTEN, on either end, inhibits MMP-2, preventing GBM proliferation [69]. The PI3K/Akt/mTOR signaling pathway has been continuously activated by EGFR and PTEN mutations, contributing to cancer [70].

mTOR is both an actuator and an appellate controller in the PI3/Akt pathway [71]. The rapamycin-sensitive mTOR complex (mTORC1) and the rapamycin-insensitive mTOR complex (mTORC2) both contain mTOR (mTORC2) [72]. mTORC2 participates in cellular metabolism, longevity, replication, and cyto-skeletal rearrangement by phosphorylating Akt at Ser-473. Tuberous sclerosis complex (TCS1/2) is inhibited by stimulated Akt, which stimulates mTORC1, which takes part in ribosomal biogenesis, protein translation, and cell growth [73, 74].

12.2.5 Hedgehog-GLI1 Pathway

Hedgehog pathways have an essential role in both tumor genesis and embryogenesis. Sonic (Shh), Indian (ihh), and Desert hedgehog (Dhh) are three types of ligands that can initiate the hedgehog pathway perfectly [75]. PTCH is a transmembrane receptor with 12 transmembrane domains. When the ligand binds to the receptor, it disables Smoothened (SMO), a 7-transmembrane receptor protein [76]. GLI1, which localizes to the nucleus and modulates multiple genes, including GLI1, PTCH1, cyclin D, Bcl-2, and VEGF, is prevented from being degraded by SMO [77]. Additional routes, such as PI3/Akt and MEK, can also trigger GLI1. Tyrosine kinase receptors such as EGFR and PDGF-R were found to regulate these above pathways [78] (Fig. 12.2).

GLI1, GLI2, and GLI3 transcription factors are members of the GLI family. These substances function as Shh network effectors. GLI1's alternate isoform, tGLI1, has also been linked to breast cancer and GBM [79]. The tGLI mutation has not been found in normal brain cells, although it is found in the majority of GBM instances [80, 81]. The activity of heparanase and VEGF-A is also being found to be upregulated by tGLI [81]. When compared to standard GLI variations, this results in enhanced vascularity in GBM [82]. Countless investigations have backed up these claims, and thus GLI can be an excellent benchmark for restorative medicines due to its lack of expression in cancerous cells [83].

12.3 Natural Products Useful in GBM

12.3.1 Quercetin

A God-gifted flavonoid and a unique plant-based phenolic compound, Quercetin (QCT), are extensively present in different varieties of vegetables and fruits that have many unique properties [84]. These may include antioxidant, anti-inflammatory, antihypertensive, and anticancer properties. Additionally, it promotes cell death and acts as a mighty apoptotic agent in brain, breast, and liver cancer cells [85]. The key cytokine that induces the inflammatory environment of tumor is IL-6 [86]. Its enhanced expression in patients with GBM and is also closely related to their survival. In addition, it has been shown that in several GBM cell lines, there was a constant activation of STAT3 and signal transducer by IL-6. Increased apoptosis and cell proliferation were marked by the suppression of IL-6 [87]. A recent report also quotes that in U87 and T98G cell lines, QCT undoubtedly decreased the STAT3 activation [88].

Additionally, it abolished the heat shock protein 27 thus acting precisely on U87 and U251 cell lines of GBM and promoting drug resistance [89]. In several studies, QCT has been reported to act as a promising agent in promoting apoptosis via mitochondria [90]. Besides these enormous properties, QCT also regulates the phospholipase D and PI3K signaling pathway, followed by activating MMP-2, NF-κB, and Caspase-3 thus promoting cell death in GBM cells through protein kinase A and C signaling pathways [91, 92]. Along with the antitumorigenic potential of QCT, it also provides pro-tumorigenic effects in a rat glioma model [93, 94].

12.3.2 Resveratrol

Resveratrol (RVT) is another promising polyphenolic phytoalexin agent in GBM. Several studies reported its antioxidant, neuroprotective, antitumorigenic, and anti-inflammatory properties in various diseases [95]. It also precisely penetrates the BBB thus acting as a curative agent in several neurodegenerative diseases. In several different forms of cancer, it worked as a chemopreventive and anti-oncogenic agent [96]. In T98G and U251 cell lines, RVT showed its significant action via NF-ΚB-dependent signaling. It also suppressed various anti-apoptotic proteins such as X-linked inhibitors of apoptosis protein and survivin [97].

RVT tends to cause the death of cancerous cells via apoptosis, autophagy, and senescence. Several other studies showed that RVT also enhanced the ROS generation in SHG44 cells of GBM thus accelerating toxicity by activating the AMPK pathway [98]. It is also reported that RVT inhibited the TOR signaling pathway, followed by a decline in the Bcl-2 gene assertion in GBM cells [99]. Moving forward, some researchers also reported that RVT proved to be a potent hindrance in the blooming of skin cancer in animals during several stages of carcinogenesis [100]. Beyond that, RVT also repressed mammary carcinogenesis induced by DMBA in several animal studies [101, 102].

Moving down to human studies, RVT also impeded tumor cells' growth and improved the level of Caspase-3 in cancerous liver cells [103]. A clinical dose of RVT, 5 g/day for 29 days, significantly improved the IGF-1 and IGF-BP-3 levels in healthy candidates thus providing its anti-proliferative effect [104]. With the activation of NF-kB and UPA/UPAR via TNF-α, RVT proved to be a promising molecule in U373MG glioma cells [105]. It also showed chemoprotective and anticarcinogenic properties in different phases of glioma [106, 107]. RVT also showed its cytostatic and cytotoxic properties in glioma cells by altering several phases (M/G2) of the cell cycle, independent of p53 in medulloblastoma cells [108, 109]. Another study showed the effect of RVT on the stem cells of glioma obtained from several patients of GBM. The study concluded that RVT showed its promising effects by acting upon the Wnt signaling pathways [110–114].

12.3.3 Curcumin

Another polyphenolic compound known as Curcumin (CCM) reported promising growth inhibition, blocks angiogenesis, and causes apoptosis in many cancer models [115]. The reduction in NF-kB and AP-1 activity also holds antioxidant and anti-inflammatory properties [116]. CCM has been incorporated in several clinical trials to treat high-risk cancers and GBM cells by inhibiting cell and angiogenesis development [117]. CCM has been reported to prevent intracranial tumor U87 and improve animals' survival rates [118]. A derived product of CCM called Turmeric Force (curcuminoids: 11%, turmerones: 45%, and several other compounds), showed an enhanced cytotoxic effect against the cancerous cells [119].

CCM also retards the activity of human rhabdomyosarcoma and embryonal cells [120]. It is also reported that CCM also alters the AKT signaling thus acting upon the genes of U87 cells and downregulating them precisely [121]. As known before, AKT signaling is linked with angiogenesis, cell proliferation, chemotherapeutic resistance, and apoptosis inhibition [122]. When AKT signaling is activated, it preferably inhibits apoptosis by reducing cytochrome-C liberation from mitochondria [123]. Thus, it abolishes pro-caspase-9 and BAD via phosphorylation [124, 125]. Moving further, the potency of CCM was also evaluated on U87MG, T98G, and T67 in humans and on C6 in rat cell lines [126].

It was noticed that CCM was doing a fabulous job by reducing the cell survival in p53 and caspase in an independent way [127, 128]. CCM also boosts the antitumor activity of nimustine in contrast to GBM by blocking the NF-κB/COX-2, PI3K/Akt signaling [129]. One study also reported that de-methoxycurcumin inhibited the Akt and NF-κB pathway in U87 cell lines and proved its anti-proliferative activity against the GBM cells [130].

12.3.4 Chrysin

Another class of phenolic compound that belongs to certain flavonoid-containing plants such as Passiflora incarnate, Passiflora caerula, and Oroxylum Indicum is Chrysin (CRS) (5,7-dihydroxyflavone) [131]. The pharmacological effect of flavones in CRS is also due to the presence of other flavonoids such as Baicalein and Wogonin [132]. Cellular and molecular pathways such as p38/MAPK/NF-kB, TBK1, Wnt, PPAR/AMPK/ERK/AKT are directly involved in its antitumor activity [133]. Some studies also reported that CRS retards the development of thyroid carcinoma via Notch 1 signaling cascade [134].

CRF was found to be a promising molecule in the depletion of free radicals thus maintaining the level of several oxidative stress parameters [135]. Also, in MCF-7 cancerous cell lines, CRS was noticed to induce apoptosis significantly [136]. With the initiation of MAPK/p38, CRS was retarding the cell cycle of C6 glioma cell lines [137]. Several studies also showed CRS's possible potential in inhibiting the tumor cells through ErK/Nrf2 signaling cascade [138]. It also significantly reduced the assertion of NADPH quinine oxidoreductase-1 and hemeoxygenase-1 [139]. Furthermore, CRS was used in several cell lines such as A172, U87MG, GBM 8901, GL15, and U87 GBM [140–145]. The concluding results showed that CRS had a potential role as an antitumor agent in GBM, followed by deterioration of mitochondria and ER and cell metabolism thus causing mortality in GBM cells [146–148]. CRS was also beneficial in downregulating the assertion of various proteins, such as laminin, MMP9, MMP2, and fibronectin, which were directly involved in eradicating the GBM cells [149–152].

12.3.5 Genistein

Another phyto-estrogenic isoflavone called Genistein (GST), reported to be extracted from Pueraria lobata, Glycine max, and Psoralea corylifolia, possess many miraculous properties (antineoplastic) in the treatment of prostate, breast, non-hormonal, and colonal carcinomas [153, 154]. GST tends to give its apoptotic and neuroprotective effect through the AKT/NF-kB pathways [155]. It also acted perfectly upon A549 cell lines and prostate cancer through MMP-9 and MMP-2 thus reducing cancerous cells' invasion [156, 157]. Further, it showed its effect in prostate cancer through apyrimidinic (AP) endonuclease 1 (APE1) [158]. It also altered the expression of several apoptotic markers such as Bcl-2, Bax, Caspase-3, and Caspase-9 [159]. GST was reported in some studies to give its therapeutic effects in U87 and TP53 GBM cell lines through the mTOR/AKT pathway and block the cell cycle phases, respectively [160].

GST was also reported for its chemoprotective property in A172, ONS76, KNS60, and U251MG GBM cell lines. Correspondingly, the combination of GST with carmustine showed its blocking effects in C6 and U87 GBM cell lines [161, 162]. In combination with other flavones, GST improved the efficacy of the primary molecules [163]. Furthermore, GST also gave its potent action by inducing cytotoxicity in many other neuroblastomas and GBM cell lines by blocking the topoisomerase II and telomerase thus enhancing CDK inhibitors' expression [164]. Further studies also said GST acted well upon tyrosine kinase EGFR and urokinase plasminogen activator by inhibiting cancer cells' growth [165]. In a survey on prostate cancer patients, who were administered GST at its pure, it was noticed that there was no change in any of the micronuclei or having any genotoxic effects [166, 167]. On the other hand, GST is also very safe even if used at its highest dose [168, 169]. However, the findings of several cancer studies on isoflavones are promising and have the potential for more research.

12.3.6 Biochanin A

Another bioactive isoflavone known as Biochanin A (BC-A) isolated from red clover showed its inhibitory action on LNCaP tumors' growth in several animal studies [171, 170]. Besides, it also showed its chemoprotective and anticancer action against GBM cell lines and different cancerous cells (prostate, oral, lungs, and breast) [172, 173]. With BC-A administration, prostate, breast, and colon cancer cells' growth is restricted via tyrosine kinase inhibition [174]. Previous studies reported that by impairing matrix metalloproteases, BC-A prevented the infiltration of glioblastoma cells. It has also been found that BC-A raised rapamycin's effectiveness in impeding the mTOR signaling in GBM cells, and their AKT critique upregulation induced by rapamycin [175].

12.3.7 Epigallocatechin Gallate

Camellia sinensis, a plant that gives very promising chemo sensitizing, antitumor, chemoprotective flavonoid catechin called Epigallocatechin gallate (EGG), which was reported to be very effective in malignant cancers [176]. By inhibiting the IGF-1 domain, which facilitates signaling pathways combined with insulin receptors, EGG governs MCF-7 and HeLa cells' cell transformation and is implicated in breast and lung carcinoma tumorigenesis [177]. Furthermore, in breast cancer cells and LNCaP prostate cancer cells, EGG is implicated in downregulating Wnt signaling and upregulating p53 transcription [178].

In GBM cells, EGG was involved in downregulating NF-kB, IGF-1R, and PDGF signaling pathways via restricting protein telomerase expression. In U87 MG GBM cell lines, EGG significantly reduced the neurosphere's invasion along with the movement of cancerous cells [179]. The downregulation of P-glycoprotein, Bcl-2, AKT phosphorylation, and Bax and PARP enhancement by EGG also showed its potential effect against GBM cells [180]. In T98G, U87MG, 1321N1, and U351 GBM cell lines, EGG provoked apoptosis by acting upon c-Jun N terminal kinase-1, Caspase-3, Caspase-9 via regulating the membrane potential of mitochondria [181]. Important evidence has been presented that EGG improves cancerous cells' sensitivity to chemotherapy drugs such as cisplatin and tamoxifen by blocking telomerase in U87-MG and 1321N1 cells and increasing the activity of GBM U251 and U87 cells to temozolomide cells [182].

In contrast, EGCG prevents glioma cell prevalence by downregulating the function of matrix metalloproteinases (MMP-9 and MMP-2) and retards their development by governing the signaling of MAPK [183]. Besides, EGG prevents the propagation of U87 cell lines and fights back against anti-apoptotic protein's survival effects, which is otherwise immune to ionizing radiation. Also, by improving the proliferation of CDK blockers (p27, p21) and promoting cell death in perivascular nooks of GBM stem cells, EGG enhances the impact of ionizing radiation on human microvascular endothelial cells in the human brain [184]. Even though EGG consistency in liposomes and lipid carriers is relatively higher, nanoparticles could prevent premature degradation of EGCG [185]. Furthermore, EGG-loaded nanoparticles display a pattern of continuous release that decreases the dosage and treatment duration, also the adverse side effects [186].

Furthermore, by integrating specific ligands on EGG nanoparticles' surface, specified delivery of EGG to cancerous cells can be enhanced. In addition, EGG-loaded hyaluronic acid nanoparticles directly target CD44, link to CD44 receptors, seize the G2/M stage of the cell cycle, and accelerate prostate cancer cell apoptosis [187]. In another research, by making micellar nano-complexes, EGG derivatives were used to hold and distribute Herceptin to breast cancer cells. In addition, EGG inhibits glioma cell prevalence by downregulating the production of matrix metalloproteinases (MMP-9 and MMP-2) and prohibits their expansion by implementing the signaling of MAPK [188]. In conjunction, by boosting CDK inhibitors' function (p27, p21) and promoting cell necrosis in perivascular bays consisting of therapy-repellent GBM stem cells. Ionizing radiation has a stronger impact on human microvascular endothelial cells in the brain when EGG is present.

12.3.8 Lentinan

Lentinan (LTN) is an acceptable and therapeutic medicinal polysaccharide harvested from *Lentinus edodes*, reported to have potent antitumor properties [189]. It also modulates the immune system by attaching to Dectin-1 and CR3 receptors on immune cell surfaces. It energizes the transit of cytokines like TNF-alpha, certain interleukins, and interferons, eventually activating differentiation, maturation, and proliferation of immune cells [190]. In addition, LTN has been shown as an additive that improves NK cell's and T cells' behavior and switches the orientation of Th1/2 towards Th1 by enhancing IL-121 generation [191].

In patients with stomach cancer, LTN therapy inhibits prostaglandin synthesis, which stabilizes T lymphocytes' formation and blocks the action of T regulating cells. It also significantly boosts the number of cytotoxic T lymphocytes in the spleen, promotes B-lymphocytes' recruitment, and improves cytotoxicity regulated by antibody-dependent cells [192]. It has been used widely in China as an active ingredient in the treatment of malignant tumors. It is also reported that for the therapeutic assessment of gastric cancer with marginal results, LTN was used as an active ingredient, followed by enhancing chemotherapeutic agents' toxicities. LTN is identified as restricting C-Myc in DLD-1 cancer cells lines to reduce the transcription of hTERT genes, consequently hindering telomerase's function in cancerous cells [193, 194].

Research analyzing the antiangiogenic impact of LTN on tumorigenesis revealed that generation of IFN, which refers to the suppression of tumor vascular growth in LAP0297 lung cancer cells, was mediated by LTN therapy [195]. In addition, LTN inhibited angiogenesis via suppressing various gene expressions [196]. The suppression of programmed cell death ligand (PD-L1) has shown a unique approach of LTN for the betterment of gastrointestinal cancer [197]. This safeguards tumor cells from

T cell denaturation by inducing downstream inhibitory signaling of T cell antigen receptors [198].

LTN in conjugation with oxaliplatin showed repression of NF-κB, STAT3, and survivin expression in H22 tumor. In MG63 cells (human osteosarcoma cells), LTN induced apoptosis and autophagy by inhibiting the MAPK/ERK signaling [199]. It is also reported that LTN decreased the cyclin D1 levels and increased caspase 3, 9, and Beclin-1 levels [200, 201]. Significantly, LTN inhibited the development of cell lines of rat C6 glioma, induced apoptosis, stops the cell cycle, improves the segments of cells in the G0/G1 stage, and decreases the percentage of cells in S phase [202–204].

12.3.9 Retinoids

Retinoids (RTN) are a group of chemical compounds which are fat-soluble and linked to vitamin A [205]. It has also been found that RTN theoretically increases chemotherapy and radiotherapy's effectiveness in GBM [206]. Retinol is imported from the liver as retinol-pivotal protein and is transformed to retinaldehyde, then finally to retinoic acid. Retinoids signaling pathways play a prominent part in neurogenesis, hippocampal neuronal dendritic development, and increased cognitive functions [207].

Research suggests that RTN significantly inhibits the cell migration and proliferation of human GBM in multiple tissues. Retinoids can trigger efficient segregation but cannot induce apoptosis [208]. In a related study, astrocyte proliferation and telomerase expression were induced, and the sensitiveness for interferon-α therapy was enhanced when GBM therapy is initiated with RTN [209]. Also, RTN therapy has been shown to minimize oxidative factors, rendering GBM cells vulnerable to radiotherapy [210].

12.3.10 Fungi (Bipolaris setariae)

Bipolaris is a dematiac hyphomycetes genus with hundreds of species. Ophiobolin A (OPBA), a sesquiterpenoid developed by morbific fungi, was processed by the crop extract of *Drechslera gigantea* as an important phytotoxin [211]. A wide range of pharmacological and biological properties, notably anticancer activity, were shown in additional compound investigations. Numerous studies have documented the potency of OPBA against glioblastoma and neuroblastoma cells [112].

OPBA mediated pyroptosis in GBM cells by disrupting internal potassium ion homeostasis. Furthermore, several studies found that OPBA induces mitochondrial damage and endoplasmic reticulum stress, compromises cell cycle development, and prevents several oncogenic trajectories in GBM cells [212, 213]. Thus, OPBA refers to a class of phytochemicals that could be used to treat cancer forms with various degrees of proapoptotic stimulation tolerance [214].

12.3.11 Isothiocyanates

Isothiocyanates (ITC), extracted from cruciferous plants, have anti-invasive, anti-inflammatory, anticancer, pancreatic, myeloma, and breast cancer suppression properties [215]. The neuroprotective and anti-inflammatory effects of ITC have recently been tested in different cancer cells. Further studies suggested that various activities of ITC were due to the inhibition of JNK/NF-α signaling [216].

A study revealed that in treatment with phenethyl ITC, the sensitivity of TMZ-resistant cells (U373, T98, U87) was increased by inhibiting MGMT expression through the NF-kB signaling cascade [217]. Additionally, ITC prevented the transcribing of MMP-9 by mitigating NF-kB and activator protein-1 to avoid C6 GBM cells from becoming invaded and migrated [218, 219].

12.4 Natural Products and Blood-Brain Barrier

Since GBM is relatively dangerous in essence, even when the tumor is in non-fervent areas, all microscopic diseases' ablation is not viable. While targeted therapy has received a lot of attention, the life expectancy of GBM patients has not improved because of inadequate drug penetration through the BBB [220] (Fig. 12.3). Consequently, substances proficient of altering the BBB porosity are extremely coveted to boost the bioaccessibility of tumor sensitive agents. The BBB is an essential dynamic vascular framework that controls molecules' access to the brain through paracellular or transcellular pathways [221]. It is made up of several tight junctions between endothelial cells and P-glycoprotein, enzymes, and specific receptors [222].

Although the BBB's paracellular conductivity is controlled by the phosphorylation of endothelial tight junctional (TJ) proteins (zonula occludens-1), P-glycoprotein's inactivation may boost the influx of drug to the brain. BBB functions are also affected by the BBB microenvironment, which involves pericytes, astrocytes, neurons, fibroblasts, microglia basement membrane, and extracellular matrix (ECM) adjacent cell types. The BBB tumor emanates from tumor capillaries that provide the tumor with nutrients and oxygen [223]. ECM, overrunning macrophages, tumor cells, tumor-associated microglia, and several other cancerous cells are part of the glioma microenvironment. Oddly, tumor growth in rat GBM models was blocked by targeting the glioma microenvironment of BBB [224].

Natural products are known to alter the BBB microenvironment by reducing the function of endocytosis, MMPs, and P-glycoproteins. Shikonin (SKN) is a primary naphthoquinone derived from the natural medicinal herb *Lithospermum erythrorhizon* recognized for its antioxidant and anti-inflammatory activities. SKN therapy significantly suppressed MMP-9 expression, raising Claudine-5 and BBB penetrability [225]. Furthermore, SKN therapy has been found to reduce the mobility, proliferation, and differentiation of cell lines U87 and U251 and restrict MMP-2 and MMP-9 development, probably by suppressing the PI3K/Akt signaling cascades. Procyanidin (PCD) also contributed to the microvessels endothelial cell's conductivity by modifying P-glycoproteins in rats [226]. More specifically,

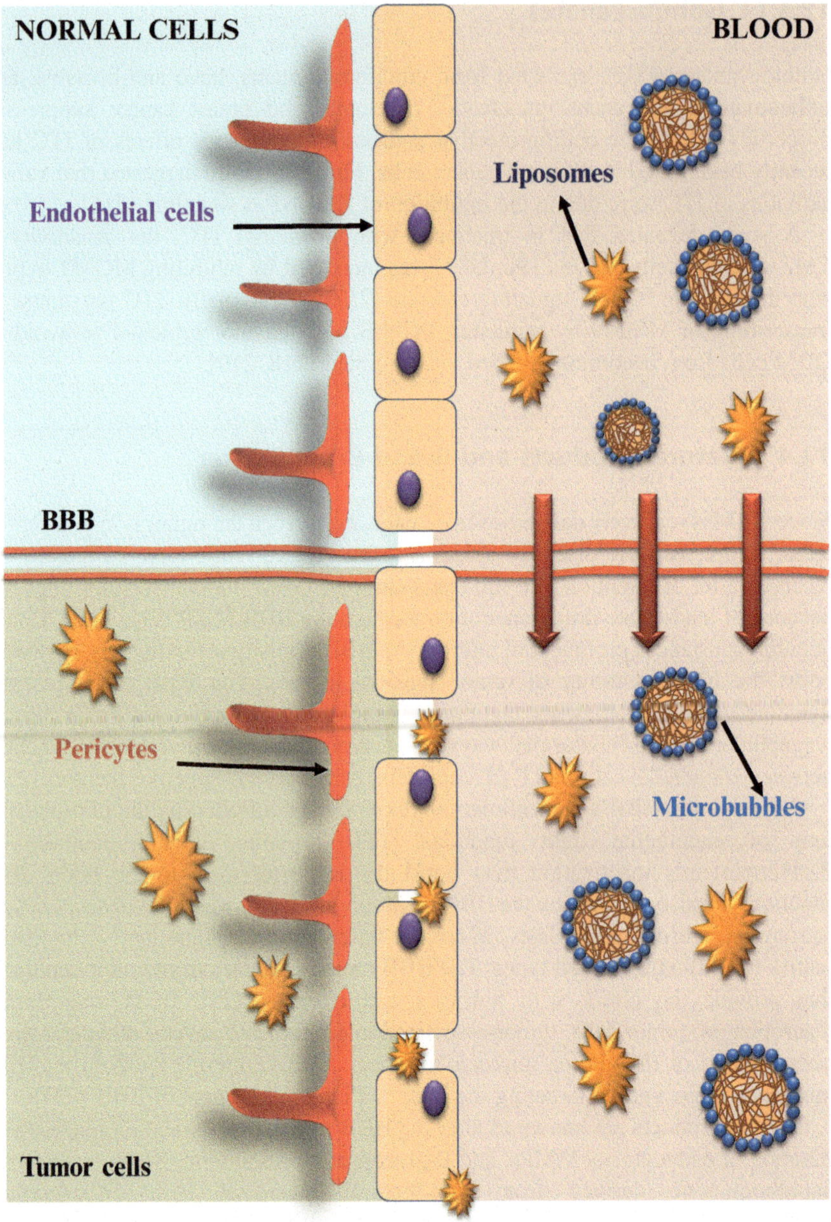

Fig. 12.3 Schematic representation of liposome influx to the tumor region

PCD also strengthened the entry of adriamycin into BBB, resulting in increased therapeutic effectiveness. Scillarenin was also shown to impede the facilitated diffusion of P-glycoprotein. Curcumin also retains the identity of BBB in hypoxic conditions and glucose depletion [227].

12.5 New Outlooks to Drug Delivery

Developments in nano-medicine have increased the possibilities of biomedical drug delivery to GBM cells [228]. Nanoparticles can solve such issues with traditional approaches, as it uses vectors for the transmission of drugs to the brain (Table 12.1) [267]. The lack of treatment for the condition complicates clinical distribution to GBM [229].

The difficulties encountered and the creative approach to the treatment of GBM reviewed, including a review of nano-biotechnology potential to support GBM drug delivery, have allowed the development of GBM's ideal nanotechnology-based drug delivery system concepts. These characteristics will be used to appraise some of the approaches mentioned thus far and influence the development of new procedures [230].

12.5.1 Drug Delivery Throughout the Blood-brain Barrier Employing Nano-Medicine

In prior decades, nano-medicine has made promising advances, specifically in the context of cancer treatment. The level and the scale of nano-related products and their functions are crucial components in the distribution of nano-drugs [231]. This means that nanostructures can engage directly, efficiently, and effectively with bioactive molecules and make people learn metabolism and molecular processes deeper. Nanoparticles with the ability to bypass or cross through the BBB could be used as a new drug delivery technology in the treatment of GBM [232].

GBM chemotherapy is also impeded as the successful delivery of chemotherapy to the desired cancerous cells is not achievable; the appearance of BBB makes the problem more challenging. Therefore, organized, effective therapeutic methodologies need to surpass the BBB and reach their brain's boundary. The efficient intrusion of lipidated medicines and the development of drugs capable of infiltrating the BBB transportation mechanism and drug-laden nano transporters are suggested solutions [233].

Several other entities need a unique transport framework to traverse the BBB except for a small number of liposoluble and micro molecules. A somewhat more reliable and personalized methodology could also be applied to incorporate unique treatments, like the nanoparticles-based system. In an effort to strengthen the obstacles, colloidal structures such as the nanoparticle system enable nano-carriers with surface properties to be built to transport the medications within the BBB

Table 12.1 Detailed analysis of nanoparticle delivery mechanisms for GBM (Data retrieved from https://clinicaltrials.gov/)

Nanoparticles	Chemical agent	Rationale	Intervention	National clinical trial identifier (NCT)	Phase	Completion date
Liposome	Rhenium	Radiation is part of traditional GBM therapy, even though it is restricted at higher concentrations due to toxicity	A stent is placed inside the tumor using stereotactic guidelines. Rhenium nanoliposomes are infused at a fixed dose via the stent. In order to show the distribution profile of Rhenium and to measure the persisted dose inside the tumor, spectroscopic imaging would then be performed at predefined times. Toxic effects and reactions to patients will be tracked for up to 90 days	NCT01906385	1/2	Ongoing–January 2020
Gold	NU-0129 (spherical nucleic acid—SNA)	NU-0129 is transferred through the BBB where it meets TME; and then the Bcl2L12 is targeted by the SNA, linked to the development of the GBM tumor	People receiving NU-0129 IV over 20–50 min and receive regular treatment tumor resection in 8–48 h. Follow-ups occur at 7, 14, 21, and 28 days and then up to 2 years every 84 days	NCT03020017	Early phase 1	Ongoing–July 2022
Albumin	ABI-009	Macrolide antibiotic rapamycin is administered to patients to stimulate immunosuppressant, antiangiogenic, and antineoplastic activity connected with NP albumin	ABI-009 administered i.v. as a single drug or in combination with Temozolomide, temozolomide + radiation, bevacizumab, and lomustine. The study will determine the number of people with drug-related adverse events	NCT03463265	2	Ongoing–June 2021

Convection-enhanced delivery (CED)	MTX110	Panobinostat preclinical effectiveness against DIPG has been demonstrated. CED is a modern technique of drug delivery that goes beyond the BBB—targeted delivery takes place when catheters have been placed inside the CNS	The purpose of the analysis is to assess the protection and tolerability of frequent administration of MTX110 co-infused with intra-tumor-convection-enhanced delivery of gadoteridol (CED)	NCT03566199	1/2	Ongoing–September 2020
Liposome	Temozolomide and SGT-53	This research will evaluate the effectiveness and protection of IV SGT-53 and standard oral temozolomide in combination in patients with confirmed GBM	Many tumors demonstrate loss of the suppressor function, p53. SGT-53 delivery aims to restore wild-type p53 function to control apoptosis, cell cycle control points, DNA repair, and angiogenesis	NCT02340156	2	Ongoing–December 2019

[234]. Nano-material interventions like dendrimers, liposomes, and polymeric micelles have been shown to bypass the BBB and reach the desired location.

Innumerable nano-material-based medications have indeed been studied for the ministrations of GBM and several other cancers [235]. GBM is highly diversified, and with various levels of stability for BBB, growing gliomas are exhibiting an unbroken BBB and diminished glioma.

Therefore, GBM techniques must be structured to identify BBB changes relating to disorders and alter nano-carrier drugs or drugs. In biological materials, transporter substances should ideally be lightweight, cationic, and inert and configured to contain heavy drug payloads to adequate systemic absorption [236]. In order to enhance the effectiveness of any GBM cancer agent, it is also important to understand the physiological and pathological state of gliomas [237].

12.5.2 Targeted Nanoparticles for Tumor Receptors

Doxorubicin (DRB), an anticancer compound attached to polysorbate-coated NPs, enters the BBB unchanged and achieves the brain's therapeutic level. In rats with 101/8 GBM tumor incorporated inside their brains, DRB formulation with coated NPs has administered, which showed potent effect than the other groups [238].

More than 20% of animals throughout this category demonstrated a prolonged regression. Tentative histopathology reported that this community has smaller tumor sizes and reduced propagation and autophagic rates. NPs can also minimize doxorubicin's systematic tolerance [239]. This analysis demonstrated that doxorubicin therapy associated with NPs provides a preventive human GBM cell opportunity [240].

12.5.3 Super-paramagnetic Particle Adducts (SPA)

SPA is being used to detect tumors quicker than recent methods and aims at the tumors quite precisely. The super-paramagnetic iron oxide NPs were assembled with a new rotating method. In order to disable NPs with modest biopolymers and aiming envoys, a basic dialysis methodology was designed that prevents the application of standard centrifugation, causing the accumulation of particles during the casting method [238].

In an attempt to optimize the binding potential of these NPs, a novel chemical framework has been developed, which combines folic acid (FA) with polyethylene glycol (PEG), which improves NP cytocompatibility. The atomic force microscopy depiction showed that the generated NPs had been well distributed with small distributional dimensions [239]. Furthermore, the biomedical section of the research revealed that PEG-FA covering of NPs substantially improved epithelial absorption of NPs by the target tissue. More research in this area is continued by introducing several biomolecules, such as tumor cells promoter target and chemotherapy envoys, into NPs. This technique holds a lot of promise for treating GBMs selectively [240].

12.5.4 Gliadel Wafers (GW)

Complications are probable after surgical excision of the GBM accompanied by radiotherapy and chemotherapy. Owing to systemic toxicity, the need for transport through the BBB successfully is a massive issue for drug delivery. GW is offering a new method for delivering chemotherapy agents to GBM cells [241, 242]. GW, recommended for the treatment of chronic glioblastoma by the FDA, is biodegradable carmustine-loaded polymers. They are implanted at the debridement site, and the medicine is progressively delivered over many weeks as the wafer polymer recedes [243].

While using GW, survival rates were much higher in a clinical trial than in placebo-controlled groups [244]. In addition, glioma patients who underwent surgery with soaked temozolomide GW were successfully treated in another study [245]. Many such studies had indicated that local drug transmission is enhanced when GW was inserted in the resection region of malignant gliomas. Clinical side effects were also decreased in ongoing glioma care [246]. Even so, there have even been records of negative impacts arising from the use of GW, including surgical inflammation, cerebral edema, interventional seizures, and rigorous death-related hydrocephalus [247, 248].

12.5.5 Biomimetic Nanoparticles Targeted to Tumors

Biomimetic (BM) NPs have also been identified to target many tumor cells. The mechanics are premised on a cyclic decapeptide (CLT), which detects coagulated plasma cells and home tumors. Iron oxide NPs and CLT-coated liposomes aggregate in tumor vessels, where further local coagulation is caused, creating new ligands of even more molecules [240]. The mechanism imitates platelets that propagate normally but aggregate at an infected position and intensify their deposition at that location. Self-enhanced homing is a new feature of NPs. The coagulation-based stimulation significantly strengthens the tumor illustration and anticipates a therapeutic agent's attachment to the molecules. While this study is still preliminary, it has a possible drug delivery connection to GBM [249].

12.5.6 Human Interleukin-13-conjugated Liposomes

Human lipid nanoparticles combined with interleukin (IL)-13 effectively adhere to GBM cancerous cells that overexpress IL-13 receptor-2 and do not bound to healthy brain cells. Liposomes containing human IL-13 perfectly bind to glioma cells through endocytosis [250]. The therapeutic efficacy and effectiveness of doxorubicin-borne IL-13-conjugated liposomes have been evaluated in vivo employing a subcutaneous glioma animal model. It was noticed that there was increased cytotoxicity and persistence of IL-13-conjugated liposomes in glioma cells containing doxorubicin collated when supplied freely. Animals receiving

IL-13 combined liposomes (*i.p.*) with doxorubicin had a substantial decrease in the tumor volume than the animals with standard drug delivery. Selectively targeted tumor cells with normal brain tissue saving suggest a viable anticancer drug delivery system for the GBM cells where tumor-specific demolition is essential [240].

12.5.7 Immunoliposomes

A study reports that an antineoplastic and antibiotic drug, daunomycin, is used for liposomal drug delivery in rats' brains. Immunoliposomes with PEG are used to improve the carriage capability of the mAb. It was also reported that the capacity was improved by up to four logarithmic magnitude orders [240]. The immunoliposome-based drug delivery mechanism has been used to target mAb mediated daunomycin in rats' brains. The immune-liposomes of the anti-EGFR show an effective and sustainable medication supply of antineoplastic compounds and can be a helpful novel approach to tumor therapy, as in GBM, the over-expressing EGFR [251].

12.5.8 Photodynamic Treatment with the PEBBLE System

PEBBLEs, a type of nanoparticle, have been designed to transport many therapeutic agents with a unique multifunction on their surface and great potential to tackle cancer. One target protein immobilized on the surface may direct PEBBLE towards a tumor; another may be used to conceit the target using MRI. In contrast, a third PEBBLE agent may provide a damaging dose of medicine or toxin in cancerous cells [240].

All three parts could be integrated to create an effective tool against cancer in a single isolated polymer sphere. The reference sample of MRI (Gd) was included in the PEBBLE system. These nanoparticles work via the circulatory system when injected intravenously into the blood. Even though it can move through the BBB and be targeted by a targeting agent, PEBBLE accumulates within the next few hours in the brain tumor that provides a convenient MRI scan [252].

Every PEBBLE carries a photo-catalyst. Once activated by a light source, the electro-catalyst transforms oxygen into one single state and efficiently destructs neighboring cells by a fiber optic probe implanted in the skull. The PEBBLE is neutral and safe before the light source is triggered. When used in conjunction with MRI, it allows wiping out cancerous cells freely while controlling scanning therapy's efficacy [253]. Focused NP therapies offer some benefits over conventional therapies. The medicines pervade cells in the body in chemotherapy to disrupt their DNA, avoid massive development, and are less toxic to healthy cells than cancerous cells.

On the other side, PEBBLE is extremely localized to the tumor location and performs relatively less work. Thus, damage to the healthy tissue is significantly less [254]. PEBBLE and other nanoparticles might also prevent creating a multidrug resistance that occurs if cancer cells mutate, then chemotherapy drugs start pumping out until they kill the cell. Thus, the cancerous cells become resistant to drug therapies. In rat models of GBM, 9L-gliosarcoma, PEBBLE therapy will substantially boost the overall survival rates [255]. The researchers eventually aim to prove the efficacy and safety of GBM care in humans. Using this approach may help prevent the emergence of drug resistance in tumors, as drug-resistant tumors are hard to treat.

12.6 Conclusion and Future Aspects

GBM appears to be a problem that is unmanageable since no existing therapy is restorative. Lateral to the quest for complete care, the supply of presently available and emerging medicines needs to be improved. Many drug delivery methodologies for brain tumors are evaluated in two forms of animal models, as brain tumors are incorporated subcutaneously or intracranially. Since glioma progression is related to numerous molecular mechanisms, a medication that can target several trails would effectively stop tumorigenesis. However, therapeutic approaches are restricting since tumor cells may build resistance to these treatments. A hybrid of targeted therapies may perhaps be the answer. Natural products are famous for their various biological modes of action at many tumorigenesis stages.

Therefore, natural products will be suitable for glioblastoma treatment, either as monotherapy or in conjunction with other antineoplastic agents (Table 12.2). Nano-biotechnology has made a massive breakthrough in this area by permitting therapeutic NPs to flow across the BBB and providing focused therapy for focused treatment of tumor cells without damaging healthy cells. Among the most promising therapeutic delivery methods for GBM are liposomal systems to deliver the therapeutic agents and super-paramagnetic iron oxide, followed by thermoablation. Aiming to increase the performance of GBM with mAbs, these are linked to boronated dendrimer thus hitting EGF receptors in the GBM.

There have been comparatively fewer clinical studies investigating the use of natural products for GBM. It was also found that Lectin from mistletoe plant extract has immune-stimulatory and immune-protective activity in GBM, along with Patupilone (epothilone B). In GBM patients, this microtubule-stabilizing endogenous cytotoxic drug proved to be surviving. Furthermore, relative to synthetic antagonists, phytochemicals have less versatility for single target proteins, which may help develop phytochemicals as potential inhibitors.

Multi-targeting phytochemicals will be an effective option for chemoprevention, considering phytochemicals' low toxicity and the requirement for long-term administration of chemotherapeutic agents. As illustrated above, there is preclinical evidence to guide yet more research with natural GBM ingredients. This awful prognosis allows us to investigate alternative therapies to enhance the patients' conditions. Putative randomized clinical trials should be carried out to investigate the usage of additional natural medication for slier target-specific drug delivery and improve standard treatments symbiotically.

Table 12.2 Involvement of natural compounds in cancer prevention by modulating different signaling pathways

S. no	Medical plants	Family	Compounds/extracts	Target molecules and additional efficacy	Dose and duration	Cell lines	Refs.
01.	*Hypericum perforatum L. (H. perforatum)*	Hypericaceae	Hyperforin, polyphenolic procyanidin B2, hypericin	Annexin V positive cells	HP 20 μM for 24 h PB-2 80 μM for 24 h	LN229	[256]
02.	*Vaccinium macrocarpon* (cranberry)	Ericaceae	Flavonoid-rich fraction 6, proanthocyanidins fraction	↑G1 phase ↓S phase cell cycle arrest (G1 phase)	Fr6 concentration: 0, 50, 100, 150, 200, 250, 300mg/L for 24 and 48 h PAC concentration: 0, 20, 40, 60, 80, 100, 120, 140, 160 mg/L for 24, 48 h	U87MG	[257]
03.	*Caesalpinia sappan*	Fabaceae	Brazilin	↑PARP ↓caspase-3, caspase-7	10 μg/ml, 15 μg/ml, 20 μg/ml for 24 h	U87 MG	[258]
04.	*Scutellaria baicalensis*	Lamiaceae	Wogonin	↑ AMPK, p53 ↓mTOR, 4E-BP1 G0/G1 phase arrest	0–100 μM for 24 h	U87 MG, U343 MG, U373 MG, T98G, MCF-10A	[259]

05.	*Andrographis paniculata*	Acanthaceae	Andrographolide	↓PI3K/AKT, caspase-3 G2/M phase arrest	10 μM	U251, U87 MG	[260]
06.	*Artemisia argyi*	Asteraceae	Jaceosidin	↑p53, Bax, Cytochrome-c, caspase-3 G2/M phase arrest	100 μM/L for 24 h	U87 MG	[261]
07.	*Angelica sinensis*	Apiaceae	(Z)-N-(2-(Dimethylamino)ethyl)-2-(3-((3-oxoisobenzofuran-1(3H)-ylidene)methyl) phenoxy) acetamide	↓Nur77, JNK	50 μg/ml for 24 h	DBTRG-05MG, GBM 8401	[262]
08.	*Spondias pinnata*	Anacardiaceae	Methyl gallate	ERK1/2 activation, apoptosis	1–30 μg/ml for 48 h	U87MG	[263]
09.	*Hedyotis diffusa* Willd	Rubiaceae	HDW extract	↓Bcl-2/Bax ratio, AKT suppression ↑caspase-3, Bcl-2, Bax and ERK S/G2-M phase arrest, MMP collapse	0, 4, 8 mg/ml for 24 h	U87MG	[264]
10.	*Olea europaea*	Oleaceae	Olea europaea leaf extract	↑ miR-153, miR-145, miR-137	1 mg/ml, 2 mg/ml for 24 h	T98G, U-138MG, U-87MG	[265]
11.	*Rhazya stricta*, *Zingiber officinale*	Apocynaceae/ Zingiberaceae	Crude alkaloid, flavonoid	↓nuclear NF-kB, p65, survivin, XIAP, cyclin-D1, ˄mitochondrial Cytochrome-c, Bax : Bcl-2 ratio, activities of caspase-3 and -9	10 μg/mL for 24, 48, 72 h	U251	[266]

References

1. Kane JR. The role of brain vasculature in glioblastoma. Mol Neurobiol. 2019;56(9):6645–53.
2. Paw I, Carpenter RC, Watabe K, Debinski W, Lo HW. Mechanisms regulating glioma invasion. Cancer Lett. 2015;362(1):1–7.
3. Wang HH, Chang TY, Lin WC, Wei KC, Shin JW. GADD45A plays a protective role against temozolomide treatment in glioblastoma cells. Sci Rep. 2017;7(1):1–5.
4. Laug D, Glasgow SM, Deneen B. A glial blueprint for gliomagenesis. Nat Rev Neurosci. 2018;19(7):393–403.
5. Desai V, Bhushan A. Natural bioactive compounds: alternative approach to the treatment of glioblastoma multiforme. Biomed Res Int. 2017;2017:9363040.
6. Koul D. PTEN signaling pathways in glioblastoma. Cancer Biol Ther. 2008;7(9):1321–5.
7. Davis ME. Glioblastoma: overview of disease and treatment. Clin J Oncol Nurs. 2016;20(5): S2.
8. Singh SK, Hawkins C, Clarke ID, Squire JA, Bayani J, Hide T, Henkelman RM, Cusimano MD, Dirks PB. Identification of human brain tumour initiating cells nature. Nature. 2004;432 (7015):396–401.
9. Aoki T, Hashimoto N, Matsutani M. Management of glioblastoma. Expert Opin Pharmacother. 2007;8(18):3133–46.
10. Gallego JM, Barcia JA, Barcia-Marino C. Fatal outcome related to carmustine implants in glioblastoma multiforme. Acta Neurochir. 2007;149(3):261–5.
11. Gromeier M, Lachmann S, Rosenfeld MR, Gutin PH, Wimmer E. Intergeneric poliovirus recombinants for the treatment of malignant glioma. Proc Natl Acad Sci. 2000;97(12):6803–8.
12. Cancer Genome Atlas Research Network. Comprehensive genomic characterization defines human glioblastoma genes and core pathways. Nature. 2008;455(7216):1061.
13. Fernandes C, Costa A, Osório L, Lago RC, Linhares P, Carvalho B, Caeiro C. Current standards of care in glioblastoma therapy. Brisbane City, QLD: Exon Publications; 2017. p. 197–241.
14. Anton K, Baehring JM, Mayer T. Glioblastoma multiforme: overview of current treatment and future perspectives. Hematol/Oncol Clin. 2012;26(4):825–53.
15. Koc K, Anik I, Cabuk BU, Ceylan SA. Fluorescein sodium-guided surgery in glioblastoma multiforme: a prospective evaluation. Br J Neurosurg. 2008;22(1):99–103.
16. Vidak M, Rozman D, Komel R. Effects of flavonoids from food and dietary supplements on glial and glioblastoma multiforme cells. Molecules. 2015;20(10):19406–32.
17. Haque A, Banik NL, Ray SK. Molecular alterations in glioblastoma: potential targets for immunotherapy. Prog Mol Biol Transl Sci. 2011;98:187–234.
18. Atiq A, Parhar I. Anti-neoplastic potential of flavonoids and polysaccharide phytochemicals in glioblastoma. Molecules. 2020;25(21):4895.
19. Lee SY. Temozolomide resistance in glioblastoma multiforme. Genes Dis. 2016;3 (3):198–210.
20. Kitange GJ, Carlson BL, Schroeder MA, Grogan PT, Lamont JD, Decker PA, Wu W, James CD, Sarkaria JN. Induction of MGMT expression is associated with temozolomide resistance in glioblastoma xenografts. Neuro Oncol. 2009;11(3):281–91.
21. Singhal N, Selva-Nayagam S, Brown MP. Prolonged and severe myelosuppression in two patients after low-dose temozolomide treatment-case study and review of literature. J Neurooncol. 2007;85(2):229–30.
22. Abbas MN, Kausar S, Cui H. Therapeutic potential of natural products in glioblastoma treatment: Targeting key glioblastoma signaling pathways and epigenetic alterations. Clin Transl Oncol. 2020;22(7):963–77.
23. Wang G, Wang J, Du L, Li F. Effect and mechanism of total flavonoids extracted from cotinus coggygria against glioblastoma cancer in vitro and in vivo. Biomed Res Int. 2015;2015:856349.
24. Clevers H. Wnt/β-catenin signaling in development and disease. Cell. 2006;127(3):469–80.

25. Nager M, Bhardwaj D, Cantí C, Medina L, Nogués P, Herreros J. β-Catenin signalling in glioblastoma multiforme and glioma-initiating cells. Chemother Res Pract. 2012;192362:2012.
26. Kaur N, Chettiar S, Rathod S, Rath P, Muzumdar D, Shaikh ML, Shiras A. Wnt3a mediated activation of Wnt/β-catenin signaling promotes tumor progression in glioblastoma. Mol Cell Neurosci. 2013;54:44–57.
27. Kamino M, Kishida M, Kibe T, Ikoma K, Iijima M, Hirano H, Tokudome M, Chen L, Koriyama C, Yamada K, Arita K. Wnt-5a signaling is correlated with infiltrative activity in human glioma by inducing cellular migration and MMP-2. Cancer Sci. 2011;102(3):540–8.
28. Pu P, Zhang Z, Kang C, Jiang R, Jia Z, Wang G, Jiang H. Downregulation of Wnt2 and β-catenin by siRNA suppresses malignant glioma cell growth. Cancer Gene Ther. 2009;16 (4):351–61.
29. Onyido EK, Sweeney E, Nateri AS. Wnt-signalling pathways and microRNAs network in carcinogenesis: experimental and bioinformatics approaches. Mol Cancer. 2016;15(1):1–7.
30. Liu Y, Yan W, Zhang W, Chen L, You G, Bao Z, Wang Y, Wang H, Kang C, Jiang T. MiR-218 reverses high invasiveness of glioblastoma cells by targeting the oncogenic transcription factor LEF1. Oncol Rep. 2012;28(3):1013–21.
31. Kohn AD, Moon RT. Wnt and calcium signaling: β-catenin-independent pathways. Cell Calcium. 2005;38(3–4):439–46.
32. Park JB, Agnihotri S, Golbourn B, Bertrand KC, Luck A, Sabha N, Smith CA, Byron S, Zadeh G, Croul S, Berens M. Transcriptional profiling of GBM invasion genes identifies effective inhibitors of the LIM kinase-Cofilin pathway. Oncotarget. 2014;5(19):9382.
33. Paw I, Carpenter RC, Watabe K, Debinski W, Lo HW. Mechanisms regulating glioma invasion. Cancer Lett. 2015;362(1):1–7.
34. Weeks A, Okolowsky N, Golbourn B, Ivanchuk S, Smith C, Rutka JT. ECT2 and RASAL2 mediate mesenchymal-amoeboid transition in human astrocytoma cells. Am J Pathol. 2012;181(2):662–74.
35. Nager M, Bhardwaj D, Cantí C, Medina L, Nogués P, Herreros J. β-Catenin signalling in glioblastoma multiforme and glioma-initiating cells. Chemother Res Pract. 2012;2012:192362.
36. Gao X, Mi Y, Ma Y, Jin W. LEF1 regulates glioblastoma cell proliferation, migration, invasion, and cancer stem-like cell self-renewal. Tumor Biol. 2014;35(11):11505–11.
37. Guo G, Kuai D, Cai S, Xue N, Liu Y, Hao J, Fan Y, Jin J, Mao X, Liu B, Zhong C. Knockdown of FRAT1 expression by RNA interference inhibits human glioblastoma cell growth, migration and invasion. PLoS One. 2013;8(4):e61206.
38. Kita D, Yonekawa Y, Weller M, Ohgaki H. PIK3CA alterations in primary (de novo) and secondary glioblastomas. Acta Neuropathol. 2007;113(3):295–302.
39. Yamini B, Yu X, Dolan ME, Wu MH, Kufe DW, Weichselbaum RR. Inhibition of nuclear factor-κB activity by temozolomide involves O6-methylguanine–induced inhibition of p65 DNA binding. Cancer Res. 2007;67(14):6889–98.
40. Nagai S, Washiyama K, Kurimoto M, Takaku A, Endo S, Kumanishi T. Aberrant nuclear factor-κB activity and its participation in the growth of human malignant astrocytoma. J Neurosurg. 2002;96(5):909–17.
41. Galvani E, Sun J, Leon LG, Sciarrillo R, Narayan RS, Sjin RT, Lee K, Ohashi K, Heideman DA, Alfieri RR, Heynen GJ. NF-κB drives acquired resistance to a novel mutant-selective EGFR inhibitor. Oncotarget. 2015;6(40):42717.
42. Takada Y, Kobayashi Y, Aggarwal BB. Evodiamine abolishes constitutive and inducible NF-κB activation by inhibiting IκBα kinase activation, thereby suppressing NF-κB-regulated antiapoptotic and metastatic gene expression, up-regulating apoptosis, and inhibiting invasion. J Biol Chem. 2005;280(17):17203–12.
43. Xia Y, Shen S, Verma IM. NF-κB, an active player in human cancers. Cancer Immunol Res. 2014;2(9):823–30.

44. Atkinson GP, Nozell SE, Benveniste ET. NF-κB and STAT3 signaling in glioma: targets for future therapies. Expert Rev Neurother. 2010;10(4):575–86.
45. Song L, Liu L, Wu Z, Li Y, Ying Z, Lin C, Wu J, Hu B, Cheng SY, Li M, Li J. TGF-β induces miR-182 to sustain NF-κB activation in glioma subsets. J Clin Invest. 2012;122(10):3563–78.
46. Roshan MK, Soltani A, Soleimani A, Kahkhaie KR, Afshari AR, Soukhtanloo M. Role of AKT and mTOR signaling pathways in the induction of epithelial-mesenchymal transition (EMT) process. Biochimie. 2019;165:229–34.
47. Salminen A, Lehtonen M, Suuronen T, Kaarniranta K, Huuskonen J. Terpenoids: natural inhibitors of NF-κB signaling with anti-inflammatory and anticancer potential. Cell Mol Life Sci. 2008;65(19):2979–99.
48. Meylan E, Burns K, Hofmann K, Blancheteau V, Martinon F, Kelliher M, Tschopp J. RIP1 is an essential mediator of Toll-like receptor 3–induced NF-κB activation. Nat Immunol. 2004;5 (5):503–7.
49. Festjens N, Berghe TV, Cornelis S, Vandenabeele P. RIP1, a kinase on the crossroads of a cell's decision to live or die. Cell Death Differ. 2007;14(3):400–10.
50. Bonavia R, Inda MM, Vandenberg S, Cheng SY, Nagane M, Hadwiger P, Tan P, Sah DW, Cavenee WK, Furnari FB. EGFRvIII promotes glioma angiogenesis and growth through the NF-κB, interleukin-8 pathway. Oncogene. 2012;31(36):4054–66.
51. Xie TX, Xia Z, Zhang NU, Gong W, Huang S. Constitutive NF-κB activity regulates the expression of VEGF and IL-8 and tumor angiogenesis of human glioblastoma. Oncol Rep. 2010;23(3):725–32.
52. Shostak K, Chariot A. EGFR and NF-κB: partners in cancer. Trends Mol Med. 2015;21 (6):385–93.
53. Dan HC, Cooper MJ, Cogswell PC, Duncan JA, Ting JP, Baldwin AS. Akt-dependent regulation of NF-κB is controlled by mTOR and Raptor in association with IKK. Genes Dev. 2008;22(11):1490–500.
54. Bai D, Ueno L, Vogt PK. Akt-mediated regulation of NFκB and the essentialness of NFκB for the oncogenicity of PI3K and Akt. Int J Cancer. 2009;125(12):2863–70.
55. Kapoor GS, Zhan Y, Johnson GR, O'Rourke DM. Distinct domains in the SHP-2 phosphatase differentially regulate epidermal growth factor receptor/NF-κB activation through Gab1 in glioblastoma cells. Mol Cell Biol. 2004;24(2):823–36.
56. Pearson JR, Regad T. Targeting cellular pathways in glioblastoma multiforme. Signal Transduct Targeted Ther. 2017;2(1):1–1.
57. Puliyappadamba VT, Chakraborty S, Chauncey SS, Li L, Hatanpaa KJ, Mickey B, Noorani S, Shu HK, Burma S, Boothman DA, Habib AA. Opposing effect of EGFRWT on EGFRvIII-mediated NF-κB activation with RIP1 as a cell death switch. Cell Rep. 2013;4(4):764–75.
58. Robe PA, Bentires-Alj M, Bonif M, Rogister B, Deprez M, Haddada H, Khac MT, Jolois O, Erkmen K, Merville MP, Black PM. In vitro and in vivo activity of the nuclear factor-κB inhibitor sulfasalazine in human glioblastomas. Clin Cancer Res. 2004;10(16):5595–603.
59. Wieland A, Trageser D, Gogolok S, Reinartz R, Höfer H, Keller M, Leinhaas A, Schelle R, Normann S, Klaas L, Waha A. Anticancer effects of niclosamide in human glioblastoma. Clin Cancer Res. 2013;19(15):4124–36.
60. Pelloski CE, Lin E, Zhang L, Yung WA, Colman H, Liu JL, Woo SY, Heimberger AB, Suki D, Prados M, Chang S. Prognostic associations of activated mitogen-activated protein kinase and Akt pathways in glioblastoma. Clin Cancer Res. 2006;12(13):3935–41.
61. Li X, Wu C, Chen N, Gu H, Yen A, Cao L, Wang E, Wang L. PI3K/Akt/mTOR signaling pathway and targeted therapy for glioblastoma. Oncotarget. 2016;7(22):33440.
62. Ogiso H, Ishitani R, Nureki O, Fukai S, Yamanaka M, Kim JH, Saito K, Sakamoto A, Inoue M, Shirouzu M, Yokoyama S. Crystal structure of the complex of human epidermal growth factor and receptor extracellular domains. Cell. 2002;110(6):775–87.
63. Koul D, Fu J, Shen R, LaFortune TA, Wang S, Tiao N, Kim YW, Liu JL, Ramnarian D, Yuan Y, Garcia-Echevrria C. Antitumor activity of NVP-BKM120—a selective pan class I

PI3 kinase inhibitor showed differential forms of cell death based on p53 status of glioma cells. Clin Cancer Res. 2012;18(1):184–95.
64. Pitz MW, Eisenhauer EA, MacNeil MV, Thiessen B, Easaw JC, Macdonald DR, Eisenstat DD, Kakumanu AS, Salim M, Chalchal H, Squire J. Phase II study of PX-866 in recurrent glioblastoma. Neuro Oncol. 2015;17(9):1270–4.
65. Ma DJ, Galanis E, Anderson SK, Schiff D, Kaufmann TJ, Peller PJ, Giannini C, Brown PD, Uhm JH, McGraw S, Jaeckle KA. A phase II trial of everolimus, temozolomide, and radiotherapy in patients with newly diagnosed glioblastoma: NCCTG N057K. Neuro Oncol. 2015;17(9):1261–9.
66. Kubiatowski T, Jang T, Lachyankar MB, Salmonsen R, Nabi RR, Quesenberry PJ, Litofsky NS, Ross AH, Recht LD. Association of increased phosphatidylinositol 3-kinase signaling with increased invasiveness and gelatinase activity in malignant gliomas. J Neurosurg. 2001;95(3):480–8.
67. O'Reilly KE, Rojo F, She QB, Solit D, Mills GB, Smith D, Lane H, Hofmann F, Hicklin DJ, Ludwig DL, Baselga J. mTOR inhibition induces upstream receptor tyrosine kinase signaling and activates Akt. Cancer Res. 2006;66(3):1500–8.
68. Martini M, De Santis MC, Braccini L, Gulluni F, Hirsch E. PI3K/AKT signaling pathway and cancer: an updated review. Ann Med. 2014;46(6):372–83.
69. Gulati N, Karsy M, Albert L, Murali R, Jhanwar-Uniyal M. Involvement of mTORC1 and mTORC2 in regulation of glioblastoma multiforme growth and motility. Int J Oncol. 2009;35(4):731–40.
70. Wu SH, Bi JF, Cloughesy T, Cavenee WK, Mischel PS. Emerging function of mTORC2 as a core regulator in glioblastoma: metabolic reprogramming and drug resistance. Cancer Biol Med. 2014;11(4):255.
71. Dowling RJ, Topisirovic I, Fonseca BD, Sonenberg N. Dissecting the role of mTOR: lessons from mTOR inhibitors. Biochim Biophys Acta. 2010;1804(3):433–9.
72. Hay N, Sonenberg N. Upstream and downstream of mTOR. Genes Dev. 2004;18(16):1926–45.
73. Fonović M, Turk B. Cysteine cathepsins and extracellular matrix degradation. Biochim Biophys Acta. 2014;1840(8):2560–70.
74. Frame MC, Brunton VG. Advances in Rho-dependent actin regulation and oncogenic transformation. Curr Opin Genet Dev. 2002;12(1):36–43.
75. Clement V, Sanchez P, De Tribolet N, Radovanovic I, i Altaba AR. HEDGEHOG-GLI1 signaling regulates human glioma growth, cancer stem cell self-renewal, and tumorigenicity. Curr Biol. 2007;17(2):165–72.
76. Rimkus TK, Carpenter RL, Qasem S, Chan M, Lo HW. Targeting the sonic hedgehog signaling pathway: review of smoothened and GLI inhibitors. Cancer. 2016;8(2):22.
77. Bigelow RL, Chari NS, Undén AB, Spurgers KB, Lee S, Roop DR, Toftgård R, McDonnell TJ. Transcriptional regulation of bcl-2 mediated by the sonic hedgehog signaling pathway through gli-1. J Biol Chem. 2004;279(2):1197–205.
78. Zhu H, Lo HW. The human glioma-associated oncogene homolog 1 (GLI1) family of transcription factors in gene regulation and diseases. Curr Genomics. 2010;11(4):238–45.
79. Xie J, Aszterbaum M, Zhang X, Bonifas JM, Zachary C, Epstein E, McCormick F. A role of PDGFRα in basal cell carcinoma proliferation. Proc Natl Acad Sci. 2001;98(16):9255–9.
80. Cao X, Geradts J, Dewhirst MW, Lo HW. Upregulation of VEGF-A and CD24 gene expression by the tGLI1 transcription factor contributes to the aggressive behavior of breast cancer cells. Oncogene. 2012;31(1):104–15.
81. Dikshit B, Irshad K, Madan E, Aggarwal N, Sarkar C, Chandra PS, Gupta DK, Chattopadhyay P, Sinha S, Chosdol K. FAT1 acts as an upstream regulator of oncogenic and inflammatory pathways, via PDCD4, in glioma cells. Oncogene. 2013;32(33):3798–808.
82. Lo HW, Zhu H, Cao X, Aldrich A, Ali-Osman F. A novel splice variant of GLI1 that promotes glioblastoma cell migration and invasion. Cancer Res. 2009;69(17):6790–8.

83. Zhu H, Carpenter RL, Han W, Lo HW. The GLI1 splice variant TGLI1 promotes glioblastoma angiogenesis and growth. Cancer Lett. 2014;343(1):51–61.
84. Hong DS, Angelo LS, Kurzrock R. Interleukin-6 and its receptor in cancer: implications for translational therapeutics. Cancer. 2007;110:1911–28.
85. Chang CY, Li MC, Liao SL, Huang YL, Shen CC, Pan HC. Prognostic and clinical implication of IL-6 expression in glioblastoma multiforme. J Clin Neurosci. 2005;12(8):930–3.
86. Rahaman SO, Harbor PC, Chernova O, Barnett GH, Vogelbaum MA, Haque SJ. Inhibition of constitutively active Stat3 suppresses proliferation and induces apoptosis in glioblastoma multiforme cells. Oncogene. 2002;21(55):8404–13.
87. Bischoff SC. Quercetin: potentials in the prevention and therapy of disease. Curr Opin Clin Nutr Metab Care. 2008;11(6):733–40.
88. Perez-Vizcaino F, Duarte J, Andriantsitohaina R. Endothelial function and cardiovascular disease: effects of quercetin and wine polyphenols. Free Radic Res. 2006;40(10):1054–65.
89. Chen SF, Nieh S, Jao SW, Liu CL, Wu CH, Chang YC, Yang CY, Lin YS. Quercetin suppresses drug-resistant spheres via the p38 MAPK–Hsp27 apoptotic pathway in oral cancer cells. PLoS One. 2012;7(11):e49275.
90. Russo M, Palumbo R, Tedesco I, Mazzarella G, Russo P, Iacomino G, Russo GL. Quercetin and anti-CD95 (Fas/Apo1) enhance apoptosis in HPB-ALL cell line. FEBS Lett. 1999;462 (3):322–8.
91. Michaud-Levesque J, Bousquet-Gagnon N, Béliveau R. Quercetin abrogates IL-6/STAT3 signaling and inhibits glioblastoma cell line growth and migration. Exp Cell Res. 2012;318 (8):925–35.
92. Sang DP, Li RJ, Lan Q. Quercetin sensitizes human glioblastoma cells to temozolomide in vitro via inhibition of Hsp27. Acta Pharmacol Sin. 2014;35(6):832–8.
93. Kim H, Moon JY, Ahn KS, Cho SK. Quercetin induces mitochondrial mediated apoptosis and protective autophagy in human glioblastoma U373MG cells. Oxid Med Cell Longev. 2013;2013:596496.
94. Zamin LL, Filippi-Chiela EC, Vargas J, Demartini DR, Meurer L, Souza AP, Bonorino C, Salbego C, Lenz G. Quercetin promotes glioma growth in a rat model. Food Chem Toxicol. 2014;63:205–11.
95. El-Readi MZ, Eid S, Abdelghany AA, Al-Amoudi HS, Efferth T, Wink M. Resveratrol mediated cancer cell apoptosis, and modulation of multidrug resistance proteins and metabolic enzymes. Phytomedicine. 2019;55:269–81.
96. Vervandier-Fasseur D, Latruffe N. The potential use of resveratrol for cancer prevention. Molecules. 2019;24(24):4506.
97. Jiao Y, Li H, Liu Y, Guo A, Xu X, Qu X, Wang S, Zhao J, Li Y, Cao Y. Resveratrol inhibits the invasion of glioblastoma-initiating cells via down-regulation of the PI3K/Akt/NF-κB signaling pathway. Nutrients. 2015;7(6):4383–402.
98. Westhoff MA, Zhou S, Nonnenmacher L, Karpel-Massler G, Jennewein C, Schneider M, Halatsch ME, Carragher NO, Baumann B, Krause A, Simmet T. Inhibition of NF-κB signaling ablates the invasive phenotype of glioblastoma. Mol Cancer Res. 2013;11(12):1611–23.
99. Huang H, Lin H, Zhang X, Li J. Resveratrol reverses temozolomide resistance by downregulation of MGMT in T98G glioblastoma cells by the NF-κB-dependent pathway. Oncol Rep. 2012;27(6):2050–6.
100. Li F, Sethi G. Targeting transcription factor NF-κB to overcome chemoresistance and radioresistance in cancer therapy. Biochim Biophys Acta. 2010;1805(2):167–80.
101. Hegi ME, Diserens AC, Gorlia T, Hamou MF, De Tribolet N, Weller M, Kros JM, Hainfellner JA, Mason W, Mariani L, Bromberg JE. MGMT gene silencing and benefit from temozolomide in glioblastoma. N Engl J Med. 2005;352(10):997–1003.
102. Arepalli SK, Choi M, Jung JK, Lee H. Novel NF-κB inhibitors: a patent review (2011–2014). Expert Opin Ther Pat. 2015;25(3):319–34.

103. Sehdev V, Lai JC, Bhushan A. Biochanin A modulates cell viability, invasion, and growth promoting signaling pathways in HER-2-positive breast cancer cells. J Oncol. 2009;2009:121458.
104. Jang M, Cai L, Udeani GO, Slowing KV, Thomas CF, Beecher CW, Fong HH, Farnsworth NR, Kinghorn AD, Mehta RG, Moon RC. Cancer chemopreventive activity of resveratrol, a natural product derived from grapes. Science. 1997;275(5297):218–20.
105. Gill C, Walsh SE, Morrissey C, Fitzpatrick JM, Watson RW. Resveratrol sensitizes androgen independent prostate cancer cells to death-receptor mediated apoptosis through multiple mechanisms. Prostate. 2007;67(15):1641–53.
106. Patel KR, Brown VA, Jones DJ, Britton RG, Hemingway D, Miller AS, West KP, Booth TD, Perloff M, Crowell JA, Brenner DE. Clinical pharmacology of resveratrol and its metabolites in colorectal cancer patients. Cancer Res. 2010;70(19):7392–9.
107. Howells LM, Berry DP, Elliott PJ, Jacobson EW, Hoffmann E, Hegarty B, Brown K, Steward WP, Gescher AJ. Phase I randomized, double-blind pilot study of micronized resveratrol (SRT501) in patients with hepatic metastases—safety, pharmacokinetics, and pharmacodynamics. Cancer Prev Res. 2011;4(9):1419–25.
108. Brown VA, Patel KR, Viskaduraki M, Crowell JA, Perloff M, Booth TD, Vasilinin G, Sen A, Schinas AM, Piccirilli G, Brown K. Repeat dose study of the cancer chemopreventive agent resveratrol in healthy volunteers: safety, pharmacokinetics, and effect on the insulin-like growth factor axis. Cancer Res. 2010;70(22):9003–11.
109. Gangemi RM, Griffero F, Marubbi D, Perera M, Capra MC, Malatesta P, Ravetti GL, Zona GL, Daga A, Corte G. SOX2 silencing in glioblastoma tumor-initiating cells causes stop of proliferation and loss of tumorigenicity. Stem Cells. 2009;27(1):40–8.
110. Ryu J, Ku BM, Lee YK, et al. Resveratrol reduces tnf-alpha-induced u373mg human glioma cell invasion through regulating nf-kappa b activation and upa/upar expression. Anticancer Res. 2011;31:4223–30.
111. Filippi-Chiela EC, Thomé MP. e Silva MM, Pelegrini AL, Ledur PF, Garicochea B, Zamin LL, Lenz G. Resveratrol abrogates the temozolomide-induced G2 arrest leading to mitotic catastrophe and reinforces the temozolomide-induced senescence in glioma cells. BMC Cancer. 2013;13(1):1–3.
112. Cilibrasi C, Riva G, Romano G, Cadamuro M, Bazzoni R, Butta V, Paoletta L, Dalprà L, Strazzabosco M, Lavitrano M, Giovannoni R. Resveratrol impairs glioma stem cells proliferation and motility by modulating the wnt signaling pathway. PLoS One. 2017;12(1): e0169854.
113. Paul I, Bhattacharya S, Chatterjee A, Ghosh MK. Current understanding on EGFR and Wnt/β-catenin signaling in glioma and their possible crosstalk. Genes Cancer. 2013;4 (11–12):427–46.
114. Götze S, Wolter M, Reifenberger G, Müller O, Sievers S. Frequent promoter hypermethylation of Wnt pathway inhibitor genes in malignant astrocytic gliomas. Int J Cancer. 2010;126 (11):2584–93.
115. Duvoix A, Blasius R, Delhalle S, Schnekenburger M, Morceau F, Henry E, Dicato M, Diederich M. Chemopreventive and therapeutic effects of curcumin. Cancer Lett. 2005;223:181–90.
116. Perry MC, Demeule M, Régina A, Moumdjian R, Béliveau R. Curcumin inhibits tumor growth and angiogenesis in glioblastoma xenografts. Mol Nutr Food Res. 2010;54(8):1192–201.
117. Anand P, Kunnumakkara AB, Newman RA, Aggarwal BB. Bioavailability of curcumin: problems and promises. Mol Pharm. 2007;4(6):807–18.
118. Suresh D, Srinivasan K. Tissue distribution & elimination of capsaicin, piperine & curcumin following oral intake in rats. Indian J Med Res. 2010;131(5):682–91.
119. Ramachandran C, Resek AP, Escalon E, Aviram A, Melnick SJ. Potentiation of gemcitabine by Turmeric Force™ in pancreatic cancer cell lines. Oncol Rep. 2010;23(6):1529–35.

120. Ramachandran C, Nair SM, Escalon E, Melnick SJ. Potentiation of etoposide and temozolomide cytotoxicity by curcumin and turmeric force in brain tumor cell lines. J Complement Integr Med. 2012;9(1):Article 20.
121. Ji M, Choi J, Lee J, Lee Y. Induction of apoptosis by ar-turmerone on various cell lines. Int J Mol Med. 2004;14(2):253–6.
122. Ramachandran C, Quirin KW, Escalon EA, Lollett IV, Melnick SJ. Therapeutic effect of supercritical CO2 extracts of Curcuma species with cancer drugs in rhabdomyosarcoma cell lines. Phytother Res. 2015;29(8):1152–60.
123. Ramachandran C, Portalatin G, Quirin KW, Escalon E, Khatib Z, Melnick SJ. Inhibition of AKT signaling by supercritical CO2 extract of mango ginger (Curcuma amada Roxb.) in human glioblastoma cells. J Complement Integr Med. 2015;12(4):307–15.
124. Bellacosa A, Kumar CC, Di Cristofano A, Testa JR. Activation of AKT kinases in cancer: implications for therapeutic targeting. Adv Cancer Res. 2005;94:29–86.
125. Hanahan D, Weinberg RA. The hallmarks of cancer cell. 2000;100(1):57–70.
126. Arlt A, Gehrz A, Müerköster S, Vorndamm J, Kruse ML, Fölsch UR, Schäfer H. Role of NF-κ B and Akt/PI3K in the resistance of pancreatic carcinoma cell lines against gemcitabine-induced cell death. Oncogene. 2003;22(21):3243–51.
127. Cheng JQ, Jiang X, Fraser M, Li M, Dan HC, Sun M, Tsang BK. Role of X-linked inhibitor of apoptosis protein in chemoresistance in ovarian cancer: possible involvement of the phosphoinositide-3 kinase/Akt pathway. Drug Resist Updat. 2002;5(3–4):131–46.
128. Falasca M. PI3K/Akt signalling pathway specific inhibitors: a novel strategy to sensitize cancer cells to anti-cancer drugs. Curr Pharm Des. 2010;16(12):1410–6.
129. Whang YE, Yuan XJ, Liu Y, Majumder S, Lewis TD. Regulation of sensitivity to TRAIL by the PTEN tumor suppressor. Vitam Horm. 2004;67:409–26.
130. Downward J. PI 3-kinase, Akt and cell survival. In: Seminars in cell & developmental biology, vol. 15. Cambridge, MA: Academic Press; 2004. p. 177–82.
131. Naz S, Imran M, Rauf A, Orhan IE, Shariati MA, Shahbaz M, Qaisrani TB, Shah ZA, Plygun S, Heydari M. Chrysin: Pharmacological and therapeutic properties. Life Sci. 2019;235:116797.
132. Morissette M, Litim N, Di Paolo T. Natural phytoestrogens: a class of promising neuroprotective agents for Parkinson disease. In: Discovery and development of neuroprotective agents from natural products. Amsterdam: Elsevier; 2018. p. 9–61.
133. Narayana KR, Reddy MS, Chaluvadi MR, Krishna DR. Bioflavonoids classification, pharmacological, biochemical effects and therapeutic potential. Indian J Pharm. 2001;33(1):2–16.
134. Mehdi SH, Nafees S, Zafaryab M, Khan MA, Alam Rizvi MM. Chrysin: a promising anticancer agent its current trends and future perspectives. Eur J Exp Biol. 2018;8:16.
135. Sun LR, Zhou W, Zhang HM, Guo QS, Yang W, Li BJ, Sun ZH, Gao SH, Cui RJ. Modulation of multiple signaling pathways of the plant-derived natural products in cancer. Front Oncol. 2019;9:1153.
136. Siddiqui A, Badruddeen, Akhtar J, Uddin MS S, Khan MI, Khalid M, Ahmad M. A naturally occurring flavone (Chrysin): chemistry, occurrence, pharmacokinetic, toxicity, molecular targets and medicinal properties. J Biol Active Prod Nat. 2018;8(4):208-227.
137. Santos BL, Oliveira MN, Coelho PL, Pitanga BP, da Silva AB, Adelita T, Silva VD, de FD Costa M, El-Bachá RS, Tardy M, Chneiweiss H. Flavonoids suppress human glioblastoma cell growth by inhibiting cell metabolism, migration, and by regulating extracellular matrix proteins and metalloproteinases expression. Chem Biol Interact. 2015;242:123–38.
138. Hong TB, Rahumatullah A, Yogarajah T, Ahmad M, Yin KB. Potential effects of chrysin on MDA-MB-231 cells. Int J Mol Sci. 2010;11(3):1057–69.
139. Yang F, Jin H, Pi J, Jiang JH, Liu L, Bai HH, Yang PH, Cai JY. Anti-tumor activity evaluation of novel chrysin–organogermanium (IV) complex in MCF-7 cells. Bioorg Med Chem Lett. 2013;23(20):5544–51.

140. Weng MS, Ho YS, Lin JK. Chrysin induces G1 phase cell cycle arrest in C6 glioma cells through inducing p21Waf1/Cip1 expression: involvement of p38 mitogen-activated protein kinase. Biochem Pharmacol. 2005;69(12):1815–27.
141. Wang J, Wang H, Sun K, Wang X, Pan H, Zhu J, Ji X, Li X. Chrysin suppresses proliferation, migration, and invasion in glioblastoma cell lines via mediating the ERK/Nrf2 signaling pathway. Drug Des Dev Ther. 2018;12:721.
142. Souza LC, Antunes MS, Borges Filho C, Del Fabbro L, de Gomes MG, Goes AT, Donato F, Prigol M, Boeira SP, Jesse CR. Flavonoid Chrysin prevents age-related cognitive decline via attenuation of oxidative stress and modulation of BDNF levels in aged mouse brain. Pharmacol Biochem Behav. 2015;134:22–30.
143. Gülden M, Appel D, Syska M, Uecker S, Wages F, Seibert H. Chrysin and silibinin sensitize human glioblastoma cells for arsenic trioxide. Food Chem Toxicol. 2017;105:486–97.
144. Markiewicz-Żukowska R, Borawska MH, Fiedorowicz A, Naliwajko SK, Sawicka D, Car H. Propolis changes the anticancer activity of temozolomide in U87MG human glioblastoma cell line. BMC Complement Altern Med. 2013;13(1):1–9.
145. Liao CL, Chen CM, Chang YZ, Liu GY, Hung HC, Hsieh TY, Lin CL. Pine (pinus morrisonicola hayata) needle extracts sensitize GBM8901 human glioblastoma cells to temozolomide by downregulating autophagy and O 6-methylguanine-DNA methyltransferase expression. J Agric Food Chem. 2014;62(43):10458–67.
146. Borawska MH, Naliwajko SK, Moskwa J, Markiewicz-Żukowska R, Puścion-Jakubik A, Soroczyńska J. Anti-proliferative and anti-migration effects of Polish propolis combined with Hypericum perforatum L. on glioblastoma multiforme cell line U87MG. BMC Complement Altern Med. 2016;16(1):1–9.
147. Mani R, Natesan V. Chrysin: Sources, beneficial pharmacological activities, and molecular mechanism of action. Phytochemistry. 2018;145:187–96.
148. Eatemadi A, Daraee H, Aiyelabegan HT, Negahdari B, Rajeian B, Zarghami N. Synthesis and characterization of chrysin-loaded PCL-PEG-PCL nanoparticle and its effect on breast cancer cell line. Biomed Pharmacother. 2016;84:1915–22.
149. Zheng H, Li S, Pu Y, Lai Y, He B, Gu Z. Nanoparticles generated by PEG-Chrysin conjugates for efficient anticancer drug delivery. Eur J Pharm Biopharm. 2014;87(3):454–60.
150. Sabzichi M, Mohammadian J, Bazzaz R, Pirouzpanah MB, Shaaker M, Hamishehkar H, Chavoshi H, Salehi R, Samadi N. Chrysin loaded nanostructured lipid carriers (NLCs) triggers apoptosis in MCF-7 cancer cells by inhibiting the Nrf2 pathway. Process Biochem. 2017;60:84–91.
151. Anari E, Akbarzadeh A, Zarghami N. Chrysin-loaded PLGA-PEG nanoparticles designed for enhanced effect on the breast cancer cell line. Artif Cells Nanomed Biotechnol. 2016;44 (6):1410–6.
152. Mohammadian F, Pilehvar-Soltanahmadi Y, Mofarrah M, Dastani-Habashi M, Zarghami N. Down regulation of miR-18a, miR-21 and miR-221 genes in gastric cancer cell line by chrysin-loaded PLGA-PEG nanoparticles. Artif Cells Nanomed Biotechnol. 2016;44 (8):1972–8.
153. Kikuta S. The cytotoxic effect of genistein, a soybean isoflavone, against cultured tribolium cells. Insects. 2020;11(4):241.
154. Kaufman PB, Duke JA, Brielmann H, Boik J, Hoyt JE. A comparative survey of leguminous plants as sources of the isoflavones, genistein and daidzein: implications for human nutrition and health. J Altern Complement Med. 1997;3(1):7–12.
155. Ahmad IU, Forman JD, Sarkar FH, Hillman GG, Heath E, Vaishampayan U, Cher ML, Andic F, Rossi PJ, Kucuk O. Soy isoflavones in conjunction with radiation therapy in patients with prostate cancer. Nutr Cancer. 2010;62(7):996–1000.
156. Surh YJ. Cancer chemoprevention with dietary phytochemicals. Nat Rev Cancer. 2003;3 (10):768–80.

157. Singh-Gupta V, Joiner MC, Runyan L, Yunker CK, Sarkar FH, Miller S, Gadgeel SM, Konski AA, Hillman GG. Soy isoflavones augment radiation effect by inhibiting APE1/Ref-1 DNA repair activity in non-small cell lung cancer. J Thorac Oncol. 2011;6(4):688–98.
158. Sobhy MM, Mahmoud SS, El-Sayed SH, Rizk EM, Raafat A, Negm MS. Impact of treatment with a protein tyrosine kinase inhibitor (Genistein) on acute and chronic experimental Schistosoma mansoni infection. Exp Parasitol. 2018;185:115–23.
159. Puli S, Jain A, Lai JC, Bhushan A. Effect of combination treatment of rapamycin and isoflavones on mTOR pathway in human glioblastoma (U87) cells. Neurochem Res. 2010;35(7):986–93.
160. Khoshyomn S, Nathan D, Manske GC, Osler TM, Penar PL. Synergistic effect of genistein and BCNU on growth inhibition and cytotoxicity of glioblastoma cells. J Neurooncol. 2002;57 (3):193–200.
161. Ravindranath MH, Muthugounder S, Presser N, Viswanathan S. Anticancer therapeutic potential of soy isoflavone, genistein. Adv Exp Med Biol. 2004;546:121–65.
162. Schmidt F, Knobbe CB, Frank B, Wolburg H, Weller M. The topoisomerase II inhibitor, genistein, induces G2/M arrest and apoptosis in human malignant glioma cell lines. Oncol Rep. 2008;19(4):1061–6.
163. Wang HK. The therapeutic potential of flavonoids. Expert Opin Investig Drugs. 2000;9 (9):2103–19.
164. Myers DE, Sicheneder A, Clementson D, Dvorak N, Venkatachalam T, Sev AR, Chandan-Langlie M, Uckun FM. Large scale manufacturing of B43 (anti-CD19)-genistein for clinical trials in leukemia and lymphoma. Leuk Lymphoma. 1998;29(3-4):329–38.
165. Mendes LP, Gaeti MP, de Ávila PH, de Sousa VM, dos Santos RB, de Ávila Marcelino RI, Dos Santos LC, Valadares MC, Lima EM. Multicompartimental nanoparticles for co-encapsulation and multimodal drug delivery to tumor cells and neovasculature. Pharm Res. 2014;31(5):1106–19.
166. Chuan LI, Zhang J, Yu-Jiao ZU, Shu-Fang NI, Jun CA, Qian WA, Shao-Ping NI, Ze-Yuan DE, Ming-Yong XI, Shu WA. Biocompatible and biodegradable nanoparticles for enhancement of anti-cancer activities of phytochemicals. Chin J Nat Med. 2015;13(9):641–52.
167. de Azambuja CR, dos Santos LG, Rodrigues MR, Rodrigues RF, da Silveira EF, Azambuja JH, Flores AF, Horn AP, Dora CL, Muccillo-Baisch AL, Braganhol E. Physico-chemical characterization of asolectin–genistein liposomal system: An approach to analyze its in vitro antioxidant potential and effect in glioma cells viability. Chem Phys Lipids. 2015;193:24–35.
168. Phan V, Walters J, Brownlow B, Elbayoumi T. Enhanced cytotoxicity of optimized liposomal genistein via specific induction of apoptosis in breast, ovarian and prostate carcinomas. J Drug Target. 2013;21(10):1001–11.
169. de Azambuja Borges CR, Silva NO, Rodrigues MR, Marinho MA, de Oliveira FS, Cassiana M, Horn AP, Parize AL, Flores DC, Clementin RM, de Lima VR. Dimiristoylphosphatidylcholine/genistein molecular interactions: a physico-chemical approach to anti-glioma drug delivery systems. Chem Phys Lipids. 2019;225:104828.
170. Puli S, Lai JC, Bhushan A. Inhibition of matrix degrading enzymes and invasion in human glioblastoma (U87MG) cells by isoflavones. J Neurooncol. 2006;79(2):135–42.
171. Ahmad IU, Forman JD, Sarkar FH, Hillman GG, Heath E, Vaishampayan U, Cher ML, Andic F, Rossi PJ, Kucuk O. Soy isoflavones in conjunction with radiation therapy in patients with prostate cancer. Nutr Cancer. 2010;62(7):996–1000.
172. Goodman M, Bostick RM, Kucuk O, Jones DP. Clinical trials of antioxidants as cancer prevention agents: past, present, and future. Free Radic Biol Med. 2011;51(5):1068–84.
173. Banerjee S, Li Y, Wang Z, Sarkar FH. Multi-targeted therapy of cancer by genistein. Cancer Lett. 2008;269(2):226–42.
174. Singh-Gupta V, Joiner MC, Runyan L, Yunker CK, Sarkar FH, Miller S, Gadgeel SM, Konski AA, Hillman GG. Soy isoflavones augment radiation effect by inhibiting APE1/Ref-1 DNA repair activity in non-small cell lung cancer. J Thorac Oncol. 2011;6(4):688–98.

175. Puli S, Jain A, Lai JC, Bhushan A. Effect of combination treatment of rapamycin and isoflavones on mTOR pathway in human glioblastoma (U87) cells. Neurochem Res. 2010;35(7):986–93.
176. Kim KH, Seol HJ, Kim EH, Rheey J, Jin HJ, Lee Y, Joo KM, Lee J, Nam DH. Wnt/β-catenin signaling is a key downstream mediator of MET signaling in glioblastoma stem cells. Neuro Oncol. 2013;15(2):161–71.
177. Zhang Y, Wang SX, Ma JW, Li HY, Ye JC, Xie SM, Du B, Zhong XY. EGCG inhibits properties of glioma stem-like cells and synergizes with temozolomide through downregulation of P-glycoprotein inhibition. J Neurooncol. 2015;121(1):41–52.
178. Chen TC, Wang W, Golden EB, Thomas S, Sivakumar W, Hofman FM, Louie SG, Schönthal AH. Green tea epigallocatechin gallate enhances therapeutic efficacy of temozolomide in orthotopic mouse glioblastoma models. Cancer Lett. 2011;302(2):100–8.
179. Nihal M, Ahsan H, Siddiqui IA, Mukhtar H, Ahmad N, Wood GS. (-)-Epigallocatechin-3-gallate (EGCG) sensitizes melanoma cells to interferon induced growth inhibition in a mouse model of human melanoma. Cell Cycle. 2009;8(13):2057–63.
180. Chen H, Landen CN, Li Y, Alvarez RD, Tollefsbol TO. Epigallocatechin gallate and sulforaphane combination treatment induce apoptosis in paclitaxel-resistant ovarian cancer cells through hTERT and Bcl-2 down-regulation. Exp Cell Res. 2013;319(5):697–706.
181. Lee HK, Xiang C, Cazacu S, Finniss S, Kazimirsky G, Lemke N, Lehman NL, Rempel SA, Mikkelsen T, Brodie C. GRP78 is overexpressed in glioblastomas and regulates glioma cell growth and apoptosis. Neuro Oncol. 2008;10(3):236–43.
182. Singh BN, Shankar S, Srivastava RK. Green tea catechin, epigallocatechin-3-gallate (EGCG): mechanisms, perspectives and clinical applications. Biochem Pharmacol. 2011;82 (12):1807–21.
183. Liang G, Tang A, Lin X, Li L, Zhang S, Huang Z, Tang H, Li QQ. Green tea catechins augment the antitumor activity of doxorubicin in an in vivo mouse model for chemoresistant liver cancer. Int J Oncol. 2010;37(1):111–23.
184. Li C, Zhou C, Wang S, Feng Y, Lin W, Lin S, Wang Y, Huang H, Liu P, Mu YG, Shen X. Sensitization of glioma cells to tamoxifen-induced apoptosis by Pl3-kinase inhibitor through the GSK-3β/β-catenin signaling pathway. PLoS One. 2011;6(10):e27053.
185. Bettuzzi S, Brausi M, Rizzi F, Castagnetti G, Peracchia G, Corti A. Chemoprevention of human prostate cancer by oral administration of green tea catechins in volunteers with high-grade prostate intraepithelial neoplasia: a preliminary report from a one-year proof-of-principle study. Cancer Res. 2006;66(2):1234–40.
186. Jatoi A, Ellison N, Burch PA, Sloan JA, Dakhil SR, Novotny P, Tan W, Fitch TR, Rowland KM, Young CY, Flynn PJ. A phase II trial of green tea in the treatment of patients with androgen independent metastatic prostate carcinoma. Cancer. 2003;97(6):1442–6.
187. Shanafelt TD, Lee YK, Call TG, Nowakowski GS, Dingli D, Zent CS, Kay NE. Clinical effects of oral green tea extracts in four patients with low grade B-cell malignancies. Leuk Res. 2006;30(6):707–12.
188. Manero F, Gautier F, Gallenne T, Cauquil N, Grée D, Cartron PF, Geneste O, Grée R, Vallette FM, Juin P. The small organic compound HA14-1 prevents Bcl-2 interaction with Bax to sensitize malignant glioma cells to induction of cell death. Cancer Res. 2006;66(5):2757–64.
189. Meng Y, Lyu F, Xu X, Zhang L. Recent advances in chain conformation and bioactivities of triple-helix polysaccharides. Biomacromolecules. 2020;21(5):1653–77.
190. Jiao G, Yu G, Zhang J, Ewart HS. Chemical structures and bioactivities of sulfated polysaccharides from marine algae. Mar Drugs. 2011;9(2):196–223.
191. Bae IY, Kim HW, Yoo HJ, Kim ES, Lee S, Park DY, Lee HG. Correlation of branching structure of mushroom β-glucan with its physiological activities. Food Res Int. 2013;51 (1):195–200.
192. Li GH, Shen YM, Zhang KQ. Nematicidal activity and chemical component of Poria cocos. J Microbiol. 2005;43(1):17–20.

193. Cheng JJ, Chang CC, Chao CH, Lu MK. Characterization of fungal sulfated polysaccharides and their synergistic anticancer effects with doxorubicin. Carbohydr Polym. 2012;90(1):134–9.
194. Zen K, Liu Y, Cairo D, Parkos CA. CD11b/CD18-dependent interactions of neutrophils with intestinal epithelium are mediated by fucosylated proteoglycans. J Immunol. 2002;169(9):5270–8.
195. Atashrazm F, Lowenthal RM, Woods GM, Holloway AF, Dickinson JL. Fucoidan and cancer: a multifunctional molecule with anti-tumor potential. Mar Drugs. 2015;13(4):2327–46.
196. Zhang Y, Li S, Wang X, Zhang L, Cheung PC. Advances in lentinan: isolation, structure, chain conformation and bioactivities. Food Hydrocoll. 2011;25(2):196–206.
197. Zhou Z, Han Z, Zeng Y, Zhang M, Cui Y, Xu L, Zhang L. Chinese FDA approved fungal glycan-based drugs: an overview of structures, mechanisms and clinical related studies. Transl Med. 2014;4(141):1.
198. Yoshino S, Tabata T, Hazama S, Iizuka N, Yamamoto K, Hirayama M, Tangoku A, Oka M. Immunoregulatory effects of the antitumor polysaccharide lentinan on Th1/Th2 balance in patients with digestive cancers. Anticancer Res. 2000;20(6C):4707–11.
199. Wang XE, Wang YH, Zhou Q, Peng M, Zhang J, Chen M, Ma LJ, Xie GM. Immunomodulatory effect of lentinan on aberrant T subsets and cytokines profile in non-small cell lung cancer patients. Pathol Oncol Res. 2020;26(1):499–505.
200. Xie JH, Jin ML, Morris GA, Zha XQ, Chen HQ, Yi Y, Li JE, Wang ZJ, Gao J, Nie SP, Shang P. Advances on bioactive polysaccharides from medicinal plants. Crit Rev Food Sci Nutr. 2016;56(sup1):S60–84.
201. Deng S, Zhang G, Kuai J, Fan P, Wang X, Zhou P, Yang D, Zheng X, Liu X, Wu Q, Huang Y. Lentinan inhibits tumor angiogenesis via interferon γ and in a T cell independent manner. J Exp Clin Cancer Res. 2018;37(1):1–2.
202. Higashi D, Seki K, Ishibashi Y, Egawa Y, Koga M, Sasaki T, Hirano K, Mikami K, Futami K, Maekawa T, Sudo M. The effect of lentinan combination therapy for unresectable advanced gastric cancer. Anticancer Res. 2012;32(6):2365–8.
203. Zhou B, Fu Q, Song SS, Zheng HL, Wei YZ. Inhibitory effect of schizophyllan on rat glioma cells. Bangladesh J Pharmacol. 2015;10(4):759–64.
204. Ina H, Yoneda M, Kanda M, Kodera Y, Kabeya M, Yuasa S. Lentinan, a shiitake mushroom beta-glucan, stimulates tumor-specific adaptive immunity through PD-L1 down-regulation in gastric cancer cells. Med Chem. 2016;6:710–4.
205. Mawson AR. Retinoids in the treatment of glioma: a new perspective. Cancer Manag Res. 2012;4:233.
206. Haar CP, Hebbar P, Wallace GC, Das A, Vandergrift WA, Smith JA, Giglio P, Patel SJ, Ray SK, Banik NL. Drug resistance in glioblastoma: a mini review. Neurochem Res. 2012;37(6):1192–200.
207. Lippman SM, Lotan R. Advances in the development of retinoids as chemopreventive agents. J Nutr. 2000;130(2):479S–82S.
208. Das A, Banik NL, Ray SK. N-(4-Hydroxyphenyl) retinamide induced both differentiation and apoptosis in human glioblastoma T98G and U87MG cells. Brain Res. 2008;1227:207–15.
209. Mellai M, Caldera V, Patrucco A, Annovazzi L, Schiffer D. Survivin expression in glioblastomas correlates with proliferation, but not with apoptosis. Anticancer Res. 2008;28(1A):109–18.
210. George J, Banik NL, Ray SK. Survivin knockdown and concurrent 4-HPR treatment controlled human glioblastoma in vitro and in vivo. Neuro Oncol. 2010;12(11):1088–101.
211. Tian W, Deng Z, Hong K. The biological activities of sesterterpenoid-type ophiobolins. Mar Drugs. 2017;15(7):229.
212. Bury M, Novo-Uzal E, Andolfi A, Cimini S, Wauthoz N, Heffeter P, Lallemand B, Avolio F, Delporte C, Cimmino A, Dubois J. Ophiobolin A, a sesterterpenoid fungal phytotoxin, displays higher in vitro growth-inhibitory effects in mammalian than in plant cells and displays in vivo antitumor activity. Int J Oncol. 2013;43(2):575–85.

213. Bury M, Girault A, Megalizzi V, Spiegl-Kreinecker S, Mathieu V, Berger W, Evidente A, Kornienko A, Gailly P, Vandier C, Kiss R. Ophiobolin A induces paraptosis-like cell death in human glioblastoma cells by decreasing BKCa channel activity. Cell Death Dis. 2013;4(3): e561.
214. Morrison R, Lodge T, Evidente A, Kiss R, Townley H. Ophiobolin A, a sesterpenoid fungal phytotoxin, displays different mechanisms of cell death in mammalian cells depending upon the cancer cell origin. Int J Oncol. 2017;50(3):773–86.
215. Brunelli D, Tavecchio M, Falcioni C, Frapolli R, Erba E, Iori R, Rollin P, Barillari J, Manzotti C, Morazzoni P, D'Incalci M. The isothiocyanate produced from glucomoringin inhibits NF-kB and reduces myeloma growth in nude mice in vivo. Biochem Pharmacol. 2010;79(8):1141–8.
216. Prawan A, Saw CL, Khor TO, Keum YS, Yu S, Hu L, Kong AN. Anti-NF-κB and anti-inflammatory activities of synthetic isothiocyanates: effect of chemical structures and cellular signaling. Chem Biol Interact. 2009;179(2–3):202–11.
217. Subedi L, Venkatesan R, Kim SY. Neuroprotective and anti-inflammatory activities of allyl isothiocyanate through attenuation of JNK/NF-κB/TNF-α signaling. Int J Mol Sci. 2017;18 (7):1423.
218. Guo Z, Wang H, Wei J, Han L, Li Z. Sequential treatment of phenethyl isothiocyanate increases sensitivity of Temozolomide resistant glioblastoma cells by decreasing expression of MGMT via NF-κB pathway. Am J Transl Res. 2019;11(2):696.
219. Lee CS, Cho HJ, Jeong YJ, Shin JM, Park KK, Park YY, Bae YS, Chung IK, Kim M, Kim CH, Jin F. Isothiocyanates inhibit the invasion and migration of C6 glioma cells by blocking FAK/ JNK-mediated MMP-9 expression. Oncol Rep. 2015;34(6):2901–8.
220. Kreuter J. Influence of the surface properties on nanoparticle-mediated transport of drugs to the brain. J Nanosci Nanotechnol. 2004;4(5):484–8.
221. Peer D, Karp JM, Hong S, Farokhzad OC, Margalit R, Langer R. Nanocarriers as an emerging platform for cancer therapy. Nat Nanotechnol. 2007;2(12):751–60.
222. Begley DJ, Brightman MW. Structural and functional aspects of the blood-brain barrier. Peptide transport and delivery into the central nervous system. 2003; pp. 39-78.
223. Deeken JF, Löscher W. The blood-brain barrier and cancer: transporters, treatment, and Trojan horses. Clin Cancer Res. 2007;13(6):1663–74.
224. Pardridge WM. Blood-brain barrier drug targeting: the future of brain drug development. Mol Interv. 2003;3(2):90.
225. Egleton RD, Davis TP. Development of neuropeptide drugs that cross the blood-brain barrier. NeuroRx. 2005;2(1):44–53.
226. Pardridge WM. Molecular Trojan horses for blood-brain barrier drug delivery. Discov Med. 2009;6(34):139–43.
227. Woodworth GF, Dunn GP, Nance EA, Hanes J, Brem H. Emerging insights into barriers to effective brain tumor therapeutics. Front Oncol. 2014;4:126.
228. Kim SS, Rait A, Rubab F, Rao AK, Kiritsy MC, Pirollo KF, Wang S, Weiner LM, Chang EH. The clinical potential of targeted nanomedicine: delivering to cancer stem-like cells. Mol Ther. 2014;22(2):278–91.
229. Panyam J, Labhasetwar V. Sustained cytoplasmic delivery of drugs with intracellular receptors using biodegradable nanoparticles. Mol Pharm. 2004;1(1):77–84.
230. Allard E, Passirani C, Benoit JP. Convection-enhanced delivery of nanocarriers for the treatment of brain tumors. Biomaterials. 2009;30(12):2302–18.
231. Li Y, He H, Jia X, Lu WL, Lou J, Wei Y. A dual-targeting nanocarrier based on poly (amidoamine) dendrimers conjugated with transferrin and tamoxifen for treating brain gliomas. Biomaterials. 2012;33(15):3899–908.
232. Hendricks BK, Cohen-Gadol AA, Miller JC. Novel delivery methods bypassing the blood-brain and blood-tumor barriers. Neurosurg Focus. 2015;38(3):E10.
233. Lai JC, Ananthakrishnan G, Jandhyam S, Dukhande VV, Bhushan A, Gokhale M, Daniels CK, Leung SW. Treatment of human astrocytoma U87 cells with silicon dioxide nanoparticles

lowers their survival and alters their expression of mitochondrial and cell signaling proteins. Int J Nanomedicine. 2010;5:715.

234. Bobyk L, Edouard M, Deman P, Vautrin M, Pernet-Gallay K, Delaroche J, Adam JF, Estève F, Ravanat JL, Elleaume H. Photoactivation of gold nanoparticles for glioma treatment. Nanomed Nanotechnol Biol Med. 2013;9(7):1089–97.
235. Aryal M, Park J, Vykhodtseva N, Zhang YZ, McDannold N. Enhancement in blood-tumor barrier permeability and delivery of liposomal doxorubicin using focused ultrasound and microbubbles: evaluation during tumor progression in a rat glioma model. Phys Med Biol. 2015;60(6):2511.
236. Kim SS, Harford JB, Pirollo KF, Chang EH. Effective treatment of glioblastoma requires crossing the blood–brain barrier and targeting tumors including cancer stem cells: the promise of nanomedicine. Biochem Biophys Res Commun. 2015;468(3):485–9.
237. Juillerat-Jeanneret L. The targeted delivery of cancer drugs across the blood–brain barrier: chemical modifications of drugs or drug-nanoparticles? Drug Discov Today. 2008;13 (23-24):1099–106.
238. Steiniger SC, Kreuter J, Khalansky AS, Skidan IN, Bobruskin AI, Smirnova ZS, Severin SE, Uhl R, Kock M, Geiger KD, Gelperina SE. Chemotherapy of glioblastoma in rats using doxorubicin-loaded nanoparticles. Int J Cancer. 2004;109(5):759–67.
239. Zhang Y, Sun C, Kohler N, Zhang M. Self-assembled coatings on individual monodisperse magnetite nanoparticles for efficient intracellular uptake. Biomed Microdevices. 2004;6 (1):33–40.
240. Eldridge B. Preclinical development of carbon nanotube mediated thermal therapy for treatment of glioblastoma multiforme: Determining the effects of nanomaterial properties, dose, and irradiation parameters on the efficacy and potential negative repercussions of treatment (Doctoral dissertation, Wake Forest University).
241. Bregy A, Shah AH, Diaz MV, Pierce HE, Ames PL, Diaz D, Komotar RJ. The role of Gliadel wafers in the treatment of high-grade gliomas. Expert Rev Anticancer Ther. 2013;13 (12):1453–61.
242. Panigrahi M, Das PK, Parikh PM. Brain tumor and Gliadel wafer treatment. Indian J Cancer. 2011;48(1):11.
243. Miglierini P, Bouchekoua M, Rousseau B, Hieu PD, Malhaire JP, Pradier O. Impact of the per-operatory application of GLIADEL wafers (BCNU, carmustine) in combination with temozolomide and radiotherapy in patients with glioblastoma multiforme: efficacy and toxicity. Clin Neurol Neurosurg. 2012;114(9):1222–5.
244. Westphal M, Hilt DC, Bortey E, Delavault P, Olivares R, Warnke PC, Whittle IR, Jääskeläinen J, Ram Z. A phase 3 trial of local chemotherapy with biodegradable carmustine (BCNU) wafers (Gliadel wafers) in patients with primary malignant glioma. Neuro Oncol. 2003;5(2):79–88.
245. Brem H, Piantadosi S, Burger PC, Walker M, Selker R, Vick NA, Black K, Sisti M, Brem S, Mohr G, Muller P. Placebo-controlled trial of safety and efficacy of intraoperative controlled delivery by biodegradable polymers of chemotherapy for recurrent gliomas. Lancet. 1995;345 (8956):1008–12.
246. McGirt MJ, Than KD, Weingart JD, Chaichana KL, Attenello FJ, Olivi A, Laterra J, Kleinberg LR, Grossman SA, Brem H, Quiñones-Hinojosa A. Gliadel (BCNU) wafer plus concomitant temozolomide therapy after primary resection of glioblastoma multiforme. J Neurosurg. 2009;110(3):583–8.
247. Gallia GL, Brem S, Brem H. Local treatment of malignant brain tumors using implantable chemotherapeutic polymers. J Natl Compr Canc Netw. 2005;3(5):721–8.
248. Weber EL, Goebel EA. Cerebral edema associated with Gliadel wafers: two case studies. Neuro Oncol. 2005;7(1):84–9.
249. Simberg D, Duza T, Park JH, Essler M, Pilch J, Zhang L, Derfus AM, Yang M, Hoffman RM, Bhatia S, Sailor MJ. Biomimetic amplification of nanoparticle homing to tumors. Proc Natl Acad Sci. 2007;104(3):932–6.

250. Madhankumar AB, Slagle-Webb B, Mintz A, Sheehan JM, Connor JR. Interleukin-13 receptor–targeted nanovesicles are a potential therapy for glioblastoma multiforme. Mol Cancer Ther. 2006;5(12):3162–9.
251. Mamot C, Drummond DC, Noble CO, Kallab V, Guo Z, Hong K, Kirpotin DB, Park JW. Epidermal growth factor receptor–targeted immunoliposomes significantly enhance the efficacy of multiple anticancer drugs in vivo. Cancer Res. 2005;65(24):11631–8.
252. Lee YE, Kopelman R. Polymeric nanoparticles for photodynamic therapy. In: Biomedical nanotechnology. Totowa, NJ: Humana Press; 2011. p. 151–78.
253. Jain KK. Potential of nanobiotechnology in the management of glioblastoma multiforme. In: Glioblastoma. New York, NY: Springer; 2010. p. 399–419.
254. Koo YE, Reddy GR, Bhojani M, Schneider R, Philbert MA, Rehemtulla A, Ross BD, Kopelman R. Brain cancer diagnosis and therapy with nanoplatforms. Adv Drug Deliv Rev. 2006;58(14):1556–77.
255. Gupta AH, Kathpalia HT. Recent advances in brain targeted drug delivery systems: a review. Int J Pharm Pharm Sci. 2014;6(2):51–7.
256. Hostanska K, Reichling J, Bommer S, Weber M, Saller R. Hyperforin a constituent of St John's wort (Hypericum perforatum L.) extract induces apoptosis by triggering activation of caspases and with hypericin synergistically exerts cytotoxicity towards human malignant cell lines. Eur J Pharm Biopharm. 2003;56(1):121–32.
257. Ferguson PJ, Kurowska EM, Freeman DJ, Chambers AF, Koropatnick J. In vivo inhibition of growth of human tumor lines by flavonoid fractions from cranberry extract. Nutr Cancer. 2006;56(1):86–94.
258. Lee DY, Lee MK, Kim GS, Noh HJ, Lee MH. Brazilin inhibits growth and induces apoptosis in human glioblastoma cells. Molecules. 2013;18(2):2449–57.
259. Lee DH, Lee TH, Jung CH, Kim YH. Wogonin induces apoptosis by activating the AMPK and p53 signaling pathways in human glioblastoma cells. Cell Signal. 2012;24(11):2216–25.
260. Li Y, Zhang P, Qiu F, Chen L, Miao C, Li J, Xiao W, Ma E. Inactivation of PI3K/Akt signaling mediates proliferation inhibition and G2/M phase arrest induced by andrographolide in human glioblastoma cells. Life Sci. 2012;90(25-26):962–7.
261. Khan M, Yu B, Rasul A, Al Shawi A, Yi F, Yang H, Ma T. Jaceosidin induces apoptosis in U87 glioblastoma cells through G2/M phase arrest. Evid Based Complement Alternat Med. 2012;2012:703034.
262. Chang LF, Lin PC, Ho LI, Liu PY, Wu WC, Chiang IP, Chang HW, Lin SZ, Harn YC, Harn HJ, Chiou TW. Overexpression of the orphan receptor Nur77 and its translocation induced by PCH4 may inhibit malignant glioma cell growth and induce cell apoptosis. J Surg Oncol. 2011;103(5):442–50.
263. Chaudhuri D, Ghate NB, Singh SS, Mandal N. Methyl gallate isolated from Spondias pinnata exhibits anticancer activity against human glioblastoma by induction of apoptosis and sustained extracellular signal-regulated kinase 1/2 activation. Pharmacogn Mag. 2015;11 (42):269.
264. Zhang Y, Xie RF, Xiao QG, Li R, Shen XL, Zhu XG. Hedyotis diffusa Willd extract inhibits the growth of human glioblastoma cells by inducing mitochondrial apoptosis via AKT/ERK pathways. J Ethnopharmacol. 2014;158:404–11.
265. Tezcan G, Tunca B, Bekar A, Budak F, Sahin S, Cecener G, Egeli U, Taskapılıoglu MO, Kocaeli H, Tolunay S, Malyer H. Olea europaea leaf extract improves the treatment response of GBM stem cells by modulating miRNA expression. Am J Cancer Res. 2014;4(5):572.
266. Elkady AI, Hussein RA, Abu-Zinadah OA. Effects of crude extracts from medicinal herbs Rhazya stricta and Zingiber officinale on growth and proliferation of human brain cancer cell line in vitro. Biomed Res Int. 2014;2014:260210.
267. U.S. National Library of Medicine. ClinicalTrials.gov [Internet]. U.S. National Institute of Health. 2020 [cited 2020 Dec 2]. Available from: https://clinicaltrials.gov/ct2/home

Printed by Printforce, the Netherlands